Official Journal of the 'Mediterranean League ag[...]olic Diseases'

Pathophysiology of Haemostasis and Thrombosis

Formerly 'Haemostasis'

KARGER

Printed in Slovenia
by Litterapicta, Ljubljana

Guidelines for Authors

Pathophysiology of Haemostasis and Thrombosis

Submission

Only original papers written in English that communicate novel findings in the field of haemostasis and thrombosis are considered. Both contributions to the basic understanding of these processes and reports on clinical management of disorders in this field are acceptable. Manuscripts should be sent to:

Editorial Office
'Pathophysiology of Haemostasis and Thrombosis'
attn. Mrs. T. Camphuisen-Engel
Maastricht University
Department of Biochemistry
Faculty of Medicine II, Level 4
P.O. Box 616
NL–6200 MD Maastricht (The Netherlands)
Tel. +31 43 388 1678/1674
Fax +31 43 388 4159
E-Mail T.Camphuisen@bioch.unimaas.nl

Manuscripts should be submitted in triplicate (with three sets of illustrations of which one is an original), typewritten double-spaced on one side of the paper, with a wide margin.

Conditions

All manuscripts are subject to editorial review. A manuscript is to be considered rejected when an author does not return a revised manuscript within 3 months of receiving the suggestions for revision, unless the author explains further delay. Manuscripts are received with the explicit understanding that they are not under simultaneous consideration by any other publication. Submission of an article for publication implies the transfer of the copyright from the author to the publisher upon acceptance. Accepted papers become the permanent property of 'Pathophysiology of Haemostasis and Thrombosis' and may not be reproduced by any means, in whole or in part, without the written consent of both the author and the publisher. It is the author's responsibility to obtain permission to reproduce illustrations, tables, etc. from other publications.

Arrangement

Title page: The first page of each paper should indicate the title, the authors' names, and the institute where the work was conducted. A short title for use as running head as well as the full address of the author to whom correspondence should be sent are also required.

Full address: The exact postal address complete with postal code must be given at the bottom of the title page. Please also supply phone and fax numbers, as well as your e-mail address.

Key words: For indexing purposes, a list of 3–10 key words in English is essential.

Abstract: Each paper needs an abstract of up to 10 lines.

Footnotes: Avoid footnotes. When essential, they are numbered consecutively and typed at the foot of the appropriate page.

Tables and illustrations: Tables and illustrations (both numbered in Arabic numerals) should be prepared on separate sheets. Tables require a heading and figures a legend, also prepared on a separate sheet. For the reproduction of illustrations, only good drawings and original photographs can be accepted; negatives or photocopies cannot be used. Due to technical reasons, figures with a screen background should not be submitted. When possible, group several illustrations on one block for reproduction (max. size 180 × 223 mm) or provide crop marks. On the back of each illustration, indicate its number, the author's name, and 'top' with a soft pencil.

Color illustrations: Up to 6 color illustrations per page can be integrated within the text at the reduced price of CHF 660.–/USD 545.00 per page. Color illustrations are reproduced at the author's expense.

References: In the text identify references by Arabic numerals [in square brackets]. Material submitted for publication but not yet accepted should be noted as 'unpublished data' and not be included in the reference list. The list of references should include only those publications which are cited in the text. Do not alphabetize; number references in the order in which they are first mentioned in the text. The surnames of the authors followed by initials should be given. There should be no punctuation other than a comma to separate the authors. Cite all authors, 'et al' is not sufficient. Abbreviate journal names according to the Index Medicus system. (Also see International Committee of Medical Journal Editors: Uniform requirements for manuscripts submitted to biomedical journals. N Engl J Med 1997;336:309–315.)

Examples:
(a) Papers published in periodicals: Sun J, Koto H, Chung KF: Interaction of ozone and allergen challenges on bronchial responsiveness and inflammation in sensitised guinea pigs. Int Arch Allergy Immunol 1997;112:191–195.
(b) Monographs: Matthews DE, Farewell VT: Using and Understanding Medical Statistics, ed 3, revised. Basel, Karger, 1996.
(c) Edited books: Parren PWHI, Burton DR: Antibodies against HIV-1 from phage display libraries: Mapping of an immune response and progress towards antiviral immunotherapy; in Capra JD (ed): Antibody Engineering. Chem Immunol. Basel, Karger, 1997, vol 65, pp 18–56.

Page charges

There are no page charges for papers of 4 or fewer printed pages (including tables, illustrations and references). Each additional complete or partial page is charged to the author at CHF 275.–/USD 196.00. The allotted size of a paper is equal to approx. 12 manuscript pages (including tables, illustrations and references).

Galley proofs

Unless indicated otherwise, galley proofs are sent to the first-named author and should be returned with the least possible delay. Alterations made in galley proofs, other than the correction of printer's errors, are charged to the author. No page proofs are supplied.

Reprints

Order forms and a price list are sent with the galley proofs. Orders submitted after the issue is printed are subject to considerably higher prices.

KARGER
Fax +41 61 306 12 34
E-Mail karger@karger.ch
www.karger.com

The Guidelines for Authors are available at:
www.karger.com/pht_Guidelines

General Information

Pathophysiology of Haemostasis and Thrombosis

Publication data: 'Pathophysiology of Haemostasis and Thrombosis' is published 6 times a year. Volume 33 with 6 issues appears in 2003.

Subscription rates: Subscriptions run for a full calendar year. Prices are given per year.

Personal subscription:

Print or Online	**Print/Online combined**
CHF 480.50	CHF 519.50
EUR 343.50	EUR 371.50
USD 370.00	USD 400.00
postage and handling	(added to print and print/online)
CHF 30.20 Europe,	CHF 44.90 Overseas
EUR 21.60	
USD 30.20	

Institutional subscription:

Print or Online	**Print/Online combined**
CHF 961.–	CHF 1038.–
EUR 687.–	EUR 741.–
USD 740.00	USD 798.00
postage and handling	(added to print and print/online)
CHF 37.80 Europe,	CHF 56.10 Overseas
EUR 27.–	
USD 37.80	

Airmail surcharge: CHF 37.80 / USD 31.50

Discount subscription prices:
Deutsche Arbeitsgemeinschaft für Blutgerinnungsforschung; International Society of Hematology; Mediterranean League against Thromboembolic Diseases

Microforms: Please direct all enquiries and orders to:
University Microfilms Inc.
300 North Zeeb Road, P.O. Box 1346
Ann Arbor, MI 48106-1346 (USA)

Subscription orders: Orders can be placed at agencies, bookstores, directly with the Publisher
S. Karger AG, P.O. Box
CH–4009 Basel (Switzerland)
or with any of the following distributors:
Deutschland: S. Karger GmbH, Postfach
D–79095 Freiburg
France: Librairie Luginbühl
36, bd de Latour-Maubourg
F–75007 Paris
Great Britain, Ireland: S. Karger AG
4 Rickett Street
London SW6 1RU, UK
USA: S. Karger Publishers, Inc.
26 West Avon Road, P.O. Box 529
Farmington, CT 06085, USA
India, Bangladesh, Sri Lanka:
Panther Publishers Private Ltd.
33, First Main
Koramangala First Block
Bangalore 560 034, India
Japan: Karger Japan, Inc.
Yushima S Bld. 3F
4-2-3, Yushima, Bunkyo-ku
Tokyo 113-0034, Japan

Change of address: Both old and new address should be sent to the subscription source.

Single issues and back volumes: Information can be obtained through the Publisher.

Advertising: Correspondence and rate requests should be addressed to the Publisher.

Bibliographic indices: This journal is regularly listed in bibliographic services, including *Current Contents*® and Index Medicus/MEDLINE.

Copying: This journal has been registered with the Copyright Clearance Center (CCC), as indicated by the code appearing on the first page of each article. For readers in the US, this code signals consent for copying of articles for personal or internal use, or for the personal or internal use of specific clients, provided that the stated fee is paid per copy directly to
Copyright Clearance Center Inc.
222 Rosewood Drive
Danvers, MA 01923 (USA)
A copy of the first page of the article must accompany payment. Consent does not extend to copying for general distribution, for promotion, for creating new works, or for resale. In these cases, specific written permission must be obtained from the copyright owner,
S. Karger AG,
P.O. Box, CH–4009 Basel (Switzerland).

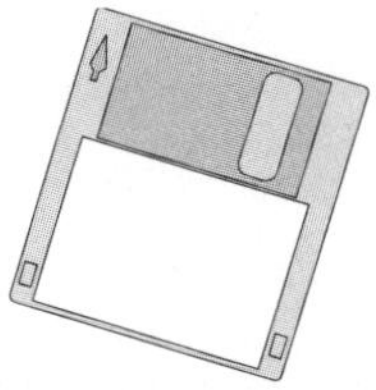

Disk Submission

A **comprehensive version** of these guidelines for the **submission of manuscripts and illustrations on disk** can be accessed online under **www.karger.com/disksubmission** or requested as a leaflet from the editorial department.

Please follow the general rules on style and arrangement in the **'Guidelines for Authors'** of the journal. Submit a **double-spaced printout** of your manuscript matching the file on disk exactly.

Technical Information

Store only data pertinent to this manuscript. Include your fonts (screen and printer fonts for Macintosh). For a **text only** manuscript, use a 3.5-inch disk. For **text and illustrations,** use 3.5 or 5.25 Magneto Optical Disc; CD-ROM (DOS or hybrid); iomega Zip/DOS (100 MB), or 44 MB, 88 MB or 200 MB SyQuest. Compress extensive data using ZIP format.

Data Description

Label your disk with the **title of the journal or book** for which it is submitted; a **short version** of the paper's title; your **name,** postal and e-mail address, fax and phone number; **hard- and software** used, including the version; and the **complete list of the file names.** File names consist of eight characters before the dot identifying the file and three characters after the dot identifying the application.

Text and Format

The **preferred word-processing package is MS-Word.** Other commonly used PC text programs and ASCII formats are accepted.
Update your data when you revise subsequent to the reviewer's or editor's decision and mark revisions clearly. Manuscripts accepted for publication are subject to **copy editing:** changes and/or questions will be marked in the manuscript, which will be returned to you with your disk and the galley proofs for checking.
Enter your text continuously flush left. Do not use any layout functions. Do not split words at the end of a line. **Do not use indentations.** Use a blank line before and a hard return at the end of paragraphs.
Arrange headings flush left. Insert only **one space after punctuation marks.** Insert Greek letters, mathematical symbols etc. with your word-processing program. Use **boldface and italics** as well as sub- and superscript where appropriate.
Tables are part of the text and should be placed at the end of the text file. Separate the individual parts of a table by lines. Use the tabulator instead of spaces. Format operation data on one line in the same column.

Legends to illustrations are part of the text and should also be listed at the end of the text file.

Illustrations

Store illustrations as separate files: do not integrate them in your text. Export **line drawings/vector graphics** as TIF, EPS or WMF format. Use Photoshop for processing and retouching **scanned half-tone images.** Save the original scan and the processed version. Export **black and white or color images** as TIF or EPS format in their anticipated size in print. **For detailed information** on how to submit illustration data on disk please consult the leaflet or **www.karger.com/disksubmission.**

KI 02 DISK

KARGER

Fax +41 61 306 12 34
E-Mail karger@karger.ch
www.karger.com

The Journal Home Page is available at:
www.karger.com/pht

Pathophysiology
of Haemostasis
and Thrombosis

18th International Congress on Thrombosis

Abstracts

Ljubljana, Slovenia, June 20–24, 2004

Guest Editors
Mojca Stegnar, Ljubljana
Mojca Bozic, Ljubljana
Matija Kozak, Ljubljana
Polona Peternel, Ljubljana
Nina Vene, Ljubljana

KARGER

Basel · Freiburg · Paris · London · New York ·
Bangalore · Bangkok · Singapore · Tokyo · Sydney

S. Karger
Medical and Scientific Publishers
Basel • Freiburg • Paris • London
New York • Bangalore • Bangkok
Singapore • Tokyo • Sydney

Drug Dosage
The authors and the publisher have exerted every effort to ensure that drug selection and dosage set forth in this text are in accord with current recommendations and practice at the time of publication. However, in view of ongoing research, changes in government regulations, and the constant flow of information relating to drug therapy and drug reactions, the reader is urged to check the package insert for each drug for any change in indications and dosage and for added warnings and precautions. This is particularly important when the recommended agent is a new and/or infrequently employed drug.

Printed in Switzerland on acid-free paper by
Reinhardt Druck, Basel
ISBN 3–8055–7798–2

KARGER

Fax +41 61 306 12 34
E-Mail karger@karger.ch
www.karger.com

Contents

ORAL COMMUNICATIONS

Emerging prognostic factors in coronary artery disease OC002
Brogi D, Sofi F*, Fatini C, Lenti M, Valente S, Lombardi A, Lucarini L, Sticchi E, Abbate R, Gensini GF

Increased plasma concentration of platelet-derived microparticles in young survivors of myocardial infarction OC003
Michelsen A*, Brodin E, Brosstad F, Hansen J

Gene-gene interaction of the ABCA1 transporter and paraoxonase genes in inherited predisposition to myocardial infarction in young men OC004
Pchelina S*, Sheydina A, Taraskina A, Rodygina T, Schwarzman A

Circulating endothelial cells predict outcomes in patients with acute coronary syndrome: relationship to plasma von Willebrand factor and interleukin-6 OC005
Lee W*, Lıp G

High ambulatory pulse pressure is associated with abnormal thrombogenesis and endothelial damage/dysfunction in patients with coronary heart disease OC006
Lee W*, Lıp G

Hematological malignanices

Thrombosis of splanchnic veins in patients with silent myeloproliferative disorders OC007
Miljic P*, Sefer D, Sretenovic M, Suvajdzic N, Colovic M

A prospective observational study on catheter-related complications in patients with hematological malignancies (CATHEM) OC008
Falanga A*, Moia M, Cortelezzi A, Pogliani E, Boccadoro M, Gallo E, Nosari A, Rizzoli V, Rodeghiero F, Gussoni G

Proteolysis of von Willebrand factor increases in children during the induction therapy for acute lymphoblastic leukemia OC009
Perutelli P, Amato S, De Mattia D, Del Vecchio G, Giordano P, Saracco P, Russo G, Molinari A*

Factor XIII activity levels in acute leukemia OC010
Stemmelin G, Dubboscq C, Shanley C, Ceresetto JM*, Rabinovich O, Gutierrez M, Mendizabal G, Doti C, Vicente M, Bullorsky E

Alterations of coagulation pathway parameters in children with acute lymphoblastic leukaemia (ALL) OC011
Hatzipantelis E*, Athanassiou-Metaxa M, Tzimouli V, Kleta D, Gombakis N, Garipidou V, Athanasiadou-Piperop F, Sidi-Fragandrea V, Koliouskas D

Coordinated dysregulation of cellular receptors, proangiogenic factors and intracellular pathways in acute leukemia OC012
Barbarroja N, Lopez-Pedrera C*, Buendia P, Siendones E, Capote M, Montiel-Duarte C, Dorado G, Torres A, Velasco F

Animal experimental models

Platelets migrate in response to allergen in vivo and in vitro: role of IgE OC013
Pitchford S*, Momi S, Casali L, Gresele P

Successful inhibition of venous thrombus growth after oral administration of BAY 59-7939, a direct Factor Xa inhibitor in rabbits OC014
Biemond BJ*, Friederich PW, Levi M, Perzborn E, Buetehorn U, Büller H

Increased pulmonary expression of thrombin receptor in rabbits with endotoxin-induced acute lung injury OC015
Gando S*, Jesmin S, Sakuma I, Kobayashi S, Sakuraya F, Matsuda N, Hattori Y

PPAR-alpha deficiency does not modify age dependent but prevents high fat diet increase in plasma PAI-1 as well as insulin resistance OC016
Mavri A, Bastelica D, Steals B, El Ayachi S, Juhan-Vague I, Alessi MC

Differential expression patterns of proteins in the ischemic myocardium OC017
Jang Y*, Hwang K, Sohn Y, Seung K, Chung KH

Suitability of selected clotting assays to explain anitithrombotic potential of LK732, argatroban and nadroparin in rat venous thrombosis model OC018
Peternel L*, Drevenšek G, Budihna M, Zega A, Božič M, Stegnar M, Černe M, Urleb U

VTE prophylaxis

Ximelagatran for the secondary prevention of venous thromboembolism: a complementary follow-up analysis of the THRIVE III Study OC019
Schulman S*, Lundström T, Wåhlander K, Billing Clason S, Eriksson H, for the THRIVE III

Long-term follow-up of 122 patients with inferior vena cava filters - non-randomised, retrospective comparison with 120 patients treated for venous th OC020
Hajduk B*, Małek G, Oniszh K, Burakowski J, Wawrzyńska L, Tomkowski W

The development in attitudes towards thromboprophylaxis in Danish surgical departments during a twenty year period OC021
Rasmussen M*, Wegner L, Wille-Jørgens P

A comparison of venous thromboembolism prophylaxis practice patterns in acutely ill medical patients; IMPROVE versus clinical trial populations OC022
Anderson F, Tapson V, Decousus H*, Spyropoulos A, Turpie A, FitzGerald G

Practice variation in USA and Europe for the prevention of venous thromboembolism in hospitalized medical patients: Findings from IMPROVE OC023
Pini M, Froehlich J, Bergmann JF, Monreal M*, Piovella F, Huang W, Anderson F

Cancer and thrombosis

Fibrinolysis

Cardiovascular disease

Platelets I

Aspirin resistance and prognosis in the setting of non st elevation acute coronary syndromes OC047
Perdiou A*, Zairis M, Tsiribis V, Patsourakos N, Lyras A, Foussas S, Tsoukanas K

Application of the cone and plate(let) Analyzer for testing the response to aspirin treatment OC048
Spectre G*, Brill A, Gural A, Turetzky N, Mosseri E, Savion D, Varon D

Antiphospholipid syndrome

Regulation of NF-kB activation in the anti-phospholipid syndrome: involvement of ERK1/2 and p38 MAP kinase pathways OC049
Buendia P, Lopez-Pedrera C*, Barbarroja N, Montiel-Duarte C, Siendones E, Dorado G, Aguirre MA, Cuadrado M, Torres A, Velasco F

Platelet deposition under flow condition is increased in patients with antiphospholipid syndrome who experient thrombotic events OC050
Shenkman B, Levi Y, Tamarin I, Savion N, Shoenfeld Y, Varon D

Laboratory diagnosis of antiphospholipid syndrome: difficulties and possibilities OC051
Makatsaria A*, Khizroeva D, Bitsadze VO, Baimuradova SM

Elevated levels of prothrombin fragment 1+2 in patients with antiphospholipid antibodies but without clinical signs of antiphospholipid syndrome OC052
Ambrožič A*, Božič B, Rozman B

Detection of antiphospholipid antibodies (APAs) in patients with autoimmune and thrombotic diseases OC053
Nagy E*, Sallai K, Gergely P, Bodó I

A survey on diagnosis of lupus anticoagulant among laboratories of the Italian Federation Of Anticoagulation Clinics (FCSA) OC054
Biasiolo A*, Tripodi A, Chantarangkul V, Gresele P, Marongiu F, Barcellona D, Erba N, Veschi F, Ghirarduzzi A, Pengo V

VTE – Clinical aspects I

Objective assessment of deep vein thrombosis and pulmonary embolism can be deferred without increased risk of thrombosis OC055
Siragusa S*, Anastasio R, Porta C, Falaschi F, Pirrelli S, Malato A, Bonifacio G, Palmieri P, Bressan MA, Mariani G

Value of D-dimer, for the exclusion of deep venous thrombosis, in the low-moderate and high pre-test probability groups OC056
El Kheir D*, Gerdes V, Büller HR

Residual post treatment ultrasound detected thrombosis is associated with an increased risk of recurrence OC057
Young L, Ockelford P*, Rolfe-Vyson V, McKelvie S, Harper P

The long-term clinical course of acute deep vein thrombosis of upper extremities. A prospective cohort study OC058
Prandoni P, Bernardi E*, Marchiori A, Lensing A, Prins M, Sartor D, Piccioli A, Simioni P, Pagnan A, Girolami A

Chronic renal failure: thrombotic events and relation with the levels of thrombomodulin, TFPI and von Willebrand factor OC059
Sioulis A, Grekas D, Boutou A, Girtovitis F, Tasiopoulou K, Avdelidou A, Makris P

Venous thromboembolism and spinal surgery OC060
Fletcher J*, Hitos K, Dexter M, Cree A, Dandie G, Saker K, Butler G

Direct thrombin inhibitors

Efficacy and safety of ximelagatran for prevention of thromboembolism using the EXPRESS regimen across different orthopaedic surgery patient groups OC061
Eriksson BI*, Agnelli G, Cohen AT, Dahl OE, Lassen M, Mouret P, Rosencher N, Kälebo P, Panfilov S, Andersson M

Dabigatran etexilate, new oral direct thrombin inhibitor, in the prevention of thromboembolic events after total hip/knee replacement: BISTRO-2 Study OC062
Eriksson BI*, Dahl OE, Büller HR, Hettiarachchi R, Rosencher N, Bravo ML, Ahnfelt L, Piovella F, Stangier J, Kälebo P

Influence of time of first dose on the efficacy and safety of postoperative ximelagatran for prevention of thromboembolism after orthopaedic surgery OC063
Dahl OE*, Eriksson BI, Agnelli G, Cohen AT, Mouret P, Rosencher N, Panfilov S, Andersson M

Timing of initiation of thromboembolism prophylaxis in total hip/knee replacement with dabigatran etexilate, a new oral direct thrombin inhibitor OC064
Dahl OE*, Eriksson BI, Büller HR, Hettiarachchi R, Rosencher N, Bravo ML, Ahnfelt L, Piovella F, Stangier J, Kälebo P

Ximelagatran/melagatran versus LMWH in major orthopedic surgery: relationship between efficacy and safety and timing of initial administration OC065
Zufferey P, Laporte S, Quenet S, Molliex S, Auboyer C, Decousus H, Mismetti P*

LMWH or ximelagatran versus VKA in the prevention of VTE after major knee surgery: a meta-analysis of randomized controlled trials OC066
Iorio A*, Ferrante F, Nenci G

Haemophilia

A familial multi-vitamin K-dependent syndrom associated with compound heterozygosity in the gamma-glutamyl carboxylase gene OC067
Darghouth D, LeRicousse S, Mrad A, Gharbi Y, Maherzi A, Kastally R*, Rosa J

VTE – Clinical aspects II

Inherited protein S deficiency type I, but not type III is a risk factor for venous, but not arterial thrombosis; a study in 81 families OC091
Brouwer JLP*, Veeger N, van der Schaaf W, Kluin-Nelemans H, van der Meer J

Markers of inflammation, D-dimer and recurrences after a first episode of venous thromboembolism OC092
Cosmi B*, Legnani C, Guazzaloca G, Coccheri S, Palareti G

Success of initiatives to familiarize vascular physicians in Germany with outpatient treatment of deep venous thrombosis OC093
Werner B*, Jürgen D, Horst E G

Cost-effectiveness of bemiparin in the acute and long-term treatment of deep vein thrombosis OC094
Rocha E, Gómez-Outes A*, Martínez-González J*, Kakkar V

Outpatient tinzaparin therapy in 102 patients with pulmonary embolism - final results OC095
Olsson*, Bajc M, Bitzén U, Carlsson MS, Elf J, Jönsson K, Magnusson P, Olsson B, Jonson B

Analysis of predisposing factors and 6 month outcomes of DVT management in 668 patients treated with LMWH(tinzaparin) as outpatients OC096
Rhodes S, Bond S*, Green E

Genetic Polymorphisms

Haplotypes of the EPCR gene, plasma sEPCR levels and the risk of deep venous thrombosis OC097
Uitte de Willige S*, van Marion V, Rosendaal F, Vos H, de Visser M, Bertina R

Expression and characterization of a new factor V mutation (R1698W) found in combination with FV Leiden OC098
Lunghi B, Scanavini D, Ulazzi L, Busani C, Redaelli R, Tagariello G, Bernardi F*

Genetic markers of inflammation and sensitivity to activated protein C (APC) OC099
González-Ordóñ A*, Macias D, Arias A, Fernández-Carreira JM, Morán M, Peliz M, Martín L

Frequency of cytochrome CYP2C9 polymorphism in Russian Population and it effects in 62 patients treated by warfarin OC100
Vavilova T*, Sirotkina O, Ulitina A, Kadinskaya M, Schwarzman A

TNFR1 +36 G/G genotype and the metabolic syndrome both predispose obese women to higher levels of soluble TNFRs, PAI-1 and liver enzymes OC101
Mavri A, Bastelica D, Saut N, Verdier M, Renucci J, Juhan-Vague I, Alessi MC

Fibrinogen polymorphisms Taq I, Hae III and Bcl I are not major risk factors for deep-vein thrombosis OC102
Božič M*, Teran N, Peterlin B, Stegnar M

Ischaemic stroke

Inherited risk factors for ischemic stroke OC103
Sirotkina O*, Tcherkas Y, Elchaninov A, Merkulova A, Chukhlovina M, Denisenko A, Schwarzman A

Inherited prothrombotic risk factors (factor V G1691A, factor II G20210A, MTHFR C677T and platelet polymorphisms) in pediatric ischemic stroke OC104
Oliveira L, Ozelo M, Rossi F, Annichino-Bizzacchi JM*, Moura-Ribeiro M, Castro V

Congenital thrombophilia in patients with cerebral ischemia and patent foramen ovalis (PFO) OC105
Pengo V*, Zanchetta M, Pedon L, Carrozza A, Bison E, Biasiolo A, Maiolino P, Iliceto S

Lipoprotein(a) and C-reactive protein in children with cerebrovascular Events OC106
Zrinski Topić R, Coen D*, Fuček M, Miloš M, Leniček-Krleža J, Dodig S

Genetic determinants of hyperhomocysteinemia in ischemic stroke: The role of MTHFR (C677T and A1298C), TSER and MTR A2756G OC107
Kim N*, Oh D, Park S

Is thrombin activatable fibrinolysis inhibitor a contributing factor for development of thrombotic complications in patients with ischemic stroke? OC108
Antovic J*, Rooth E, Wallen H, Kaponides G, von Arbin M, Wahlgren N, Stenmark J, Blombäck M

Oral anticoagulant treatment I

Bleeding complications of oral anticoagulation therapy: a prospective audit OC109
Bond S*, Rhodes S, Green E, James R, Taylor M, Rose P, Emmas C

The relationship of D-dimer and residual vein thrombosis as risk factors for recurrent venous thromboembolism after anticoagulation withdrawal OC110
Cosmi B*, Legnani C, Cini M, Guazzaloca G, Palareti G

Drug interactions and risk of acute bleeding leading to hospitalisation or death in patients with chronic atrial fibrillation treated with warfarin OC111
Gasse C*, Hollowell J, Meier C, Troost J, Schneider V, Haefeli W

The effect of vitamin K substitution on anticoagulant treatment OC112
Rombouts E*, Van der Meer F, Rosendaal F

Telemedicine for managing patients on oral anticoagulant therapy OC113
Testa S*, Alatri A, Morstabilini G, Denti N, Martellenghi E, Mazzei G, Negri D, Pani A, Camaiora A, Lari B

Absolute risk of venous and arterial thromboembolism associated with mild hyperhomocysteinemia OC136
van de Poel M*, Libourel E, Bank I, Middeldorp S, Hamulyak K, Prins M, Büller HR, van der Meer J

Methionine loading test affects thrombin generation in high risk patients OC137
Domagala TB*, Undas A, Celińska-Lowenhoff M, Rybak M, Szczeklik A

Hyperhomocysteinemia in cancer patients with thrombosis is independent of methylene tetrahydrofolate reductase gene mutation OC138
Cunanan J*, Tobu M, Iqbal O, Demir M, Fareed J, Deitcher S

Metalloproteinases

Circulating tissue inhibitor of metalloproteinase-1 elevation correlates with impaired diastolic relaxation in patients with hypertension OC139
Tayebjee M*, Nadar S, MacFadyen R, Lip G

Circulating MMP-9, TIMP-1 and TIMP-2 in gestational hypertension OC140
Tayebjee M*, Karalis I, Nadar S, Beevers DG, MacFadyen R, Lip G

Matrix metalloproteinase-9 and tissue inhibitor of metalloproteinase-1 in hypertension: Relationship to cardiovascular risk and treatment OC141
Tayebjee M*, Nadar S, Blann AD, Beevers DG, MacFadyen R, Lip G

Correlation of protein and mRNA expression of fibrinolytic and matrix metalloproteinase systems in endometriosis OC142
Ramón L, Gilabert-Estellés J, Castelló R, Gilabert J, España F, Chirivella M, Romeu A, Aznar J, Estellés A*

Popliteal arterial aneurysm - the role of proteolytic enzymes OC143
Kozak M*, Štalc J, Tominc U

The roles of serum matrix metalloproteinases in patients with post myocardial infarction to heart failure OC144
Jong G*, Ma T, Kuo S

Heparins

Managed hemostasis "point-of-care" testing in a large hospital: a three-year experience and the assessment of clotting tests OC145
Paniccia R*, Costanzo M, Tronchin M, Messeri G, Gazzini A, Coviello S, Antonucci E, Abbate R, Gensini G, Prisco D

Once-daily LMWH versus UFH for the treatment of acute venous thromboembolism: a non-inferiority meta-analysis OC146
Assante C*, Cucherat M, Laporte S, Rivron-Guillot K, Decousus H, Mismetti P

Therapeutic implications of product individuality in commercially available low molecular weight heparins and their generic versions OC147
Maddineni J*, Walenga J, Jeske W, Hoppensteadt D, Fareed J, Messmore H

Evaluation of the effectiveness and safety of bemiparin, a second-generation low-molecular-weight heparin, in several orthopaedic settings OC148
Otero-Fernández R, Gómez-Outes A, Martínez-González J*, Maeso R, Fontcuberta J

Bemiparin prospective observational study on the prevention of venous thromboembolism in medical patients OC149
Gómez-Outes A, Martínez-González J*, Maeso R, García-Hernández A

Low-molecular-weight heparin causes less heparin-induced antibodies than unfractionated heparin: A prospective study in neurologic patients OC150
Harbrecht U*, Andrea K, Britta B, Peter H, Thomas K, Christoph P

Thrombophilia

Factors I, VII, VIII, IX, X and XI levels and the risk of deep venous thrombosis OC151
Mello T, Machado T, Ozello M, Annichino-Bizzacchi JM*

High factor VIII (FVIII) levels in venous thromboembolism: role of the unbound component of FVIII OC152
Schambeck C*, Großmann R, Schwender S, Teuchert K, Walter U

The relationship between inherited thrombophilia and residual vein thrombosis as risk factors for recurrent venous thromboembolism OC153
Cosmi B*, Legnani C, Cini M, Guazzaloca G, Palareti G

Retinal vein thrombosis and thrombophilic risk factors OC154
Barillari G*, Roman D, Giacomello R, Dello Russo P, De Stasio G, Bandello F, Biffoni F

Risk factors for CNS thrombosis in neonates and children OC155
Pergantou H*, Kapsimali Z, Adamtziki E, Platokouki H, Vranou M, Aronis S

Coagulation activation in patients with and without thrombophilia during anticoagulant treatment for venous thrombosis OC156
Vižintin Cuderman T*, Božič M, Peternel P, Stegnar M

TAFI

A new TAFI antigen assay independent of polymorphism 325Thr/Ile and147 Ala/Thr OC157
Cost H, Grimaux M, Grosley M, Woodhams B*

Influence of the Thrombin Activatable Fibrinolysis Inhibitor (TAFI) Thr325Ile polymorphism on TAFI levels determined with three new assays OC158
Frère C, Aillaud MF, Saut N, Grosley M, Beltran J, Juhan-Vague I, Alessi MC*

TAFI levels in patients with acute myocardial infarction treated with thrombolysis OC159
Frère C*, Renard S, Grosley, Beltran J, Gils A, Declerck P, Chandler W, Van De Werf F, Juhan-Vague I, Alessi MC

Mediation of fibrinolytic deficit in cancer patients by plasminogen activator inhibitor-1 and thrombin activatable fibrinolytic inhibitor OC160
Florian-Kujawski M*, Hoppensteadt D, Iqbal O, Demir M, Tobu M, Fareed D, Fareed J

Modulation of thrombin activatable fibrinolytic inhibitor (TAFI) by heparins: Variation among normal and patient populations OC161
Florian-Kujawski M*, Maddineni J, Hoppensteadt D, Janssen M, Wilmer M, Bick R, Iqbal O, Tobu M, Fareed J

Does thrombin activatable fibrinolysis inhibitor (TAFI) contribute to hemostatic complications in patients with different types of brain injury? OC162
Antovic J*, Rooth E, Wallen H, Hannerz J, Nekludov M, Kaponides G, von Arbin M, Wahlgren N, Antovic A, Blombäck M

FEATURED POSTERS

Cardiovascular disease I

Abnormal heart rate variability is associated with platelet activation in stable coronary disease during recovery from myocardial infarction FP01
Hamaad A*, Blann AD, Lip G, MacFadyen R

Abnormalities in heart rate variability is associated with platelet activation in acute ST-elevation myocardial infarction FP02
Hamaad A*, Blann AD, Lip G, MacFadyen R

EPCR 23 bp Insertion in Atherosclerosis and Early MI FP03
Ulu A*, Akar R, Emiroglu O, Ucanok K, Akar E, Akar N

Soluble tissue factor in plasma from patients with acute myocardial infarction is not microvesicle associated FP04
Seljeflot I*, Lyberg T, Arnesen H

The effects of home-based versus hospital-based cardiac rehabilitation on plasma haemostatic markers in patients with coronary heart disease FP05
Lee W*, Jolly K, Lip G

Anticoagulant therapy

Hemostatic markers in patients with chronic atrial fibrillation - relationship to thromboembolic risk FP06
Vene N*, Mavri A, Košmelj K, Stegnar M

Anticoagulation in conventional versus transesophageal echocardiography guided cardioversion of atrial fibrillation FP07
Dokler Glavnik A*, Žohar P*, Gunzek R*, Bervar M*, Marinšek M*, Škrabl Močnik F*

Low molecular weight heparin limits prothrombotic reactions and may shorten in-hospital stay of patients with heart failure FP08
Wachnicka-Truty R*, Birkholz-Gołaszewska A, Korzeniowski A, Flasiński J, Górski J

Replacing acenocoumarol with the low molecular weight heparin Tinzaparin sodium in patients undergoing general surgery operations: a pilot study FP09
Volteas S*, Bossinakou I, Kotsopoulou M, Mattheou S, Kalatzopoulos D, Nicolakeas M, Sikiotis K

Oral Anticoagulant Therapy Management In Patient Self-Testing FP10
Testa S*, Alatri A, Morstabilini G

Methods in coagulation

Anti-Xa activity monitoring of the synthetic pentasaccharide Fondaparinux FP11
Van Dreden P*, Fontaine S, Woodhams

The Ecarin Chromogenic Assay (ECA) for quantitative determination of direct thrombin inhibitors-From a routine method to a point-of-care test FP12
Lange U*, Frische I, Olschewski A, Nowak G, Bucha E

A novel assay for tissue factor pathway inhibitor (TFPI) anticoagulant activity in plasma FP13
Dahm A*, Andersen T, Rosendaal F, Sandset P

A novel coagulation assay used to detect procoagulant phospholipid correlates with microparticle numbers in resting and collagen-stimulated samples FP14
Connor D*, Exner T, Ma D, Joseph J*

Von Willebrand factor cleavage in vitro at room temperature occurs without the need for divalent ions FP15
Perutelli P*, Amato S, Molinari A

Cardiovascular disease II

Dietary habits and their role on the occurrence of coronary artery disease: is the Italian a real Mediterranean-diet? FP16
Sofi F*, Giuliani G, Vecchio S, Martinelli F, Fedi S, Cellai A, Gori A, Ferrini S, Abbate R, Gensini GF

Oxidative stress-a link between endothelial injury, coagulation activation and atherosclerosis in haemodialysis patients FP17
Pawlak K*, Naumnik B, Brzosko S, Pawlak D, Mysliwiec M

Platelets

VTE

Lipoproteins

Direct thrombin inhibitors

Cancer

Effect of combination antı-angiogenesis therapy on markers of coagulation, platelet activation and angiogenesis in patients with advanced cancer FP41
Caine G, Harris A, Christodoulos K, Lip G, Blann AD

Intrinsic "tenase" and prothrombinase activity of t-lymphoblastoid cells is enhanced by lipid peroxidation FP42
Pickering W*, Gray E, Goodall A, Barrowcliffe T

Upregulation of monocyte chemotactic protein-1 and CD40 ligand in cancer patients and their modulation by subcutaneous enoxaparin FP43
Fareed J*, Tobu M, Demir M, Hoppensteadt D, Deitcher S

Platelet-derived vegf, flt-1, angiopoietın-1 and p-selectin in breast and prostate cancer FP44
Caine G, Lip G, Blann AD*

Optimal dosing of bemiparin for the prevention of venous thromboembolism in surgery for cancer FP45
Gómez-Outes A, Martínez-González J*, del Campo J, Rocha E*

POSTERS

Cardiovascular disease

Ischaemic cardiopathy and associated risk factors in two elderly women groups of low socio-economic condition PO001
Narváez I*, Saez de Lafuente J, Sáez Y, Vacas M, Molinero E, Sagastagoitia J, Magro A, Santos M, Sabino E, Iriarte J

Factors that may influence in the adequate control of arterial hypertension PO002
Narváez I*, Caso R, Martinez B, Molinero E, Sagastagoitia J, Vacas M, Saez Y, Saez de Lafuente J, Iriarte J, Iriarte M

Coronary heart disease estimation in an elderly population PO003
Vacas M*, Martinez B, Caso R, Narváez I, Saez Y, Iriarte M, Iriarte J, Molinero E, Sagastagoitia J, Gandarias JM

Prothrombotic risk in white coat hypertensives PO004
Theodossiades G*, Vyssoulis G, Karpanou E, Zervoudaki A, Tsevrenis V, Kokkinos D, Stefanadis C

Pathogenetic role of nitric oxide in thomboembolic complications in patients with chronic hart failure PO005
Mirsamatova G

A comparison of off-pump and on-pump coronary-artery bypass surgery by sonoclot analysis PO006
Paniccia R*, Caciolli S, Palmarini M, Costanzo M, Pretelli P, Stefano P, Attanasio M, Abbate R, Gensini GF, Prisco D

A comparison between inthima-media thickness and coronary artery disease PO007
Liva S, Pegoraro C, Cucchini U, Andriani C, Pelliccioni S, Maiolino G, Napodano M, Ramondo A, Pengo V, Iliceto S

The effects of incremental shuttle walking on activation of haemostatic and haemorheologic markers in patients with coronary heart disease PO008
Lee W*, Ingram J, Jolly K, Lip G

Use of low-molecular-weight-heparin in early cardioversion PO009
Dokler Glavnik A*, Škrabl Močnik F, Žohar P, Bervar M, Marinšek M, Gunzek R

Left ventricular diastolic dysfunction is associated with abnormal haemorheology, thrombogenesis and endothelial damage/dysfunction PO010
Lee W*, Lip G

Plasma vascular endothelial growth factor (VEGF) and the angiopoietin/Tie2 System in proliferative sickle retinopathy PO011
Mohan J, Lip P, Bareford D, Blann AD*, Lip G

Fluid shear stress, blood coagulation and epigenome topography of granulocytes nuclei at atherosclerosis: what is evident? PO012
Teplyakov A

New polymorphism in the first intron of the ABCA1 transporter gene PO013
Sheydina A*, Pchelina S, Demina E, Schwarzman A

Enhanced level of tissue-type plasminogen activator antigen in hypertensive small deep infarcts PO014
Ionova V*, Suslina Z, Maximova M, Tanashian M, Klimovich L

Hyperhomocysteinemia is significant risk factor for cerebral arterial occlusive diseases in North West Russia PO015
Shmeleva V*, Kapustin S, Papayan L

Oral methionine load induces von Willebrand factor changes in women with peripheral occlusive disease PO016
Peutelli P*, Amato S, Bottini F, Minniti G, Cerone R, Molinari A

Analysis of 5 SNPs of the ABCA1 gene in patients with ischemic stroke PO017
Taraskina A, Sheydina A*, Sirotkina O, Elchaninov A, Pchelina S

ASO titer and efficacy of streptokinase in acute myocardial infarction patients PO018
Ostovan M*, Hooshmand S

Lymphocyte platelet adhesion in acute coronary syndrome PO019
Solpov A*, Govorin A, Gorbunov V, Vitkovsky Y

Different molecules of endothelial origin - master of cytokines network balance: new evidence of lymphocytes functioning at atherosclerosis PO020
Teplyakov A*

Haemorheological alterations in patients with previous myocardial infarction and angiographically normal coronary arteries (MINC) PO021
Mannini L*, Paniccia R, Cecchi E, Giuello A, Bruschettini A, Margheri M, Giglioli C, Comeglio M, Abbate R, Gensini GF

Long-term clinical outcomes of a platelet glycoprotein IIb/IIIa receptor blocker (Abciximab: ReoPro®) coated stent in coronary artery disease PO022
Jeong M*, Kim W, Kim J, Ahn YK, Cho JG, Park J, Kang J

Coagulation factors and inhibitors

Protein C as diagnostic marker in early diagnosis severe intra-abdominal infections PO023
Vukosavljević D*, Vodnik T, Majkić-Singh N, Karamarković A

Is factor VII deficiency predisposing to foetal loss? (Study of a large family) PO024
Lo Pinto G*, Perroni L, Cusano R, Barbaresi M, Costa M, Malatesti V

The relationship between ABO blood subgroups, von Willebrand factor, factor VIII and ristocetin cofactor PO025
Sousa N, Anicchino-Bizzacchi JM*, Siqueira L, Leite E, Locatelli M, Barjas-Castro ML

A proteomic approach for the resolution of vitamin K dependent proteins PO026
Uras F*, Salman Dilgimen A, Uras A

Factor XIII Val34Leu polymorphism as a modulator of resistance to fibrinolysis in subjects treated with aspirin PO027
Undas A*, Brożek J, Iwaniec T, Szczeklik A

Factor VII activity and blood coagulation at the site of microvascular injury PO028
Brzezinska B, Undas A, Padjas A*, Iwaniec T, Musiał J

Role of fibrin in thrombin behavior PO029
de Bosch N

Factor XIII level and prevalence of FXIII-A Val34Leu polymorphism in patients with peripheral arterial disease and Raynaud's disease PO030
Shemirani A*, Csiki Z, Szomják E, Katona É, Bereczky Z, Muszbek L

Factor XIII subunit B: a protein A-binding protein PO031
Kerényi A*, Haramura G, Muszbek L

Effect of short wave frequency electromagnetic radiation on lymphocyte-platelet adhesion and tissue factor expression by leukocytes PO032
Nardina I*, Vitkovsky Y

FVIII Levels During Attacks of Familial Mediterranean Fever PO033
Akar N*, Ekim M, Gürman C

Successful use of recombinant activated factor VII (rFVIIa) in a patient with severe bleeding during transabdominal retropubic prostatectomy PO034
Monteiro C*, Jorreto M, Gonçalves L, Fraga M, Pereira R

Tensile strength of blood clot PO035
Savushkin AV*

Blood clot: hydraulic resistance and its changing PO036
Savushkin AV*

Erythrocyte desert out the blood clot phenomenon (filtration "back to front") PO037
Savushkin AV*

Anticoagulant therapy

Warfarin is superior to Acenocoumarol in the management of patients requiring low doses of oral anticoagulants PO038
Ceresetto JM*, Rabinovich O, Stemmelin G, Shanley C, Duboscq C, Gutierrez M, Mendizabal G, Doti C, Vicente M, Bullorsky E

Validation of CoaguChek S on samples of patients on stable oral anticoagulation PO039
Laszlo P*

Dental surgery in patients treated with oral anticoagulants PO040
Dimova C*, Kostovska S, Dejanova V, Kovacevska I, Andonovska B

Evaluating the interaction of allopurinol with the oral anticoagulants PO041
Rodrigues*, Martins R, Viegas E

Recurrence of deep vein thrombosis in a patient with combined thrombophilic disorder, complicated by warfarin-induced liver damage PO042
Hirmerová J*, Mecová E, Chudáček Z

Ambulatory programme of monitoring oral anticoagulant therapy in the Basque country: Evaluation of the point of-care device ProTime PO043
Vacas M*, Santos M, Longa M, Martin S, Lafuente P, Iriarte J, Gandarias JM

Patient relationship to the oral anticoagulant therapy with regard to the age, level of education and duration of treatment PO044
Vukelic-Damijani N*, Caser L, Skalamera R, Vujaklija-Stipanovic K

Self-management of anticoagulation: a randomised trial (SMART) PO045
Fitzmaurice D*, Murray E, McCahon D, Jowett S, Sandhur H, Hobbs R

Importance of continuous education in anticoagulated patients PO046
Iriarte J*, Longa M, Zorraquin A, Santos M, Vacas M, Narvaez I, Sabino E, Gandarias JM, Saez Y, Saez de Lafuente J

Animal experimental models

Cancer and thrombosis

Endothelial cells

Gene expression profiling of endothelial cells from normal and systemic sclerosis patients PO069
Giusti B*, Fibbi G, Rossi L, D'Alessio S, Poggi F, Margheri F, Del Rosso A, Matucci-Cerinic M, Abbate R, Del Rosso M

Comparison of platelets' and endothelium function between diabetics and normal subjects PO070
Makris P*, Koukourikou M, Girtovitis F, Boutou A, Giannoulis E, Pithara E, Spartali A, Karamitsos D

The evaluation of disfunction of endothelium in patients with hypertensive small deep infarcts PO071
Maximova M*, Suslina Z, Ionova V, Tanashian M

Direct thrombin inhibitors

The influence of melagatran on thrombin generation, comparison with other anticoagulant drugs PO072
Al Dieri R*, Hemker H, Béguin S

Melagatran is efficiently eliminated by hemodialysis in uremic patients PO073
Eriksson UG, Samuelsson O, Attman PO, Lepkowska M, Ohlsson L, Carlsson S, Fager G

No influence of food on the pharmacokinetics, pharmacodynamics, or tolerability of the 36mg oral tablet formulation of ximelagatran PO074
Ersdal E*, Schutzer K, Eriksson UG, Lönnerstedt C, Ohlsson L, Wall U

Efficacy and safety of postoperative ximelagatran for prevention of thromboembolism across different orthopaedic surgery patient groups PO075
Dahl OE*, Eriksson BI, Agnelli G, Cohen AT, Mouret P, Rosencher N, Panfilov S, Andersson M

Effect of the oral, direct Factor Xa inhibitor, BAY 59-7939, on thrombin generation after tissue factor pathway activation PO076
Gerotziafas G*, Depasse F, Chakroun T, Elalamy I, Samama M

Studies on the mechanism of action of BAY 59-7939 - an oral, direct Factor Xa inhibitor PO077
Fareed J*, Hoppensteadt D, Maddenini J, Schultz C, Nevelle B, Iqbal O, Perzborn E, Misselwitz F

Effects of BAY 59-7939, an innovative, oral, direct Factor Xa inhibitor, on thrombin generation in healthy volunteers PO078
Harder S, Graff J*, v. Hentig N, Misselwitz F, Kubitza D, Zuehlsdorf M, Wensing G, Mueck W, Becka M, Breddin HK

Biochemical and pharmacologic properties of BAY 59-7939, an oral, direct Factor Xa inhibitor PO079
Perzborn E*, Strassburger J, Wilmen A, Lampe T, Pernerstorfer J, Pohlmann J, Roehrig S, Schlemmer K, Straub A

Multiple dose escalation study investigating BAY 59-7939 - an oral, direct Factor Xa inhibitor - in healthy male subjects PO080
Kubitza D*, Becka M, Wensing G, Voith B, Zuehlsdorf M

Single dose escalation study of BAY 59-7939 - an oral, direct Factor Xa inhibitor - in healthy male subjects PO081
Kubitza D*, Becka M, Wensing G, Voith B, Zuehlsdorf M

The oral direct thrombin inhibitor ximelagatran shows bioequivalence when administered as whole or crushed tablets or in solution via nasogastric tube PO082
Schützer K*, Lönnerstedt C, Wall U, Ohlsson L, Sarich T, Teng R, Eriksson UG

The pharmacokinetics and pharmacodynamics of the oral direct thrombin inhibitor ximelagatran when administered with erythromycin PO083
Dorani H*, Schützer K, Sarich T, Wall U, Ohlsson L, Eriksson UG

Lipoproteins and haemostasis

Effect of malondialdehyde modified low density lipoproteins on platelet adhesion PO084
Suttnar J*, Otahalova E, Dyr JE, Cermak J

Lipoprotein (a) as a marker of diffuse coronary artery disease in young survivors of myocardial infarction PO085
Zorio E, Falcó C, Palencia M, Arnau MA, España F, Ramón L, España F, Castelló R, Almenar L, Estellés A*

The effect of the new Russian food supplement "Eiferol" on the hemostasis and lipid metabolism in patients with disease of the liver PO086
Vjacheslav I*, Valentina P, Galina A, Margarita K, ludmila L

Atorvastatin affects thrombosis/fibrinolysis system during the acute phace of unstable angina PO087
Kotsopoulou M*, Bosinakou E, Tousoulis D, Antoniades C, Fostira E, Pitsavos C, Stefanadis C

Effects of atorvastatin on thrombosis/fibrinolysis system and endothelial function, in patients with heart failure PO088
Kotsopoulou M*, Antoniades C, Tousoulis D, Bosinakou E, Cheimona A, Pitsavos C, Stefanadis C

Fibrinolysis

The t-PA and PAI-1 activities under treatment by thrombolytic and anticoagulant medicaments in patients with acute myocardial infarction PO089
Krasnobryzha I*, Savchuk O

Relationship between global fibrinolytic capacity and cardiovascular risk factors in obese patients PO090
Turgut B, Guldiken S, Demir M*, Ugur-Altun B, Gerenli M, Vuralo O, Tugrul A

Tissue plasminogen activator plasma levels is an independent predictor of in-hospital major events in patients with unstable angina PO091
Gougopoulou D*, Theodoridis T, El Ali M, Koulouris S, Karabinos I, Gianoulis T, Exadaktylos N, Christopoulou-Cokkin V

D-dimer promotes endothelial dysfunction in diabetes mellitus PO092
Yevdokimova N*, Lugovskij E, Komisarenko S

Pretreatment PAI-1 levels and streptokinase thrombolysis in Iranian patients with acute MI in spite of negligible antistreptokinase antibodies PO093
Shemirani H*, Tajmirriahi, Rezaei A, Oresi A

Elevated levels of methylglyoxal may contribute to the development of thrombotic complications in diabetes mellitus PO094
Léránt I*, Kolev K, Machovich R

Plasma flow velocity and fibrin specificity of thrombolytic agent promote thrombolysis of non-retracted and retracted whole blood clots PO095
Tratar G*, Blinc A, Štrukelj M, Mikac U, Serša I

Coagulation/fibrinolysis system parameters are affected by smoking cessation PO096
Hatzizacharias A*, Makris T, Krespi P, Stavroulakis G, Paizis J, Tsoukala C, Mandalaki T, Votteas V

Plasminogen Activator Inhibitor (PAI) 4G/5G polymorphism in patients with coronary artery disease PO097
Apergis G*, Bellia M*, Bratsas A*, Pavlou E*, Brilli S*, Gagou A*, Georgopoulos J*, Andrioti E*

The relationship between Ins/Del (I/D) polymorphism in ACE gene with t-PA I/D and PAI-1 4G/5G polymorphisms in PE PO098
Altinok B*, Oner F, Numanoglu N, Oguzulgen K, Ekim N, Akar N

PAI-1 levels, 4G/5G genotype and insulin resistance in severe and morbid obesity. Effect of weight loss and influence of 4G/5G genotype PO099
Solá E, Vayá A, Castelló R, España F, Hernández A, Aznar J, Estellés A*

Haemostasis activation markers

Poster withdrawn PO100

Troponin concentration in NSTEMI patients depends on intensity of prothrombotic reactions PO101
Wachnicka-Truty R*, Korzeniowski A, Birkholz-Gołaszewska A, Kliz J, Flasiński J, Dmochowska-Wróblewsk W

D-dimer and soluble fibrin at ischemic heart disease and acute impairment cerebral circulation PO102
Lugovskoy E*, Kolesnikova I, Gritsenko P, Lugovskaya N, Komisarenko S

D-dimer levels in long term anticoagulated patients PO103
Gafou A*, Tsevrenis V, Nomikou E, Bellia M, Paulou E, Andrioti E

A normal Wells´s score and a normal D-dimer test safely exclude pulmonary embolism PO104
Söderberg M*, Brohult J

D- dimer in the diagnosis of pulmonary embolism PO105
Škrgat-Kristan S*, Meško Brguljan P*, Košnik M, Šorli J

The usefulness of D-dimer in hospitalized patients with lung diseases PO106
Fijalkowska A*, Piwek A, Wiatr E, Kurzyna M, Kuca P, Burakowski J, Kober J, Szturmowicz M, Tomkowski W, Torbicki A

The characteristic of the soluble fibrin-monomer complexes fraction PO107
Savchuk O*, Volodymyr C, Tatyana P

Management of coagulopathy and associated severe bleeding in immediate post-partum period PO108
Gonçalves L*, Oliveira G, Pereira R, Cunha-Ribeiro L

Increased thrombin-antithrombin III levels in preeclampsia and disseminated intravascular coagulation on two different ELISAs PO109
Simpson D, Whittier A, Andrews J, Fink C, Lopez L

Heparins and related drugs

Effect of parnaparin, a low molecular weight heparin, on platelet-leukocyte interaction PO110
Maugeri N*, de Gaetano G, Donati MB, Cerletti C

Paradoxical action of the synthetic pentasaccharide (Arixtra®) PO111
Makris P*, Boutou A, Tsoukas D, Papmichos S, Sarridou D, Triantafyllou A, Psatha V, Chasilidis A, Anestakis D, Girtovitis F

Influence of the original low molecular weight heparin on the rabbits plasma anticoagulant activity PO112
Drozd N*, Bannicova G, Sukhanova P, Miphtakhova N, Makarov V, Varlamov V, Vikhoreva G

Different response of bone turnover markers during venous thromboembolic prophylaxis with LMWH or oral anticoagulants PO113
Wawrzyńska L*, Przedlacki J, Hajduk B, Tomkowski W, Torbicki A

Inflammation

Lupus anticoagulants

Methods in coagulation

Perinatal and paediatric haemostasis

Platelets

Poly-APS induced thrombocyte aggregation is partly blocked by the combination of acetylsalicylic acid, clopidogrel and abciximab PO165
Šuput D, Bunc M*

Influence of platelet activation agonists on lymphocyte-platelet adhesion PO166
Solpov A*, Vitkovsky Y, Kuznik B

Influence of recombinant interleukin 2 on platelet aggregation and lymphocyte-platelet adhesion PO167
Vitkovsky Y*, Solpov A, Kuznik B

The severity of peripheral arterial disease can influence plasma platelet microparticle levels PO168
Tan K, Tayebjee M, Blann AD*, Lynd C, Lip G*

Patients with stable ischaemic heart disease have increased levels of platelet microparticles PO169
Tan K, Tayebjee M, Blann AD*, Lip G*

Prevalence of aspirin resistance in cardiovascular patients using the PFA-100 diagnostic system PO170
Narvaez I*, Vacas M, Saez Y, Caso R, Martinez B, Sagastagoitia J, Molinero E, Santos M, Saez de Lafuente J, Iriarte J

Clinical effects of combined tirofiban with LMWH in patients with acute coronary syndrome PO171
Kim J, Jeong M*, Kim W, Ahn YK, Cho JG, Park J, Kang J

Thrombocytopenia in the intensive care unit. Case series PO172
Duarte P*, Grand B, Egozcue J, Fernandez J, Cacchione R, Riveros D

Salvage plasmapheresis in case of pulmonary embolism caused by heparin-induced thrombocytopenia type II resistant to danaparoid sodium and lepirudin PO173
Antonijevic N*, Savic N, Perunicic J, Mikovic D, Kovac M, Stanojevic M, Calija B, Obradovic S, Milosevic R, Vasiljevic Z

Pregnancy, menopause, hormones

Prospective study of coagulability in pregnancy - a new approach to the early detection of preeclampsia and cardiovascular complications PO174
Sylvest Andersen A*, Berthelsen JG, Breindahl M, Fareed J, Rud Lassen M

No need for laboratory monitoring during low dose LMMH thromboprophylaxis during pregnancy PO175
van Rooijen M*, Nord E, Lampén Mondzo K, Bremme K

Factor VIII levels in the early postpartum period PO176
Procházka M*, Slavík L, Procházková J, Hrachovec P, Krčová V, Zielina P

Polymorphism of gene PAI-1 4G/4G and preembrionic losses PO177
Bitsadze VO*, Baimuradova SM, Makatsaria A

Acute vascular violations in pregnant women with thrombophilias PO178
Bitsadze VO*, Baimuradova SM, Stuleva N, Makatsaria A

The effects of oral hormone replacement therapy on C-reactive protein and other inflammatory markers in women with previous venous thromboembolism PO179
Eilertsen A*, Høibraaten E, Sandvik L, Opstad Andersen T, Mowinckel M, Sandset P

Estrogen receptors and venous thrombosis PO180
Aléssio AM, Höehr N, Nogueira C, Mansur A, Ozello M, Siqueira L, Annichino-Bizzacchi J M*

The effect of norethisterone acetate on inflammatory markers in postmenopausal women receiving estradiol PO181
Žegura B*, Gužič-Salobir B, Šebeštjen M, Keber I, Koenig W

The influence of hormone replacement therapy (HRT) on factor VIIa/antithrombin (FVIIa/AT) complex PO182
Dahm A*, Hoibraaten E, Morrissey J, Andersen T, Sandset P

Thrombophilic mutations as inherited risk factors for myocardial infarction in postmenopausal women PO183
Sirotkina O*, Smirnova N, Rodygina T, Toperverg O, Churina S, Schwarzman A

Thrombophilia

Heterozygous Factor V Leiden deficiency with venous thrombosis and pulmonary embolism in a woman with breast cancer PO184
Kotsopoulou M*, Apergis G, Bosinakou E, Sklabou S, Paylou E, Mantzourani A, Andrioti E

Coagulation studies in patients with thrombosed prosthetic heart valves and intracardiac clots PO185
Saour J*, Saour T, Shereen A, Al hamed M, Hawari S, Saour B, Shoukri M, Mamo L

Thrombosis and familial thrombophelia registry, preliminary report PO186
Mammo L*, Saour T, Hawari S, Sidiqui K, Shereen A, Saour B, Saour J

Frequency of hereditary thrombophilia in Egypt population PO187
Ulu A*, Elsayed S, Yildiz Z, Cin S, Elsobky E, Akar N

Prothrombin G20210A mutation in patients with cerebrovascular disease PO188
Ulutin T, Altinisik J, Somay G, Buyru N

Prothrombin G20210 mutation and association with severe life threatening thrombosis among thrombophilic patients PO189
Bellia M*, Sklavou S, Theodosiadis G, Gafou A, Georgopoulos J, Andrioti E

VTE

PLENARY LECTURES

PL01

"Resistance" to aspirin and other antiplatelet drugs

Patrono C

University of Rome "La Sapienza", Rome, Italy

Acetylation of platelet COX-1, inhibition of TXA_2 production and prevention of thrombotic complications share two rather unique features: they are measurable effects of a once daily regimen of aspirin administration, despite a 20-min half-life of the drug, and they show saturability of the effect at low doses. The amount of daily aspirin currently recommended by all international guidelines represents a 3- to 10-fold excess over the minimum amount of the drug necessary and sufficient to fully inactivate platelet COX-1 upon repeated daily dosing (20-30 mg). This excess can easily accommodate interindividual variations in drug absorption, body weight, platelet count and turnover. Thus, it is not surprising that the interindividual variability in the degree of suppression of platelet TXA_2 production is quite limited, even in the presence of a high platelet count. In view of the remarkable consistency in the platelet TXA_2-suppressing effect of aspirin, both the American College of Chest Physicians Consensus Conference on Antithrombotic Therapy and the European Society of Cardiology Task Force on Antiplatelet Agents recommend that no test of platelet function be performed to assess the antiplatelet effect of aspirin in the individual patient. As with any drug (antithrombotic, lipid lowering or antihypertensive) used to prevent atherothrombosis, treatment 'failure' can occur with aspirin - perhaps not surprisingly, given the multifactorial nature of atherothrombosis. Thus, there is no scientific basis to change antithrombotic, lipid-lowering or antihypertensive therapy in the face of a treatment 'failure', as we cannot be sure whether a second vascular event occurring in the same patient reflects the same pathophysiological event that led to the first. Moreover, we have no controlled evidence that changing therapy is a more effective strategy than maintaining an evidence-based therapy. Given the size of the relative risk reduction (typically, 15 to 25%) associated with long-term aspirin prophylaxis, studies aiming to detect an attenuation or loss of this effect as a function of 'resistance' should have both the sensitivity and specificity necessary to detect such a small 'signal'. None of the studies published so far meets these requirements.

PL02

Cancer and cardiovascular disease: does a common soil exist?

Donati MB

Center for High Technology and Education in Biomedical Sciences, Campobasso, Italy

Cardiovascular disease (CVD) and cancer are considered the major killers of westernized countries and more and more also of emerging countries. Evidence is accumulating that ischemic CVD and some forms of tumors (particularly hormone-dependent tumors and tumors of the gastrointestinal tract) share some common mechanisms and could therefore benefit from similar preventive and therapeutic strategies. The pieces of evidence for a possible "common soil hypothesis" in the pathogenesis of ischemic CVD and of the above mentioned tumors can be grouped schematically as follows: **Cellular/molecular level**: common mechanisms have been recognized in the growth and migration of tumor and vascular cells and crucial mediators have been identified, such as adhesion molecules of the selectin and integrin families or metalloproteases; in this context, inflammatory mediators (cytokines, growth factors) are able to amplify both proliferative and migratory responses. We are presently running experiments aiming at verifying whether the pathogenetic sequence leading to leukocyte recruitment at inflammatory sites may recapitulate the events occurring during extravasation of tumor cells during hematogenous dissemination. **Pharmacological level**: there is ample experimental evidence that some antithrombotic agents have anti-metastatic and anti-invasive properties; these data, produced by several groups including ours 10-20 years ago, are getting presently clinical confirmation, at least in some settings (see early stage tumors as in the FAMOUS or the MALT studies). Also the cancer preventive effects of aspirin, the most widely used antithrombotic agent in the secondary prevention of CVD, deserve careful consideration. **Epidemiological level:** it is noteworthy that the above mentioned tumors and CVD share common risk/ protection factors, such as the metabolic syndrome, insulin-resistance, obesity, sedentary life and may be markedly influenced by dietary components. There is strong evidence for a geographical gradient for both types of disease and for the significant protective effect of a strict adherence to the Mediterranean diet against both cancer and cardiovascular mortality. Several experimental models and cellular studies have offered recently a biological plausibility to these epidemiological observations (see f.i. the cancer preventive and antithrombotic effects of anti-oxidant components of vegetables, wine and olive oil, the main ingredients of the Mediterranean diet).

PL03

Angiogenesis: A link to thrombosis in atherothrombotic disease

Conway E

Center for Transgene Technology & Gene Therapy, University of Leuven, Belgium
Flander Interuniversity Institute for Biotechnology, Belgium

Introduction: New insights to explain the clinical manifestations of atherosclerosis have resulted in a paradigm in which thrombosis is the major cause of acute coronary syndromes, peripheral vascular disease and stroke. Major efforts have been directed toward developing drugs to reduce thrombin and fibrin formation. Recent studies support a central role for angiogenesis of the atherosclerotic plaque in promoting atherothrombosis. The findings, in the face of efforts to use angiogenic agents to enhance vascular function, underline the challenge in treating atherothrombotic disease. **Aim**: The goal is to review the current model of atherosclerosis, the development of plaques and atherothrombosis, highlighting the mechanistic links between angiogenesis, inflammation and coagulation. Summary: Atherosclerosis is a complex, chronic inflammatory disorder characterized first, by dysfunctional endothelium, which results in enhanced adhesion molecule expression, release of cytokines/chemokines, and recruitment of monocytes/macrophages into the intima. These cells internalize oxLDL, and help perpetuate the atherogenic/thrombotic process by inducing accumulation of more macrophages and smooth muscle cells, synthesizng extracellular matrix, promoting formation of a fibrous-capped plaque, and releasing cytokines, growth factors and matrix metalloproteinases which contribute to plaque disruption and thrombus formation. Several cellular and biochemical events promote the expression and release of tissue factor, facilitating further thrombus formation. Closely linked, is a prominent neovascular response in the atheromatous arteries, associated with increased expression of angiogenic factors, including VEGF, bFGF and Plgf. The vasa vasorum become plentiful in the plaque, forming plexi in the vessel wall, enabling leukocyte trafficking into the lesions, thus sustaining plaque growth. In this context, VEGF may also promote inflammation, plaque rupture, hemorrhage and thrombosis. A vicious circle ensues, as thrombin and tissue factor may promote angiogenic factor release and plaque growth. **Conclusion**: Progress in elucidating the molecular pathways regulating atherogenesis support a role for angiogenesis in promoting atherothrombosis. Advances in our understanding of these pathways set the stage for the evaluation of novel approaches to prevent thrombogenicity, and thereby decrease morbidity and mortality of atherosclerotic disease.

PL04

Antiphospholipid syndrome: association between laboratory tests and clinical practice

Galli M

Division of Hematology, Ospedali Riuniti, Bergamo, Italy

The combination of thromboembolic events, obstetric complications, and antiphospholipid antibodies defines the antiphospholipid syndrome. Two forms have been described: the "primary" syndrome, where there is no evidence of an underlying disease, and the "secondary" syndrome, mainly in the setting of systemic lupus erythematosus. In 1998, an international panel of experts met in Sapporo to establish the classification criteria for definite antiphospholipid syndrome. To support the inclusion of lupus anticoagulants and anticardiolipin antibodies as laboratory criteria for the antiphospholipid syndrome in relation to thrombosis, we made a systematic computer-assisted (MEDLINE) search of the literature published in the English language from 1988 through 2001. Twenty-five prospective, ambispective, cross-sectional, and case-control studies on more than 7,000 patients and controls provided or enabled us to calculate the odds ratio (OR) with 95% confidence interval (CI) of lupus anticoagulants and anticardiolipin antibodies for arterial and/or venous thrombosis. The review formally established that lupus anticoagulants are strong risk factors for thrombosis, irrespective of the site (arterial or venous) and type (first event or recurrence), the presence of systemic lupus erythematosus, and the coagulation tests used to detect them. Anticardiolipin antibodies were not such strong risk factors, and less than half of their associations with thrombosis (16 out of 33) were significant, unless the G isotype and medium or high titers were considered. Separate analysis of the different types of thrombosis showed anticardiolipin antibodies were associated with cerebral stroke and myocardial infarction, but not with deep vein thrombosis. Five studies directly compared lupus anticoagulants and anticardiolipin antibodies for their OR for thrombosis in a few hundred patients and controls: the former, but not the latter, antibodies were significantly associated with thrombosis. Work in the 1990s made it clear that the true antigenic targets of antiphospholipid antibodies are not the phospholipids *per se*, but plasma proteins bound to an anionic (not necessarily phospholipid) surface. Antibodies to β2-glycoprotein I and prothrombin are the two most frequent and best-studied antiphospholipid antibodies. Since their first description, the relationship between anti β2-glycoprotein I and antiprothrombin antibodies and thrombosis have been amply studied. Investigators are now inclined to consider them good candidate laboratory criteria for the antiphospholipid syndrome, together with or possibly in replace of lupus anticoagulants and anticardiolipin antibodies. To contribute to this issue, we extended our computer-assisted search of the literature (MEDLINE) to studies on anti β2-glycoprotein I and antiprothrombin antibodies. Thirty-two articles were retrieved: cross-sectional and case-control studies gave information on 1,324 patients and 1,973 controls, and retrospective studies contributed another 3,778 patients. All but four studies employed home made assays, mostly ELISA. Systemic lupus erythematosus, the antiphospholipid syndrome, and the presence of lupus anticoagulants and/or anticardiolipin antibodies were the enrolment criteria in 26 studies. This makes it difficult to establish the relative roles of antiβ2-glycoprotein I and antiprothrombin antibodies as independent risk factors of thrombosis. Only 11 studies did multivariate analysis using logistic regression, which allows a summary of the risk assessment, given the joint contribution of each risk factor. The OR with 95% CI for thrombosis were available or could be calculated in 27 studies on 4,394 patients and 1,973 controls for anti β2-glycoprotein I antibodies, and in 17 studies on 2,339 patients and 613 controls for antiprothrombin antibodies. Thirty-four of 60 associations with thrombosis (57%) were significant for anti β2-glycoprotein I antibodies, particularly when the G isotype was considered. Regarding antiprothrombin antibodies, statistical significance was found for only 17 of 46 available associations (37%). In conclusion, we reviewed a wide selection of clinical studies on antiphospholipid antibodies, and formed the opinion that they are, at best, inconclusive. Only lupus anticoagulants were consistently associated with thrombosis, which implies that measuring them is helpful to define the patients' risk of arterial and venous thrombosis, and to guide therapeutic management. The results of studies on anticardiolipin and anti β2-glycoprotein I antibodies are less convincing and partly controversial, but they leave open the possibility that their measurement too may be practical and useful, at least in some situations. At present, there does not seem to be any role for measurement of antiprothrombin antibodies. We foresee the need for well-designed clinical trials, to help establish which, if any, among the various antibodies, are risk factors for the antiphospholipid syndrome. To accomplish this, standardization or at least harmonization of the methods used to detect the antiphospholipid antibodies is mandatory. Without it, any clinical study will be criticisable and unable to reach firm conclusions.

PL05

Coronary heart disease and inflammation -the lessons from therapeutic trials

Čerček B

Cedars-Sinai Medical Center, Los Angeles, California, U.S.A., University of California, Los Angeles (UCLA) CA., U.S.A.

An inflammatory response in the atherosclerotic arteries accompanying the accumulation of the lipids in fibrous material may be triggered by oxidized lipids, infection, mechanical stress. Chlamydia pneumoniae infects macrophages that infiltrate the vessel wall secreting cytokines and growth factor causing plaque growth and rupture. Early studies with anti-chlamydial antibiotics (roxithromyin, azithromycin) indicated beneficial effect of treatment in prevention of recurrent clinical events in patients with acute coronary syndrome (ACS) and also chronic coronary artery disease (CAD). Larger trials did not show an effect on clinical endpoints in patients admitted with ACS (AZACS) or in patients with chronic CAD (WIZARD). Both studies did indicate an early positive effect that was lost after few months. The short-term treatment with antibiotics may not confer beneficial long-term effect due to inadequate duration. Another possibility is that a total "infection burden" of several chronic infections predisposes to CAD progression and plaque destabilization. Several studies have indicated that subjects with high c-reactive protein (CRP) have a high risk for subsequent ACS. Aspirin has been shown in the primary prevention trial to neutralize the risk of increased CRP. In the patients with CAD (PRINCE, MIRACLE trials) the therapy with statins reduced the subsequent event rate that was paralleled by reduction in the CRP concentration. CRP reduction with statins is independent of the LDL lowering. Currently the proven clinical effects of statins are primarily related to the reduction of LDL cholesterol and there has been no study to demonstrate independent beneficial effect of anti-inflammatory pleotropic properties of statins in CAD patients.

PL06

Assessment of endothelial dysfunction: focus on atherothrombotic disease

Blann AD

Haemostasis, Thrombosis and Vascular Biology Unit, University Department of Medicine, City Hospital, Birmingham, UK

A fully functioning endothelium is essential if the development and progression of atherosclerosis is to be resisted. Indeed, damage to the endothelium is the link between health, risk factors such as diabetes, and the presence of clear disease as suggested by stroke and myocardial infarction. Our current approach to endothelial dysfunction considers firstly normal endothelial cell functioning which promotes anti-coagulation, minimises the flow of tissue fluid out of the blood, and helps maintain vascular tone by the release of vasoconstrictors and vasodilators. A healthy response to inflammation is the transient increase in the expression of adhesion molecules. Thus a dysfunctional endothelium fails in these tasks and instead (respectively) promotes thrombosis, oedema, hypertension and leukocyte adhesion. Assessment of endothelial dysfunction therefore follows these leads. Regarding anticoagulation and thrombosis, dysfunction is assessed by the release of specific vascular products such as von Willebrand factor and tissue plasminogen activator. Dysfunction leading to the loss of correct blood pressure regulation is assessed by flow mediated dilatation (FMD), and excess cytokine stimulation of the endothelium leading to damage may be assessed by soluble adhesion molecules such as E-selectin. However, the most unequivocal demonstration of severe endothelial damage is the appearance of circulating endothelial cells in the blood, as are present in acute myocardial infarction and chronic heart failure. Of these methods, increased plasma markers and impaired FMD predict adverse events although the time consuming and difficult assessment of FMD leaves von Willebrand factor measurement by ELISA as the most convenient in large epidemiological studies.

PL07

Different locations of atherosclerosis – different risk factors, different therapies?

Lowe G

University of Glasgow, Glasgow, UK

During the 1960's and 1970's, pathological and epidemiological studies showed significant associations between atherosclerosis (and its thrombotic complications) in the heart, brain and legs. Over the past 40 years, smoking, blood pressure, cholesterol and diabetes have been established as causal risk factors for coronary, cerebral and peripheral arterial disease. Their predictive value for cardiovascular events has been underestimated, due to the regression – dilution bias. The weak association of cholesterol with (ischaemic) stroke has delayed evaluation of cholesterol reduction as secondary prevention in patients with stroke: however a recent Heart Protection Study meta-analysis (Lancet 2004) shows that statins significantly reduce the risk of cardiovascular events in such patients. Conversely, statins reduce the risk of stroke (as well as coronary heart disease) in patients with coronary or peripheral arterial disease. Furthermore, the benefit of statins is unrelated to baseline cholesterol. Hence, statins are indicated in all patients with coronary heart disease, ischaemic stroke or peripheral arterial disease, regardless of baseline cholesterol. Cholesterol level is therefore a poor predictor of benefit from its reduction. In addition to statins, patients with clinical disease at any site benefit from reductions in smoking, blood pressure, weight, glucose and immobility; as well as aspirin or other antiplatelets. Emerging risk predictors (e.g. homocysteine, fibrinogen, C-reactive protein) appear to predict cardiovascular events at all sites. In conclusion, the prevention of atherothrombosis at all sites is similar in patients presenting with disease at any site. However, treatment of acute thrombosis (e.g. heparin, thrombolysis) differs between the soft brain and the harder heart and leg.

PL08

Do platelets trigger atherosclerosis?

Gawaz M

1. Medizinische Klinik, Klinikum rechts der Isar und Deutsches Herzzentrum, Technische Universität Muenchen, Muenchen, Germany

Platelets play a key role in thrombotic vascular occlusion at the atherosclerotic plaque leading to acute thrombotic episodes that result in acute coronary syndrome and stroke. After the prolonged process of silent plaque evolution, atheromas become susceptible to plaque rupture, leading to platelet adhesion and subsequent activation on the exposed, highly thrombogenic subendothelial surface, which initiates the dreaded clinical complications of thromboischemic episodes. Enhanced responsiveness of the atherosclerotic plaque to platelets can be triggered, for example by changes in the shear forces supporting platelet recruitment to the vulnerable plaque. Furthermore, biological changes in the form of chemotaxis of monocytes towards the plaque region, transmigration through the endothelial barrier, macrophage differentiation, phagocytosis, and secretion of proteolytic enzymes (plasminogen activator system, metalloproteinases) appear to substantially contribute to the instability of the plaque. Over the past few years platelets have been recognized to play a critical role in chemotaxis and migration of monocytes, thus promoting inflammation and progression of atherosclerosis. Experimental evidences indicate that platelets might significantly contribute to the inflammatory processes that promote atherosclerotic lesion formation. Platelets can adhere directly to the intact endothelial monolayer even in the absence of endothelial disruption. During adhesion platelets are activated and release proinflammatory cytokines and chemoattractants (such as interleukin-1□, platelet factor 4 (PF4), CD40 ligand). *In vitro* interactions between platelets and endothelial cells trigger the secretion of chemokines and the expression of adhesion molecules and promote the adhesion of leukocytes. In this manner, the adhesion of platelets to the endothelial surface might generate signals that lead to the recruitment and extravasation of monocytes during atherosclerotic plaque progression, a process of paramount importance for atherogenesis. Moreover, platelets have been found to substantially alter the pericellular proteolytic activity of endothelial cells (activation of metalloproteinases) resulting in extracellular matrix degradation and fibrous cap thinning of a vulnerable lesion. Thus, in areas of platelet accumulation at lesion prone sites, an enhanced release of platelet-derived proatherogenic compounds favors atherogenetic changes within the arterial wall and the development of atherosclerotic plaques. Platelet express several adhesion receptors, including integrins, cell adhesion molecules of the immunoglobulin superfamily, leucine-rich glycoproteins, and selectins that have been shown to mediate platelet adhesion to endothelial cells *in vitro* and *in vivo* . The integrin GPIIb-IIIa and the von Willebrand factor receptor GPIb have been demonstrated to largely contribute to endothelial-platelet adhesion which makes them classic candidates for inhibition. Only recently it was shown that chronic platelet activation accelerates atherosclerosis and that long-term treatment with a blocking anti-GPIb□ monoclonal antibody substantially limited atherosclerotic lesion formation in ApoE deficient mice compared to control animals. This decrease in atherosclerotic lesions was paralleled by a reduction of leukocyte adhesion and intimal infiltration. The question arises why current anti-platelet treatment strategies do not effectively prevent development or progression of atherosclerosis in human. Although there is *in vivo* evidence that administration of a high dosage of aspirin limits atheroprogression in mice, to date there is no clinical data showing that an intensified anti-platelet therapy that combines aspirin, clopidogrel, and GPIIb-IIIa inhibitors in high-risk patients can prevent atheroprogression or restenosis after percutaneous coronary interventions. However, none of the current anti-platelet drugs used in the clinical setting effectively inhibited adhesion and subsequent degranulation of platelets because they all target subsequent and late events of platelet-mediated thrombus formation. Moreover, drug resistance is increasingly recognized in patients treated with aspirin or clopidogrel. Pharmacological developments that are directed against the very early events of platelet adhesion to endothelial cells may be the key link to prevent platelet-mediated pro-atherogenic alterations of the arterial wall and thus atherosclerosis.

STATE-OF-THE-ART LECTURES

SA01

Thrombosis and stroke in neonates, infants and children

Nowak-Göttl U

Abstract not available

SA02

Metalloproteinases in development and progression of vascular disease

Lijnen H

Center for Molecular and Vascular Biology, University of Leuven, Belgium

Remodeling of the vascular wall plays a role in the pathogenesis of major cardiovascular diseases such as restenosis and atherosclerosis. Remodeling requires proteolytic activity that can be generated by the fibrinolytic (plasminogen/plasmin) and/or matrix metalloproteinase (MMP) systems. The availability of transgenic mice with inactivation or over-expression of specific MMP system components has allowed studying its in vivo role in processes requiring cell migration and extracellular matrix degradation. The temporal and topographic expression patterns of several MMPs after vascular injury in mice are compatible with a role in neointima formation. Furthermore, smooth muscle cell migration and neointima formation after vascular injury is significantly enhanced in mice with deficiency of TIMP-1, the main physiologic MMP inhibitor. In atherosclerotic lesions, plasmin generated via macrophage-secreted u-PA can activate several proMMPs. Studies in mice with combined deficiency of apolipoprotein E and MMP-3 (stromelysin-1) or TIMP-1 strongly suggest that active MMPs may contribute to plaque destabilisation by degrading extracellular matrix components, but may also promote aneurysm formation by proteolytic degradation of the elastic lamina. Thus, the MM system may represent a therapeutic target for treatment of restenosis or atherosclerosis.

SA03

Atrial fibrillation and the hypercoagulable state: from basic science to clinical practice

Lip G

Haemostasis Thrombosis and Vascular Biology Unit, University Department of Medicine, City Hospital, UK

The reasons for stroke occurring in atrial fibrillation (AF) are complex, but most strokes represent embolism of thrombus formed within the left atrium, predominantly within the left atrial appendage (LAA). Over 150 years ago, Virchow proposed a triad of abnormalities that predisposes to thrombus formation (thrombogenesis), that is, flow abnormalities, abnormalities of vessel wall and abnormal blood constituents. 'Flow abnormalities' are evident in AF, as the loss of atrial systole and irregular ventricular response promotes stasis within the LAA, which can be witnessed by transoesophageal echocardiographic (TOE) studies as reduced Doppler flow velocities within the LAA and an increase in spontaneous echo contrast (SEC). Both SEC and reduced LAA flow velocities have been shown to associate with presence of intra-atrial thrombus and stroke. Furthermore, 'abnormalities of the vessel wall' (or atrial wall or endocardium) are present in AF, with evidence of anatomical, microscopic and molecular-level abnormalities in the endocardium of the LAA in patients with AF, as well as an increase in levels of circulating markers of platelet activation, fibrin deposition/turnover and endothelial damage/dysfunction in patients with AF ('abnormal blood constituents'), thus fulfilling the third component of Virchow's triad. These indices are not related to structural heart disease or aetiology of AF, and have recently been shown to have prognostic value. Thus, AF satisfies Virchow's triad of thrombogenesis and can be regarded as a true 'pro-thrombotic' or hypercoagulable state. Clinical correlations of thromboembolism in atrial fibrillation the presence of non-valvular AF increase the risk of stroke approximately fivefold. The presence of mitral stenosis and AF results in an approximately eighteenfold increase in stroke risk, but the declining prevalence of rheumatic heart disease means that non-valvular AF represents the greatest public health problem. The risk of thromboembolic stroke due to AF also rises with age, and thus AF becomes the predominant independent risk factor for stroke in the age group of 80-89 years, with an attributable risk of 23.5% of all strokes. Indeed, AF is present in approximately 20% of all stroke patients, and stroke associated with AF carries an increase in mortality, morbidity and healthcare costs. The risk of stroke in AF is not homogeneous, and the presence of certain additional clinical and echocardiographic features are also associated with an increase in AF-related stroke risk, and may be useful to identify patients at greatest risk in order to target appropriate therapy, allowing risk stratification for thromboprophylaxis.

SA04

Adipose tissue and atherothrombosis

Alessi MC (1), Lijnen H (2), Bastelica D (1), Juhan-Vague I (1)*

(1) Laboratoire d'Hématologie, INSERM UMR626, UFR de Médecine, Université de la Méditerranée, Marseille, France
(2) Center for Molecular and Vascular Biology, KU Leuven, Belgium,

Obesity is associated with increased cardiovascular mortality and morbidity mainly through insulin resistance. Dysregulation of proteins secretion by adipose tissue contributes to obesity-related diseases such as vascular disease and type II diabetes. Leptin, a satiety signal for the central nervous system is also related to insulin and glucose metabolism and may play an important role in regulating vascular tone. Adiponectin acts as an anti-inflammatory and anti-atherogenic plasma protein and appears a biologically relevant endogenous modulator of vascular remodeling. Resistin is involved in glucose metabolism and promotes endothelial cell activation. Adipose tissue contributes also to create a subinflammatory status, which could induce chronic insulin insensitivity and explain the disturbances in the haemostatic and fibrinolytic systems observed in obesity. Obese subjects have higher values of circulating fibrinogen, factor VIII, von Willebrand factor, factor IX and plasminogen activator inhibitor (PAI-1) compared to non-obese subjects. Elevated plasma levels of PAI-1 demonstrated the strongest association with the degree of insulin resistance and could be an underlying mechanism for the thrombotic tendency and the progression of atherosclerosis during obesity. PAI-1 is mainly expressed by the stromal part of the adipose tissue. During adipocyte differentiation, in contrast to leptin, PAI-1 secretion does not follow human adipocyte maturation, and in situ hybridization in culture did not reveal PAI-1 mRNA in lipid-filled cells. Multiple regulatory pathways have been proposed to explain the increased synthesis of PAI-1 during insulin-resistance, a major one being the TNF pathway. The role of elevated PAI-1expression during the metabolic syndrome is not fully understood. Its contribution to tissue remodeling makes PAI-1 a good candidate for controlling weight gain during obesity and thus for participating in the development of insulin resistance. Indeed, increased PAI-1 levels predict type 2 diabetes independent of insulin resistance. The effect of PAI-1 was examined on adipose tissue growth in several mouse models as well as on adipocyte differenciation in vitro. Most of the data indicate that PAI-1 can effectively modulate weight gain and may be a potential therapeutic target for controlling cardiovascular morbidity in obese subjects. Anti PAI-1 counpounds are under investigation in animal models.

SA05

Hormone replacement therapy: influence on cardiovascular disease and venous thromboembolism

Conard J

Hemostasis-Thrombosis Unit, Hotel-Dieu hospital, Paris, France

Hormone replacement therapy (HRT) generally includes an estrogen (conjugated equine estrogen or estradiol by oral or non-oral route, patch, gel, intra-nasal) and a progestagen (progesterone or other). **Hemostasis.** Conjugated equine estrogens (CEE) as well as estradiol by oral route induce changes in hemostasis that are similar to those observed during combined oral contraception: increase in clotting factors, decrease in antithrombin and protein S, acquired APC resistance, profibrinolytic effect. In contrast, no significant changes have been observed with estradiol administered by non-oral route. **Risk of coronary heart disease (CHD) or stroke**. A cardiovascular protection was observed in case-control studies with CEE. In contrast, in the recent randomized trials (HERS, WHI estrogen plus progestin), the risk of CHD was significantly elevated the first year and HRT was not beneficial thereafter. In the WHI estrogen-alone trial, a non-significant increased risk was observed the first year but the cumulative effect suggests a possible modest benefit with long-term use. In addition, an increased risk of stroke has been observed in the HERS (relative risk RR 1.23), in the WHI estrogen plus progestin (RR 1.41) and also in the WHI estrogen-alone trial (HR 1.39, CI95% 1.10-1.77), leading to the early termination of the trial. **Risk of venous thromboembolism (VTE).** Estrogens by oral route are associated with an increased risk of VTE close to 2 in most studies. The risk is higher the first year of use and it is further increased in women with hereditary thrombophilia (demonstrated in factor V Leiden carriers). In contrast, estradiol by transdermal route was not associated with an increased risk in the ESTHER case-control study. **Conclusion.** The use of HRT with oral estrogens is presently recommended only for menopausal symptoms at the smallest effective dose for the shortest possible time. It is contra-indicated in women with history of VTE, CHD or stroke, or with thrombophilia. More studies are needed to evaluate the safety of estradiol by transdermal route in women with thrombophilia and/or history of VTE.

SA06

Restenosis: lessions from therapy

Binder BR

Department of Vascular Biology and Thrombosis Research, Medical University Vienna, Austria

Percutaneous transluminal balloon angioplasty is currently the treatment of choice for obstructive atherosclerotic vascular disease. Still, more than 40% of initially successfully treated patients develop 'restenosis' within 6 months after the intervention severely hampering the overall success of this therapeutic measure. The proposed mechanisms underlying the process of restenosis have led to respective therapeutic strategies ranging from the use of anti-platelet drugs and antioxidants to radiotherapy. None of the several strategies, however, could decrease the number of patients suffering from restenosis significantly. Inflammation has been implicated as an early step in the development of atherosclerosis and post angioplasty restenosis. The contribution of NF-kB to restenosis could be demonstrated in animal experiments using adenoviral based gene therapy overexpressing the inhibitor of NF-kB, I-kB. This treatment resulted in significantly reduced inflammatory response, increased apoptosis, positive remodeling and significantly less lumen loss but no significant change in neointima formation. Inhibition of restenosis could also be achieved by overexpression of tissue factor pathway inhibitor likely mediated by suppressed monocyte chemoattraction also indicating participation of an inflammatory mechanism. There is also a crosstalk between the NF-kB pathway and the EGR-1/NAK-1 pathways. Modulation of the NAK-1/EGR-1 pathway resulted in reduced neointima formation but no lumen gain because of lack of positive remodelling. This indicates that inflammation participates in 'restenosis' via two distinct and independent pathways.

SA07

Asymptomatic carotid stenosis: natural history and management

Coccheri S

Chair of Angiology, University of Bologna, Italy

Stroke is a major cause of death and disability in the western World. About 40 % of all strokes are atherothrombotic; half of them are due to stenosing plaques in the extracranial part of the supra-aortic arteries. Symptomatic Carotid Stenosis (SCS) is so defined when associated with ipsilateral hemispheric or retinal neurological deficit. Studies have shown that yearly risk of ipsilateral stroke in SCS is as high as 14 to 25 %. Thromboendoarterectomy (TEA) markedly reduces the risk in SCS greater than 70 %. Asymptomatic carotid stenosis (ACS) has a high prevalence (> 10 % over age 75) and is associated with a low yearly risk for stroke (2 %) and a similar risk for myocardial infarction (AMI). TEA halves the risk of stroke, but the absolute reduction is low and the advantage over medical treatment uncertain. Medical therapy remains necessary to prevent AMI. In order to identify a population with ACS at higher risk of stroke, the ACSRS study was undertaken, in which the main predictors of stroke were morphology of plaque, degree of stenosis, and the presence and duration of hypertension. These factors identify a population of ACS at higher risk in which TEA appears health and cost-effective. All patients with ACS should anyway receive medical treatment. Antiplatelet agents, statins, antihypertensive drugs, dietary counselling, smoking cessation, and reduction of other risk factors as diabetes, obesity, and probably homocysteine levels, are essential measures in prevention of stroke and AMI in ACS patients.

SA08

Do haemostatic markers that predict cardiovascular disease exist?

Stegnar M

University Medical Centre, Department of Angiology, Ljubljana, Slovenia

Recognition of the central role of thrombosis in the pathogenesis of cardiovascular diseases has prompted growing interest in the association of haemostatic variables with cardiovascular diseases. In the investigation of predictive value of haemostatic markers in cardiovascular disease two main types of measurements exist: determination of levels of haemostatic factors and measurement of haemostasis activation products. In the first type of measurements the most useful factors identified have been fibrinogen, factor VIII, von Willebrand factor and fibrinolytic variables: tissue-type plasminogen activator (t-PA) and t-PA inhibitor-1 (PAI-1), but the evidence if increase in these factors is causal for cardiovascular disease needs to be proven. The second promising type of measurement is that of activation products of coagulation cascade and fibrinolysis: prothrombin fragment 1+2 (F1+2) released by factor Xa, fibrinopeptides A and B released from fibrinogen by thrombin, soluble fibrin being formed through polymerization of fibrin monomers with fibrin/fibrinogen degradation products, thrombin-antithrombin (TAT) and plasmin/antiplasmin (PAP) complexes and D-dimer, the specific degradation product of crosslinked fibrin. Measurement of haemostasis activation markers has several weaknesses: the assays are not standardized, and most activation markers are sensitive to in vitro artefacts. Consequently, great care is necessary in the pre-analytical phase. D-dimer was most extensively studied because the assay is widely available and D-dimer is relatively stable in plasma. D-dimer, but not F1+2, TAT, and PAP, is associated with a history of cardiovascular events. There is substantial evidence from several prospective studies that D-dimer is a strong, consistent predictor of cardiovascular events in patients with or without arterial disease. High level of D-dimer is also a significant predictor of combined cardiovascular events in patients with atrial fibrillation on oral anticoagulant treatment. On this basis, D-dimer could be a useful additional marker of cardiovascular risk in such patients. A small number of soluble fibrin assays has entered clinical evaluation and since they detect different structural or functional properties of soluble fibrin little correlation between different assays exists.

SYMPOSIA

SY01

Extended versus rapid analysis of the leg vein system: A multicenter ultrasound study (The ERASMUS study) - An interim analysis

Bernardi E on behalf of the Erasmus investigators' group

Emergency Department Padua University Hospital, Italy

Introduction: serial compression ultrasonography (CUS) is a reliable method for the diagnosis of proximal deep venous thrombosis (DVT) in symptomatic (out) patients. Similarly, the safety of combined strategies (e.g. CUS + D-dimer or pretest clinical probability) introduced to limit the number of repeat CUS, has been convincingly demonstrated. Nonetheless, CUS-based approaches have not gained widespread application. Echo-color-Doppler (ECD), because of its ability to investigate the calf-vein system is adopted by most vascular laboratories as first line test in case of clinically suspected DVT, although time-consuming and technically demanding. In addition, the specificity of calf veins imaging is uncertain, as is the negative predictive value of a normal ECD workup. To date, no direct comparisons of these strategies isare available in the literature. **Aim of the Study**: to compare the safety and feasibility of two diagnostic approaches: a compound CUS strategy ("rapid"), and the ECD evaluation of the whole-leg ("extended"). **Methods**: randomised, prospective, multicenter study, with independent and blind adjudication of thromboembolic events and independent safety monitoring. All consecutive symptomatic patients referred to the study centres with clinically suspected DVT (first episode) will be eligible for inclusion; informed patients without exclusion criteria will be enrolled. *Rapid strategy*: CUS will be performed first; if normal, patients will have D-dimer testing. Those with abnormal results will undergo repeat CUS at 1 week; those with normal workup will be discharged without further investigation, and followed-up for 3 months. *Extended strategy*: patients with normal whole-leg ECD workup at baseline will be discharged without further testing, and followed-up for 3 months. All patients with normal workup will be instructed to immediately return to the study centres should symptoms suggesting venous thromboembolic events (VTE) arise during the study period, to undergo objective confirmation of the disease. *Primary Outcome*: rate of symptomatic VTE during a 3-months follow-up, after a normal diagnostic workup with either of the two proposed strategies. All events will be adjudicated by a blind and independent committee, based on the results of objective testing, as follows: CUS, ECD or venography (suspected DVT); ventilation-perfusion lung scan, (helical) spiral CT scan, or pulmonary angiography (suspected PE). Suspected fatal PE will be adjudicated on the findings of autopsy or on clinical grounds, according to an independent physician. **Results**: an interim data analysis will be presented during the congress session.

SY02

Can we safely exclude DVT without instrumental testing?

Palareti G

Dept. Angiology & Blood Coagulation, University Hospital S. Orsola-Malpighi, Bologna, Italy

Objective testing for leg DVT is necessary since clinical assessment alone is unreliable. The prevalence of true DVT among patients with a suspected DVT of a leg is less than 20%. The currently adopted non-invasive and cost-effective diagnostic strategies are based on a) venous compression ultrasonography (CUS), with different algorythms using repeated CUS 1 week after an initially normal CUS to detect proximalization of an isolated calf DVT; b) assessment of clinical probability to evaluate the individual risk of DVT presence; and c) measurement of plasma D-dimer levels (DD) that, when normal, may contribute to rule out DVT. Strategies for DVT diagnosis differ in in- and out-patients, and if the suspected event is the first or a recurrence. In cases of suspected recurrent DVT an instrumental testing is usually mandatory, even though normal DD may help in excluding the event. In-patients with suspected DVT are very often at high clinical probability and rarely have normal DD. In these patients is rarely possible to safely exclude DVT without an instrumental testing. On the other hand, it is currently considered that CUS can be safely avoided in out-patients with suspected DVT who have a low clinical probability and normal DD. In this regard a measure of caution is required in order to consider the possibility of false normal DD and of a variability in the assessment of clinical probability. First, the high negative values of both these diagnostic tools in clinical studies may also be the results of the low DVT prevalence in the examined populations. With regards to DD, it is well known that false normal results can be expected in case of low sensitivity of the used method, incorrect cut-off values, very small thrombotic burden (that however can suddenly increase), long interval from initiation of symptoms and when patients are already treated with anticoagulants. Normal DD have recently been reported in the first few days after trauma in patients who subsequently develop thrombosis. In our experience normal DD are found at the first examination in about 4% of patients with diagnosed DVT. With regards to the clinical probability, it should be considered that: a) some important risk factors (such as pill use, presence of personal or familial thrombophilia and previous thrombotic events) are not included in the most widely adopted score (Wells) and that b) the great relevance given to the possible alternative diagnosis (-2 points) increases the risk of a non negligible inter-observer variability. With these cautions in mind regarding both the value of DD and the assessment of clinical probability, we believe that outpatients with suspected DVT, with very low clinical probability (considering all the risk factors) and normal DD (preferably using a sensitive method) can safely be excluded from further examination with instrumental testing.

SY03

The role of helical CT in the diagnosis of pulmonary embolism

Huisman M

Department of General Internal Medicine Leiden University Medical Centre Leiden, The Netherlands

Pulmonary embolism (PE) is a common disorder. However, because of the signs and symptoms of the disease are non-specific, the clinical diagnosis is problematic. Accurate diagnosis of PE is essential, since appropriate diagnosis and treatment will decrease morbidity. Chest radiograph, ventilation-perfusion (V/Q) scanning, helical CT, and pulmonary angiography, and D-dimer and clinical probability tests are currently commonly used tests in diagnosing VTE. In the last decade, with improving helical CT imaging, CT for the diagnosis of pulmonary embolism (PE) has gained widespread acceptance and in many hospitals, helical CT is used as a first-line study in the evaluation of clinically suspected PE. In the first evaluation studies versus gold standard angiography, it was demonstrated that the accuracy of CT was better for lobar and segmental arteries, with overall sensitivities ranging from 64 to 100 % and specificities ranging from 89 to 100 %. Careful follow-up studies, combining normal helical CT with repeated normal compression ultrasonography of the leg veins, however showed acceptable failure rates during three months follow-up, ranging from 0.8 to 1.8 %. More recently, with multirow detector CT improvement in visualization of subsegmental arteries is possible and, although no formal long term follow-up study has been performed, management using helical CT alone, seems potentially feasible. Whether this will lead to insurmountable logistic problems during out of office hours or unacceptable costs is yet unknown. It might well be that different algorithms of PE diagnosis will prevail depending on whether a patient presents during daily hours – in which helical CT will be easily available - or during nights or weekends – where a combination of clinical prediction rules and D-dimer tests might triage whether a patient should undergo further invasive testing.

SY04

Receptor cooperation and protein phosphorylation are regulatory mechanisms of platelet recruitment. Modulatory role of erythrocytes

Santos M (1), Valles J (1), Moscardo A (1), Aznar J (2), Piñon M (1)*

(1) Research Center, University Hospital La Fe, Valencia, Spain.
(2) Department of Clinical Pathology, University Hospital La Fe, Valencia, Spain

Platelet activation induces the release of granular components and metabolic products. This platelet releasate is a complex physiological agonist that upon interaction with other platelets induces platelet recruitment and thrombus growth. The agonistic potency of the platelet releasate is increased when platelets are stimulated in the presence of intact erythrocytes (RBCs) (1,2). This results in a greater extent of recruitment, $\alpha_{IIb\beta 3}$ receptor activation and P-selectin exposure on recruiting platelets. These effects are markedly higher in diabetic patients, which may contribute to their tendency toward atherothrombosis. Due to the clinical implications of recruitment, it seems of interest to study the biochemical mechanisms and its pharmacological regulation. Protein tyrosine phosphorylation is an important signaling pathway of platelet recruitment, which is amplified by RBCs. In contrast, PKC-associated mechanisms do not have an essential role. ADP, TXA_2 and 5HT are known components of the platelet releasate, that signaling through specific receptors via Gq (P2Y1 of ADP, TXA_2 5HT) or Gi (P2Y12 of ADP) have an individual contribution to the final response of recruiting platelets. The cooperation between the TXA_2 and P2Y12 receptors is particularly relevant concerning protein tyrosine phosphorylation, cytoskeletal reorganization and incorporation of signaling molecules to the cytoskeleton. The available data reveal that platelet recruitment is a complex and highly regulated process in which platelet-erythrocyte interactions play a relevant role. More knowledge about this process could provide new therapeutic targets for antithrombotic therapy. (Grants FIS01/1208/ FIS03/0270/GRUPOS03/005). 1-Santos MT et al. J. Clin Invest 1991; 87: 571-580. 2- Vallés J et al Blood 2002;99:3978-84.

SY05

ERK2 activation in collagen platelet aggregation requires cotimulation of Gi-coupled ADP receptor and Gq-coupled TXA2 receptor

*Roger S, Mazharian A, Bryckaert M**

INSERM U.348 - Hôpital Lariboisière – PARIS, France

The stimulation of platelets by low doses of collagen induces ERK2 activation. In this report, we demonstrate that collagen-induced ERK2 activation depends on thromboxane A_2 (TXA_2) formation and ADP release. The collagen-induced ERK2 activation was inhibited by indomethacin (88%) and by AR-C69931MX (70%), a specific antagonist of P2Y12, a Gi-coupled ADP receptor. AR-C69931MX (10 μM) inhibition was overcome by epinephrine (1 μM), an agonist of the Gi-coupled α_{2A}-adrenergic receptor, suggesting that the Gi-coupled receptor was necessary for ERK2 activation by collagen. By contrast, MRS 2179 (10 μM) a specific antagonist of P2Y1, a Gq-coupled ADP receptor, did not affect collagen-induced ERK2 activation. Little or no ERK2 activation was observed with ADP alone (10 μM). By contrast, U46619 (10 μM), a stable analog of TXA_2, induced ERK2 activation in an ADP-dependent manner, via the P2Y12 receptor. These results suggest that the Gi-dependent signaling pathway, stimulated by ADP or epinephrine, was not the only pathway required for ERK2 activation by collagen. Costimulation of the specific $G_{12/13}$-coupled TXA_2 receptor with a low dose of U 46619 (10 nM) and of Gi- and Gq-coupled ADP receptor (10 μM) induced very low levels of ERK2 activation, similar to those observed with ADP alone, suggesting that $G_{12/13}$ is not involved or not sufficient to induce the additional pathway necessary for ERK2 activation. The Gq-coupled TXA_2 receptor was required for ERK2 activation by U 46619 (10 μM) and low doses of collagen, clearly showing that a coordinated pathway through both Gq from TXA_2 and Gi from ADP was necessary for ERK2 activation. Finally, we demonstrate that ERK2 activation is involved in collagen-induced aggregation and secretion.

SY06

Lysosomal b-N-acetylhexosaminidase is a primer of platelet activation

Rossi R (1), Giannini S (1), Mencarelli S (2), Falcinelli E (1), Orlacchio A (2), Emiliani C (2), Gresele P (1)*

(1) Department of Internal Medicine, Section of Internal and Cardiovascular Medicine, University of Perugia, Perugia, Italy
(2) Department of Biochemical Sciences and Molecular Biotechonology, University of Perugia, Perugia, Italy

Introduction: Platelets contain, besides alfa- and delta-granules, lysosomes which store mainly acid hydrolases. Human platelets release their lysosomal content both *in vitro*, after stimulation with strong agonists, and *in vivo* at a localised site of vessel wall damage (Ciferri et al, 2000). Beta-N-acetylexosaminidase (Hex) is the main lysosomal glycohydrolase in human platelets and about 30% of it is released *in vivo* upon activation. The two major forms of Hex, Hex A and Hex B, can hydrolyse the glucidic moiety from the non reducing end of the oligosaccharide chain of glycoproteins, glycolipids and glycosaminoglycans, but a role for extracellular Hex has not been established yet. **Aim**: We studied the effect of Hex on platelet activation and the platelet signal trasduction pathways. **Materials and methods**: Hex from a human placenta extract, was fractionated in its two isoforms by DEAE-cellulose, and further purified; in some selected experiments, Hex was purified from human platelets. Gel-filtered platelets were pre-incubated for two minutes at 37°C with purified Hex, at a concentration (2mU/ml) similar to that previously found to be released *in vivo*, or with its vehicle and tested for aggregation, P-Sel release and GPIIb/IIIa activation after stimulation with subthreshold doses of thrombin. For p47 phosphorylation experiments ^{32}P-labeled platelets were used. **Results**: Unfractionated purified Hex did not induce platelet activation by itself but it did enhance platelet aggregation (+190.8%±64.9%), P-sel release (+64.1%±15.5%) and GPIIb/IIIa activation (+138%±20.8%) induced by subthreshold doses of thrombin; Hex enhanced p47 phosphorylation (+20% vs ctrl) too. Preincubation with the PKC inhibitor, RO 31-8220, the PLA_2 inhibitor, aristolochic acid, the LOX inhibitor, NDGA and the Ca^{++} influx inhibitor, $NiCl_2$, completely abolished the Hex potentiation; the PTKs inhibitor, tyrphostine and the PI3-K inhibitor, wortmannin partially reduced the Hex priming, while the COX inhibitor, aspirin, the p38-MAPK inhibitor, SB 203580, and the MAPK inhibitor, PD 169316, did not affect the Hex potentiating activity. Concerning the Hex isoforms: both Hex A (alfa /beta structure) and Hex B (beta/ beta) were found to prime platelet activation. **Conclusions**: Lysosomal Hex acts as a proaggregatory agent with an activity involving PKC, PLA_2 and LOX dependent mechanisms and Ca^{++} influx.

SY07

Gene-gene and gene-environment interactions in mild hyperhomocysteinemia

D'Angelo A, Mazzola G, Fermo I*

Coagulation Service and Thrombosis Research Unit, IRCCS H S. Raffaele, Milano, Italy

Mild/moderate hyperhomocysteinemia (HHcy), a highly prevalent condition, is independently associated with an increased risk of arterial and venous thromboembolic diseases. Early reports of the association of mild/moderate HHcy with juvenile venous thromboembolism have shown familiarity for HHcy in relatives of index cases with thrombosis. Similar to inherited thrombophilia defects, inheritance of the HHcy phenotype was accordingly retained important for the definition of HHcy as an independent risk factor for thrombosis. Current knowledge recognizes a number of determinants of the HHcy phenotype, including genetic as well as environmental factors. MTHFR thermolability accounts for a 10-fold increase in the risk of mild/moderate HHcy. HHcy in MTHFR 677TT subjects is dependent on folate and, to a lesser degree, vitamin B12 status. Still, it is common experience that MTHFR 677TT subjects with similar borderline low plasma folate (and cobalamin) show very different, unexplained, fasting (and PML) tHcy levels. This observation led to the hypothesis that coexistence of MTHFR thermolability with additional gene defects in the enzyme involved in homocysteine metabolism may be responsible for the phenotype variability. Accordingly, a number of relatively common polymorphisms in MTHFR (A2981C), methionine synthase (A2756G), methionine synthase reductase (A66G), and cystathionine-β-synthase (844ins68) have been explored as potentially involved in the HHcy phenotype, isolated or in association with MTHFR thermolability. Transcobalamin (TC) delivers vitaminB12 to peripheral tissues. A common genetic polymorphism that may influence homocysteine levels is the transcobalamin (TC) codon 259 genetic polymorphism that results in the substitution of proline for arginine and is the major determinant of the TC phenotypic variability in the population. With the possible exception of the cystathionine-β-synthase insertion, we found no evidence for an increased risk of HHcy for any of these polymorphisms, isolated or in association with MTHFR thermolability. Available evidence suggests that environmental factors and MTHFR thermolability are main determinants of the HHcy phenotype. Among environmental factors, vitamin status and renal function appear to play a major role. Gender and age are also major determinants of tHcy levels, but the gender effect tends to disappear with increasing age. If mild/moderate HHcy is a pathogenetic risk factor for thrombosis, intervention aimed to improve the vitamin status appears of major importance, irrespective of common gene polymorphisms of the homocysteine metabolism.

SY08

Homocysteine, vitamin B6 and the risk of recurrent venous thromboembolism

*Eichinger S**

Dept. of Internal Medicine I, Div. of Hematolgoy/Hemostasis, Medical Unviversity of Vienna, Vienna, Austria

Hyperhomocysteinemia (HHC) is an independent risk factor for cardiovascular disease, and even mildly to moderately elevated homocysteine levels have been associated with a heightened risk for a first venous thromboembolism (VTE). HHC is caused either by genetic defects and/or by a deficiency of the vitamins (B12, B6 and folic acid) involved in the homocysteine metabolism. The mechanisms by which HHC might contribute to atherogenesis and thrombogenesis are still incompletely understood. Within the frame of a large prospective cohort study (Austrian Study on Recurrent Venous Thromboembolism), we have shown that patients with a first spontaneous VTE and HHC (> 95th percentile of controls) have a 3-times higher risk of recurrent VTE compared with patients with lower levels. Low plasma levels of pyridoxal-5`-phosphate (PLP), the coenzyme form of vitamin B6, are associated with an increased risk for are a first venous thrombosis independently of established thrombotic risk factors including HHC. We therefore investigated whether or not low levels of PLP are also a risk factor of recurrent VTE. In 766 patients with a first spontaneous VTE the adjusted relative risk of recurrence was 1.5 (95th% CI 0.92-2.5) in patients with PLP levels below the 15th percentile of thrombosis patients compared with those with higher levels. Supplementation of folic acid, alone or in combination with vitamin B12 and vitamin B6, reduces plasma homocysteine concentrations by 25-30% both in healthy subjects and in patients with venous thrombosis. In a randomized, placebo-controlled, double-blind trial the effects of vitamin supplementation (5 mg folic acid, 50 mg pyridoxine, 0.4 mg hydroxycobalamin) on the risk of recurrent thrombosis after discontinuation of standard oral anticoagulant therapy was studied in 701 patients with a first spontaneous VTE. After 2.5 years, the relative risk of recurrence was 0.84 (95%CI 0.56-1.26) in patients receiving vitamins compared with those receiving placebo. Thus, in patients with VTE and HHC a significant effect on the risk of recurrence by vitamin supplementation could not be shown. Further and larger studies are needed to show whether vitamin supplementation might be beneficial in subgroups of patients with VTE.

SY09

Homocysteine lowering by B vitamins and the prevention of deep-vein thrombosis and pulmonary embolism: The VITRO trial

Willems H (1), den Heijer M (2), Blom H (3), Gerrits W (1), Cattaneo M (4), Eichinger S (5), Rosendaal F (6), Bos G (7)*

(1) Dep Hematology, Leyenburg Hospital, The Hague, The Netherlands
(2) Dep Endocrinol and Dep Epidemiol. Biostat, Univ Med Ctr Nijmegen, NL
(3) Lab Pediat and Neurol, Univ Med Ctr Nijmegen, Nijmegen, The Netherlands
(4) Unit Hematol Thromb, Dep Med, Surg and Dentistry, Univ of Milano, Italy
(5) Div Hematol and Hemost, Vienna University Hospital, Vienna, Austria
(6) Dep Epidemiol and Dep Haematol, Leiden Univ Med Ctr, Leiden, NL
(7) Dep Intern Med, Univ Hospital Maastricht, Maastricht, The Netherlands

Background*:* Hyperhomocysteinemia is a risk factor for venous thrombosis and arterial vascular disease. Supplementation with folic acid, vitamin B12 and vitamin B6 reduces homocysteine concentrations by 25-30% in healthy subjects and in patients with venous thrombosis. Until now, there are no results of clinical trials whether homocysteine lowering by B-vitamins indeed lowers the risk for venous thrombosis. **Methods***:* In the VITRO (VItamins and ThROmbosis) study, we investigated the effect of daily supplementation of 5 mg folic acid, 50 mg of pyridoxin and 0.4 mg hydroxycobalamin (high-dose multivitamin) as secondary prevention of deep-vein thrombosis and pulmonary embolism. Consecutive patients with primary deep-vein thrombosis or pulmonary embolism, who were admitted to an anticoagulation clinic, were asked to participate. Patients between 20 to 80 years old, with objectively confirmed proximal deep-vein thrombosis or pulmonary embolism in absence of other major risk factors for deep-vein thrombosis (malignancy, surgery, pregnancy and child-bed, long-term immobility) and a homocysteine concentration in the top quartile entered the study. They were randomised to high-dose multivitamin supplementation or placebo and were followed for 2.5 years. End-points in the study were recurrent DVT or recurrent PE, as diagnosed by the own physician of the patient. Parallel to this study a similar study was conducted in a random sample of patients in the lowest three homocysteine quartiles. **Results***:* Patients were selected through anticoagulation centers and Thrombosis Centers. Subjects were divided according to their homocysteine level in a hyperhomocysteinemic (n=360) and a normohomocysteinemic group (n=341). The number of recurrent events of venous thrombosis was 43 out of 348 in the vitamin group and 50 out of 353 in the placebo group. The relative risk in hyperhomocysteinemic group was 1.14 (95%CI 0.65-1.98) and in the normohomocysteinemic group 0.58 (95%CI 0.31-1.07). The overall relative risk was 0.84 (95%CI 0.56-1.26). ***Conclusions****:* The results of our study do not support the early hypothesis of a 50% reduction. The precision of our estimates does not allow distinguishing between 'no effect' or a modest effect as expected on the base of genetic studies on the effect of MTHFR 677TT genotype. Large scale trials are needed to establish or exclude a modest beneficial effect of vitamin supplementation.

SY10

Is hyperhomocysteinemia an important risk factor for cardiovascular disease?

Cattaneo M

Unit of Hematology and Thrombosis. Ospedale SanPaolo. Dept. of Medicine, Surgery and Dentistry, University of Milan, Milan, Italy

Case-control, cross-sectional and prospective studies have clearly proven that there is a graded association between the plasma levels of total homocysteine (tHcy) and the risk for occlusive arterial and venous disease. Despite this, hyperhomocysteinemia has not been universally accepted yet as an established cardiovascular risk factor. The scepticism of some physicians and investigators stems from the lack of proof that hyperhomocysteinemia causes cardiovascular diseases and that lowering tHcy reduces the cardiovascular risk. However, the association between a risk factor and a disease is not necessarily causal. By definition, risk factors are nothing more than statistical predictors of the risk for a disease. The demonstration of their causal association with that disease is strictly dependent on the demonstration, within proper randomized trials, that their modification alters the risk. The evidence of the association of hyperhomocysteinemia with cardiovascular diseases is overwhelming and was demonstrated not only by case-control studies, but was also confirmed by the majority of prospective studies. Hyperhomocysteinemia fulfils all the minor criteria for causality, including the demonstration of the association between cardiovascular risk and the mutant 677T allele of the gene encoding for methylene-tetrahydrofolate reductase (MTHFR), which is associated with decreased enzymatic activity and predisposes to hyperhomocysteinemia. Finally, although it is true there is no demonstration yet that correction of mild/moderate hyperhomocysteinemia reduces the cardiovascular risk, one should not disregard the clear evidence that the very high cardiovascular risk of patients with homocystinuria is decreased by the supplementation of vitamins that lower their very high plasma tHcy levels. Based on the above considerations, I think that hyperhomocysteinemia should be considered a proven cardiovascular risk factor, and that its causal role is not unlikely. Hyperhomocysteinemia is not a major risk factor for cardiovascular disease. A recent meta-analysis showed that the strength of the association between homocysteine and the risk for ischemic heart disease or stroke is lower than that reported by previous summary analysis. It showed that a decrease of tHcy level of about 3 μmol/L would be associated with an 11% lower risk for ischemic heart disease and 19% lower stroke risk. Despite the fact that hyperhomocysteinemia is not a major risk factor, if the ongoing clinical trials eventually show that decreasing tHcy with vitamin supplementation is indeed associated with a reduction in cardiovascular risk, then the potential implication for public health would still be very important, considering the high worldwide incidence of cardiovascular diseases. As a consequence, hyperhomocysteinemia will have to be considered a very important risk factor for cardiovascular diseases. Its importance will not derive from the strength of its association with the disease, but, rather, from the fact that its correction is easy, inexpensive and safe. No other cardiovascular risk factor could boast these very important characteristics, including quitting smoking, which, although cheap and safe is certainly not easy.

SY11

Risk factors for recurrent venous thromboembolism: the role of persistent venous obstruction

Prandoni P

Department of Medical and Surgical Sciences, 2nd Chair of Internal Medicine, University of Padua, Italy

Among factors associated with an increased risk for recurrent venous thromboembolism (VTE) in patients with deep-vein thrombosis (DVT) of the lower extremity the persistence of vein thrombosis, as shown by repeated ultrasonography over time, has been advocated. To estimate the risk for recurrent VTE in patients with and without residual vein thrombosis, repeat ultrasound was performed over time in 313 consecutive patients with proximal DVT who were followed prospectively for up to six years after a 3 to 6-month period of anticoagulation. 124 patients (39.6%) had an idiopathic DVT, 109 (35.2%) had a thrombosis associated with transient risk factors, and 80 (25.6%) were carriers of thrombophilic defects. Venous ultrasonography showed a full vein recanalization at three months in 61 (19.5%) patients. The cumulative incidence of normalized ultrasonography was 38.8% at 6 months, 58.1% at one year, 69.3% at two years, and 73.8% at three years. Of the 313 patients, 58 experienced a recurrent VTE, of whom 41 occurred while the patient still had residual thrombosis. Using a time dependent univariate Cox proportional hazard model, the hazard ratio (HR) for a recurrent event was 2.9 (95% CI, 1.6 to 5.2; p=0.001) during the time that residual thrombosis was present. Using a multivariate stepwise Cox proportional hazards model with persistent residual thrombosis as a time-dependent variable, the HRs in this multivariate model were 2.4 (95% CI, 1.3 to 4.4; p= 0.004) for persistent residual thrombosis, 2.5 (95% CI, 1.4 to 4.4; p=0.003) for spontaneous versus secondary thrombosis, and 3.1 (95% CI, 1.8 to 5.2; p<0.001) for thrombophilia versus no thrombophilia. In conclusion, persistent venous obstruction is a powerful and independent risk factor for recurrent VTE in patients with venous thrombosis.

SY12

Low-dose warfarin

Palareti G

Dept. Angiology & Blood Coagulation, University Hospital S. Orsola-Malpighi, Bologna, Italy

Several studies have shown that full-dose warfarin (targeted therapeutic range 2.0-3.0 INR) is highly effective in reducing the risk of recurrent VTE. Usual care includes this treatment for up to 12 months after a first idiopathic VTE. Full-dose warfarin for longer than one year was shown more effective than placebo. However, the rates of major bleeding episodes are higher during this extended treatment. A low-intensity warfarin therapy may be an attractive option for a prolonged secondary prophylaxis of VTE, provided that it proves effective in reducing VTE without an excess of bleeding complications. In a recent study (Ridker et al NEJM 2003;348:1425) patients with both a first episode or two or more episodes of VTE were randomized to receive placebo or low-intensity warfarin (INR range: 1.5-2.0) after receiving a full dose of anticoagulant therapy for a median of 6.5 months. The trial was terminated after 508 patients had been enrolled and followed up for a mean of 2.1 years. Low-intensity warfarin produced a risk reduction of 64% (hazards ratio: 0.36; 95% confidence intervals: 0.19-0.67) when compared to placebo without a significant difference in major hemorrhage or death. Risk reductions were similar for all subgroups including those with and without inherited thrombophilia. A direct comparison of low-intensity (INR 1.5-1.9) with conventional-intensity (INR 2.0-3.0) warfarin therapy for long-term prevention of recurrent VTE has been recently published (Kearon et al. NEJM 2003;349:631). In that double-blind study patients with a first unprovoked VTE were all treated with conventional-intensity for at least 3 months and then randomized to prolong warfarin treatment at low- or conventional-intensity for an average of 2.4 years. The rates of recurrences were 1.9% and 0.7% in low- and conventional-intensity patients, respectively (hazard ratio 2.8; 95% CI 1.1-7.0). No differences were recorded in major and all bleeding events between the two groups. From these data it can be concluded that conventional-intensity warfarin therapy is more effective than low-intensity without carrying an increased risk of clinically important bleeding. It has been calculated that low-intensity anticoagulation reduces the risk of VTE recurrence by about 75%, whereas conventional-intensity reduces the risk by over 90% with no differences in the risk of bleeding.

SY13

Duration of warfarin

Agnelli G

Abstract not available

SY14

TAFI at the interface between coagulation and fibrinolysis

Bouma B (1 and 2)

(1) Dept of Molecular and Experimental Medicine, The Scripps Research Institute, La Jolla CA, USA
(2) Dept of Haematology, University Medical Center Utrecht, The Netherlands

TAFI (Thrombin-Activatable Fibrinolysis Inhibitor) is a carboxypeptidase B-like enzyme that preferentially hydrolyzes C-terminal basic aminoacids. It is a single chain plasma glycoprotein of 55 kDA and circulates in plasma at a concentration of 4 -15 μg/ml. Activation of TAFI by thrombin occurs by a single cleavage at Arg-92. Activated TAFI (TAFIa) is unstable; its inactivation is caused by conformational instability, which is highly sensitive to temperature. TAFIa down-regulates fibrinolysis by the removal of C-terminal lysines from fibrin. These C-terminal lysines are exposed upon limited proteolysis of fibrin by plasmin and act as a ligand for the lysine-binding sites of plasminogen and t-PA. Elimination of these lysines by TAFIa abrogates the fibrin cofactor function of t-PA-mediated plasminogen activation, resulting in a down-regulation of fibrinolysis. The thrombin needed for the activation of TAFI is generated by the intrinsic coagulation system in a factor XI dependent way. This implies that the coagulation system plays a role in the regulation of fibrinolysis and that any disturbance in the generation of thrombin will result in an increased rate of fibrinolysis. Such a mechanism may explain the bleeding abnormalities of factor XI-deficient patients. These patients are prone to bleeding from tissues with a high fibrinolytic activity and it is at these sites that the down-regulation of fibrinolysis is not provided for by the factor XI-dependent generation of thrombin and subsequent activation of TAFI. A defective activation of TAFI might also contribute to bleeding disorders such as haemophilia A and B. At low tissue factor concentrations, these patients have a reduced thrombin generation via the extrinsic pathway and a reduced secondary burst via the intrinsic pathway. Because of this, the activation of TAFI and thus the down-regulation of fibrinolysis by the intrinsic pathway is defective. This results not only in an inadequate haemostatic response but also, where fibrin has already been formed, in its more rapid dissolution leading to destabilization of the haemostatic plug. Increased levels of TAFI or an increased rate of activation of TAFI were reported to be associated with a mild increased risk for venous thrombosis. In vivo evidence for a role of TAFI has been obtained from TAFI knockout mice. Although homozygous TAFI-gene deficient mice did not exhibit haemostatic abnormalities, an abnormality in the wound-healing process was detected. Histological examination of cutaneous wounds revealed inappropriate organization of skin wound closure in the TAFI knockout mice, including an altered pattern of epithelial migration. Although the time required for heal the cutaneous wounds was only slightly delayed, TAFI appears to be important for appropriate organization of the healing process.

SY15

TAFI in human ischaemic stroke

Monasterio J

Vascular Biology and Haemostasis Unit, University Hospital Vall d'Hebro, Barcelona

Standardization of thrombin activable Fibrinolysis inhibitor (TAFI) levels in a healthy Caucasian population and in vascular disease patients: Carboxy peptidase U (CPU 35KDa) or thrombin activated fibrinolysis inhibitor (TAFIa) is generated from its zymogene (proCPU 55KDa) by enzymatic activation and exerts an antifibrinolytic action. A great variability in TAFI Ag levels has been reported in healthy population. Our aim is to determine whether variability is due to physiologic variations or to insufficient standardization of the method, and to allow a better interpretation of the results in patients with vascular diseases. We performed a method validation of an immunoabsorbent assay (Zymutest TAFI Ag Hyphen Biomed) in healthy controls and in patients with sepsis and MOF, in ischaemic stroke patients in acute and chronic phase and in women receiving hormones replacement therapy (HRT). After validation of TAFI assay, its values in healthy population were x=114.29;SD=29.62% and neither age nor gender influenced the results (p=0.284 and p=0.117). Basal values in patients with sepsis with MOF were higher than in the septic ones without MOF (p<0.01). In patients with ischaemic stroke in both acute and chronic phase, TAFI levels were higher than in healthy group (p<0.01). No differences were found in women receiving HRT. After method was validated in optimal conditions, we found lesser variability of TAFI Ag values than in previous publications, and a relationship between TAFI Ag over expression and ischaemic stroke. **Thrombin-activable fibrinolysis inhibitor levels in acute phase of Ischaemic Stroke:** The purpose of our work was to study TAFI levels in the acute phase of ischaemic stroke and to know whether there is a relationship with ischaemic stroke clinical evolution. Method: In 30 consecutive ischaemic stroke patients, TAFI plasma levels were measured by means of enzyme-linked immunosorbent assay (Zymutest TAFI Ag Hyphen Biomed). Results are expressed as a percentage of the pooled plasma reference and expressed as mean (± SD) and compared with the values obtained in 30 healthy control subjects. All patients samples were drawn within the first 24 hours after symptom onset (mean 4.6 hours) and before any treatment was started. Results: TAFI plasma concentration was significantly higher (p<0.001) in stroke patients (158.4±53.2 %) than in healthy control subjects (105.6±30.2%). The highest TAFI levels were found in cases of neurological deterioration (worsening, 198.1±63.0 %; stable, 130.5±39.3%; improving, 173.9±52.0%; P=0.057). Conclusions: High levels of TAFI values are found in the acute phase of ischaemic stroke and particularly in those patients with worsening prognostic. Thrombin-Activable Fibrinolysis inhibitor levels related to t-PA induced recanalization resistance of the middle cerebral artery (MCA) in human ischaemic stroke. Our present interest is to know whether Thrombin-activable fibrinolysis inhibitor (TAFI) levels are related to t-PA recanalization of the MCA in human ischaemic stroke. An endogenous resistance produced by endogenous fibrinolysis inhibitor (TAFI) might decrease the benefit of thrombolysis-induced recanalization in stroke patients, treated with tPA, blocking several residues from partially degraded fibrin, eliminating plasminogen-binding sites. Methods and results: Thrombin-activable fibrinolysis inhibitor (TAFI) ELISA: was measured in 41 stroke patients involving MCA territory, before t-PA administration and 12h and 24h after symptoms onset. Recanalization was diagnosed by transcraneal Doppler performed at arrival and at the end of t-PA infusion. At arrival, 64 % of patients had a proximal CMA occlusion and 36 % a distal one. Significant baseline high levels of TAFI were found, (178.8 ±54.6 %) versus 141.8±45.6 %; p=0.034 in cases in which recanalization was achieved at the end of t-PA infusion (44 %). In a selected group with proximal MCA occlusion lower baseline circulant TAFI levels were found in those who remained occluded as compared with patients with total or partial recanalization (135.0±41.6 versus 184.6±51.3 %; p=0.018). Lowest levels of TAFI antigen were found when recanalization was not achieved at the end of t-PA. Baseline TAFI cut point values below 160 %, obtained from OR 7.78 (1.2-50.4;p=0.031), was the only variable associated to recanalization resistance. This study demonstrates that low baseline plasmatic TAFI levels below 160% predict t-PA induced recanalization resistance with a sensitivity of 77% and specificity of 70 % and we hypothesize that this is probably due to TAFI consumption that, when activated at clot surface, blocks plasminogen binding sites and consequently recanalization by tPA thrombolysis.

SY16

TAFI: Molecular forms of an emerging potential risk factor for thrombotic diseases

Juhan-Vague I, Frère C, Morange P, Alessi MC*

Lab Haematology, CHU Timone. Inserm UMR 626. Marseille, France

The role of TAFI in the balance between coagulation and fibrinolysis suggests its involvement in the development of atherothrombotic diseases. Controversial results have recently emerged which could be related to the methods used for quantification of circulating TAFI. We have previously shown, using an ELISA based on polyclonal antibodies (PC), a very large interindividual variability of TAFI Ag levels, strongly associated with some polymorphisms in the TAFI gene, in strong linkage desequilibrium with each other, such as the Ala147Thr , the Thr325Ile and several polymorphisms in the 5' or 3' region. It was shown more recently that variations in TAFI concentration may account for the existence of specific TAFI isoforms (Thr or Ile at 325) rather than « true » difference of TAFI levels. This leads to re-examine the properties of the available TAFI assays. Functional assays which quantify the amount of "activatable TAFI" were compared with several ELISA. We could distinguish assays greatly sensitive to the TAFI 325Ile isoform or to the TAFI after activation whereas one ELISA recognizes just as well all these TAFI forms. Interestingly, the results of all the assays demonstrated an association with TAFI genotypes. This allows to conclude that both quantitative and qualitative modifications of circulating TAFI are associated with TAFI gene polymorphisms. In clinical studies we have conducted, patients who suffered from an acute myocardial infarction, exhibited an increase in TAFIa levels and a decrease in the proform levels, indicating an activation of TAFI during the acute thrombotic event. Thrombolysis with rt-PA induced an increase in TAFIa levels whereas staphylokinase, which is not associated with systemic lysis, did not lead to TAFI level variations. In the prospective PRIME study, patients who developed stable angina, exhibited higher baseline TAFI levels than controls, whatever the sensitivity of the TAFI assay used towards the Ile325 isoform, therefore angina patients exhibit « true » high circulating TAFI levels. Interestingly, whereas the allele frequency of Thr325Ile did not differ between patients and controls, a significant difference was observed for the Ala147Thr, the increasing allele Thr147 having the higher frequency in patients, indicating that Ala147Thr is associated with quantitative changes of TAFI levels. In the retrospective HIFMECH study, as well as and in the prospective PRIME study, very high TAFI levels (>90th percentile- PC ELISA) were protective against myocardial infarction, with a higher frequency of the increasing allele Thr147 in control compared to patients (HIFMECH). The significance of these results needs to be further investigated. These results indicate that, in clinical studies, a battery of well characterized tests is necessary, in order to describe the behaviour of TAFI in the atherothrombotic process.

SY17

Venous thromboembolism as a 'marker' for cancer: to screen or not to screen

Prins M

Clinical Epidemiology, Academic Hospital Maatricht

The increased incidence of cancer among patients with a recent diagnosis of venous thromboembolism has been firmly established on the basis of population studies, as well as clinical studies. Studies in patients with thrombosis clearly indicate that the risk of cancer during 12 to 24 months is increased among those who do not have a clear explanation for the cause of their thrombosis ('idiopathic thrombosis'). Recent studies indicate that extensive screening can detect unknown cancer among patients with a recent episode of thrombosis and that these cancers are in a earlier stage. However, in the SOMIT-study, cancer related mortality during the 2 year follow-up period was 2.0% in the extensive screening group versus 3.9% in the control group (absolute difference, 1.9%; 95% CI, -5.5 to 10.9). Although early detection of occult cancers may be associated with improved treatment possibilities, it remains uncertain whether this improves the prognosis.

SY18

Therapy of VTE in different cancer patients

Kakkar AK

Abstract not available

SY19

Biological and clinical aspects of anticancer effects of antithrombotics

Falanga A

Hematology-Oncology Dept, Ospedali Riuniti, Bergamo, Italy

Hemostatic mechanisms play a role not only in cancer-associated thrombotic diathesis but also in tumor growth and dissemination. The early observations of fibrin deposition around blood-borne malignant cells and circulating fibrin-tumor-cell-platelet microthrombi were interpreted since the beginning as means for the transport and dissemination of tumor cells. Hence, inhibition of fibrin formation has been considered a possible tool against malignant disease progression. An antineoplastic effect of antithrombotic agents (anticoagulant and antiaggregating drugs) in tumor cells in vitro, experimental animal models, and cancer patients has often been suggested. Anticoagulant drugs such as heparins and vitamin K antagonists have been repeatedly tested in this context. However, heparins have been more extensively studied. Several reports in animal models demonstrate that heparin can reduce the primary tumor growth or metastatic spread. It is known that heparin inhibits adhesive properties of tumor cells and their migration trough the vascular endothelium. A synergistic effect of heparin with conventional antineoplastic agents has also been shown. In the last twenty years, many retrospective analyses have been conducted to evaluate survival in cancer patients prospectively enrolled in clinical studies of peri-operative thromboprophylaxis with unfractionated heparin (UFH) or low-molecular-weight heparin (LMWH) or in clinical trials of initial therapy of thrombosis with LMWH versus UFH. These studies have shown a beneficial effect of heparins, particularly LMWH, on mortality in these patients. More recently a number of prospective randomized clinical trials of LMWH for survival as a primary end-point in cancer patients have been conducted, showing promising results, particularly in the early stages of the disease. The proposed mechanisms for antitumor effects of heparins are numerous and include: 1. Inhibition of fibrin formation; 2. Interference with cell membrane adhesion molecules; 3. Inhibition of neo-angiogenesis and endothelial cell proliferation; 4. Induction of apoptosis; 5. Inhibition of heparanase activity; 6. Modulation of inflammatory cytokine activity.

SY20

Circulating endothelial cells: realities and promises in vascular disorders

Dignat-George F

INSERM U 608, Laboratoire d'Hématologie et d'immunologie UFR de Pharmacie, Marseille, France

Endothelial contribution to human vascular disorders is difficult to investigate, owing to the paucity of non-invasive methods and of specific endothelial markers. Circulating endothelial cells (CECs) might be used as a surrogate non-invasive marker for the study of vascular alterations. To address this problem, we produced an antibody against the endothelial molecule CD146 (S-Endo1) and developed, in the nineties, an original and sensitive immuno-magnetic separation assay. Using this approach, we demonstrated that an elevated number of CECs could be considered as a novel marker of vascular injury in pathological settings like heart catherization, sickle cell anaemia, bacterial infection, thrombotic thrombocytopenic purpura or acute coronary syndromes. CECs correspond to very rare cells present in blood since levels in the range of 3 cells/ml are measured in healthy individuals whereas levels from 5 to 1000 cells / ml are detectable in these pathologies. Several clinical interests of CECs will be discussed in the field of acute coronary syndromes, including their relevance as marker of disease activity, severity or treatment efficacy, or their use in diagnostic tests. The origin of endothelial cells present in peripheral blood is difficult to establish. They could correspond to endothelial cells dislodged from the vessels in response to injury. It was subsequently shown that a subset of CECs comprised a population of bone marrow-derived endothelial progenitors that participate to angiogenesis. Identification of the origin and characteristics of CECs provides fascinating insights into endothelial cell pathobiology. Moreover, CECs constitute original and promising tools for diagnosis, prognosis and therapy of vascular disorders.

SY21

Circulating endothelial cells and markers of vascular damage: prognostic value

Blann AD

Thrombosis, Haemostasis and Vascular Biology Unit, University Department of Medicine, City Hospital, Birmingham, UK

Circulating endothelial cells (CECs), defined by immuno-magnetic beads bearing mAb to CD146, are increased in the plasma of a diverse group of diseases, implying damage to the endothelium that may reflect pathophysiology. Endothelial dysfunction is marked by increased plasma von Willebrand factor (vWf) and by impaired physiological flow-mediated dilatation (FMD), and there is an inverse relationship between the two. However, the relationship of vWf and FMD to CECs is unknown. We hypothesised relationships between vWf, CECs and FMD in two groups of patients (a) with chronic heart failure (CHF) and (b) others with an acute coronary syndrome (ACS). In 30 patients with CHF we found abnormalities in FMD, CECs and vWf compared to 20 healthy controls with significant inverse correlations between FMD and vWf ($p=0.001$), FMD and CECs ($p=0.002$) and a positive correlation between CECs and vWf ($p=0.032$). In multivariate analysis only FMD ($p<0.001$) independently associated with CHF. In 39 patients with ACS, similarly, FMD correlated with vWf ($p<0.05$), FMD with CECs ($p<0.001$) and CECs with vWf ($p<0.001$). These data confirm hypothesised relationships and indicate that CECs truly mark endothelial damage. In a third study we measured CECs and vWf at baseline and 48 hrs after admission for ACS in 156 patients. Major cardiovascular end points (MACE) were sought after 30 days and at 1 year follow up. 48hr CECs ($p<0.001$) were the strongest independent predictor of MACE, followed by ΔvWf ($p=0.048$) but 48hr CECs were the only independent predictor of death ($p=0.007$). At 1 year's follow-up any MACE was predicted by 48hr CECs ($p<0.001$) but age ($p=0.046$) and 48hr CECs ($p<0.001$) were the only independent predictors of death. These data point to the value of assessing endothelial damage with CECs as predictors of severe endothelial damage and risk of major cardiovascular disease.

SY22

Circulating endothelial cells in vasculitis and transplantation

Woywodt A, Haller H, Haubitz M*

Division of Nephrology, Department of Medicine, Hannover Medical School, Germany

Circulating endothelial cells have been established as markers of vascular disease. In this talk, we will provide a short review on our data in ANCA-associated vasculitis and transplantation Vasculitis: We were able to demonstrate that cell numbers in excess of 25/ml have a high positive predictive value for active vasculitis whereas patients with other glomerulonephritides and infection had normal values. Moreover, we found that cell numbers correlated with disease activity and declined during six months of successful immunosuppressive therapy. Finally, we detected a necrotic and pro-coagulant cell phenotype. Transplantation: We first studied circulating endothelial cells in renal transplant recipients with or without rejection. Not surprisingly, patients with vascular rejection displayed grossly elevated cell numbers. Surprisingly, however, all renal transplant recipients had slightly elevated cell numbers when compared to controls. We speculated that immunosuppressive drugs, such as calcineurine inhibitors, might be responsible. We therefore studied cell numbers in renal transplant recipients who did not receive calcineurine inhibitors and compared them to matched controls. Indeed, these patients had significantly lower cell numbers when compared to their matched counterparts. These results provide further evidence for endothelial damage by calcineurine inhibitors. Very recently, we studied cell numbers in patients undergoing allogeneic hematopoietic stem-cell transplantation. Endothelial disease, such as veno-occlusive disease of the liver, capillary leak and graft-versus-host disease, is common in these patients. We were able to demonstrate a marked and intensity-dependent elevation of cell numbers during the early conditioning period. This finding may provide a novel marker for endothelial disease in these patients.

SY23

Circulating endothelial cells in preclinical cancer models and in cancer patients

Mancuso P (1), Paul S (1), Calleri A (1), Cassi C (1), Pruneri G (1), Monestiroli S (1), Gobb A (1), Shultz L (2), Bertolini F (1)*

(1) European Institute of Oncology and FIRC Institute of Molecular Oncology, Milan, Italy
(2) The Jackson Laboratory, Bar Harbor, ME, USA

At the present time, there is a clear lack of markers able to describe the angiogenic activity of a tumor type and to predict the clinical impact of anti-angiogenic drugs. We recently demonstrated that circulating endothelial cells (CEC) are 5-7 fold increased in preclinical cancer models and in breast cancer and lymphoma patients. We further investigated the origin of increased CEC in cancer by investigating NOD/SCID beta-2 microglobulin knockout mice transplanted with human purified bone marrow or peripheral blood CD34+ or CD133+ cells. Mice showing human engraftment 2 months after transplant were injected with Namalwa lymphoma cells. Before tumor cell injection, most CEC were murine, expressed a mature phenotype, and expressed markers of apoptosis, thus suggesting that steady-state CEC may derive from turnover of vessel endothelium. When chimeric mice were injected with tumor cells, the frequency of human CEC increased, the percentage of cells showing a progenitor (CD133+) phenotype increased to 3-8% of all CEC and cells showing markers of apoptosis decreased to less than 40%. These data underscore the relevant contribution of marrow-derived endothelial progenitors to CEC increase in cancer. In a second series of studies, we prospectively evaluated CEC kinetics and viability in more than 200 patients undergoing chemotherapy for hematological malignancies or solid tumors and in lymphoma-bearing mice treated with different chemotherapy (CT). At diagnosis, patients had a significant CEC increase, and a 2-3 fold reduction of apoptosis markers. Although the impact of different CT regimens on CEC kinetics was variable, in patients and in preclinical models low-dose, daily CT regimens were associated with a more consistent and profound decrease of CEC number and viability when compared to regimens based upon maximum tolerable drug dosage. In most patients achieving complete remission (but not in patients with progressive disease) CEC were reduced to normal values. We also observed a CEC increase preceding overt clinical relapse in some leukemia and lymphoma patients. Taken together, our data indicate that i) in normal subjects most CEC derive from vessel cell turnover, ii) cancer development is associated with mobilization of marrow-derived CEC progenitors and profound changes in CEC viability, proliferation and differentiation patterns, iii) the evaluation of kinetics and viability of this non-invasive surrogate angiogenesis marker is promising to assess the anti-angiogenic activity of different drug regimens, iv) metronomic CT is associated with profound CEC decrease.

SY24

Genetics of thrombophilia

*Castoldi E (1), Marchetti G (2), Bernardi F (2)**

(1) Department of Biochemistry, Maastricht University, Cardiovascular Research Institute Maastricht, The Netherlands
(2) Department of Biochemistry and Molecular Biology, University of Ferrara, Italy

The pathogenesis of thrombotic disorders recognises, besides environmental factors, clear genetic components. Family-based study has estimated that more than 60% of the variation in susceptibility to thrombosis between individuals is attributable to genetic factors. Although numerous genetic risk factors for thrombosis have already been detected, a large fraction of all thrombophilic families are not accounted for by the known defects, suggesting the existence of additional genetic factors that contribute to thrombotic risk. Investigations of the genetic bases of thrombosis have traditionally focused on the coagulation cascade and its regulatory pathways, which offer well-defined and easily measurable phenotypes amenable to the candidate-gene approach. In the last 50 years several genetically determined alterations in coagulation factors and their physiological inhibitors have been reported to contribute to the risk of venous and arterial thrombosis. These defects permanently shift the haemostatic balance in the procoagulant direction, a condition known as (familial) thrombophilia and associated with a life-long increased thrombotic risk. With respect to venous thrombosis, the first genetic defects to be recognised were quantitative and/or functional deficiencies of the natural anticoagulants antithrombin, protein C and protein S which represented a common finding in probands of thrombophilic families as well as in other affected family members. The deficiencies of the natural anticoagulants account only for a minor fraction of all cases of thrombosis. More recently it was recognised that increased amounts or the "improved" function of procoagulant factors can also induce a thrombophilic state. This is the case for resistance to activated protein C, mainly due to the factor V Leiden mutation, and elevated levels of prothrombin associated with the PT 20210 G/A mutation. Other emerging hypercoagulable states, whose genetic bases have not been elucidated yet, are high plasma levels of coagulation factors VIII, IX, XI, lipoprotein (a) and possibly thrombin activatable fibrinolysis inhibitor (TAFI). Low plasma levels of TFPI could constitute a DVT risk factor. These abnormalities are relatively common in the general population and are found in a large proportion of thrombotic patients. Moreover, on account of their prevalence, they are likely to be co-inherited with either AT, PC or PS deficiency, leading to a significantly increased risk of thrombosis in carriers of double defects. Several examples of interaction between thrombophilic defects have indeed been described which i) provide an explanation for the variable clinical phenotype observed among carriers of the same abnormality, even within the same family; and ii) demonstrate that thrombosis is a complex genetic trait. As for other multifactorial disorders, the susceptibility to thrombosis is the result of the complex interplay of several genetic and acquired/environmental factors, each contributing mildly or moderately to the overall risk. Thrombotic susceptibility can be thought as a continuous variable, which shows a normal distribution in the general population: most individuals have an intermediate risk of thrombosis, whereas few have either a very low or a very high risk. An individual's susceptibility to thrombosis may vary over time due to variable exposure to acquired/environmental risk factors. When susceptibility exceeds a certain threshold value, thrombosis occurs. Identification of all (major) genetic determinants of thrombosis and full appreciation of their mechanisms of action will eventually make it possible to develop new strategies, and design selective drugs for the personalised prevention and treatment of thrombotic disorders, tailored to the specific characteristics and needs of each particular patient.

SY25

Elevated clotting factor levels and venous thrombosis

Bertina R

Hemostasis and Thrombosis Research Center, LUMC, Leiden, The Netherlands

During the past years an increasing number of coagulation proteins has been implicated to play a role in the development of venous thromboembolism (VTE). Increased plasma levels of Fibrinogen, Factor VIII (FVIII), Factor IX (FIX), Factor XI (FXI) and Prothrombin (FII) all were reported to be independent risk factors of VTE. There is limited information on the molecular basis of these plasma phenotypes. In addition some of these plasma phenotypes may form clusters, which may point to defects in common pathways affecting biosynthesis or clearance. In combination with uncertainties as to what should be considered the cut-off for an elevated level and in some cases (FIX, FXI) the lack of published confirmatory and/or prospective studies, this has delayed the incorporation of these parameters in thrombophilia screening procedures. Elevated FVIII levels (>P90 of normal distribution) are associated with a 2.2-fold increased risk of first VTE, and in some studies also with an increased risk of recurrent thrombosis. The effect on the thrombosis risk is related to the actual FVIII concentration. Via its effect on plasma VWF levels blood group is an important genetic determinant of plasma FVIII levels, but other loci (inside and outside the genes coding for FVIII and VWF) might also be involved. A few studies have addressed the role of receptor mediated stimulation of VWF release, inflammation, acute phase and LRP-mediated clearance in the regulation of plasma VWF/FVIII levels, some of these with promising results. Elevated FII (>P90 of normal distribution) is associated with a 2.2-fold increased risk of first VTE. 14 % of individuals with FII in the highest quartile also carry the 20210A allele of the prothrombin gene, a genetic variation, which is associated with about 30% higher plasma FII levels. Sequencing of prothrombin genes in individuals with isolated elevated FII did not reveal any novel sequence variations except for the 19911G/A, which is a polymorphism in intron 13 associated with a 8 % increase in FII level. Elevated FIX and elevated FXI levels (>P90 of normal distribution) have been reported to be associated with about 2-fold increased risk of first VTE. Also here the actual thrombosis risk seems to be related to the plasma level of FIX and FXI. However, there are only a few published studies on this subject. Family studies show that heritability of FIX and FXI levels is considerable, suggesting that genetic factors might be involved. So far there is no evidence for a contribution of the FIX and FXI genes themselves. Sequencing of these genes in individuals with an isolated elevated FIX or FXI did not reveal any novel gene variations.

SY26

Management of thrombophilia: who to screen

Baglin T

Addenbrooke's Hospital, Cambridge, UK

Testing for laboratory evidence of heritable thrombophilia is now common. This practice undoubtedly arose in response to association studies, which revealed the influence of heritable thrombophilic defects on the development of VTE. Now that high quality clinical outcome studies are being reported it is becoming apparent that despite association, testing has limited predictive value for the majority of unselected symptomatic patients. Clearly, there is a difference between the ability of a test to explain why one individual is more likely to suffer a thrombosis than another and the ability of the same test to predict which patients who have already had thrombosis are likely to suffer a recurrence. In the absence of grade A recommendations, it is inevitable that practice will vary. Decisions will be influenced by local resources, competing demands for clinical and laboratory services and not least the professional interest of the haematologist. If thrombophilia testing is performed there is a strong case for selecting patients for testing as in most cases decisions regarding intensity and duration of anticoagulant therapy can be made purely in relation to clinical criteria. The polygenic basis of venous thrombosis and the influence of environmental factors make it difficult to predict from laboratory test results the likelihood of recurrent VTE. Furthermore, clinical outcome studies, which estimate risk due to one or more specified mutations, may be flawed due to the contribution of additional but unidentified genetic factors. It is possible that most patients who suffer a thrombotic event, particularly an unprecipitated event, have an underlying hypercoagulable state. As it is impossible at present to identify the multiple individual factors affecting thrombosis risk it might be more beneficial to use a "global" test to identify hypercoagulability, rather than search for thrombophilic defects. Measures of hypercoagulability, such as D-dimer and the thrombin potential, should now be evaluated and their predictive value compared with conventional measures of thrombophilia.

SY27

New developments in diagnosis and treatment of heparin-induced thrombocytopenia

Lubenow N

Greifswald University, Dept. of Transfusion Medicine, Greifswald, Germany

Heparin-induced thrombocytopenia (HIT) is a drug induced prothrombotic syndrome. New findings relevant for diagnosis and treatment of HIT have been made recently. Diagnosis: Using the criterion '50% platelet count fall' rather than a threshold of <150,000/µL improves the sensitivity of HIT-diagnosis in postoperative orthopaedic patients and possibly in other patient groups. The recommended frequency of platelet count monitoring for early detection of HIT depends on the heparin used (unfractionated heparin (UFH) vs. low molecular weight heparin (LMWH)) and the patient population - a general recommendation is not useful. In the same patient population, LMWH will cause HIT less often than UFH (about 10%). In children the two groups at main risk for HIT seem to be newborns and infants < 4 years undergoing cardiac surgery and teenagers treated with heparin for thrombosis. Treatment: New data show that lepirudin (0.10 mg/kg/h i.v. infusion, no bolus, aPTT adjusted) effectively prevented new TECs in patients with HIT and thrombocytopenia only ('isolated HIT') compared to a control group (p=0.0058). In danaparoid treatment of isolated HIT, patients seem to benefit from 'therapeutic' anticoagulation, rather than the 'prophylactic' dose. While fondaparinux does not seem to induce HIT-antibodies, there are only few data on treatment of HIT patients with this compound. Lepirudin, argatroban or danaparoid should therefore be used as the primary treatment in HIT. Anaphylaxis following treatment with lepirudin can occur, but is rare (approximately 0.015% on first exposure and 0.16% on reexposure), furthermore it seems to be IgG, rather than IgE-mediated. In lepirudin treatment of HIT-patients we recommend omission of the bolus unless there are limb- or life threatening thromboses. This will avoid overdosing as well as probably lessen the the severity of anaphylaxis. Reexposure of HIT patients with heparin is possible in certain situations, such as cardiopulmonary bypass, provided no HIT antibodies are detectable. This is usually the case about 100 days after stopping heparin.

SY28

Thrombocytopenia as marker of disseminated intravascular coagulation

ten Cate H

Dept. of Internal Medicine, Laboratory for Clinical Thrombosis and Haemostasis, Slotervaart Hospital, Amsterdam, The Netherlands

Disseminated intravascular coagulation (DIC) is a complex syndrome arising in the course of severe underlying morbidity. It either develops gradually in the course of protracted diseases, particularly malignancies, or second to acute severe diseases, including sepsis. The diagnosis of DIC has improved since the international society for thrombosis and haemostasis (ISTH) reached consensus on uniform criteria, adopted from criteria published by the Japanese Ministry of Health and Welfare. The present definition of DIC includes criteria that signal both overt DIC and impeding DIC, and are based on rather simple, conventional laboratory methods. The main advantage of this approach is that the diagnosis of DIC remains possible in virtually all countries since the use of sophisticated laboratory tools is avoided. One of the hallmarks of DIC is thrombocytopenia and platelet counts $\leq 100 \times 10^3/\mu l$ and $\leq 50 \times 10^3/\mu l$ add 1 and 2 points respectively, to the ISTH DIC score. Although the general impression is that thrombocytopenia is an important characteristic of DIC, its accuracy as a marker has not been established. The list of causes of thrombocytopenia is extensive and includes an array of disorders that have one of four effects: decreased platelet production by the marrow (viral infections, toxins); increased destruction due to immune and non-immune causes; dilutional or distributional causes; and spurious causes (such as EDTA agglutination). Thus, the *specificity* of thrombocytopenia as single marker of DIC is probably low. It is for this reason that the diagnosis of DIC has to rely on a panel of laboratory tests that quantify (changes in) different aspects (underlying disease, platelets, coagulation and fibrinolysis). The other issue is the *sensitivity* of platelet changes due to DIC. Elegant studies from Fletcher Taylor's group in sepsis models have demonstrated that platelet counts, like white cells do not show a dose dependent behaviour upon increasing E. coli challenge. Both in sub lethal and lethal E. coli studies platelet counts reached a level of about $165 \times 10^3/\mu l$ after 6 hours, further dropping during the total 48 hour period of study, remaining low while other markers such as fibrinogen and white cell counts had returned to baseline or higher levels. In contrast, markers of coagulation activation typically rise in the first 6 hours. These data suggest that thrombocytopenia is probably not an *early* marker of DIC, but most likely a significant indicator of *ongoing*, overt DIC. Clinically, the use of platelet counts for detecting DIC should always be used in combination with other markers according to ISTH criteria and should be followed in time to reflect changes in clinical course.

SY29

The von Willebrand factor-cleaving protease (ADAMTS-13) and the diagnosis of thrombotic thrombocytopenic purpura

Kremer Hovinga J

Severe deficiency of the von Willebrand factor (VWF)-cleaving protease, now denoted as ADAMTS (a disintegrin and metalloprotease with thrombospondin type 1 domains)-13 of <5% of the normal is a specific finding for thrombotic thrombocytopenic purpura (TTP), a life-threatening disorder presenting with thrombocytopenia, microangiopathic hemolytic anemia with schistocytes on the blood smear, often accompanied by organ dysfunctions such as neurological abnormalities or renal insufficiency, and fever. Until the late seventies of the 20th century TTP remained an almost universally fatal disorder. The introduction of plasma exchange therapy (PE) with replacement of fresh frozen plasma has dramatically improved the survival of patients with acute TTP from less than 10% to about 80-90% and is now considered the therapy of choice. Upon vascular injury endothelial cells release extremely adhesive ultralarge vWf multimers into the circulation, where they are slowly but continuously attacked by plasma protease(s). Deficiency of ADAMTS-13 prevents normal processing of ultralarge VWF multimers, and it is assumed that persistence of unusually large VWF multimers is responsible for the formation of platelet thrombi under high shear stress, a pathophysiological hallmark of TTP. The reported sensitivity rates of severe ADAMTS-13 deficiency for the clinical diagnosis of TTP range from 33 to 100%. Therefore, some researchers argue that only severe ADAMTS-13 deficiency defines acute TTP, whereas others find a considerable proportion of patients with acute TTP without severe ADAMTS-13 deficiency. Today, two forms of classical TTP are distinguished. Hereditary TTP, also known as Upshaw-Schulman syndrome is caused by severe constitutional ADAMTS-13 deficiency due to homozygous or compound heterozygous mutations of the ADAMTS13 gene, which is located on chromosome 9q34 and contains 29 exons. On the other hand, the acquired or sporadic form of TTP is caused by circulating autoantibodies inhibiting ADAMTS-13 activity, mainly IgG. Relapses are frequent among these patients and occur in about 35-50% of the survivors of an acute bout of acquired TTP. Reappearance of the inhibitor resulting in severe ADAMTS-13 deficiency may precede a clinical relapse. However, severe ADAMTS-13 deficiency is not inevitably associated with or followed by microvascular platelet clumping and other clinical signs of TTP, as asymptomatic subjects with prolonged severe acquired or constitutional ADAMTS-13 deficiency have been reported. Although severe ADAMTS-13 deficiency is a very strong risk factor for TTP, additional, hitherto unknown triggers may be necessary for the onset of an acute TTP episode, at least in some patients. Although, recent discoveries have answered some eminent questions in the field of TTP, they generated even more new ones. It will be interesting to see how they will inspire further research and hopefully lead to a better management of patients with TTP, as mortality and morbidity rates are still considerably high.

SY30

What is forthcoming in the treatment of hemophilia and von Willebrand disease

Lee C

Abstract not available

SY31

The value of factor VIII and von Willebrand factor as risk factors for arterial and venous thrombosis

Martinelli I

A. Bianchi Bonomi Hemophilia & Thrombosis Ctr, IRCCS Maggiore Hospital, University of Milan, Italy

Von Willebrand factor (vWF) serves as carrier for factor VIII (FVIII) in plasma. This carrier function may provide for the delivery of FVIII to sites of arterial injury, but data *in vitro* suggest that vWF supports thrombosis independent of its function as a carrier for factor VIII. In arterial thrombosis vWF is crucial, and experimental studies showed that animals with severe deficiency of vWF were normally susceptible to atherosclerosis, while they were protected from the formation of platelet-rich thrombi on the atherosclerotic lesions and the consequent clinical complications, such as myocardial infarction. In contrast, FVIII does not play an important role in arterial thrombosis, whereas in venous thrombosis both vWF and FVIII play a role. The risk of venous thrombosis increases with increasing vWF or FVIII concentrations and is higher in subject of non-0 blood groups than in those of group 0. Evidence has suggested that also inflammation may be involved in the pathogenesis of thrombosis, being FVIII an acute phase protein. However, the stability in FVIII levels when measured repeatedly over time after thrombosis was demonstrated, as well as the persistence of elevated levels after adjustment for levels of fibrinogen and C-reactive protein. Moreover, elevated FVIII levels are highly predictive of recurrent venous thromboembolism and are correlated with markers of thrombin generation (prothrombin fragment 1+2 and thrombin-antithrombin complex). Elevated levels of FVIII within families have also been associated with an increased risk of venous and arterial thrombosis. Although elevated FVIII is a clear risk factor for venous thrombosis and its inclusion in the laboratory work-up of patients with the disease has been advised, future studies of genetic and external determinants may resolve the question of how to integrate FVIII measurement into clinical practice. Additional work is also required to understand the interplay of inflammation in thrombotic processes. As concerning vWF in the pathogenesis of arterial thrombosis, the definition of its exact role must rely on the results of clinical trials evaluating the antithrombotic efficacy of molecules inhibiting the interaction between vWF and its platelet receptors.

SY32

ADAMTS13 deficiency: a new mechanism for arterial thrombosis?

Scheiflinger F

Baxter BioScience, Biomedical Research Center, A-2304 Orth, Austria

Increased plasma von Willebrand factor (VWF) levels have been identified as a risk factor for myocardial infarction and may be associated with increased risk of death after stroke. Recent investigations underscored the importance of VWF in arterial thrombosis and established a critical role of VWF for the development of platelet thrombi under arterial blood flow conditions. At high shear rates, the binding of the VWF A1 domain to the platelet receptor GPIb/IX/V complex is essential for an efficient tethering of platelets to a surface. Because of the inverse relation between adhesive activity and molecular size of VWF, high molecular weight VWF multimers are more active in supporting platelet aggregation under high shear stress conditions than smaller ones. On the other hand, accumulation of high molecular weight VWF may increase the risk of unwanted VWF-platelet interaction, platelet aggregation and microvasular thrombosis. Recent work on the etiology of thrombotic thrombocytopenic purpura (TTP), a life threatening disease characterized by microangiopathic hemolytic anemia, thrombocytopenia and multiorgan failure, lead to the identification of a protease involved in the regulation of VWF molecular weight. TTP is strongly associated with the presence of unusually large VWF (ULVWF) molecules in plasma. It was known for some time that VWF is specifically cleaved within the A2 domain, however, it was discovered only recently that a low abundant plasma enzyme controls the VWF multimeric size in a shear stress dependent fashion. The protease showed a high degree of homology to a family of multi domain Zn metalloproteinases and was named ADAMTS13 (a disintergin and metalloproteinase with thrombospondin type 1 motives). Increased ADAMTS13 activity has been associated with increased proteolysis of VWF and may eventually lead to a bleeding tendency. Conversely, decreased VWF proteolysis due to ADAMTS13 deficiency may result in an increase of the relative amount of high molecular weight VWF multimers in the plasma and therefore increase the risk of arterial thrombosis. Although firm data are still missing, it is tempting to speculate that ADAMTS13 deficiency could represent a new risk factor for the development of arterial thrombosis.

SY33

Predictive value of D-dimer in recurrent deep venous thrombosis or is it time to tailor anticoagulant therapy according to values of D-dimer?

Palareti G

Dept. Angiology & Blood Coagulation, University Hospital S. Orsola-Malpighi, Bologna, Italy

After a first episode of venous thromboembolism (VTE) the risk of recurrence is relatively high and clinical consequences important. While long-term treatment with oral anticoagulants is indicated to reduce this risk, the incidence of treatment-associated major bleeding can be expected in about 2%. Though in recent years a number of clinical studies have investigated the effects of treatment periods of different length, the optimal duration of oral anticoagulant therapy (OAT) is still a matter of controversy. Since the risk of recurrence differs from patient to patient, a major problem is the absence of reliable markers of risk prediction, which would facilitate selection of those patients at higher risk of recurrence for long-term treatment. D-dimer levels (DD) tend to increase after OAT is stopped. When measured after OAT discontinuation DD were found to be significantly higher in patients who subsequently had VTE recurrence (Palareti et al., Thromb Haemost 2002). In line with these results a more recent study confirmed that the rate of VTE recurrence was significantly lower in subjects whose DD were normal when obtained one month after anticoagulation was stopped (Palareti et al. Circulation 2003). Subgroup analysis showed that this was also the case in subjects with identified heritable thrombophilia. In the hypothesis that the test may be relevant for the management of anticoagulant treatment in VTE patients we believe that results obtained a few weeks after OAT withdrawal can be clinically relevant as criteria to decide whether or not OAT should be resumed. Another debated issue is whether residual venous abnormalities are predictive of recurrent VTE. It has recently been shown (Piovella et al., Haematologica 2002) that normalisation of ultrasound findings predict lower risk of recurrence. As regards the relationship between DD and the degree of recanalisation, our recent data suggest that high DD levels do not seem to relate to poorer recanalisation, although the highest recurrence rates were in the subgroup with no complete recanalisation and raised

DD. In conclusion, normal DD examined after OAT discontinuation have a high NPV for VTE recurrence.

SY34

Clinical usefulness of D-dimer in different groups of patients with suspected venous thromboembolism

Bounameaux H

Division of angiolgy and hemostasis, University Hospital of Geneva, Geneva, Switzerland

During the past decade, D-dimer measurement has become a widely used diagnostic tool in patients with clinically suspected venous thromboembolism. While the sensitivity of the ELISA assays and many automated turbidimetric tests is excellent (98 to 100%), its specificity varies widely in function of age, presence of cancer, in or outpatient status, and a priori clinical probability, which results in wide variations of the test utility in different populations. These characteristics will be reviewed on the basis of the Geneva Venous Thromboembolism Database, which contains over 1400 patients who were submitted to standardized, sequential diagnostic strategies.

SY35

D-Dimer testing in pregnancy

Eichinger S

Dept. of Internal Medicine I, Div. of Hematology/Hemostasis, Medical University of Vienna, Vienna, Austria

Normal pregnancy is associated with various alterations of the hemostatic system. While the levels of factors VII, VIII, X and von Willebrand antigen increase, protein S, factor XI and platelets tend to decrease throughout pregnancy. Elevated markers of coagulation activation, such as prothrombin fragment F1+2 and D-Dimer, indicate an increased thrombin activity and an increased fibrinolysis following fibrin formation. Overall, the balance of pro- and anticoagulant forces seems to be altered towards a hypercoagulable state. Testing for D-Dimer during pregnancy could be useful for the diagnosis and prediction of a venous thromboembolic event (VTE) or pregnancy-related complications, and for monitoring antithrombotic treatment. This approach, however, is hampered by the fact that even an uncomplicated pregnancy in healthy women is accompanied by a substantial increase of D-Dimer that is not necessarily indicative for a VTE or other pregnancy-related complications. Thus, prior clinical application reference values for D-Dimer during pregnancy need to be established. To evaluate the monitoring of antithrombotic treatment during pregnancy by D-Dimer, we prospectively followed 61 women who received low molecular weight heparin (LMWH) thromboprophylaxis and 113 healthy pregnant women who did not receive any antithrombotic treatment, and measured D-Dimer throughout pregnancy in both groups. Pregnant women who received LMWH at thromboprophylactic dosages still had significantly higher D-Dimer levels than healthy pregnant controls. The activation of the coagulation system occurred already during the early course of pregnancy. Further studies are needed to investigate the optimal beginning and dosage of LMWH thromboprophylaxis in pregnant women.

SY36

Thrombolysis in submassive pulmonary embolism

Büller HR

Department of Vascular Medicine, Academic Medical Center, University of Amsterdam, the Netherlands

Thrombolytic agents have profoundly changed the clinical management of patients with acute myocardial infarction. Their efficacy in restoring patency and minimizing damage to the myocardium has been proven in many large randomized trials. It should be realized that the actual thrombus in the coronary arteries is relatively small (millimetres) and that due to the specific symptoms and widely available coronary care units, the time between onset of the clot and the infusion of thrombolytic agents is well known and can be shortened to several hours by acute intervention. It is also well known that infusions after 6-12 hours are less effective. In pulmonary embolism the situation is quite different. The onset is usually not known and there is circumstantial evidence that before pulmonary embolism becomes symptomatic days or even weeks may go by. These older clots are less amendable to lysis. Furthermore the thrombi in this situation may be several centimetres long both in the lungs and the place of origin (i.e. the deep leg and pelvic veins). It is surprising that in contrast to cardiology the number of good clinical studies on thrombolysis in pulmonary embolism is limited with usually small number of patients studied. Although there appears to be a marked defect on surrogate markers, such as perfusion lung scanning and hemodynamic measurements, the results on clinical outcomes, such as all cause mortality, pulmonary embolism related mortality and venous thromboembolism recurrences are not convincingly in favour of thrombolytic therapy as compared to heparin. The pooled relative risk of 8 randomized studies with a total of 453 patients are 1.3 (0.6-2.5); 1.7 (0.6-5.0) and 1.4 (0.6-3.3) for total, pulmonary embolism related mortality and recurrences, respectively. On the other hand there is a clear twofold increase in major bleeding (RR 1.8; 1.04-3.1). Whether patients with echocardiographically detected right ventricular failure represents a specific subgroup of pulmonary embolism, which may require more aggressive therapy, such as thrombolysis, is heavily debated. The clinical evidence will be reviewed. Given the considerable doubt about the usefulness of thrombolytic therapy in submassive pulmonary embolism this treatment regimen should be considered experimental and be avoided in clinical practice.

SY37

The fibrinolytic system and thrombotic tendency

Kluft C

Gaubius Laboratory, TNO-PG, Leiden, The Netherlands

The observation that plasminogen deficiency is not a major risk factor for thrombosis can only lead to the conclusion that plasminogen/plasmin participation in fibrinolysis can be buffered by other mechanisms in most situations. This apparent redundancy is not unique and can be viewed as an argument for the importance of the effects achieved by plasminogen/plasmin as well. Major questions are where locally the other mechanisms are stronger or weaker and in which situations such as treatment, disease or trauma or in the case of abnormal fibrin structures the full power of multiple pathways is required. A major issue is how many and which buffering pathways exist. Thrombolytic treatment with plasminogen activators is an obvious area for concern about plasminogen concentrations. The symptoms in plasminogen deficiency of lignous conjunctivitis indicate poor back-up in these soft tissues. The association of the hyperresponsive variant (4G) of the PAI-1 gene with persisting fibrin and increased mortality in traumatic situations where PAI-1 is strongly increased indicate a clear role for the plasminogen/plasmin route in coping with thrombi and organ failure in such conditions. The effective treatment of oral bleeding problems indicates a high fibrinolytic power at those locations. It is suggested that the role of fibrinolysis in thrombosis and bleeding requires a careful evaluation of clinical phenotypes to identify the exact situations where weaknesses and increased activity of the fibrinolytic system are of clinical relevance. In addition the buffering mechanisms should be identified to clarify where the plasminogen-plasmin system becomes sufficiently important to take its share in buffering.

SY38

Fibrin stabilization, fibrin structure and the risk of thrombosis

Muszbek L, Bereczky Z, Shemirani A, Katona É*

University of Debrecen, Medical and Health Science Center, Department of Clinical Biochemistry and Molecular Pathology, Debrecen, Hungary

Unless protective mechanisms prevent its proteolytic degradation, freshly formed fibrin is promptly eliminated by the powerful mechanism of fibrinolysis. Blood coagulation factor XIII (FXIII) plays a key role in mechanically stabilizing the fibrin network by cross-linking glutamine and lysine residues of fibrin chains through isopeptide bonds. Several lines of evidence clearly indicate that cross-linking of fibrin and covalently attaching a2-plasmin inhibitor (a2-PI) to fibrin a-chains by activated FXIII (FXIIIa) provides significant protection against plasmin-induced fibrinolysis. It seems that the cross-linking of a2-PI is more important in the early protection of newly formed fibrin clot, while the formation of highly cross-linked fibrin a-chain polymers contribute to the high fibrinolytic resistance of aged thrombi. FXIII-induced cross-linking also occurs extravasally, at the site of inflammation or in the tumor stroma. FXIII released from inflammatory or tumor associated macrophages might contribute to this process. The persistence of extravasally formed and cross-linked fibrin might be important in the pathomechanism of a number of inflammatory diseases. The presence of FXIII in the bronchoalveolar lavage fluid suggests that such a mechanism operates in chronic inflammatory disease of the lung. Protection of fibrin from plasmin by cross-linked a2-PI has also been demonstrated in the lymph nodes with Hodgkin's disease. The role of elevated FXIII level in the risk for thromboembolic diseases has not been investigated previously. Most recently we have demonstrated that in myeloproliferative diseases with high platelet count FXIII level is elevated and high FXIII levels observed in certain patients are related to increased risk for venous thrombosis. We have also demonstrated a significant increase of plasma FXIII level in patients with peripheral artery disease. In the last couple of years a polymorphism in the FXIII-A gene that results in Val34Leu replacement created a lot of interest. The first reports demonstrated its protective effect against arterial and venous thrombosis. However, part of the follow-up studies reached different conclusions concerning protection against myocardial infarction. It seems that the concomitant presence of certain other genetic and/or environmental factors is required for the appearance of significant protection by the Leu34 allele. Meta-analysis of eight different studies showed only marginal (OR: 0.9?0.1) protective effect, against venous thrombosis. The polymorphism has been shown to accelerate the proteolytic step of FXIII activation and also seem to influence the structure of fibrin. However, these biochemical findings could not be causatively related to any anti-thrombotic mechanism.

SY39

New aspects in thrombosis research: possible role of complement and mast cells as profibrinolytic and antithrombotic cells

Wojta J (1), Kaun C (1), Zorn G (1), Ghannadan M (2), Hauswirth A (2), Sperr W (2), Binder BR (3), Maurer G (1), Huber K (1), Valent P (2)*

(1) Department of Internal Medicine II, Medical University of Vienna
(2) Department of Internal Medicine I, Medical University of Vienna
(3) Department of Vascular Biology and Thrombosis Research, Medical University of Vienna

We have recently shown that resting human mast cells (MC) produce tissue-type plasminogen activator (t-PA) without simultaneously expressing plasminogen activator inhibitor 1 (PAI-1). We will present data showing that the anaphylatoxin rhC5a is as a potent inducer of PAI-1 expression in human MC and basophils. In primary human skin MC and primary blood basophils, exposure to rhC5a was followed by an increase from undetectable to significant levels of PAI-1. In addition rhC5a induced a concentration-and time-dependent increase in PAI-1 antigen in the MC line HMC-1 and the basophil cell line KU-812 and increased the expression of PAI-1 mRNA in HMC-1. In conditioned media of HMC-1 treated with rhC5a active PAI-1 could be detected. A simultaneous loss of t-PA activity in conditioned media from the same cells indicated that rhC5a-induced PAI-1 was capable of inhibiting the enzymatic activity of co-produced t-PA. Correspondingly, the levels of t-PA-PAI-1 complexes increased in rhC5a treated cells. When HMC-1 cells were incubated with pertussis toxin or anti C5a receptor antibodies the effect of rhC5a on PAI-1 production was completely abolished. Treatment of C5a with plasmin resulted in loss of its ability to induce PAI-1 production in MC. Considering the suggested role for MC and components of the complement system in the development of cardiovascular diseases we hypothesize that MC by producing t-PA in a resting state and by expressing PAI-1 when activated by C5a might participate in the modulation of the balance between proteases and protease inhibitors regulating tissue injury and repair in such disease processes.

SY40

Will pharmacogenetics of antithrombotic drugs modify our approach to clinical (mega)trials?

Iacoviello L, de Gaetano G*

Center for High Technology Research and Education in Biomedical Sciences, Catholic University, Campobasso, Italy

Therapeutic indications are generally derived from large epidemiologic studies or groups of patients who are seldom representative of the general population. The beneficial effect of anti-thrombotic drugs usually ranged between 20% and 40%: though statistically significant, such an effect could also be read as limited to relatively small groups of "responders". As an example, out of 100 patients with acute myocardial infarction, 10 would suffer another infarction or die within one year; if given aspirin (or another anti-thrombotic drug), only 3 would benefit from the treatment ("responders"), while 7 would not ("non-responders") and 90 would be treated unnecessarily. This would correspond to a drug-induced 30% reduction of clinically relevant end-points. As ischemic cardiovascular disease is a complex, multi-factorial entity, the existence of "responders" and "non-responders" to therapy could be expected. The rapid development of techniques for genetic polymorphisms has allowed, in the past decade, to investigate the possible relations between genotypes and phenotypes. In particular, candidate genes were identified and tested not only for their protective or deleterious influence on ischemic cardiovascular disease but also as a way to identify individuals with different sensitivity to drugs. This approach, referred to as "pharmacogenetics", would also allow to recognize for instance possible genetic regulations of "aspirin resistance" as a biochemical phenotype. The glycoprotein IIb/IIIa complex acts as a receptor for fibrinogen and other adhesive molecules on the surface of platelets and is required for their aggregation. Polymorphism $P1^{A2}$ is a variant of the gene encoding for glycoprotein IIIa and is present in 25% of the white population This polymorphism has been associated with an increased risk of coronary heart disease, especially at young age and in patients undergoing coronary bypass. It has been recently shown that the $P1^{A2}$ allele is associated with an increased reactivity of platelets to aggregation and with an altered integrin-mediated function of adhesion, spreading and clot retraction. Moreover, the presence of the $P1^{A2}$ polymorphism might influence the anti-aggregatory effect of aspirin and affect safety and efficacy of anti IIb/IIIa antagonists. Considering genetic categories related to platelet function or other hemostatic factor activity in clinical trials could provide a model to predict drug efficacy and risk of bleeding of patients and ultimately the choice of the antithrombotic drug.

SY41

Cytochrome P450 2C9 (CYP2C9) polymorphism and warfarin dose requirement

Peternel P (1), Herman D (2), Globokar T (2), Stegnar M (1), Dolžan V (2)*

(1) Department of Angiology, University Medical Centre, Ljubljana, Slovenia
(2) Institute of Biochemistry, Faculty of Medicine, Ljubljana, Slovenia

Background. The adjustment of warfarin treatment is strictly individual, its effective dosage varies among patients up to 100 times. Cytochrome P450 2C9 (CYP2C9) is largely responsible for the anticoagulant effect of warfarin. Genetic polymorphisms of the CYP2C9 gene, which give rise to proteins with decreased catabolic activity, have been described. The variant alleles include CYP2C9*2 with a point mutation in exon 3 causing an Arg144Cys exchange, and CYP2C9*3 with a point mutation in exon 7 resulting in an Ile359Leu exchange. **Aim.** The aim of this study was to asses the influence of CYP2C9 polymorphism on the warfarin dose requirement in cardiac patients. **Methods.** 157 patients receiving warfarin from 6 months to 14 (average 3.5) years due to atrial fibrillation (n=145) and mechanical heart valves (n=12) were included. The patients were divided into low (<2.15 mg/day, n=38), medium (2.5-7 mg/day, n=103) and high (>7 mg/day, n=16) warfarin dose requirement group. CYP2C9 polymorphisms were analysed by PCR amplification of genomic DNA followed by restriction enzyme analysis. **Results.** In the low dose group 13 patients (34.2 %) were homozygous for the wild-type allele (*1/*1), 20 patients (52.6 %) were heterozygous and 5 patients (13.2 %) were homozygous for polymorphic alleles. In the medium dose group 74 patients (71.8 %) had*1/*1 genotype, 27 patients (26.2 %) were heterozygous and 2 patients (2.0 %) were homozygous for polymorphic alleles. In the high dose group all the patients were homozygous for wild-type allele. The frequencies of CYP2C9*3 polymorphic alleles were significantly higher in low dose as compared to the medium dose (26.3 % vs 4.9 %, p 0.01). The average warfarin dose was the highest among patients with*1/*1 genotype (4.42 mg/day) and was decreasing with the number of polymorphic alleles. Co-morbid states, body mass index and drug inhibitors of CYP2C9 did not significantly affect dose, stability and complications of warfarin treatment. **Conclusions.** Polymorphism CYP2C9 had major influence on warfarin dose requirement, while contribution of clinical factors was of minor importance. CYP2C9 polymorphism occurred in 34 % of individuals, suggesting its potential clinical importance when aiming for rational and individualised anticoagulant therapy with warfarin.

SY42

Antithrombotic efficacy of aspirin and genetic polymorphisms in the hemostatic system

Musial J, Szczeklik A, Undas A, Sanak M*

Dept. of Medicine, Jagiellonian Univ. School of Medicine, Krakow, Poland

Despite high prophylactic efficacy of aspirin in secondary prevention of ischemic heart disease, some patients still experience recurrent cardiovascular episodes. At least part of this so called "aspirin resistance" may depend on platelet glycoprotein (GP) polymorphisms leading to changed platelet response and hemostatic system activation following ingestion of antiplatelet drugs. PlA1/PlA2 polymorphism in the beta3 subunit of GPIIb/IIIa has been reported to be a risk factor for myocardial infarction. We report here on the influence of this polymorphism on the activation of hemostatic system and platelet function following aspirin and clipidogrel therapy in healthy subjects and patients with ischemic heart disease. We show that PlA1/PlA2 polymorphism may infuence the efficacy of antiplatelet drugs as antithrombotic agents. This way genetic analysis may help to choose the best antiplatelet therapy for subgropus of patients with ischemic heart disease.

SY43

The blood vessel wall

Blann AD

Haemostasis, Thrombosis and Vascular Biology Unit, Birmingham, UK

The blood vessel consists of a number of layers of different cells, each performing different functions. The innermost layer of these cells, the intima, is that which interfaces directly with the blood, and is composed entirely of endothelial cells. These cells do not merely form a passive layer between the blood and the rest of the blood vessel, but perform vital functions in haemostasis and in regulating vascular tone. With an anticoagulant nature, the healthy endothelium secretes factors such as tissue plasminogen activator, ADPase, and expresses membrane thrombomodulin. However, when damaged, it releases pro-coagulants such as von Willebrand factor. Similarly, the healthy endothelium uses nitric oxide, prostacyclin and other molecules to help maintain normal blood pressure, and these molecules also inhibit platelet activity. But a dysfunctional endothelium fails to produce these vasodilators so that hypertension and impaired flow mediated dilatation can result. Like any cell, any individual endothelial cell has a defined life span, and when it dies probably is sloughed off into the blood. It follows that high numbers of the circulating endothelial cells seem likely to reflect excess cell death, or at least severe damage, that we would expect to have pathophysiological consequences. Thus the (damaged) endothelium can contribute to Virchow's triad by failing to maintain an anti-coagulant service and in failing to correctly regulate blood pressure. These should predispose to thrombosis and hypertension.

SY44

Virchow's triad revisited: Blood constituents

Lip G

Haemostasis Thrombosis and Vascular Biology Unit, University Department of Medicine, City Hospital, Birmingham, UK

In 1856, Virchow published his classical triad of the factors that lead to the development of thrombosis (thrombogenesis). The three components are abnormalities of blood vessel wall, abnormalities of blood constituents, and abnormalities of blood flow. Whilst Virchow originally referred to venous thrombosis, the concepts can also be applied to arterial thrombosis. The latter is pertinent as thrombogenesis and atherogenesis are intimately related. The constituents of the blood are many and varied, but soluble coagulation factors (such as fibrinogen and tissue factor) and cells (such as platelets) are also clearly important. Indeed, platelets have long been implicated in the pathogenesis of atherosclerosis as major components of thrombosis, or as constituents of atheroma. Platelet function (or dysfunction) has been be quantified by parameters such as an increased tendency to aggregate, but also by measuring the levels of platelet metabolic products in both the plasma and urine, including the alpha granule constituents (beta thromboglobulin and platelet factor 4 (PF4)) and the soluble form of the adhesion molecule P-selectin (i.e. sPsel) in the plasma. Indices such as sPsel have also been shown to have prognostic significance. Coagulation and fibrinolytic factors are also important. For example, increased fibrinogen is associated with many different forms of cardiovascular and inflammatory disease, with prognostic implications for cardiovascular events. The mechanism(s) for these relationships are unclear, but it seems likely that increased levels of fibrinogen may promote platelet aggregation, as well as providing a ready source of fibrin. Fibrin D-dimer is representative of thrombogenesis and fibrin turnover, the latter also influenced by levels of plasmin/plasminogen, tissue plasminogen activator (tPA), and plasminogen activator inhibitor-1 (PAI-1). Consequently, increased levels of D-dimer are present among patients with a variety of cardiovascular diseases and atrial fibrillation. In peripheral artery disease, D-dimer levels correlate with disease severity. In some patient groups, such as peripheral artery disease and atrial fibrillation, raised D-dimer levels are not merely indicators of current disease, but can be related to prognosis. In atrial fibrillation, D-dimer levels also alter following the introduction of antithrombotic therapy and cardioversion. Blood constituents may provide information useful in identifying those at risk of accelerated disease progression, in monitoring this progression, or in clinical staging. The patients with the highest levels of the markers appear to be at the highest risk of disease progression, and if so, a panel of 'high risk' blood constituent indices (platelet and coagulation markers) may give a composite score of risk, may be a useful tool in predicting subjects at highest risk.

SY45

Virchow's triad revisited: Abnormal flow

Lowe GDO

University of Glasgow, Glasgow, UK

Virchow rightly recognised that blood flow plays an important role in thrombosis. The roles of blood flow in haemostasis, and in arterial, intra-cardiac, and venous thrombosis are reviewed. In streamline (laminar) flow, shear stresses are maximal at the vessel wall, and affect endothelial cell morphology and function (e.g. secretion of NO, prostacyclin, t-PA and vWF). Platelets are also concentrated at the vessel wall (due to axial concentration of red cells) where they can be activated by high shear stresses and are well-placed to interact with vWF and subendothelium, resulting in platelet adhesion and the initial stages of haemostasis. On the other hand, increasing wall shear forces increase removal of thrombin and fibrin monomer, hence stasis (induced by internal or external pressure) is required to allow fibrin formation and secondary haemostasis. Atherogenesis occurs in areas of arterial flow separation, which promotes platelet, leucocyte, LDL and fibrinogen adhesion and wall infiltration. Rheological variables (e.g. wall shear stress, viscosity, haematocrit, fibrinogen, LDL) have been correlated with the extent of ultrasonic carotid intima-media thickening. Arterial thrombosis usually follows rupture of atherosclerotic plaques and intra-plaque haemorrhage: high intra-stenotic shear stresses may activate platelets, promoting the initial platelet-rich "white-head" of arterial thrombi, while low post-stenotic shear stresses may promote the subsequent, fibrin – and red cell-rich "red tail". Blood viscosity, platelet microemboli, and activated leucocytes may each reduce post-stenotic microcirculatory blood flow, promoting infarction. Such mechanisms may explain the associations of increased levels of blood and plasma viscosity, haematocrit, white cell count, fibrinogen and vWF with risk and outcome of myocardial, cerebral and limb infarction. Areas of recirculating blood flow under low shear stresses predispose to intracardiac thromboembolism (e.g. atrial fibrillation, in which elevated fibrin D-dimer levels are normalised after cardioversion) and venous thromboembolism (fibrin D-dimer levels are associated with most risk factors). There is good evidence that reduction of venous stasis in the legs reduces the risk of venous thromboembolism. There is increasing evidence that regular exercise and avoidance of immobility reduces the risk of both arterial and venous thrombosis and also has systemic antithrombotic and anti-inflammatory effects. So: "Go with the flow!"

SY46

Assessment of the risk for prophylactic treatment of venous thrombo-embolism in medical patients

Samama MM, Gertotziafas G, Horellou M, Elalamy I, Conard J*

Service d'Hématologie Biologique, Hôpital Hôtel-Dieu de Paris, France

An increase in awareness of the risk for venous thromboembolism (VTE) in medical patients is expected since 3 different randomized studies have shown that the incidence of VTE can be reduced by 50% to 66% in hospitalized patients with acute medical illness (Medenox, Prevent, Artemis trials). One of the reasons of the under-utilization of antithrombotic prophylaxis in these patients is the inadequate identification of populations at risk. Recent work has clearly identified a long list of risk factors and has evaluated the weight of each one. The overall risk of VTE for an individual patient is determined by taking into consideration the presence of the predisposing and the exposing risk factors in this specific patient. A computer-based program called "Decision Matrix" has been developed by a large group of experts under the auspice of the RAND/ULCA methodology. It can be used today, as an educational tool, but a prospective study is planned to evaluate its appropriateness in acutely ill medical patients. Moreover, it could suggest recommendations for prophylaxis in a large spectrum of patients with different characteristics. Thus, identifying the medical patients at risk for thrombosis is important in order to reduce the burden of VTE disease.

SY47

Assessment of the risk and the prophylaxis of venous thromboembolism in surgical patients

Bergqvist D

University Hospital, Department of Surgery, Uppsala, Sweden

In patients undergoing surgery often two or three of the pathophysiological cornerstones in Virchow's triad are altered in a thrombogenic direction: venous stasis during anaesthesia, changes in the haemostatic system with activation of the coagulation and inhibited fibrinolysis and sometimes – as in orthopaedic surgery – endothelial damage. Several risk factors have been reported such as type of surgery, increasing age, malignancy, immobilization, previous venous thromboembolism, hyperestrogenemia, varicose veins, biochemical thrombophilic alterations, preoperative trauma. According to the ACCP consensus conference (2204) there are four levels of thromboembolism risk in surgical patients without prophylaxis (low, moderate, high and highest risk). Laparoscopic cholecystectomy belongs to the low risk group where no specific prophylaxis is indicated whereas patients undergoing hip surgery or surgery for abdominal/pelvic cancer belong to the highest risk group, where also modern prophylactic methods leave some patients without effective prevention. To optimise prophylaxis it is probably of value to have written instruction when to use it and what to use. What to use? The prophylactic methods with documented effects against venous thromboembolism and approval by health care authorities (at least in some countries) are low molecular weight heparins (dominating), unfractionated heparin (rarely used today), vitamin K antagonists (theoretically possible, effective but problematic both concerning logistics and side effects), dextran (rarely used but does prevent fatal pulmonary embolism), the factor Xa inhibitor fondaparinux (effective in orthopaedic surgery) and selective thrombin inhibitors (most documentation on ximelagatran/melagatran in orthopaedic surgery with a possibility for oral administration). Mechanical methods may be a choice in patients with higher risk of bleeding. When to start? Most documentation is on preoperative start. However, an increasing number of studies confirm the possibility of postoperative start. There seems to be an optimal starting window from a prophylactic point of view between two hours preoperatively to ten hours postoperatively. When to stop? Most documentation is on duration of prophylaxis for around one week. In patients undergoing elective hip surgery and probably in patients undergoing hip fracture surgery and surgery for abdominal/pelvic malignancies evidence is accumulating that extended prophylaxis for around one month postoperatively significantly decreases the frequency of clinically relevant venous thromboembolism.

SY48

Assessment of the risk and prophylactic treatment of venous thromboembolism in pregnancy

Conard J, Horellou M*

Hemostasis-Thrombosis Unit, Hotel-Dieu hospital, Paris, France

Pregnancy is associated with an increased risk of venous thrombo-embolism. In the general population, the estimated risk is less than 1 thrombosis per 1 000 pregnancies. Risk factors are the following: age above 35 years, unplanned cesarean section, bed rest, history of venous thrombosis, multiparity, gemellarity, severe ovarian hyperstimulation. In addition, women with thrombophilia have an increased risk. The magnitude of the risk depends on the type of thrombophilia: high risk: AT deficiency, antiphospholipid syndrome; intermediate risk: PC deficiency, homozygous FV Leiden or FII 20210A carriers, combined thrombophilias; moderate risk: heterozygous FV Leiden or FII 20210A, PS deficiency. In the different recommendations (ACCP, American College of Obstetricians and Gynecologists and French recommendations from ANAES), there is a consensus to consider the risk is high in the post-partum and women with thrombophilia and/or history of VTE should receive prophylaxis for at least 6 weeks. During pregnancy, recommendations are unclear and grades of evidence are low, established from observational, often small-sized studies. Low molecular weight heparin (LMWH) is commonly used but the doses are not well-defined. It could be simple to recommend a prophylaxis throughout pregnancy in all women at risk of VTE due to history of VTE and/or thrombophilia. However, although the safety of LMWH is considered as satisfactory, the risk of developing a heparin-induced thrombocytopenia exists and the prophylactic treatment may be a burden for the pregnant woman. Prophylaxis throughout pregnancy is required in high-risk pregnant women (4 to 6 000 iu twice a day). In contrast, LMWH prophylaxis may not be recommended ante-partum in women at moderate risk with no history of VTE. In other women, the prophylaxis is often decided on a case-by-case basis. A prophylaxis (4 to 6 000 iu once a day) during part of pregnancy may be considered in some cases. Informations are missing concerning the risk of thrombosis during each trimester of pregnancy in the different thrombophilias. Elastic compression stockings are frequently recommended during pregnancy and post-partum.

SY49

Assessment of the risk and prophylactic treatment of venous thromboembolism in the elderly

Couturaud F

Abstract not available

SY50

Warfarin management in difficult situations

Palareti G

Dept. Angiology & Blood Coagulation, University Hospital S. Orsola-Malpighi, Bologna, Italy

An unexpected condition of over-anticoagulation is not a rare finding during treatment with OAT. Since it is known that the risk of bleeding increases sharply in association with very high INR values patients with very high INR values (>7.0) or with more moderately high INR values but at high risk of bleeding should receive orally one or two mg of vitamin K; the INR will be measured the following day and oral vitamin K given again if necessary. In patients with an INR of 4.5-6.9 withholding warfarin for one or two days followed by a reduction of the weekly dose is usually sufficient. All patients with minor bleeding and an INR over the therapeutic range should receive intravenous vitamin K that will correct the INR values within 6-8 hours. In cases with a major though not life threatening bleeding a complete reversal of anticoagulation is advisable. A complete and rapid reversal of anticoagulation is recommended in patients with life threatening bleeding. PCC infusion will completely correct the coagulopathy within 5-10 minutes. A dose of 5-10mg of vitamin K should also be administered intravenously. The management of OAT in patients undergoing invasive procedures requires the careful evaluation of three elements: a) the thromboembolic risk of in case of OAT interruption; b) the bleeding risk of the procedure per se and in case anticoagulation is continued; c) the necessity of alternative anticoagulation (bridging therapy) and its possible risks. The substantial difference between the consequences of major bleeding events and thromboembolic complications should also be taken into account. Permanent disability and death are common after arterial thromboembolism, especially in case of cerebrovascular events (70-75%), while they are less frequent in case of venous thromboembolic complications (4-10%) or major post-operative haemorrhage (1-6%). In case of invasive procedures, the management of OAT has three possible choices: a) continuation of treatment; b) temporary discontinuation of OAT without alternative treatment; c) temporary discontinuation of therapy with alternative treatment (bridging therapy). In the absence of certain indications, even if OAT can be continued it is advisable to negotiate OAT management with the specialist who will perform the procedure.

SY51

Computer assisted anticoagulant therapy

Manotti C

Thrombosis Center Azienda Ospedaliera Di Parma, Italy

The number of patients receiving oral anticoagulant therapy is constantly increasing worldwide. This has led to the development of computerised decision support systems (CDSS) for a better management of patient care. Many computerised programs have been developed and introduced in clinical practice first in the Netherlands in Leiden since 1972 and later in UK and also in Italy since 1986 by means of the "Parma" system, this program is now widely used by anticoagulant clinics in Italy on the basis of good results observed in local experience. CDSS to be useful must provide a database of information about patients and clinical and follow-up data, which must be available on-screen for easy consultation during dosage prescription. Most of these systems use main modules: for suggesting confirmation of previous dosage (stable patients) or a dose variation on the basis of logical criteria derived from rules usually applied by physician in the dosage prescription and by a mathematical equation derived from regression slopes for variation of INR values on dose of anticoagulant for a range of weekly dosages. Only two randomised multicenter studies have been recently published: one by Poller in 1998 using DAWN program and another by our group in 2001 with PARMA system. Both the study demonstrated the effectiveness of computer-assisted dosage in improving the time spent into therapeutic range in comparison with traditional (manual) method. Both concluded that CDSS gives a better INR control than experienced physician did but clinical out come (haemorrhagic and thromboembolic events) remain to be assessed together with cost effectiveness To definitely assess the real benefit of CDSS as stated by multicentre studies large specifically designed trials are necessary. In 2002 a European project totally supported by the European Commission will started, 40 European centres will be involved in the project co-ordinated by Prof. Poller. 8 thousand patients will be randomised to receive dosage though traditional method, while 8 thousand will be randomised in CDSS, 20 Centres will use DAWN program and the other 20 PARMA System. The first trial objective is to determine whether a significant clinical benefit results from CDSS or not. Finally it will be investigated if CDSS may prevent bleeding and thromboembolic events that would have considerable cost-saving implications. The future scenario for CDSS must be considered. In fact the constant increase of patients' number and their pressure on thrombosis centre had led to the development of alternative models for delivery OAT: Primary care, General Practitioner, Patient self testing and self management. The use of CDSS has been central to the decentralisation process and may be useful in maintain the efficacy and quality of anticoagulant control.

SY52

Self adjustment of oral anticoagulant therapy

Watzke H

Department of Internal Medicine I, University of Medicine, Vienna, Austria

Patient self-management (PSM) of oral anticoagulant therapy has been investigated for many years now as a possible alternative method of controlling anticoagulant therapy. It consists of two integral parts: patient self-testing of the intensity of oral anticoagulation (PST) and patient self-dosing of vitamin K antagonists. This model of care provides a convenient opportunity for increased frequency of testing and thus has the potential to improve outcome of patients with long-term anticoagulant therapy. Self-testing is usually carried out with the use of a portable prothrombin time monitor. Several point of care (POC) monitors have been approved. They all use capillary whole blood. There correlation with laboratories methods is excellent (r-value between 0.86 and 0.97) with a reasonable coefficient of variation within the tests (CV between 4%-6%). Nevertheless, measures are still needed to ensure correct performance of the instruments in daily life, as the WHO calibration procedure is not practicable on the monitors and methods based on lyophilized plasma or plasma standards have not been established. The feasibility of PST using these instruments has been studied using surrogate endpoints (such as time in therapeutic range (TTR)) and clinical endpoints (such as recurrent thromboembolism or hemorrhage) and has come out favorable compared with conventional care. PSM, the combination of patient self-testing with patient self-dosing, has been compared with conventional therapy in several prospective randomized studies including selected or consecutive patients. All of these studies used surrogate endpoints such as TTR as primary outcome measures. PSM compared equally good or favorably with conventional management in these studies, depending on the quality of the conventionally monitored control group. PSM compared equally good when compared with high-quality management delivered by anticoagulation clinics. Both management modalities have a TTR which is between 80% -90%. PSM generally is superior to conventional management, when the latter is delivered by routine medical care (RMC), which has a TTR of 40% to 60%. These data suggest, that patients who are willing to self manage their therapy with oral anticoagulation after having undergone adequate training of testing and dosing are able to do so safely. Their quality of anticoagulation is equal to the one delivered by ACS and superior to the one delivered by RMC.

SY53

Mediterranean diet: is all the secret in oil?

Serra-Majem L

Foundation for the Advancement of Mediterranean Diet, Barcelona, Spain

Objective: The purpose of this study was to analyze the association of food, nutrient and energy intakes with olive oil consumption in Spain, and to review the importance in other foods like fish, nuts, in Mediterranean diet. **Design:** Cross sectional study by face to face interview in a population based random sample of 1600 individuals between 18 and 60 years of age derived from the Catalan Nutrition Survey. Two 24-hour recalls were administered to measure food and nutrient intakes. Food consumption and nutrient intakes were analysed comparing the highest and lowest quartiles of olive oil consumption. **Results:** Those with the highest consumption of olive oil (greater than 13.5% of total calories, 4th quartile) consumed less cereal, baked goods, whole milk, sausages, candy, fruit juice and soft drinks, but more fish, eggs, vegetables and added fats, as compared to those with the lowest olive oil consumption (less than 6.8% of total calories, 1st quartile). The group with the greatest olive oil consumption also demonstrated high total fat intake, although saturated fats showed a lower percentage of total energy intake. Vitamin intake was more adequate in those with the highest consumption of olive oil. **Conclusion:** Olive oil is a key contributor to the healthy aspects attributed to the Mediterranean diet, and as such, nutritional objectives in Mediterranean countries should address reducing saturated fats, without modifying quantities of olive oil. Other foods like nuts, fish and fruits and vegetables are also crucial.

SY54

The Mediterranean lecture: wine and thrombosis – from epidemiology to physiology and back

de Gaetano G

Research Laboratories, Center for High Technology Research and Education in Biomedical Sciences, Campobasso, Italy

The protective effect of moderate alcohol consumption on the risk of cardiovascular disease has been consistently shown in many epidemiological studies. Anti-atherogenic alterations in plasma lipoproteins, particularly increase in high-density lipoprotein (HDL) cholesterol, are considered as the most plausible mechanism of the protective effect of alcohol consumption on coronary artery disease (CHD). Other potential mechanisms contributing to the cardio-protective effect of moderate alcohol consumption include anti-thrombotic down regulation of blood platelet function, as well as of the coagulation and fibrinolysis balance. Since the proposal of a "French paradox" in the early Nineties, the possibility that consuming alcohol in the form of wine might confer a protection against CHD above that expected from its alcohol content, has made the topic "wine and health" more and more popular. Many epidemiological studies have explored such a possibility, by comparing specific alcoholic beverage types (wine, beer, liqueur) in respect to their relative capacity to reduce the risk of CHD. In parallel, experimental studies have been done, in which wine and wine-derived products have been tested for their capacity to interfere with molecular and cellular mechanisms relevant to the pathogenesis of CHD. Wine might indeed conceivably have other non-ethanol related beneficial effects. The biological rationale for such a hypothesis has been intrinsically linked to the enrichment in grape-derived, non-alcoholic components that possibly make it peculiar in respect to other alcoholic beverages. In fact, while the mechanisms underlying the effects of alcohol on cardiovascular disease have been limited to lipid metabolism and the haemostatic system, those related to wine consumption have also been extended to specific anti-inflammatory, antioxidant and nitric oxide-related vaso-relaxant properties of its polyphenolic constituents. The effect of wine consumption has been carefully investigated to account for potential confounding of several conditions (inappropriate use of abstainers as control population, correlation between wine or total alcohol consumption and markers of healthy lifestyle and socioeconomic factors, diet, etc.). Strong evidence indicates that moderate wine consumption rather than confounders reduces both fatal and non fatal CHD events. In spite of the fact that the healthy effect of moderate intake of wine is by now well accepted, important issues remain about the relationship between wine, alcohol and CHD. Among these are the differences in types of alcoholic beverages, the optimal amount of alcohol intake in men and women, the individual or environmental modulation of the alcohol-related effect and the pattern of drinking. Some of these issues have been recently addressed in a large meta-analysis, in which the relationship between wine or beer consumption and CHD risk was quantitatively evaluated. The purpose of this presentation is to summarize the experimental and epidemiological studies with wine or wine-derived products aimed at finding biological explanations for the supposed superior cardio-protective effects of wine consumption and to discuss some open questions about wine and vascular disease as approached in epidemiological studies.

SY55

Adherence to Mediterranean diet and coronary heart disease

Trichopoulou A

Department of Hygiene and Epidemiology, Medical School, University of Athens, Athens, Greece

While several investigations have focused on the association between individual foods and nutrients upon the development of chronic diseases, few have examined the role that entire dietary patterns may play in health and disease. An important reason for this paucity of evidence is the difficulty to assess or even define a dietary pattern. Yet, dietary patterns have the ability to integrate complex or subtle interactive effects of many dietary exposures and resolve problems generated by multiple testing and the high correlations that regularly exist among several of these exposures. A dietary pattern generally considered to have beneficial health effects is that of the Mediterranean diet. The traditional diet of the Mediterranean people is characterized by high intake of vegetables, legumes, fruits, nuts and unrefined cereals, high intake of olive oil but low intake of saturated lipids, moderately high intake of fish, moderate intake of dairy products mostly in the form of cheese or yogurt, low intake of meat and poultry, and regular but moderate intake of ethanol, primarily in the form of wine and generally during meals. By reviewing cohort studies exploring the association of Mediterranean diet with overall mortality and, hence, longevity a number of conclusions can be drawn. Firstly, there appears to exist sufficient evidence that diet does indeed influence longevity. Secondly, an optimal diet for the prevention of both coronary heart disease and cancer is likely to extensively overlap with the traditional Mediterranean diet. It is not yet clear which components in the Mediterranean diet are more important for its apparent health effects, but olive oil, plant foods and moderate wine consumption are likely candidates.

SY56

Platelet proteomics: identification of potential therapeutic targets

Maguire P, Fitzgerald D*

Dept of Clinical Pharmacology, Royal College of Surgeon's in Ireland, Dublin 2, Ireland

Newly developed proteomic technologies now permit the routine identification of hundreds or even thousands of proteins in a single experiment. However, the global study of any proteome has unique challenges that set it apart from comprehensive studies of genes and transcripts. The detection of low-abundance, biologically relevant, proteins poses a particular challenge, especially given that the dynamic range of proteins in cells is estimated to be 10^6 or greater. Nevertheless, the incorporation of proteomics into functional biochemical and biological investigation has proved to be a powerful tool when applied to platelet biology. We have analysed specific platelet subproteomes in an effort to capture proteins of low abundance including the characterisation of the phosphotyrosine proteome and the proteins released from activated platelets. These approaches have revealed a wealth of relevant platelet proteins, which may in the future prove suitable as therapeutic targets in atherothrombosis.

SY57

Peptidomimetic inhibitors of thrombin

Kikelj D

University of Ljubljana, Faculty of Pharmacy, Ljubljana, Slovenia

Thrombin, a trypsin-like serine protease, which is is formed by the cleavage of prothrombin by the serine protease Factor Xa, is the final enzyme of the blood coagulation cascade. The primary function of thrombin is to catalyse the transformation of fibrinogen to fibrin which after polymerization forms the matrix of the developing clot. Thrombin is responsible for the stabilization of the growing clot by activation of Factor XIII to XIIIa which covalently cross-links the fibrin strands. Thrombin is also a potent activator of platelet aggregation via the thrombin receptor and regulates its own generation by activating coagulation Factors V, VIII and XI. Limitations imposed by the well established anticoagulant agents acetylsalicylic acid as well as indirect thrombin inhibitors heparin and warfarin, associated with a risk of bleeding, the need of routine coagulation monitoring and/or parenteral administration has stimulated the research towards the discovery of small-molecule inhibitors of the coagulation cascade enzymes. The key position of thrombin in the coagulation cascade has made it a popular target for discovery of novel antithrombotic agents. A major advantage of small-molecule direct thrombin inhibitors is their potential to inhibit also clot-bound thrombin. Starting with hirudin, a natural peptide isolated from the medicinal leech, its shorter synthetic analogue hirulog and argatroban, the first therapeutically used synthetic small-molecule thrombin active site inhibitor, hundreds of direct thrombin inhibitors have been discovered over the last 20 years. Most of them are peptidomimetic compounds, based on the amino acid sequence of fibrinogen, which binds into the thrombin active site. Since elucidation of the crystal structure of human thrombin in 1989, the structure-based design of small molecule peptidomimetic thrombin inhibitors has been greatly aided by the use of x-ray crystallographic analysis of thrombin-inhibitor complexes. The ultimate goal of most research programmes and drug optimization strategies is to develop an orally bioavailable small-molecule direct thrombin inhibitor that would be suitable for once or twice daily dosing. The lecture will give an overview of discovery of peptidomimetic small-molecule direct thrombin inhibitors culminating in registration of ximelagatran in late 2003 as the first peroral thrombin inhibitor to be introduced in the therapy.

SY58

Antithrombotic effects of statins

Tremoli E, Colli S, Mussoni L, Sironi L, Banfi C, Camera M*

Department of Pharmacological Sciences, University of Milan and Centro Cardiologico Monzino, IRCCS, Milan, Italy

Clinical trials have shown that 3-hydroxy-3-methylglutaryl coenzyme A (HMG-CoA) reductase inhibitors or statin therapy reduce the levels of total and low-density cholesterol in plasma and the incidence of atherothrombotic events. The beneficial effects of statins on clinical events may involve both lipid and nonlipid mechanisms that modify endothelial function, inflammatory responses, plaque stability, and thrombus formation. In particular, statins have been shown to reduce in vitro the expression of tissue factor protein and activity in macrophages and endothelial cells. Administration of statins to rabbits fed cholesterol-rich diet results in a dramatic reduction in the accumulation of macrophages in the aortic arch accompanied by marked reduction in the expression of tissue factor. In this experimental model also the thrombogenicity of the aortic wall is markedly reduced. In addition, administration of statins to patients undergoing carotid endoatherectomy results in a reduction of inflammatory and procoagualnt markers in carotid plaques. Statins may favourably influence also the fibrinolytic balance, reducing the expression of plasminogen activator inhibitor type 1 (PAI-1) and increasing that of tissue plasminogen inhibitor (t-PA) in endothelial cells exposed to a variety of stimuli. However, the in vivo effects of statins on fibrinolysis in different clinical settings are not straightforward. This discrepancy can be explained if the different metabolic factors influencing the fibrinolytic system are taken into account. Controversial data are also available concerning a potential effect of statins on platelet aggregation and thromboxane formation. A beneficial effect of statins is observed on vascular endothelium, and in particular on nitric oxide production, as a consequence of increased expression of eNOS. Overall these data sustain the concept that the beneficial affect of statins involves a direct effect on prothrombotic variables. Moreover, in vitro and in vivo data indicate that statins significant decrease in the levels of inflammation markers, such as C-reactive protein, interleukin 6, and tumor necrosis factor alpha. Thus, interrelated inhibition of inflammation and thrombosis may largely contribute to clinical benefits from statin therapy.

SY59

Synthetic Factor Xa inhibitors

Samama MM, Gerotziafas G*

Service d'Hématologie Biologique, Hôpital Hôtel-Dieu de Paris, France

Heparins and vitamin K antagonists are the landmarks of the antithrombotic treatment. Both of them were discovered by serendipity, they are multi-targeted drugs and share several limitations. New molecules have been designed in order to be both more selective concerning their biological target and more homogeneous in their biochemical structure aiming to an improved benefit/risk ratio in the treatment of thrombotic disease. We will present a review of the pharmacological characteristics of the new synthetic direct or antithrombin dependent inhibitors of FXa in the light of the modern concept of blood coagulation process. We will also present the most recent data from the clinical trials with synthetic inhibitors of FXa. Among them fondaparinux, is the first synthetic and specific FXa inhibitor, which has been approved by health authorities in Europe and in the USA for the prophylaxis of venous thromboembolism in major orthopedic surgery and its approval for the treatment of pulmonary embolism and DVT as a single daily subcutaneous injection is in process. The phase II dose –finding trial of the "meta-pentasaccharide" idraparinux administered subcutaneously once weekly in the secondary prevention of VTE has been completed and a phase III trial has been started. The DX-9065a is the first direct synthetic inhibitor, which has been studied in a dose-finding trial in patients with coronary disease. Fondaparinux, idraparinux and DX-9065a are only active by parenteral route. Orally active direct FXa inhibitors are very attractive antithrombotics. Among them, razaxaban, BAY59-7939, ZK-807834 and JTV-803 are being studied in phase II trials in the prevention of VTE in major orthopedic surgery. The encouraging results from these phase II trials allow full clinical development of these specific anti-Xa agents. Several other synthetic direct inhibitors of FXa (such as the FXV673, YM60828, KFA-1411) are in a pre-clinical stage of research. From a clinical point of view, the results from the recent trials with the synthetic specific FXa inhibitors clearly show that the inhibition of FXa is a good target in the antithrombotic strategy and that although these agents have no antithrombin activity they exert in man antithrombotic activity by inhibiting thrombin generation.

SY60

Role of transfusion programs in stroke prevention in susceptible sickle cell children

Fontes E, Amorim L, Azevedo F, Leite A, Moura P, Lobo C*

Inst.Est.Hematol. A.S.C - HEMORIO, Rio de Janeiro - Brazil

Introduction: Sickle cell disease (SCD) is a group of hereditary hemoglobinopathies associated with a clinical syndrome characterised by chronic haemolysis and anaemia, susceptibility to infections, organ dysfunction and painful crisis. The painful crises are related to micro-thrombosis due to erythrocyte hyperaggregation. One of the most serious complications of sickle cell disease is stroke. The disease has a high prevalence in Brazil, where it is considered as a major public health problem. **Aims**: We present here the results of the interventions used to prevent strokes in sickle cell patients. **Material and methods:** All patients with SCD that presented a stroke were prospectively followed up, and they were included in a chronic transfusion program, whose aims were to maintain S-haemoglobin below 40-50%. All the SCD children (2-5 years) were submitted to a transcranial Doppler; those whose cerebral flow speed was over 170 cm/s, were also assigned to be included in chronic transfusion program. The patients included on the program were submitted to a partial exchange-transfusion at 3-weeks interval; the initial and subsequent evaluations included S-haemoglobin level, ferritin, anti-erythrocyte antibody screening, and screening for transfusion-transmitted diseases. **Results:** From 1999 through 2003, 85 patients were included on the program. The global rate of stroke recurrence was 5.9%; in the group included on the program due to abnormal results on transcranial Doppler this rate was 0%. The ferritin level was maintained below 1,000 mcg/μL in 81% of the patients, and the rate alloimmunisation was 7%. There was no case of seroconversion. **Conclusions:** The transfusion approach used for preventing stroke was effective, and was associated to a very low frequency of complications.

SY61

Haemostatic cardiovascular risk factors: differential effects of red wine and diet on healthy young population

Mezzano D (1), Leighton F (2)**

(1) Department of Haematology, School of Medicine, P. Catholic University of Chile
(2) Department of Molecular and Cell Biology, Faculty of Biological Sciences, P. Catholic University of

Aims: We compared prospectively the effects of a Mediterranean-type diet (MD) and a high-fat diet (HFD), with/without red wine supplementation, on plasma concentration of emergent haemostatic cardiovascular risk factors (HCVRF) and on variables of primary haemostasis: bleeding time (BT), plasma von Willebrand factor (VWF:Ag) and platelet aggregation/secretion. **Study design**: Two groups (21 healthy male each) received either MD or HFD during 90 days. Between days 30-60, both diets were supplemented with 240 ml/day of red wine. **Results**: MD was associated with: lower plasma fibrinogen ($p = 0.03$), factor VIIc ($p=0.034$) and factor VIIIc ($p=0.0057$); higher levels of protein S ($p=0.013$); longer BT ($p=0.017$); and marginal increases in platelet serotonin aggregation and secretion after stimulation with epinephrine. Red wine supplementation, in both diets, resulted in lower plasma fibrinogen ($p=0.001$) and factor VIIc ($p=0.05$), and in increased t-PA ($p=0.01$) and PAI-1 ($p=0.0003$). The effects of wine on antithrombin III ($p=0.01$) were divergent: there was a decrease in the HFD group but it increased slightly in the MD group. No effects of diet or wine were detected in plasma proteins C and S. With regard to primary haemostasis, neither BT nor VWF:Ag changed significantly as a consequence of wine intake. Wine supplementation also resulted in a significant increase in *ex vivo* platelet aggregation and secretion after stimulation with collagen (1 and 2 μg/ml, $p \leq 0.01$). **Conclusion**: MD and moderate consumption of red wine have complementary, mostly beneficial effects on haemostatic CV risk factors. The longer BT in individuals on MD, independently of red wine, would denote less interaction of platelets with the vascular wall, which would be beneficial from the point of view of CV risk. However, the increased platelet aggregation/secretion, a possible "rebound" phenomenon, would be a risk factor for thrombosis.

SY62

Management of patients with acute venous thromboembolism: Findings from the RIETE Registry

Monreal M, Suárez C, González Fajardo J, Barba R, Uresandi F, Valle R, Rondón P*

Servicio de Medicina Interna, Hospital Universitari Germans Trias i Pujol, Badalona, Spain

Background: Guidelines for the treatment of venous thromboembolism (VTE) are mainly based on randomized controlled trials, but a number of patients with VTE are excluded from trials due to co-morbidities. Thus, treatment regimens derived from clinical studies may not be suitable for all patient groups. Objectives The Registro Informatizado de la Enfermedad TromboEmbólica (RIETE) will collate VTE management and outcomes data for at least 12,000 patients over 3 years, providing "real-world" comparisons of treatments. Its aim is to provide information on the Internet to help physicians to evaluate treatment options in different patient groups, aiding treatment selection. **Methods:** Centers enroll all patients with symptomatic, objectively confirmed VTE. Treatment and outcome data are recorded. A minimum 3-month follow-up period is required. **Results:** 6,855 patients have so far enrolled in RIETE. 1,635 of them (24%) had at least one reason to be excluded from clinical trials: recent bleeding (2.6%); renal insufficiency (13.6%); thrombocytopenia (2.5%); abnormal prothrombin time (9.1%) and pregnancy (0.7%). During the 3-month follow-up period the rates of fatal pulmonary embolism (odds ratio: 3.3; 95% CI: 2.5-5.2); minor bleeding (odds ratio: 1.8; 95% CI: 1.3-2.2); major bleeding (odds ratio: 3.1; 95% CI: 2.3-4.1) and fatal bleeding (odds ratio: 4.1; 95% CI: 2.1-8.0) were significantly higher in these patients than in the remaining 5,220 patients. **Conclusions:** The expanding RIETE database of "real-world" outcomes may lead to improved treatment of VTE, especially for those patients not usually included in randomized clinical trials.

ORAL COMMUNICATIONS

OC001

Polymorphisms on thrombospondin genes and premature acute myocardial infarction: a controversy to settle

Peyvandi F (1), Palla R (1), Menegatti M (1), Merlini P (2), Marziliano N (3), Bernardinelli L (4,5), Mannucci P (1)*

(1) A. Bianchi Bonomi Hemophilia and Thrombosis Centre, Fondazione Luigi Villa, IRCCS Maggiore Hospital, Italy
(2) Division of Cardiology, Ospedale Niguarda, Milan, Italy
(3) Applera Italia, Molecular Biology Lab, Monza, Italy
(4) Dipartimento di Scienze Sanitarie Applicate, University of Pavia, Italy
(5) MRC Biostatistics Unit, Institute of Public Health, University Forvie Site, Cambridge, UK

Introduction: In the last decade research efforts have focused on the search of genetic risk factors in complex diseases such as myocardial infarction (MI) by means of association studies based upon single nucleotide polymorphisms (SNPs) of genes encoding proteins involved in thrombogenesis. In general these studies yielded results of little or no clinical impact, usually because the size sample populations were too small. This situation is epitomised by two recent studies (TheGeneQuest Study, *Circulation* 2001 and Boekholdt *et al*., *ATVB* 2002) that analysed three SNPs in the thrombospondins genes THSB1 (N700S), THSB2 (T/G in the 3'UTR) and THSB4 (A387). The first study, on 352 white American patients and 418 healthy individuals, reports a high association between N700S SNP in the homozygous state and risk of MI (Odd Ratio [OR]=8.7, 95%CI 0.96-78.1), a protective effect of THSB2 gene SNP (OR=0.4, 95%CI 0.16-0.97), and a smaller relative risk of A387P SNP (OR=1.6, 95%CI 0.75-3.6). The same SNPs analysed by Boekholdt *et al*. in 503 Dutch cases and 1071 healthy controls gave strikingly different results: N700S showed no significant association, while both T/G of the 3' UTR (OR=0.44, 95%CI 0.24-0.84) and A387P (OR=0.43, 95%CI 0.22-0.85) showed a reduced risk of premature MI. **Aims**: Our study was carried out in the attempt to solve this controversy by analysing a sample of sufficiently large size to have a 0.80 power to find a difference. **Material and methods**: 1539 Italian patients who survived a first MI at less than 45 years, fully characterised in terms of non-genetic risk factors and extent of coronary artery stenosis and 1539 healthy controls (matched for sex, age and geographical origin) were analysed. Genotype was performed by PCR followed by SNPs detection using wild type and mutant TaqMan fluorescinated probes on the ABI Prism 9700 sequence detection system (Applied Biosystems). **Results**: Allele frequency and the ORs, estimated using a conditional logistic regression model are shown in the Table (statistically significant results are showed in bold).

	cases	controls	unadjusted or (c.i. 95%)	p value	adjusted or (c.i. 95%)	p value
THSB1 (A/G => N700S)						
Allele A frequency	90,04%	92,39%	1,33 (1,11-1,60)	0,002	1,39 (1,07-1,81)	0,013
Allele G frequency	9,56%	7,61%				
THSB2 (T/G in 3'UTR)						
Allele T frequency	74,42%	73,44%	0,95 (0,84-1,07)	0,382	0,99 (0,83-1,19)	0,929
Allele G frequency	25,58%	26,56%				
THSB4 (G/C => A387P)						
Allele G frequency	78,81%	80,00%	1,07 (0,94-1,22)	0,267	1,20 (0,99-1,44)	0,058
Allele C frequency	21,19%	20,00%				

Conclusion: This study found that N700S SNP on THSB1 is associated with a significant increased risk of premature MI, providing a stronger evidence of association because of a narrower 95% CI than the *Circulation* study. The T to G SNP in THSB2 was not associated with MI, while in both *Circulation* and *ATVB* studies it was associated to a decreased risk of MI. No significant association with MI was found for A387P SNP on THSB4. This study assesses the importance of a well characterised population with an adequate sample size to reach sufficient statistical power in genotype analysis in order to obtain significant results.

OC002

Emerging prognostic factors in coronary artery disease

Brogi D, Sofi F, Fatini C, Lenti M, Valente S, Lombardi A, Lucarini L, Sticchi E, Abbate R, Gensini GF*

Department of Medical and Surgical Critical Care, University of Florence, Thrombosis Centre, Aziend

Recent data indicate that emerging haemostasis-related factors have an important role in the pathogenesis of coronary artery disease (CAD) but their prognostic value in CAD patients have not been defined yet. Aim of our study was to evaluate the prognostic value of emerging genetic and metabolic haemostasis-related risk factors in a group of consecutive patients with angiographic diagnosis of CAD who were referred to the Coronary Intensive Therapy Unit of the University of Florence. We investigated, at the time of admission, the presence of Factor V Leiden and prothrombin G20210A mutations, homocysteine (Hcy), lipoprotein (a) [Lp(a)] and plasminogen activator inhibitor 1 (PAI-1) plasma levels in 416 patients and in 300 healthy subjects recruited from the blood donors of our hospital. Hyperhomocysteinemia, defined as a concentration of Hcy above the 95th percentile of controls, was diagnosed in 85/416 patients (20.4%) and in 10/300 controls (3.3%); Lp(a) levels above 300 mg/L, cut-off of cardiovascular risk, were present in 146/416 patients (35.1%) and in 41/416(13.7) controls and PAI-1 >15 IU/L in 204/416 patients (49%) and in 41/300 controls (13.7%). No statistically significant difference concerning the presence of the 2 investigated mutations in patients compared to controls was observed. Patients were followed up for a mean period of 14.7±4.7 months: 80/416 had a major cardiac event (MACE: 46/80 deaths and 34/80 target lesion revascularization). Hyperhomocysteinemia was present in 25/80 (31.3%) patients with MACE compared to 56/316 (17.9%) patients without MACE (p<0.05), elevated PAI-1 levels in 26/80 (63.4%) compared to 150/316 (47.5%) (p<0.05) and Lp(a)>300 mg/L in 27/80 (33.8%) compared to 111/316 (35.4) (p n.s.). At the multivariate analysis, adjusted for traditional and haemostasis-related risk factors and also for the number of vessels with a stenosis > 75%, hyperhomocysteinemia and high PAI-1 levels resulted independent predictive factors for MACE (hyperhomocysteinemia: OR= 2.1, 95%CI 1.2-3.8, p<0.01; PAI-1: OR= 1.1 95%CI 1.03-2.09, p=0.004). This study reveals that elevated homocysteine plasma levels and high levels of PAI-1 could be predictors for MACE in patients with established CAD.

OC003

Increased plasma concentration of platelet-derived microparticles in young survivors of myocardial infarction

Michelsen A (1), Brodin E (2), Brosstad F (1), Hansen J (2)*

(1) Research Institute for Internal Medicine, University of Oslo, Oslo, Norway
(2) Center for Atherothrombotic Research in Tromsø, University of Tromsø, Tromsø, Norway

Introduction: Prothrombotic mechanisms are of major importance for the formation of an occlusive thrombus in young patients with myocardial infarction (MI). Experimental studies have shown that platelet-derived microparticles (PDMP) possess procoagulant properties suggesting a pivotal role in the pathogenesis of arterial thrombotic diseases. **Aims:** To determine the concentrations of PDMP in plasma from young MI patients and study their relation to coagulation activation, assessed by thrombin-antithrombin (TAT) complexes. **Material and methods:** A population based case (n=61)-control (n=61) study matched for age and gender was conducted in MI-patients between 40 and 60 years of age and more than a year after the coronary event. An ELISA assay was developed to quantify PDMP by the concentration of activated GPIIb/IIIa in plasma and plasma was filtered (0.1 μm size exclusion) to discriminate between small (< 0.1 μm) and large (≥ 0.1 μm) PDMP. **Results**: Young survivors of MI had significantly higher mean platelet volume (MPV) (p=0.012) and PDMP (314.3 μg/L, 273.1-361.4 vs. 225.8 μg/L, 186.8-273.1, p=0.009) (geometric mean and 95%CI) than age- and gender matched healthy controls. In simple regression analysis, the total amount of PDMP positively associated with platelet count (r=0.44, p<0.001) and soluble CD40L (r=0.50, p<0.001), whereas large PDMP was correlated with platelet count (r=0.28, p<0.05), sCD40L (r=0.37, p<0.01) and TAT (r=0.35, p<0.01). To study the predictive role of PDMP for MI, logistic regression models were conducted. In simple regression models, MPV (1.70, 1.09-2.67) (OR, 95%CI), total PDMP (2.39, 1.20-4.78), small PDMP (2.52, 1.10-5.74) and large PDMP (1.65, 1.06-2.72) were significant predictors for MI. The predictive role of total, small and large PDMP for MI, remained significant even after adjustment for age, sex, BMI and main serum lipids. **Conclusions**: The present study suggests that PDMP is an independent risk factor for MI. The positive correlation found between large PDMP and thrombin generation support the concept that formation of PDMP is of crucial importance for increased coagulation activation in MI patients.

OC004

Gene-gene interaction of the ABCA1 transporter and paraoxonase genes in inherited predisposition to myocardial infarction in young men

Pchelina S (1,2), Sheydina A (2), Taraskina A (2), Rodygina T (2), Schwarzman A (2)*

(1) Pavlov's State Medical University, St.Petersburg, Russia
(2) Petersbusg Nuclear Physics Institute RAS, St.Petersburg, Russia

Introduction. Oxidative modification of low-density lipoproteins (LDLs) is a major contributor to atherosclerosis. High–density lipoproteins (HDLs) can protect LDLs from oxidative damage. The mechanism of this protective effect may involve paraoxonase (PON1), an HDL-associated enzyme. On the other hand, the efflux of the intracellular cholesterol and its subsequent uptake by HDL particles is now thought to be catalyzed by an enzyme that is a member of ATP-binding cassette transporter family, known as the ABCA1 enzyme (ABCA1). **Aims.** To investigate the genotype distribution of the C(-108)T, L54M and Q191R polymorphisms of the PON1 gene and the G(-191)C, C69T, C(-17)G and 319insG polymorphisms of the ABCA1 gene in men, survived after myocardial infarction (MI) at the age under 45 (204 subjects) and in the control group (170 subjects without cardiac vascular pathology) and to estimate the gene-gene interaction of these genes in the development of MI. **Materials and methods.** Genotypes were determined by PCR with restriction analysis described earlier. **Results.** The R191 allele frequency was significantly higher in patients than in controls (P<0.0003). Odds ratio (OR) for the RR genotype carriers was 3.8 (95%CI: 1.8-8.2), compared to the RQ and QQ genotypes carriers. The C(-108) allele frequency was increased among controls compared with patients (P<0.05). OR for the high expressor CC genotype carriers was 0.5 (95%CI:0.7-0.4). No significant association was found between the L54M

PON1 allele, all studied ABCA1 alleles and the risk of MI in young men. At the same time the frequencies of "atherogenic" alleles of the ABCA1 gene (C69T, G(-191)C) were twice increased in Russian population compared with the population of Netherlands (p<0.0001). The risk of MI was 6.2 times higher in the concurrent carriers of the RR 191 genotype of the PON1 gene and the C(-191) allele of the ABCA1 gene (OR=6.2[95%CI:2.0-19.6]). **Conclusions.** The simultaneous genotyping of allelic variants of the PON1 and ABCA1 genes might be extremely useful for forming the risk group of MI in young men.

OC005

Circulating endothelial cells predict outcomes in patients with acute coronary syndrome: relationship to plasma von Willebrand factor and interleukin-6

Lee W, Lip G*

Haemostasis, Thrombosis and Vascular Biology Unit, University Department of Medicine, City Hospital, Birmingham, UK

Background: It is well recognised that markers of inflammation and coagulation cascade as well as endothelial perturbation are altered in patients with acute coronary syndrome (ACS). The aim of this study was to compare the short-term prognostic value of interleukin-6 (IL-6, an inflammatory marker), von Willebrand factor levels (vWf, an index of endothelial damage/dysfunction) and circulating endothelial cells (CECs, indicating endothelial damage) in patients presenting with ACS. **Methods:** 156 patients (107 male, 64 ± 12 yrs) consecutively admitted to the coronary care unit with ACS were included. Blood was drawn within 24 hrs of admission (T1) and 48 hrs thereafter (T2) for plasma levels of vWf and IL-6 (ELISA). CECs were quantified using epifluorescence microscope after immunomagnetic separation. Baseline values were compared with 35 matched patients with stable coronary heart disease (CHD) and 35 matched healthy controls. **Results:** Levels of vWf, IL-6 and CECs were significantly higher in ACS patients compared with stable CHD and controls (all p<0.01). CECs, vWf and IL-6 were highly correlated with each other (all p<0.001). 48 patients had a major adverse clinical event (MACE; 10 deaths, 33 had refractory angina, 5 readmitted with ACS) at 30 days. On univariate analysis, CECs and IL-6 levels at T1 and T2, vWf levels at T2 and changes (T2 minus T1) of CECs, vWf and IL-6 levels over 48hrs of admission were strongly and significantly correlated with 30-day MACE (all p ≤0.002). On stepwise logistic regression analysis, CECs at T2 (Odd ratio [OR], 1.04 [95% CI, 1.02 – 1.06], p<0.001) was the strongest independent predictor for 30-day MACE, followed by the changes of IL-6 (OR, 1.024 [1.005 – 1.04], p=0.01) and vWf levels over 48hrs (OR, 1.012 [1.0 – 1.03], p=0.048). CECs level at T2 was the only single independent predictor of death at 30 days (OR, 1.011 [95% CI, 1.003 – 1.02], p=0.007). **Conclusions:** Raised plasma levels of vWf, IL-6 and numbers of CECs during the first 48 hrs of ACS were strongly associated with MACE at 30 days. CECs levels at 48hrs were the only independent predictor of both death and MACE at 30 days, indicating the crucial role of endothelial/vascular damage in the pathogenesis of ACS.

OC006

High ambulatory pulse pressure is associated with abnormal thrombogenesis and endothelial damage/dysfunction in patients with coronary heart disease

Lee W, Lip G*

Haemostasis, Thrombosis and Vascular Biology Unit, University Department of Medicine, City Hospital, Birmingham, UK

Background: Both pulse pressure (PP) and mean arterial blood pressure (MAP) have been implicated as independent predictors of cardiovascular (CV) risk. PP measures the pulsatile component, whereas MAP measures the steady component of BP. We hypothesized that high 24-h ambulatory PP in patients with coronary heart disease (CHD) is associated with an increased risk of haemostasis, which may be related to abnormal haemorheology (raised haematocrit, plasma viscosity and fibrinogen levels), endothelial damage/dysfunction (raised plasma von Willebrand factor, vWf and/or impaired flow-mediated dilatation, FMD), thrombogenesis (raised D-dimer, Dd) and platelet activation (raised soluble P-selectin, sPsel). **Methods**: We studied 73 patients with stable CHD who were in sinus rhythm and with preserved left ventricular systolic function (mean ejection fraction 61±10%). All completed a 24-h ambulatory BP monitoring. Patients were divided into 2 groups according to high (above median) or low (below median) values of the ambulatory PP (51 mmHg). Endothelium-dependent vasodilatation was assessed by FMD of the brachial artery. **Results**: The 2 groups were not different in clinical and demographic characteristics except patients with high-PP were older (p=0.002). 24-h mean PP was correlated with age (r=0.48), vWf (r=0.41), FMD (r= -0.36), sPsel (r=0.34), Dd (r=0.28) and fibrinogen (r=0.25) levels (all p<0.05), but not with plasma viscosity or haematocrit. None of hemostatic indices correlated with 24-hour MAP. On multivariate ANCOVA analysis, after controlling for age, 24-h MAP, mean systolic and diastolic blood pressures (BP), vWf, fibrinogen, Dd, sPsel levels and impaired FMD remained significantly higher in patients with high 24-h PP (all p<0.05). **Conclusions**: High 24-h PP load in patients with CHD was associated with a prothrombotic state (with higher levels of fibrinogen, Dd and sPsel) and evidence of endothelial damage/dysfunction (higher vWf and impaired FMD), independently of age and steady BP components. These may contribute to higher CV risk associated with increased PP.

OC007

Thrombosis of splanchnic veins in patients with silent myeloproliferative disorders

Miljic P, Sefer D, Sretenovic M, Suvajdzic N, Colovic M*

Thrombosis of splanchnic veins occur frequently in patients with overt myeloproliferative disorders, namely polycythaemia vera and essential thrombocythaemia. Spontaneous (endogenous) erythroid and/or megakaryocyte colonies formation (SCF) from bone marrow or peripheral blood is considered as a sensitive and reliable index of myeloproliferative state, even before onset of characteristic changes in peripheral blood. This early phase of myeloproliferation characterized by normal findings in peripheral blood, pronounced tendency to thrombosis and presence of SCF is known as silent myeloproliferative disorder (silent MPD). Recently a high incidence of silent MPD has been reported in patients with hepatic or portal vein thrombosis, but the clinical course of this disease is not well known, and the treatment of patients with thrombosis and silent MPD still represents an unresolved issue. During last 8 years we investigated 40 patients with thrombosis of splanchnic veins and revealed 14 (35%) patients (11F and 3M) with silent MPD. The patients have been diagnosed as having silent MPD if the presence of SCF from bone marrow or peripheral blood has been established, without meeting other conventional criteria for the diagnosis of an overt myeloproliferative disorder. These patients initially suffered 28 thrombotic events, majority of which were localized in portal, lienal and hepatic veins. The mean age of patients was 35 years (19-63), and the median duration of follow-up was 4,5 years (2-8). Eight out of 14 pts (57%) received oral anticoagulants, and 3 of them died during follow-up period (bleeding from oesophageal varices in 2, and pulmonary embolism in 1). Hydroxyurea was administered in 2 (14%) patients, and no thrombotic or bleeding complications were observed during follow-up. Four patients have not been treated with anticoagulants because of large oesophageal varices, and one of them died from gastrointestinal bleeding. Although our study is limited in size, the results suggest that silent MPD represents an important cause of splanhnic venous thrombosis and that administration of hydroxyurea with or without anticoagulants may be an acceptable method of treatment in these patients even if blood cell count is normal.

OC008

A prospective observational study on catheter-related complications in patients with hematological malignancies (CATHEM)

Falanga A (1), Moia M (2), Cortelezzi A (3), Pogliani E (4), Boccadoro M (5), Gallo E (6), Nosari A (7), Rizzoli V (8), Rodeghiero F (9), Gussoni G (10)*

(1) Dpt.Hematology, Bergamo, Italy
(2) Hemophilia nad Thrombosis Center, Milan
(3) Dpt. Medical Sciences, University of Milan
(4) Dpt. Hematology, University of Milan
(5) Dpt. Hematology, University of Turin
(6) Dpt. Hematology, Molinette Hosp, Tutùrin
(7) Dpt. Hematology, Niguarda Hosp, Milan
(8) Dpt. Hematology, University of Parma
(9) Dpt. Hematology, S.Bortolo Hosp, Vicenza
(10) Italfarmaco S.p.A., Italy

Introduction: Central Venous Catheter (CVC)-related thrombosis causes significant morbidity in patients with cancer, but few data are available in patients with hematological malignancies. A peculiarity of hematologic patients is thrombocytopenia, which might decrease the risk of thrombosis, but may contraindicate the use of anticoagulant drugs. **Aims**: to assess the incidence and the risk factors for symptomatic CVC-related thrombotic complications in patients with hematological malignancies and to assess the feasibility and the hemorrhagic risk of prophylaxis with anticoagulants. **Materials and methods**: prospective, observational study in 8 Italian Hematology Departments: 458 CVC in 412 patients with hematological malignancies were registered (males 50.4%, mean age 50.9 years $\pm$ 14.7). Most patients were thrombocytopenic (< 50.000 x 10^6/L in 81.2% of cases, with a mean overall duration of 19.2 days) and many had severe neutropenia (< 100 x 10^6/L in 59.8% of cases); 14.2% of patients received antithrombotic prophylaxis (LMWH in most cases). Clinical events registered up-to 3 months of follow-up were: CVC-related deep vein thrombosis (DVT) and pulmonary embolism (PE) strumentally proven, CVC-related superficial thrombophlebitis, CVC-occlusion / malfunction of thrombotic origin, major cardiovascular events, bleeding, infections and death. A composite study end-point (catheter related venous thromboembolism (VTE) + superficial thrombophlebitis + CVC occlusion / malfunction) was selected to assess a possible predictive relationship with various factors. **Results** (in brackets, percentage of patients receiving antithrombotic prophylaxis): CVC-related DVT was confirmed in 1.5% of cases (0%); total PE in 1.3% (0%); fatal PE in 0.6% (0%); CVC-related superficial thromboflebitis in 3.9% (0.2%); CVC occlusion/malfunction of thrombotic origin in 6.1% (1.1%); other major cardiovascular events 1.7% (0.4%); CVC-related bloodstream infections 4.6%; serious bleeding in 3.5% (0.4%). At multivariate logistic regression analysis thrombocytopenia was found to significantly reduce the risk of CVC-related thrombotic complications. The percentage of cases with thrombocytopenia and experiencing a CVC-related complication was however not negligible (10.2%, vs 17.4% of incidence in patients with platelet counts > 50.000 x 10^6/L. **Conclusions**: the incidence of symptomatic CVC-related thrombotic complications in patients with hematological malignancies is not negligible. Thrombocytopenia reduces thrombotic rate, which remains however consistent. Prophylaxis with anticoagulant drugs is feasible and does not appear to induce clinically relevant bleeding.

OC009

Proteolysis of von Willebrand factor increases in children during the induction therapy for acute lymphoblastic leukemia

*Perutelli P (1), Amato S (1), De Mattia D (2), Del Vecchio G (2), Giordano P (2), Saracco P (3), Russo G (4), Molinari A (1)**

(1) Thrombosis and Haemostasis Unit, Department of Hematology and Oncology, Giannina Gaslini Children&#
(2) Pediatric Clinic, School of Medicine, Bari,
(3) Department of Hematology, Regina Margherita Children's Hospital ,Turin
(4) Pediatric Clinic, School of Medicine, Catania

Introduction. Thromboembolic events may be a severe complication of acute lymphoblastic leukemia (ALL) in children. VWF is a large multimeric protein; its size is down regulated in plasma by a specific metalloprotease (ADAMTS-13). Under conditions of high shear stress, increased proteolysis occurs. **Aim.** We looked for modifications of von Willebrand factor (VWF) as a thrombophilic marker during the induction therapy of ALL. **Materials and methods.** Forty-four children (17 months to 15.2 years, median 48 months) with ALL enrolled in the pediatric centers of Bari, Catania, Genova, and Torino, participating in AIEOP (Italian Association of Pediatric Hematology and Oncology). Plasma samples were collected at the onset (T1), at day +24 (T2), +36 (T3), and +52 (T4) of the "ALL 2000" therapeutic scheme. VWF:Ag, VWF multimeric composition, and VWF proteolytic fragments were evaluated. **Results.** VWF:Ag at T4 was significantly lower than T1 (p<0.025). The larger VWF multimers (>15 multimers) decreased to a minimum at T3 (p<0.05), then raised towards the initial levels. Intermediate molecular weight multimers (6-10 multimers) increased at T2 and T3 (p<0.005). Proteolysis fragments increased at T3 (p<0.05). **Conclusions.** Our results show an increase of VWF proteolysis from T1 to T3, which leads to changes in multimeric composition and structure, whereas at T4 proteolysis has minimal effects on VWF size. The finding of a slight, but significant, increase of VWF proteolysis in ALL patients during the early phases of induction therapy is suggestive of endothelial damage. Concurrent additional prothrombotic factor might trigger thromboembolism.

OC010

Factor XIII activity levels in acute leukemia

Stemmelin G, Dubboscq C, Shanley C, Ceresetto JM, Rabinovich O, Gutierrez M, Mendizabal G, Doti C, Vicente M, Bullorsky E*

Hospital Britanico, Buenos Aires, Argentina

The A subunit of Factor XIII (FXIII), which is the active fraction of FXIII, is almost exclusively synthesized by megakariocytes and precursors of monocytes and macrophages. In a previous study we could demonstrate a significant reduction of FXIII plasma activity levels during the aplastic period after autologous and allogeneic BMT. **Objective**: To determine if the bone marrow hipoplasia in acute leukemias (AL) at diagnosis produces decrease of FXIII activity as consecuence of ineffective A subunit synthesis. Since November 2001, we prospectively studied 13 patients (4-63 years) with AL (10 AML, 2 ALL and 1 biphenotypic). FXIII plasmatic activity was determined by photometric assay (Berichrom FXIII, Dade Behring) on fixed day (basal and on days +7, +14 and +21). References values were stablished in 35 blood donors as 68-138 %. FXIII activity (mean, ±1SD) were: basal 72.3 % (± 59.5); day +7 56.9(± 44.4); day + 14 68.8 % (±27.9) and day + 21 63.2 % (±25.6). 8/13 pts (61.5 %) had low levels (<68%) of FXIII activity in basal sample.3/13 (23%) pts had lower than 10 %; only one of them presented bleeding (mild epistaxis). The correlation study between basal platelet count and FXIII activity was in the limit of statistic significance, Spearkman r=53; p 0.06. This might be considered a clear trend, considering the small number of studied patients. The hemoderivated transfusions after chemotherapy could contribute to the manteinance of FXIII activity. **In conclusion**, 1) low levels of FXIII are frequent in AL at diagnosis; 2) some pts could have subhaemostatic FXIII activity level (< 10%) and 3) a deficit of FXIII should be consider in AL pts with haemorraghic manifestation.

OC011

Alterations of coagulation pathway parameters in children with acute lymphoblastic leukaemia (ALL)

Hatzipantelis E (1), Athanassiou-Metaxa M (1), Tzimouli V (1), Kleta D (2), Gombakis N (1), Garipidou V (3), Athanasiadou-Piperop F (4), Sidi-Fragandrea V (5), Koliouskas D (5)*

(1) Thalassemia Unit, 1st Paediatric Department Of "Aristotle" University of Thessaloniki, "Hippokration
(2) General Haematologic Laboratory, "Hippokration" General Hospital, Thessaloniki, Greece
(3) 2nd Internal Medicine Department Of "Aristotle" University of Thessaloniki, "Hippokration" General H
(4) 2nd Paediatric Department Of "Aristotle" University of Thessaloniki, "AHEPA" General Hospital, Thess
(5) Pediatric Oncology Department, "Hippokration" General Hospital, Thessaloniki, Greece

Introduction: Serious dysfunction of the vascular endothelium and thromboembolic complications in children with ALL can caused from the disease itself, from therapy (asparaginase, corticosteroids), or from other conditions (sepsis, catheters). Several studies have shown the presence of endogenous thrombin generation at the time of diagnosis and persistence throughout treatment. **Aim**: Based on that knowledge, the aim of this study was to determine prospectively the alterations of coagulation pathway parameters in children with ALL during acute phase (before treatment) and 1st relapse of the disease, targeting in their possible prognostic value relating to outcome and thromboembolic complications. **Materials and methods**: Fifty patients with ALL were studied (44 B- and 6 T-cell), aged 1 to 13 years old (mean: 5,8), 18 girls and 32 boys, during acute phase and relapse. Twelve children treated with UCALL-XI and 38 with BFM-95 protocol. Three children died during acute phase of the disease. Nineteen children treated for ALL also studied (control group), 1 to 10 years after the end of therapy. In all children the levels of laboratory parameters of coagulation pathway (Platelets, PT, APTT, TT, Fibrinogen, D-dimers, ATIII, PC, PS, FVLeiden-APCR, LA, tPA, PAI-1, VWF, Plasminogen, A2-antiplasmin, A2-macroglobulin, Trombomodulin) were determined. **Results**: From all parameters determined abnormal findings were as follows: a) in patients during acute phase we found significantly increased levels of D-dimers (861,4 μg/lt, p<0,001), VWF (168,5%, p<0,001) and thrombomodulin (23,2 ng/ml, p<0,001) and significantly decreased levels of A2-antiplasmin (59,17%, p<0,05) and PS (66,69%, p<0,005), compared with control group, b) in patients during 1st relapse we found significantly increased levels of VWF (174,2%, p<0,001) and thrombomodulin (20,18 ng/ml, p<0,001) and significantly decreased levels of A2-antiplasmin (57,81%, p<0,05), PS (65,53%, p<0,005) and plasminogen (62,5%, P<0,005), compared with control group, c) the number of platelets was significantly low (p<0,001) in both groups. **Conclusion**: Abnormal values of the parameters determined during acute phase of the disease showing serious dysfunction of the vascular endothelium and coagulation pathway, results from the disease itself, while pathologic values during 1st relapse probably results from therapy.

OC012

Coordinated dysregulation of cellular receptors, proangiogenic factors and intracellular pathways in acute leukemia

Barbarroja N (1), Lopez-Pedrera C (1), Buendia P (1), Siendones E (1), Capote M (1), Montiel-Duarte C (3), Dorado G (2), Torres A (1), Velasco F (1)*

(1) Unidad de Investigacion, Hospital Reina Sofia, Cordoba, Spain
(2) Departamento de Bioquimica y Biologia Molecular, Universidad de Cordoba, Spain
(3) Servicio de Hematologia, Clinica Universitaria de Navarra, Spain

Introduction: A number of different signalling routes are triggered simultaneously in leukaemia cells, with distinct and overlapping activities. Previous studies demonstrated specific dysregulation of cellular receptors (i.e. TF or uPAR), transcription factors (i.e. AP-1 or NF-kB) and intracellular pathways (i.e. Raf/MEK/ERK or PI3K/Akt pathways) in acute leukemias. However, they did not analyse and correlate simultaneous altered signals inside the same leukemia type. **Aim**: To analyse if altered signals are coordinated into the same leukemia, and evaluate their effect on the behaviour of this disease, we have investigated the expression and activation status of the procoagulant/proangiogenic receptor TF, the angiogenic protein VEGF, and two intracellular proteins involved in their regulation: extracellular regulated kinase (ERK1/2) and nuclear factor kappa-B (NF-kB). **Patients**: Bone marrow and peripheral blood samples from 17 acute myeloid leukemia (AML) patients, 5 acute lymphoid leukemia (ALL) patients, and 10 healthy donors, were analysed. **Results**: We found significantly higher mRNA and protein VEGF and TF levels in 18 of 23 samples (mainly all subtypes of the AMLs FAB classification, except M0 and M6) compared to controls, with a significant positive correlation (p=0.0045). Almost all the blast samples showing increased TF and VEGF levels also exhibited enhanced ERK phosphorylation. Pearson's relational statistics indicated significant positive correlation between TF and phosphorylated ERK (p=0.0013) as well as VEGF and pERK (p=0.0039) levels. Increased expression of both TF and VEGF was accompanied by NF-kB activation in the same leukemia sample. Clinical studies demonstrated a higher incidence of coagulopathy, recurrence and fatal outcome among patients in which a coordinated increase in the expression and activation of the above mentioned proteins was observed. **Conclusions**: Our study establishes for the first time a coordinated dysregulation of cellular receptors, proangiogenic factors and intracellular pathways into the same leukemia type, which seems to determine a correlation with clinical features. Examining the level, nature and circumstances by which these interactions occur will be instrumental in the development of new agents designed to battle leukemia. Supported by FIS02/0215, JA61/02 and SAF2001/0918.

OC013

Platelets migrate in response to allergen in vivo and in vitro: role of IgE

Pitchford S, Momi S, Casali L, Gresele P*

Department of Internal Medicine, Section of Internal and Cardiovascular Medicine, University of Perugia, Italy

Introduction: Platelets are necessary for airway wall remodeling in a murine model of allergic inflammation, and are present in the lavage fluid of allergen sensitized and exposed animals (Pitchford *et al.* 2004.*Blood.* 103 639-647), implying that platelets can migrate into tissue. **Aims**: The migratory response of platelets from allergen sensitized mice was studied *in vitro* and their presence in lung tissue *in vivo.* **Methods**: Male C57BL/6 mice were immunised on days 0 and 7 with ovalbumin (OVA). 10µg/mouse i.p. 0.4ml in 0.1M $Al_2(OH)_3$ or Alum alone), exposed to aerosolised OVA (1%saline, 20minutes.t.i.d.) on day 15 and lungs removed for histological analysis of platelet presence at various time points. Other groups of mice were anaesthetised 7-14 days after the second immunisation, blood collected on citrate by cardiac puncture, centrifuged for platelet rich plasma (PRP) and diluted to $3x10^5$ cells/ml with assay medium. Platelet suspensions (200µl) were placed in the top wells of modified Boyden chambers, separated from the bottom wells by a 3µm micropore filter. Bottom wells were previously filled with 210µl of assay medium containing either OVA or BSA (1µg/ml). Some platelet preparations were incubated in the presence of antimouse IgE antibody (R35-92) or control antibody. After 90 minutes incubation at 37°C, the filters were washed with saline and platelets immunostained for the CD41 antigen (Santa Cruz Biotech. USA). The number of platelets per field was recorded at a depth of 0-24µm below the filter surface. 6 fields were counted on each filter using a x25 objective. Data was expressed as means±SEM of area under curve units (platelets/µµ). **Results**: significant migration occurred through the filter with OVA sensitised PRP/OVA (bottom well) (384.4±40.5) compared to OVA sensitised PRP/BSA (31.7±9.3, p<0.001) and sham sensitised PRP/OVA (30.3±7.5, p<0.001). The co-incubation of R35-92, suppressed platelet migration at concentrations of 3µg/ml (217.3±34.7 P<0.001) and 10µg/ml.(49.7±10.9 P<0.001). Lung sections from aerosol challenged mice (immunostained for CD41 antigen) revealed a significant presence of platelets emigrating to a depth of 200µm from blood vessels in OVA mice (408.8±58.2 plts/µl) compared to sham mice(99.2±22.4 plts/µl) 30 hours post exposure (p<0.001). **Conclusion**: These data demonstrate that platelets migrate towards an inflammatory stimulus *in vivo* and *in vitro*, and platelet migration to allergen can be suppressed by inhibiting the IgE pathway.

OC014

Successful inhibition of venous thrombus growth after oral administration of BAY 59-7939, a direct Factor Xa inhibitor in rabbits

Biemond BJ (1), Friederich PW (1), Levi M (1), Perzborn E (2), Buetehorn U (3), Büller H (1)*

(1) Department of Vascular Medicine, Academic Medical Center, University of Amsterdam, The Netherlands
(2) Cardiovascular Research, Bayer HealthCare AG, Wuppertal, Germany
(3) Preclinical Pharmacokinetics, Bayer HealthCare AG, Wuppertal, Germany

Introduction: The standard first-line treatment for deep vein thrombosis (DVT) is low molecular weight heparin (LMWH). Recently, clinical studies with synthetic pentasaccharide, a selective, indirect Factor Xa inhibitor, have validated Factor Xa inhibition in the treatment of DVT. **Aim**: To assess the antithrombotic properties of an oral, direct Factor Xa inhibitor, BAY 59-7939 in an experimental rabbit DVT model. **Methods**: Standard thrombi were preformed in the jugular veins of New Zealand rabbits. 125I-labelled fibrinogen was administered systemically, and thrombus growth was measured by determining the accretion of labelled fibrinogen onto the preformed clots. The effect on bleeding was analyzed by standard bleeding-time incisions in the ear. The antithrombotic properties of i.v. BAY 59-7939 were assessed at 0.3, 1.0 and 3.0 mg/kg; oral BAY 59-7939 was given at 3.0 mg/kg. The antithrombotic properties were compared with LMWH (nadroparin, 40 IE/kg bolus followed by 20 U/kg/h infusion) and pentasaccharide (fondaparinux, 40 µg/kg bolus followed by 20 µg/kg/h) and saline control. BAY 59-7939 plasma levels and anti-Factor Xa activity were determined 60 and 90 minutes after administration of the study drugs. Bleeding-time assessment was performed 90 minutes after drug administration. **Results**: Administration of i.v. BAY 59-7939 significantly reduced thrombus growth (thrombus growth: 36.3±2.7%, 36.4±2.7% and 30.1±4.6% in the low-, intermediate-, and high-dose groups vs. 46.3±4.4% in controls). The antithrombotic effect of BAY 59-7939 at the low or intermediate dose was equivalent to the antithrombotic properties of LMWH and pentasaccharide (thrombus growth: 34.5±3.5% and 35.7±3.9%, respectively). Oral BAY 59-7939 induced a significant antithrombotic effect that was similar to that of LMWH and pentasaccharide (thrombus growth: 36.9±4.5%). A consistent, strong correlation was demonstrated between plasma levels and the anti-Factor Xa activity of oral and i.v. BAY 59-7939. Interestingly, a similar antithrombotic effect was observed after oral and i.v. administration of BAY 59-7939, despite the lower plasma levels of BAY 59-7939 and anti-Factor Xa activity after oral administration. No significant differences in bleeding times were measured among the different doses of BAY 59-7939. **Conclusion**: Oral administration of BAY 59-7939 resulted in a significant antithrombotic effect that was equivalent to that of LMWH and pentasaccharide.

OC015

Increased pulmonary expression of thrombin receptor in rabbits with endotoxin-induced acute lung injury

Gando S (1), Jesmin S (2), Sakuma I (2), Kobayashi S (1), Sakuraya F (1), Matsuda N (1), Hattori Y (3)*

(1) Department of Anesthesiology and Critical Care Medicine, Hokkaido University School of Medicine, Sap
(2) Department of Cardiology, Hokkaido University School of Medicine, Sapporo, Japan
(3) Department of Pharmacology, Hokkaido University School of Medicine, Sapporo, Japan

Objectives: This study was undertaken to test the hypothesis that cross talk between coagulation and inflammation through thrombin receptor plays an important role in endotoxin-induced acute lung injury (ALI). **Materials and Methods**: Rabbits were rendered endotoxemic by an intravenous infusion of 100 ?g/kg Escherichia coli lipopolysaccharide (LPS). The control group received an equal volume of sterile saline. At 1, 3, 6, and 10 hours after LPS administration, we serially examined pulmonary expression of thrombin receptor, tumor necrosis factor- α (TNF- α), tissue factor (TF), plasminogen activator inhibitor-1 (PAI-1), and fibrin using immunohistochemistry and Western blotting. **Results**: ALI after LPS administration was confirmed by histopathological examination. Immunohistochemical analysis showed expression of thrombin receptor, TF, and PAI-1 in bronchial epithelium, alveolar pneumocytes, and vascular endothelium. On Western blots, persistently high levels of thrombin receptor protein in lung tissues up to 10 hours after LPS administration were observed. Significant increases were also found in the levels of TNF-α, TF, and PAI-1 in both lung tissue and plasma in endotoxemic rabbits compared to those in controls. In addition, we could find marked elevation of fibrin levels in lung tissue in endotoxemic rabbits. **Conclusions**: These results suggest that increased expression of molecules involved in coagulation and inflammation, including thrombin receptor play a role in LPS-induced ALI. We speculate that thrombin receptor expression would be important in the pathogenesis of ALI and acute respiratory distress syndrome in sepsis.

OC016

PPAR-α deficiency does not modify age dependent but prevents high fat diet increase in plasma PAI-1 as well as insulin resistance

Mavri A (1, 2), Bastelica D (1), Steals B (3), El Ayachi S (1), Juhan-Vague I (1), Alessi MC (1)

(1) Laboratory of Hematology, UMR 626, Faculty of Medicine, Marseille, France
(2) University Medical Centre, Dpt of Vascular disease, Ljubljana, Slovenia
(3) Unit 545, INSERM, Institut Pasteur de Lille, Lille, France

Introduction: The peroxisome proliferator activated receptor α (PPARa) controls the expression of genes involved in b-oxidation of fatty acids by interacting with specific DNA responsive elements. PPAR like responsive element was identified in the PAI-1 promoter region. This suggests that activation of PPARa by i.e. fatty acids may influence PAI-1 expression. **Aim**: To examine whether high fat diet may influence plasma PAI-1 levels in PPARa deficient mice. **Materials and methods**: Glucose, insulin (RIA), and PAI-1 (ELISA) were determined in plasma of PPARa-null mice and in wild type (WT) mice at the entry and after 16-weeks of standard diet or high fat diet. **Results and conclusions**: No significant difference was found in plasma levels of PAI-1, glucose, and insulin between PPARa-null and WT mice either at the entry or after 16-weeks of standard diet. In WT mice, 16-week of high fat diet induced obesity, hyperglycaemia, hyperinsulinaemia and elevated plasma PAI-1 levels. On contrary, PPARa-null mice gain less weight (30.9 ± 1.4 vs 39.3 ± 5.0 g, $p<0.01$), had lower glucose (121.7 ± 43.6 vs 226.3 ± 36.3 mg/dl, $p<0.01$), insulin (0.87 ± 0.36 vs 3.10 ± 1.53 mg/l, $p<0.01$) and PAI-1 (8.7 ± 12.0 vs 17.9 ± 9.5 ng/ml, $p<0.05$) levels. PAI-1 did not differ between PPARa-null mice on high fat and on standard diet (8.7 ± 12.0 vs 8.1 ± 11.3 mg/dl), but were significantly higher than at the entry (1.1 ± 0.2 mg/dl, p=0.02). In conclusion, baseline as well as age dependent increase in PAI-1 expression were not influenced by PPARa deficiency. However, high fat diet increase in plasma PAI-1 was prevented in PPARa-null mice, but this was mainly due to undeveloped state of obesity and insulin resistance. Therefore, the implication of PPARa in PAI-1 regulation is probably indirect through modulation of insulin resistance.

OC017

Differential expression patterns of proteins in the ischemic myocardium

Jang Y (1,2), Hwang K (1), Sohn Y (1), Seung K (3), Chung KH (1)*

(1) Cardiovascular Research Institute and BK21 Project for Medical Science,Yonsei University College of
(2) Cardiology Division, Department of Internal Medicine, Yonsei University College of Medicine
(3) Department of Internal Medicine, Catholic University Medical College, Seoul, Korea

Backgound: Large transmural myocardial infarction (MI) leads to maladaptive cardiac remodeling and increased risk of congestive heart failure. Angiotensin II, endothelin, and β-adrenergic receptor agonists are implicated in the development of cardiac hypertrophy, interstinal fibrosis, and heart failure after MI. The level of complexity resulting from co- and post-translational modification events can only be dissected and understood through qualitative and quantitative studies of gene expression at the level of the functional proteins themselves. **Methods and Results:** MI was produced in rats by surgical occlusion of left arterior descending coronary artery. Proteins were separated by two-dimensional polyacrylamide gel electrophoresis (2-DE) from tissue homogenate mixtures. In 2-DE, the pH 4-7 linear, 3-10 linear, and non-linear gradient strips were used. Protein detection was performed by silver staining and Brilliant Blue G-250 colloidal staining for mass spectrometry. For identification and characterization of stained protein spots, we employed tryptic digested peptide mass finger printing and matrix assisted laser desorption (MALDI) mass spectrometry for identification of protein spots. Approximately 1200 protein spots were resolved by the two-dimensional gel electrophoresis. We found that several numbers of protein spots were differentially expressed in ischemic myocardium. The Identified proteins are hemopexin, serotransferin, troponin T, aldehyde dehydrogenase and enolase. Many other proteins remained to be confirmed. **Conclusions***:* These data contribute the understanding of interplay between proteome change and the pathogenic mechanisms involved in cardiovascular diseases and are likely to result in the discovery of novel diagnostic markers and new therapeutic opportunities.

OC018

Suitability of selected clotting assays to explain anitithrombotic potential of LK732, argatroban and nadroparin in rat venous thrombosis model

Peternel L (1,2), Drevenšek G (2), Budihna M (2), Zega A (3), Božič M (4), Stegnar M (4), Černe M (1), Urleb U (1,3)*

(1) Lek Pharmaceuticals d.d., Drug Discovery, Ljubljana, Slovenia
(2) Faculty of Medicine, Inst Pharmacol Experim Toxicol, Ljubljana, Slovenia
(3) Faculty of Pharmacy, Ljubljana, Slovenia
(4) Univ Med Ctr Ljubljana, Dep Angiol, Ljubljana, Slovenia

Introduction and aim: In animal models of venous thrombosis effectiveness of antithrombotics is usually estimated by reduction of thrombus weight and by prolongation of clotting assays. The aim was to determine suitability of clotting assays to explain antithrombotic potential of three antithrombotics in rat model of venous thrombosis by means of simple correlation analysis. **Materials and methods**: In fasted male Wistar rats (290-430g, 3-4 months old) thrombus formation was achieved by a combination of thromboplastin induced hypercoagulability and complete stasis of vena cava. Before thrombus induction rats were treated by the azaphenylalanine direct thrombin inhibitor LK732 (0.3, 1 and 3mg/kg), by argatroban (0.3, 1 and 3 mg/kg) and by nadroparin (10, 30 and 100 antifX_aIU/kg). Thrombus weight was determined and blood sample was collected for determination of activated partial thromboplastin time (aPTT), thrombin time (TT) and ecarin clotting time (ECT). **Results**: In the LK732 treated rats thrombus weights correlated well with TT (R^2=0.60, $p<0.001$) and ECT (R^2=0.43, p=0.004), but much less with aPTT (R^2=0.20, p=0.072). In argatroban treated rats significant but rather low correlations were determined (TT: R^2=0.43, p=0.006; ECT: R^2=0.26, p=0.050; aPTT: R^2=0.24, p=0.047). In the nadroparin treated rats a good correlation was determined between thrombus weights and aPTT (R^2=0.40, p=0.006) or TT (R^2=0.37, p=0.009), but not between thrombus weights and ECT (R^2=0.02, p=0.574). **Conclusion**: In the LK732 treated rats total variance in thrombus weights was explained best by variation in TT and ECT, in argatroban treated rats by variation in TT and in nadroparin treated rats by variation in aPTT or TT. Thus, regardless of the mechanism of action of antithrombotic, the most suitable and universal clotting assay to assess the antithrombotic potential of selected antithrombotics in this venous thrombosis model was TT.

OC019

Ximelagatran for the secondary prevention of venous thromboembolism: a complementary follow-up analysis of the THRIVE III Study

Schulman S (1), Lundström T (2), Wåhlander K (2), Billing Clason S (2), Eriksson H (3), for the THRIVE III*

(1) Coagulation Unit, Department of Medicine, Karolinska Hospital, Stockholm, Sweden
(2) AstraZeneca R&D Mölndal, Mölndal, Sweden
(3) Department of Medicine, Sahlgrenska University Hospital/Östra, Göteborg, Sweden

Introduction: Ximelagatran (Exanta™, AstraZeneca) is an oral direct thrombin inhibitor under investigation for prevention and treatment of venous thromboembolic events (VTE). In a previously reported, international, multicentre, randomized, double-blind trial, oral ximelagatran (24 mg bid) reduced the incidence of recurrent VTE compared with placebo over 18 months in patients who had received 6 months' standard anticoagulation.(1) In the primary analysis, efficacy data were collected during 18 months of treatment or until premature study discontinuation.(1) **Aims**: A complementary intention-to-treat follow-up analysis was conducted post-study termination for the full 18-month period, regardless of whether patients discontinued study drug prematurely, to further validate the results of extended secondary prevention of VTE with ximelagatran. **Methods**: Cumulative risks of locally confirmed VTE (deep-vein thrombosis or pulmonary embolism [PE]) and death were estimated using the Kaplan-Meier procedure. Hazard ratios between treatments were estimated using a Cox proportionate hazard model. **Results**: Ximelagatran was administered to 612 patients and placebo to 611 patients. Of these, 149 patients receiving ximelagatran and 181 patients receiving placebo discontinued the study prematurely because of locally confirmed VTE, or other reasons. For recurrent VTE and/or death, 14 and 13 patients in the ximelagatran and placebo groups, respectively, were lost to further follow-up. In this analysis, the cumulative risk of VTE (3.2% vs 12.7%; hazard ratio 0.21; 95% CI 0.12-0.36; P < 0.0001), and in a separate analysis the cumulative risk of PE (0.8% vs 5.2%; hazard ratio 0.13; 95% CI 0.04-0.36; P < 0.0001), were significantly lower in the ximelagatran group than the placebo group over 18 months. Death from any cause occurred in 10 and 12 patients in the ximelagatran and placebo groups, respectively. VTE recurrence after cessation of study drug was documented in 6 and 2 patients in the ximelagatran and placebo groups, respectively. **Conclusion**: This complementary analysis confirms the results of the primary analysis and shows that oral ximelagatran 24 mg bid, administered without coagulation monitoring or dose adjustment, is effective for the long-term secondary prevention of VTE. 1. Schulman S et al. N Engl J Med. 2003;349:1713-21.

OC020

Long-term follow-up of 122 patients with inferior vena cava filters - non-randomised, retrospective comparison with 120 patients treated for venous thromboembolism

Hajduk B (1), Małek G (2), Oniszh K (2), Burakowski J (3), Wawrzyńska L (1), Tomkowski W (3)*

(1) Departemnt of Chest Medicine. National TB and Lung Diseases Research Institute, Warsaw, Poland
(2) Department of Radiology. National TB and Lung Diseases Research Institute, Warsaw, Poland
(3) Intensive Care Unit. National TB and Lung Diseases Research Institute, Warsaw, Poland

Aim: to compare rate of pulmonary embolism (PE) and recurrent deep venous thrombosis (DVT) in patients in whom insertion of inferior vena cava filters (IVCF) were performed and in patients treated without IVCF. **Material and methods**: between years 1993 - 2002, 122 IVCF were inserted in 122 patients (mean age 61,4 years + 15,2), if possible treated also with anticoagulants. Control group consisted of 120 ambulatory patients (mean age 60,6 years + 15,1) with venous thromboembolism (VTE) confirmed by objective methods and treated only with anticoagulants. Indications for filters placement were as follows: chronic thromboembolic pulmonary hypertension, massive PE, recurrent PE despite anticoagulation, severe bleeding complications of anticoagulant therapy, contraindications to anticoagulant treatment, VTE in patients with indications for surgery and high risk of massive PE. The diagnostic procedures - echocardiography and compression ultrasound examinations extended by duplex Doppler were repeated at least once a year in both groups. **Results**: recurrent PE, recurrent DVT and total caval occlusion - assessed only in the filter group - were determined as primary outcomes. In the filter group there were 6 (4,92%: 95% CI [1,82 % - 10,43%]) cases with recurrent PE and 26 (21,3%: 95% CI [14,3 to 29,8]) cases with recurrent DVT. In the control group recurrent PE and DVT were observed in 10 (8,33%: 95% CI [4,06 to 14,82]) cases and 28 (23,3%: 95% CI [16,4 to 31,8]) cases respectively. There were no statistically significant differences between both groups in the rates of PE and DVT. Only in two patients in the filter group total caval occlusion was noted (1,6%). 40 patients died in the filter group (mainly due to end-stage CTEPH and malignancy) and 7 patients in the control group. The difference between rates of deaths in both groups was statistically significant. **Conclusions**: on the contrary to other reports we found that the frequency of recurrent DVT was similar in filter and non-filter group. Total caval occlusion in the filter group was Very rare.

OC021

The development in attitudes towards thromboprophylaxis in Danish surgical departments during a twenty year period

Rasmussen M, Wegner L, Wille-Jørgens P*

Department of Surgical Gastroenterology, Bispebjerg Hospital, University of Copenhagen, Denmark

Introduction: Perioperative thromboprophylaxis has been studied over the past 35 years and effective prophylactic methods have been developed, thus lowering the incidence of venous thromboembolic complications after surgery. Implementing the results from clinical trials to daily clinical practice can although be difficult. **Aims**: To summarize and evaluate the progress in the current practice of thromboprophylaxis (TP) in Danish surgical departments over a 20 year period. **Material and Methods**: Summary of 5 questionnaires in 1981, 1985, 1990, 1995 and 2000. The questionnaires were designed in the same way through the years. **Results**: Replies was obtained from 85%-95% of the Danish surgical departments. The overall use of TP increased from 90% to100% during twenty years. The use of TP according to a written guideline increased significantly from 50% to 93% (p<0,001). Low molecular weight heparin was the drug of choice in 98% of the departments in the year 2000 and graded compression stockings in 79%. TP in emergency surgery increased from 33% to 43%. Extended prophylaxis has not gained impact in Denmark as only 17% of the orthopaedic surgery departments used TP for more than 14 days. The use of acetylsalicylic acid(ASA)as postoperative venous thromboprophylaxis has stopped, only 0,5% used ASA in 2000 as compared to 13% in 1990. **Conclusion**: The development in attitudes towards TP in Denmark complies with the scientific evolution. Methods and indications correspond with the recommendations of the literature and international consensus conference. However, the low rate of TP in emergency surgery is unsatisfactory. The authors emphasize the introduction of firm standard instructions for TP in all surgical departments. A continuous evaluation of the use of TP in Danish surgical departments by means and quality assurance studies is recommended.

OC022

A comparison of venous thromboembolism prophylaxis practice patterns in acutely ill medical patients; IMPROVE versus clinical trial populations

Anderson F (1), Tapson V (2), Decousus H (3), Spyropoulos A (4), Turpie A (5), FitzGerald G (1)*

(1) Center for Outcomes Research, University of Massachusetts Medical School, Worcester, USA
(2) Duke University Medical Center, Durham, USA
(3) Centre Hospitalier Universitaire de Bellevue, Saint-Etienne, France
(4) Lovelace Medical Center, Albuquerque, USA
(5) Hamilton Health Sciences General Hospital, Hamilton, Canada

Introduction A number of clinical trials have shown the benefits of providing acutely ill medical patients, a population at risk from venous thromboembolism (VTE), with VTE prophylaxis. However, due to the eligibility criteria of clinical trials, a large number of patients are excluded from enrolment. **Aims** To characterise prophylaxis practice patterns in hospitalised acutely ill medical patients, enrolled in IMPROVE, a prospective cohort study, who would have been eligible for inclusion in the MEDENOX, PREVENT or ARTEMIS clinical trials. **Materials and Methods** Patients ≥18 years old, and hospitalized for ≥3 days with an acute medical illness have been enrolled consecutively since July 2002. Exclusion criteria: therapeutic antithrombotic/thrombolytics at admission; major surgery/trauma during 3 months prior to admission; and VTE treatment within 24 hours of admission. A central adjudication committee reviews key clinical endpoints, including symptomatic VTE, bleeding, and death. Patients were assessed to determine if they would have been eligible for inclusion in the MEDENOX, PREVENT or ARTEMIS trials by comparing their characteristics with the inclusion/exclusion criteria from those studies. **Results** Data from 2,312 patients enrolled up to 30 September 2003 at 26 hospitals in 10 countries is presented in this analysis. For this patient population, 48% were female with a median age of 70 years, median length of hospital stay of 8 days, and 44% of patients were immobile for ≥3 days (median duration of immobility 8 days, including immobility immediately prior to hospital admission). Of all IMPROVE patients, 34% received VTE prophylaxis and 13-19% met the eligibility criteria for the MEDENOX, PREVENT or ARTEMIS trials, with advanced age, expected length of hospital stay, bleeding risk factors and renal failure being the major reasons for exclusion. Only 44-50% of patients that would have been eligible for inclusion in these trials received VTE prophylaxis. **Conclusions** Less than 20% of 'real-world' acutely ill medical patients in IMPROVE would have been eligible for inclusion in the MEDENOX, PREVENT and ARTEMIS trials. Despite consensus group recommendations that medical patients receive VTE prophylaxis, less than 50% of trial eligible patients and 34% of all IMPROVE patients received VTE prophylaxis. Increased awareness of VTE prophylaxis guidelines is therefore needed in this patient population.

OC023

Practice variation in USA and Europe for the prevention of venous thromboembolism in hospitalized medical patients: Findings from IMPROVE

Pini M (1), Froehlich J (2), Bergmann JF (3), Monreal M (4), Piovella F (5), Huang W (6), Anderson F (6)*

(1) Ospedale di Fidenza Medicina Interna, Fidenza, Italy
(2) University of Massachusetts Medical Center, Division of Cardiovascular Medicine, Worcester, USA
(3) Hôpital Lariboisiere Clinique Thérapeutique, Paris, France
(4) Hospital Germans Trias I Pujol, Badelona, Spain
(5) IRCCS Policlinico San Matteo Servizio Malattie Tromboemboliche, Pavia, Italy
(6) University of Massachusetts Medical School, Worcester, USA

Introduction The clinical practices for venous thromboembolism (VTE) prophylaxis in acutely ill hospitalized medical patients, a population at risk from VTE, are unknown. **Aims** To investigate VTE prophylaxis practice variation between Europe and USA in IMPROVE, an international prospective cohort study of acutely ill hospitalized medical patients. **Materials and Methods** Patients ≥18 years old, and hospitalized for ≥3 days with an acute medical illness have been enrolled consecutively since July 2002. Exclusion criteria: therapeutic antithrombotic/thrombolytics at admission; major surgery/trauma during 3 months prior to admission; and VTE treatment within 24 hours of admission. Data are recorded at discharge and 3 months after discharge. A central adjudication committee reviews key clinical endpoints, including symptomatic VTE, bleeding and death. **Results** Data from 1036 patients enrolled up to 30 September 2003 at 12 hospitals in 5 European countries (France, Germany, Italy, Spain and UK) and 835 patients in 7 US hospitals are presented in this analysis. European patients were less likely than US patients to be female (46% vs 54% respectively), were older (median age 71 years vs 58 years), had a longer duration of both immobility (11 days vs 6 days) and hospital stay (11 days vs 6 days) and were more likely to be immobile for ≥3 days in total (54% vs 46%). Only 49% of European and 51% of US patients received prophylaxis. In Europe, low-molecular-weight heparin was the favored prophylactic regimen, whereas in the USA, unfractionated heparin use was more common. US patients also received intermittent pneumatic compression or aspirin for VTE prophylaxis significantly more often, and elastic stockings significantly less often than European patients. Rates of suspected, but not treated, VTE were significantly higher in US patients. **Conclusions** Despite being a population at risk of VTE, only one half of IMPROVE patients in this analysis received VTE prophylaxis. Although similar rates of prophylaxis and proportions of patients receiving prophylaxis are observed, practices vary considerably between USA and Europe with UFH, IPC and aspirin being received more by US patients and LMWH and elastic stockings being given more to European patients. These remarkable geographical variations in practice patterns highlight the need for increased awareness of guideline recommendations for VTE prophylaxis in medical patients.

OC024

Deep vein thrombosis prophylaxis following arthroscopy, lower limb fractures, and in patients in plaster casts. Results of a survey

Dentali F (1), Ageno W (1), Imberti D (2)*

(1) Internal Medicine, University of Insubria, Varese, Italy
(2) Internal Medicine, Hospital of Piacenza, Italy

Background: The risk of venous thromboembolism (VTE) following non-large joint surgery or in patients with lower limb plaster cast is poorly defined. Clinical guidelines usually omit recommendations on thrombosis prophylaxis for these groups of patients. However, recent studies suggest that many of these patients are at moderate risk of VTE and that routine administration of low molecular weight heparin (LMWH) can be effective in reducing the risk of thrombosis. Because of the lack of clinical guidelines and the uncertain definition of the levels of risk, we tested the hypothesis that there is significant practice variation amongst orthopedic surgeons. **Methods**: Two hundred Italian orthopedic surgeons, representing 200 orthopedic departments throughout the country, were contacted by telephone and were asked if they routinely prescribe antithrombotic prophylaxis in patients undergoing knee arthroscopy, in patients with lower limb fractures, and in patients with lower limb plaster cast; if prophylaxis is prescribed to all patients or to selected patients; the type of prophylaxis and the timing of administration. **Results**: Following knee arthroscopy, 94% of the interviewed orthopedic surgeons prescribe pharmacologic prophylaxis of VTE. Of them, only 17% prescribe prophylaxis to selected patients based on the level of risk, 97.3% prescribe LMWH, 59% start propylaxis 12 hours before the procedure, and 59% prescribe prophylaxis for more than 10 days. In patients with lower limb fractures, 94.5% prescribe VTE prophylaxis. Of them, 6.9% select the patients, 96.8% prescribe LMWH, 74.6% start prophylaxis at the time of diagnosis, and 55% prescribe prophylaxis until complete use of the limb. In patients with plaster cast, 91% prescribe VTE prophylaxis. Of them, 25.8% select the patients, 96.2% prescribe LMWH, 41.8% start before plaster cast is applyed, and 65.4% prescribe prophylaxis until complete use of the limb. **Conclusions**: Even in the absence of clinical guidelines, prescription of VTE prophylaxis with LMWH following minor orthopedic procedures is very common, regardless of the individual level of risk. Timing and duration of prophylaxis are rather heterogenous.

OC025

Nitric oxide levels and its relevance to C-reactive Protein, CD 40L, TF and TNF-alpha in malignancy associated hypercoagulable state

Fareed J (1), Fareed D (1), Bick R (2), Bacher P (3), Iqbal O (1), Tobu M (1), Hoppensteadt D (1), Demir M (4), Saxena R (1)*

(1) Loyola University Medical Center, Maywood, IL, USA
(2) University of Texas, SW Med School, Dallas, TX, USA
(3) Abbott Laboratories, North Chicago, IL, USA
(4) Trakya University Medical School, Edrine, Turkey

Introduction: Endogenous generation of inflammatory cytokines and mediators plays an important role in the regulation of cardiovascular and inflammatory responses. One such mediator is nitric oxide (NO), which is up-regulated in several pathologic states. Increased production of NO is reported in several inflammatory disorders, such as sepsis, arthritis, immune thrombocytopenic purpura and antiphospholipid syndrome. In these conditions, NO promotes edema and vascular permeability. In addition, NO up-regulates COX-2 and the synthesis of several other inflammatory cytokines. Inflammation and thrombotic complications are often associated with malignancy. We have previously reported on the up-regulation of TNF-α, CRP, and tissue factor (TF) in patients with malignancy. **Aims:** The aim of this study is to determine the relationship between inflammatory cytokines and NO in cancer patients (CP) with hypercoagulable state. **Materials and Methods:** Baseline blood plasma samples from 160 patients with confirmed malignancy and hypercoagulable state were analyzed for NO levels. A chemical method based on chemiluminescent reaction between NO and ozone utilizing a highly sensitive gas phase NO analyzer (Model 2081, Sievers Instruments, Boulder, CO) was employed. CRP, TF, TNF-α and CD 40L were measured using commercially available ELISA methods. **Results:** Of the 160 patients plasma tested, the baseline NO levels ranged from 13.7 to 98.6 uM (63.1±15.9 uM) in contrast to age-matched control (AMC), which ranged from 9.1 to 34.6 uM (19.8± 6.2 uM, n=100). The difference in the NO levels between normal and cancer patients was statistically significant ($p<0.05$). Cancer patients also showed marked variations in the NO levels.

Eighteen of 160 cancer patients exhibited greater than 60 uM NO levels. The CRP (CP: 20.5±17.2; AMC: 5.2±1.3 ug/ml), TNF-a (CP: 38.1±66.2; AMC 0±0 pg/ml) and TF (CP: 430±160; AMC < 50 pg/ml) were also significantly elevated. A correlation between CRP (r^2=0.73) and NO levels were noted in cancer patients with malignancy. However, there was a poor correlation between NO and other inflammatory markers (r^2=<0.30). **Conclusions:** These data suggest that the pathogenesis associated with malignancy/hypercoagulable state may have a significant inflammatory component. Anticoagulant therapy with low molecular weight heparin may be useful in the management of these patients due to the antithrombotic and anti-inflammatory components in these agents.

OC026

Platelet activation, coagulation and angiogenesis in breast and prostate carcinoma

*Caine G (1), Lip G (1), Stonelake P (2), Ryan P (3), Blann AD (1)**

(1) University Department of Medicine, City Hospital, Birmingham, UK.
(2) Department of Surgery, City Hospital, Birmingham, UK.
(3) Department of Urology, City Hospital, Birmingham, UK.

Background: In health, haemostasis and angiogenesis are tightly regulated processes, but may become deregulated in cancer. Recent evidence suggests that platelet activation may link these processes as platelets can release angiogenic factors, such as vascular endothelial growth factor (VEGF). Furthermore, inflammation has also been implicated in regulating both coagulation and angiogenesis, possibly by activating platelets directly and increasing, for example, plasma fibrinogen. We hypothesized relationships between plasma markers of the processes in two common forms of cancer. **Methods**: Plasma levels of VEGF (reflecting angiogenesis), soluble P-selectin [sP-sel], marking platelet activation), tissue factor [TF], fibrinogen and fibrin D-dimer (coagulation markers), and serum levels of IL-6 (inflammation) were measured by ELISA in 30 patients with biopsy-proven breast cancer, 30 patients with biopsy-proven prostate cancer, and 30 age and sex-matched controls for each group. Prostate specific antigen was also measured in the men. Release of VEGF from IL-6 stimulated platelets was assessed by ELISA. **Results**: Plasma levels of IL-6 (P<0.02), VEGF, sP-sel, fibrinogen, and fibrin D-dimer (all p<0.01) were significantly raised in breast cancer, whereas VEGF, sP-sel, fibrin D-dimer (all p<0.01) and fibrinogen (p<0.05) were significantly raised in prostate cancer. Significant correlations were found between IL-6 and VEGF (p<0.01), and IL-6 and sP-sel (p=0.038) in breast cancer, and between PSA and sP-sel (p=0.045), and PSA and IL-6 (p<0.01) in prostate cancer. Further experiments demonstrated an in vitro IL-6 dose-dependent release of VEGF from platelets. **Conclusion**: Strong relationships between IL6 and VEGF, but not with coagulation or platelet markers, and release of VEGF from IL-6 stimulated platelets, suggest a role for inflammation and platelets in angiogenesis.

OC027

Lower APCR correlates with apoptotic activation of CD8+T cells in non-small cell lung cancer

Dworakowska D (1), Bryl E (2), Soroczyńska M (2), Witkowski J (2), Łapiński M (3), Mital A (2), Tomaszewski D (3), Dworakowski R (4), Skokowski J (3), Częstochowska E (1)*

(1) Dep. of Internal Medicine, Endocrinology and Haemostatic Disorders, Medical University of Gdansk, Po
(2) Department of Pathophysiology, Medical University of Gdansk, Poland
(3) Department if Thoracic Surgery, Medical University of Gdansk, Poland
(4) I Department of Cardiology, Medical University of Gdansk, Poland

Introduction: The relationship between thrombogenity and apoptosis was studied in various human tumor-and non-tumor cell lines and a significant correlation between thrombin generation and degree of apoptosis was found. Spontaneous apoptosis was observed in a proportion of peripheral T lymphocytes obtained from cancer patients. Since non-small cell lung cancer (NSCLC) is associated with coagulation disturbances it is important to establish whether there is a correlation between thrombogenity and apoptosis of CD3+T lymphocytes in this cancer. **Aim**: The aim of this study was to investigate a possible relation between clotting system parameters and expression of the death receptor Fas (APO-1, CD95) in circulating T lymphocytes in NSCLC. **Material and Methods**: The study group consisted of 15 healthy donors and 15 consecutive NSCLC patients, aged from 47 to 78 years (with a mean of 63 years), who underwent radical pulmonary resection. All patients' remained with no symptoms of thromboembolism, however alterations of resistance to activated protein C (APCR), protein S activity, fibrinogen and d-dimers in correlation to control group were observed. The level of expression of the death receptor Fas in various subpopulations of T lymphocytes was assessed with the use of multicolor flow cytometry. Peripheral blood mononuclear cells were obtained from patients preoperatively. **Results**: In NSCLC group we found that lower APCR was correlated with increased percentage of CD4+/CD95+ T lymphocytes (p=0.01) and with reduced percentage of CD3+/CD16+56+ and CD8+/CD16+56+ cells (p=0.02 and p=0.005, respectively). There was no correlation between proportions of all studied subpopulations of CD3+T cells and protein C and S activity, antithrombin, fibrinogen and d-dimers levels. In control group the only correlation found was that lower APCR (however still normal) correlated with increased percentage of CD4+T lymphocytes (p=0.04). **Conclusion**: These results could suggest that in NSCLC patients with no symptoms of thromboembolism, APCR alteration correlates with expression of the death receptor Fas (APO-1, CD95) in some subpopulation of CD3+ T lymphocytes; however the mechanism leading to this phenomenon remains unknown.

OC028

A double-blind placebo-controlled randomized study on enoxaparin for the prevention of upper limb DVT in cancer patients with CVC

Verso M (1), Agnelli G (1), Bertoglio S (2), Ageno W (3), Bazzzan M (4), Parise P (5), Quintavalla R (6), Naglieri E (7), Santoro A (8), Imberti D (9)*

(1) Sezione di Medicina Interna e Cardiovascolare, Dipartimento di Medicina Interna, Università d
(2) Unità Organica di Oncologia Chirurgica, Università di Genova
(3) Divisione di Medicina Interna, Ospedale di Circolo, Varese
(4) Divisione di Ematologia, Ospedale Evangelico Valdese, Torino
(5) Divisione di Medicina, Ospedale Civile di Gubbio
(6) Divisione di Medicina, Azienda Ospedaliera- Universitaria di Parma
(7) Unità Organica di Oncologia Medica e Sperimentale, IRCCO Oncologico Bari
(8) Unità Organica di Oncologia, Ospedale Humanitas, Milano
(9) Divisione di Medicina I, Ospedale di Piacenza

Background: Efficacy of prophylaxis with fixed dose of warfarin or low molecular weight heparin (LMWH) for upper limb deep vein thrombosis (UL-DVT) related to central vein catheter (CVC) has been claimed after open studies with limited sample size. The rate of bleeding in cancer patients receiving prolonged prophylaxis with LMWH is undefined. The aim of this study was to evaluate the efficacy and safety of the LMWH enoxaparin in the prevention of UL-DVT in cancer patients with CVC. **Methods**: Consecutive cancer patients with CVC for chemotherapy were included in a multicenter double blind randomized placebo-controlled study performed in 11 Italian centers. Enoxaparin, 40 mg once a day, or placebo were given subcutaneously for 6 weeks, starting 2 hours before the CVC insertion. The primary endpoint of the study was UL-DVT, as detected by venography (CVC limb) performed at 6 weeks and/or clinically overt pulmonary embolism confirmed by objective testing. The safety endpoint was major bleeding. With a postulated incidence of DVT > 30% in the placebo group and 15% in the enoxaparin group, 300 evaluable patients were required. **Results**: 385 patients were included in the study. 321 patients underwent venography (83.4%). The primary efficacy outcome was assessed in 310 patients with adequate venography. Enoxaparin reduced the incidence of UL-DVT from 18.1 % (28/155) to 14.2 % (22/155), a relative risk reduction of 21.4 % (95% CI: 0.47 to 1.31, p=0.35). Two patients in the enoxaparin group (1.0%) and 6 patients in the placebo group (3.1%) had a symptomatic venous thromboembolism. No major bleeding occurred in both treatment groups. Minor bleeding occurred in 6.3% of the patients (12/191) in the enoxaparin group and 3.6% of the patients (7/194) in the placebo group. **Conclusions**: Enoxaparin, at the dose of 40 mg daily, produced a 21% non-significant reduction in the incidence of CVC-related DVT in cancer patients. This dose was safe and well tolerated: this leaves open the option of increasing the dose of enoxaparin to optimize its efficacy in this clinical setting.

OC029

Comparison of incidence between thromboembolic events (TEs) and malignancies. An epidemiological retrospective study

Makris P, Boutou A, Papamichos S, Tsoukas D, Sarridou D, Triantafylou A, Siapera M, Boukas A, Mouratoglou S, Girtovitis F*

Haemostasis and Thrombosis Unit, A' Medical Propedeutic Clinic Aristotle University of Thessa

Introduction: Thrombosis, both venous and arterial, is a common pathologic condition and a factor of important morbidity and mortality among the general population. **Aim:** The aims of this retrospective epidemiological study are: 1) to reveal the frequency of TEs among the hospitalized patients (hosp-pts) in AHEPA University hospital of Thessaloniki, during the last forty years and to compare this frequency with the one of malignancies of any body part or organ, during the same period. 2) to find out how many people died of TEs in the west (industrialized) part of the city, during the last four decades and in the east (civil) part of the city, during the last two decades and 3) to compare this mortality with the one caused by malignancies in the same parts of the city and during the same period. **Material-Methods:** The material consisted of 108.432 file records of the same number of pts hospitalized in AHEPA Hospital (mean age=46,88±23,85). We studied the appearance of TEs and of malignancies of any body part or organ in1963, 1973, 1983, 1993 and 2002. Among the pts men were 63,75% (mean age=47,16±23) and women 36,25% (mean age=46,39±23,85). Diagnoses were confirmed by the corresponding laboratory methods that were used each period of our study. We also studied 44.117 death certificates; the 8.656 were from the west-zone of Thessaloniki and referred to the years 1960-1999, while the rest 35.461 were from the east-zone and referred to the years 1980-1999. **Results**:

Table I. The number of TEs and malignancies and their percentage rate among the total number of hosp. pts, from 1963 to 2002.

Year	number of hosp	TEs	%	Malignancies	%
1963	4509	64	1.42	337	7.5
1973	16886	515	3.05	390	2.3
1983	18284	678	3.52	431	2.4
1993	31148	2897	9.30	2000	6.4
2002	37605	3789	10.07	2583	6.9

Table II. The percentage rates of deaths caused by malignancies and by TEs in the west and in the east zone.

Years	west zone		east zone	
	Ca %	TEs%	Ca%	TEs %
1960-1969	18.4	17.4		
1970-1979	18.9	24.6		
1980-1989	19.5	31.2	18.9	15.9
1990-1999	24.3	34.4	18.4	23.4

Ca= all kind of malignancies.

Conclusions: 1)a. The total number of hosp. pts has raised about 8,34 times during the period 1963-2002. b. In the same period the total number of pts with malignancies has increased by 7,66 times, while the number of pts with TEs has raised about 59,20 times. 2) In the west zone almost 1 person out of 3 die of TEs and 1 out of 4 of cancer. For the east zone the corresponding frequencies are 1 out of 4 for TEs and less than 1 out of 5 for cancer, indicating a potential correlation of death causes with the environmental factors.

OC030

Home treatment of cancer patients with deep venous thrombosis

Limbiati S (1), Dentali F (1), Grimwood R (2), Wells P (2), Steidl L (1), Ageno W (1)*

(1) Internal Medicine, University of Insubria, Varese, Italy
(2) Ottawa Health Research Institute, Ottawa, Canada

Background: Home treatment of deep vein thrombosis (DVT) is a common practice in many centers. Cancer is frequently associated with DVT and is often considered an exclusion criterion for outpatient treatment. However, when feasible, home treatment of cancer patients with DVT improves quality of life. We performed a retrospective review of clinical practice patterns to assess the rate of cancer patients who were deemed eligible for outpatient treatment of their DVT. **Methods**: The charts of outpatients with objectively documented DVT and known cancer who were referred to the Thrombosis Unit of the Varese Hospital, Italy from February 2000 to December 2002 and to the Ottawa Hospital General Campus Thrombosis Unit, Canada from January 1999 to December 2003 were reviewed. All patients were routinely evaluated for the home treatment program at both institutions. Usually, only patients with poor clinical conditions, active bleeding or high risk of bleeding, and pain requiring parenteral narcotics were admitted to the hospital. All patients received low molecular weight heparin (LMWH) and warfarin or LMWH alone. We collected information on the rate of recurrent thrombosis, major and minor bleeding at 3 months in both groups of outpatients and inpatients. **Results**: We evaluated a total of 252 patients, their mean age was 62.1 years, 35.3% were males. Most frequent sites of cancer were breast in 21%, genitourinary in 20.6%, and gastrointestinal in 19%. The presence of metastases was known in 49.6%. Treatment with LMWH and warfarin was prescribed to 68.9%, LMWH alone to 31.1%. One hundred and sixty eight patients (66.6%) were entirely treated at home. The remaining required hospital admission, mainly because of the severity of the clinical conditions. Recurrent thrombosis occurred in 8.3% of patients treated at home and in 11.9% of hospitalized patients, major bleeding in 2.4% and in 1.2%, respectively, and minor bleeding in 6.5% and in 8.3%, respectively. **Conclusions**: The initiation of antithrombotic therapy for acute DVT in cancer patients is difficult because of an increased risk of both bleeding and recurrent thromboembolic events, but it can be entirely administered at home to at least two thirds of patients. When clinically feasible, home treatment of DVT is clearly well accepted by patients with cancer.

OC031

The influence of long-term glycemic control on fibrinolytic activity in type-1 diabetic patients

Seljeflot I (1), Larsen J (2), Dahl-Jørgense K (2), Hanssen K (3), Arnesen H (1)*

(1) Center for Clinical Research, Ullevål University Hospital, Oslo Norway
(2) Dept of Pediatrics, Ullevål University Hospital, Oslo Norway
(3) Dept of Endocrionology, Aker University Hospital, Oslo, Norway

Disturbances in the haemostatic system are well-known risk factors for atherothrombosis. Diabetic individuals are known to be prone to atherothrombosis and coronary heart disease (CDH). **Objective**: In the present study we have evaluated the relation between long-term glycemic control in insulin dependent diabetes mellitus (IDDM) patients and some fibrinolytic and inflammatory variables. The population consists of 38 type-1 diabetic patients (35-56 years, 40% women) who participated in the Oslo study from 1982. They were all regularily followed during 18 years with HbA1c measurements 3-4 times pr.year for most of the patients. **Results**: Mean HbA1c levels during 18 years were 8.2 % and correlated significantly with PAI-1 activity (r=0.497, p=0.002) and tPAag (r=0.450, p=0.005) and inversely with tPA activity (r=-0.497, p=0.004) and serum D-dimer (global test of fibrinolysis) (r=-0.371, p=0.022), all remaining statistically significant after adjustments for BMI and serum lipids which also correlated significantly with HbA1c (BMI p=0.002; triglycerides p<0.0001; HDL-C (inversely) p=0.004). HbA1c was also significantly correlated with TNFα (r=0.430, p=0.007), however not after adjustments for the highly intercorrelated variables serum lipids and BMI. No correlation with high sensitivity CRP was found. When analyzing the variables according to the tertiles of the HbA1c, the group with the highest tertile (≥8.4 %) had, compared with the two lower, significantly higher levels of PAI-1 activity (10.0 vs 6.3 U/mL), tPAag (6.7 vs 5.3 ng/mL) and TNFα (2.45 vs 1.79 pg/mL) and significantly lower levels of tPA activity (0.82 vs 1.60 IU/mL) and serum D-dimer (0.56 vs 1.53 µg/mL). **Conclusion**: Long-term glycemic control (assessed as mean HbA1c over time) was highly associated with atherothrombotic markers, especially reduced fibrinolysis.

OC032

The effects of rosiglitazone treatment on the fibrinolytic system in patients with type 2 diabetes mellitus

Guldiken S (1), Turgut B (2), Demir M (1), Arikan E (1), Kara M (1), Tugrul A (1), Vural O (1)*

(1) Trakya Unıversıty Medıcal School Deparmet of Medıcıne, Dıvısıon of Endocrınology, Edırne-Turkey
(2) Trakya Unıversıty Medıcal School Deparmet of Medıcıne, Dıvısıon of Hematology, Edırne-Turkey

Aims: Patients with type 2 diabetes mellitus (DM) are at risk for the development of cardiovascular diseases, which can in part be explained by disturbances in the haemostatic and fibrinolytic systems. Peroxisome proliferators activated receptors (PPARs) appear to play a pivotal role in the regulation of cellular proliferation and inflammation. The thiazolidinedione rosiglitazone is a PPAR-gamma agonist that was recently approved for treatment of type 2 DM. We aimed to assess the effects of rosiglitazone treatment on fibrinolytic systems and insulin sensitivity in patients with type 2 DM. **Materials and Methods:** Twenty-four patients with type 2 DM (16 females, 8 males) and 28 healthy subjects (20 females, 8 males) were enrolled in the study. BMI (kg/m^2), waist and hip circumferences, blood pressures were recorded. Fasting glucose, postprandial glucose, insulin, lipid profile, D-dimer, plasma tissue plasminogen activator (tPA), plasminogen activator inhibitor-1 (PAI-1) levels and global fibrinolytic capacity (GFC) were measured. Insulin resistance was calculated by homeostasis model assessment (HOMA-R). Patients with type 2 DM then were placed on rosiglitazone (4mg/day, for 12 weeks) in addition coexistent medication, and baseline tests were repeated. **Results:** There were no significant differences between type 2 DM and control groups regarding gender and age. Mean BMI, waist and hip measurements of type 2 diabetic patients were higher than control subjects (34.2±5.7kg/m^2, 29.9±5.4kg/m^2; 106±9cm, 91±13cm; 116±10, 106±9cm, p< 0.001, respectively). Type 2 diabetic patients had higher mean fasting glucose, postprandial glucose, fasting insulin, triglyceride HOMA-R levels (p< 0.001), whereas high-density lipoprotein cholesterol (HDL-C) levels (p< 0.01) and GFC (3.1±3.2µg/mL, 10.1±11.7µG/mL, p< 0.001) were lower in patients with type 2 DM than control subjects. There was no difference between mean plasma tPA and D-dimer levels of the two groups. Mean plasma PAI-1 level was higher in type 2 diabetic patients than control subjects (116±75 ng/mL, 57±43 ng/mL, p< 0.01). As well, type 2 diabetic patients had lower mean tPA/PAI-1 ratio than control subjects (0.12±0.16, 0.24±0.28, p< 0.05). In type 2 diabetic patients, PAI-1 levels were positively correlated with waist (r = 0.4, p< 0.05) and hip (r = 0.4, p< 0.05) circumferences. After rosiglitazone treatment, there was no difference in mean plasma levels of tPA, PAI-1, tPA/PAI-1 ratios and GFC in type 2 diabetic patients. But insulin levels and HOMA-R values were significantly different according to baseline values after the addition of rosiglitazone treatment in type 2 diabetic patients (p< 0.05, p< 0.01, respectively). **Conclusions:** We conclude that increased PAI-1 levels in type 2 diabetic patients are correlated with high waist-hip circumferences. The short term of rosiglitazone treatment of patients with type 2 diabetic patients has no effects on the fibrinolytic system although it improves insulin sensitivity. The weight loss seems to be an important factor to prevent the disturbances in the fibrinolytic systems in type 2 DM.

OC033

Phospholipids retard fibrinolysis

Kolev K (1), Váradi B (1), Tenekedjiev K (1), Machovich R (1), Longstaff C (2)*

(1) Department of Medical Biochemistry, Semmelweis University, Budapest, Hungary

(2) National Institute for Biological Standards and Control, South Mimms, United Kingdom

Introduction Whenever arterial thrombi are formed, the activated platelets release various cellular constituents. Based on the platelet content the estimated amount of phospholipids from this source can be as high as 6 – 8 g/L in large-vessel thrombi. The question rises: Does this phospholipids content affect the stability of the clots when therapeutic thrombolysis is induced with tissue-type plasminogen activator (tPA)? We have addressed this question with *in vitro* evaluation of plasminogen activation and fibrin dissolution in the presence of phospholipids. **Materials and methods** Liposomes composed of dipalmitoyl-phosphatidylcholine (PC) and dipalmitoyl-phosphatidylserine (PS) at 1:1 or 3:1 mass ratio (PCPS1:1, PCPS3:1) were prepared with extrusion through 50 nm filter. Water-soluble dihexanoyl-phosphatidylserine (DHPS) was also used. Plasminogen activation was measured in a fibrin-free assay (monitoring plasmin activity generated in a homogeneous mixture of 3 µM plasminogen and 7 nM tPA with a chromogenic plasmin substrate) and a clear fibrin-clot assay (monitoring plasmin activity generated in a two-phase system consisting of fibrin containing 0.13 – 1.2 µM plasminogen, to the surface of which 0.2 – 5 nM tPA was layered together with a chromogenic plasmin substrate). The changes in turbidity at 340 nm of opaque fibrin were used to monitor the dissolution of clots. Surface plasmon resonance (SPR), microcalorimetry and equilibrium sedimentation methods were applied for the evaluation of the interactions of phospholipids and components of the fibrinolytic system (tPA, plasminogen, plasmin). Eu-labeled tPA and plasmin (with blocked active site) were used to monitor the penetration into fibrin clots. **Results** Although neither of the used phospholipid mixtures (at concentrations up to 1 g/L) affects the plasminogen activation in the fibrin-free assay, the presence of PCPS1:1 and PCPS3:1 in the fibrin slows down the generation of plasmin in the clear clot assay (the inhibition is in the range 40 – 60 % and 20 – 40 %, respectively, for the applied range of tPA concentrations and 1 g/L phospholipids). The lysis-time of opaque fibrin containing 1 g/L of either phospholipid mixtures is prolonged by 60 %, if the dissolution is induced by tPA, and by 30 %, if plasmin is layered to the clot surface. PC liposomes have minimal effects, whereas the water-soluble DHPS has no effect in the plasminogen activation and fibrinolytic assays. Both PCPS1:1 and PCPS3:1 (1 g/L) retard the diffusion rate of Eu-tPA and Eu-plasmin into fibrin (by 75 and 50 %, respectively), whereas the PC and the DHPS have no effect on the diffusion. The binding of tPA and plasmin to PCPS1:1 and PCPS3:1 is observed with SPR and sedimentation methods, whereas microcalorimetry provides also evidence for rearrangement of the liposomes induced by these proteins. **Conclusion** Negatively charged phospholipids forming membrane-like structures retard both plasminogen activation within fibrin gels and plasmin action. The background of these effects is probably impeded protein diffusion into the clot, which is partially related to protein-phospholipid interactions.

OC034

Impaired fibrinolyis among women with premature Peripheral artery occlusive disease (PAOD)

Lindeman J (1, 2), Tanis B (2), de Maat M (1), Bloemenkamp D (3), Guimaraes A (1), Kooistra T (1), Kluft C (1), van Bockel H (2), van de Graaf Y (3)

(1) Dept. Biomedical Research, TNO Prevention and Health, Leiden, The Netherlands

(2) Dept. Vascular Surgery, LUMC, Leiden, The Netherlands

(3) Dept. Clinical Epidemiology UMC Utrecht, the Netherlands

PAOD among young women is an uncommon, albeit severe, pathology. The etiology of PAOD in this group of patients is an enigma: general risk factors in these women appear similar to those in older patients with PAOD and it is unclear whether premature PAOD reflects an early manifestation of atherosclerotic disease or whether other predisposing factors are involved as well. Impaired fibrinolysis is an independent risk factor for progression of coronary artery disease and reinfarction in patients with premature coronary artery disease but the putative role of the fibrinolytic system in the development of premature PAOD has not been studied yet. In this case-control study we investigated the association between the fibrinolytic system and the risk of PAOD among young women in The Netherlands. **Results**: Plasma fibrinogen levels were clearly higher in the patient group. No relation was found between plasma fibrinogen concentration and traditional risk factors. Fibrinogen levels were correlated with BMI in the control group but not in the patient group. Total plasma plasminogen was similar in both study groups. Levels of the tissue type plasminogen activator on the other hand were significantly higher in the patient group and were related to plasma PAI-1 (r=0.44 and 0.49 in patients and controls respectively) and the higher tPa levels in the patient group presumably reflect increased circulating t-PA-PAI-1 complexes. Plasma PAI-1 levels were higher in the patient group (33.5 [10.4-305] vs 12.7 [4.2-235] (median [range]), (p<0.001)). PAI-1 levels were related to diastolic blood pressure (r=0.49, p<0.001), CRP (r=0.37, p<0.01) and weakly related to LDL cholesterol (r=0.26, p<0.03). Such relationships were not found in the patient group, although a weak negative relationship was found between HDL cholesterol and PAI-1 levels (r=–0.35, p<0.03). TAFI activity, as assessed by a new activity assay was similar in both groups and no relationship was found between TAFI and traditional risk factors or inflammatory markers. Plasma fibrinogen degradation was assessed as a measure of on-going fibrinolysis: FDP was higher/similar in the control/both group(s). The ratio fdp/total fibrinogen was significantly lower in the patient group (p<0.002). A linear relationship was found between FDP levels and plasma fibrinogen levels in the control group (r=0.41, p<0.001) but not in the patient group. In contrast, we observed a reciprocal relationship between FDP and plasma PAI-1 levels in the patient group (r=–0.52, p<0.001). Such a relationship was not observed in the control group. **Conclusion**: these findings are consistent with impaired fibrinolyis in women with a history of premature PAOD.

OC035

Plasminogen activator ınhıbıtor-1 gene polymorphism (-675 4g/5g) associated with obesity

Özel D (1), Berberoğlu M (2), Akar E (3), Akar N (3)*

(1) Ankara University Biotechnology Institute, Ankara, Turkey
(2) Ankara University, Department of Endocrinology, Ankara, Turkey
(3) Ankara University, Department of Pediatric Molecular Genetics, Turkey

Introduction: Obesity is a multifactorial disease caused by the interaction of genetic factors with the environment is largely polygenic. A number of rare monogenic morbid human obesity have been described. And there has been a dramatic increase in the prevalence of obesity worldwide that predisposes affected persons to diseases such as, hypertension, hiperlipidemia, stroke and heart attack Also it is a major risk factor for Type II diabetes mellitus and other insulin – resistant conditions. Plasminogen activator inhibitor 1 (PAI-1) is also increases in several insulin- resistant conditions such as obesity. Besides its role in coagulation, PAI-1 seems to be involved in cell migration and angiogenesis. PAI-1 binding to the extrasellular matrix of adipose tissue could alter adipocyte function by inducing obesity. **Material and methods**: DNA was extracted by conventional methods for 133 controls, 140 obese subjects. Polymerase chain reaction of PAI-1 gene was performed according to previously reported method using primers 5'CACAGAGAGAGTCTGGCCACGT3' and 5'CCAACAGAG GACTCTTGGTCT3' which revealed a 99bp PCR product. Amplification was performed for 35 cycles with an annealing temperature of 60ºC (Biometra, Germany). The PCR products were digested with BseL1 (Fermentas,Litvania) restriction endonuclease and subjected to 3.5 % agarose gel electrophoresis. **Results**: There was a clear difference in the distribution of genotype frequency of PAI-1 gene in healthy individuals and the obese subjects; 4G was more common among obese (0.64). Frequency of 4G allele of lean subjects was 0.5. The difference between the two groups was statistically significant (p=0.004) 4G/4G homozygosity in obese cases and control group was %48 and %24 in respectively. %32 of the cases and %52 of control group carried 4G allele in heterozygote form. **Conclusion**: Our data revealed that carrying 4G/4G allele of PAI-1(-675) 4G/5G polymorphism in promoter region of the gene is somewhat associated with obesity which needs further study. (This study is supported by Ankara University Biotechnology Institute).

OC036

Expression and localization of uPA, PAI-1 and PAI-3 in primary breast cancer

*Castelló R (1), España F (1), Vázquez C (2), Fuster C (2), Almenar SM (2), Aznar J (1), Loskutoff D (3), Estellés A (1)**

(1) Hospital Universitario La Fe, Valencia, Spain.
(2) Instituto Valenciano de Oncología, Valencia, Spain.
(3) The Scripps Research Institute, La Jolla, CA, USA.

Introduction: The urokinase plasminogen activator (uPA) activity is controlled by its principal inhibitor, PA inhibitor type-1 (PAI-1), but it can also be inhibited by PAI-3. Increased levels of uPA and PAI-1 are known to be associated with a poor prognosis in cancer. However, there are no studies concerning PAI-3 expression in human breast cancer tissue. **Aims:** The objective of the present study was to determine whether PAI-3 expressed in breast cancer and analyze its relationship with uPA and PAI-1. **Material and methods:** Quantitative real-time RT-PCR assay was developed to quantify PAI-3 mRNA in 70 human breast cancer tissues. We also quantified uPA and PAI-1 mRNA levels, as well as the antigen concentration (ELISA) and localization (immunohistochemistry) of all these components. **Results:** Significant correlations between mRNA and antigen levels of uPA, PAI-1 and PAI-3 were obtained. PAI-3 mRNA and antigen concentrations were not related either to lymph node status or to TNM stage. However, both uPA and PAI-1 mRNA and antigen levels were positively correlated to TNM stage, and were significantly higher in node-positive patients. Significantly higher PAI-3 antigen levels were obtained in early relapse-free patients than in patients who suffered a relapse. Immunohistochemical analysis revealed that PAI-3 antigen was localized in stromal cells, whereas both the PAI-1 and uPA antigen were observed in cancer, endothelial and stromal cells. Moreover, higher antigen levels of uPA, PAI-1 and PAI-3, determined by ELISA, were associated with a higher immunostaining. **Conclusions:** Quantitative real-time RT-PCR, ELISA and immunohistochemistry assays have been developed to show the presence of PAI-3 mRNA and antigen in human breast cancer tissue, for the first time. PAI-3 immunostaining was observed in the stroma of breast cancer tissue, which suggests that it could inhibit stromal uPA activity and prevent tumor invasion. (FPI00-05-281, FIS PI020125 and PI020136, EVES 02/016).

OC037

Serum osteoprotegerin (OPG) levels are decreased in subjects with calcified carotid artery plaques

Mathiesen E (1), Vik A (2), Sveinbjørnsso B (3), Notø A (2), Hansen J (2)*

(1) Institute of Community Medicine, University of Tromsø, Tromsø, Norway
(2) Center for Atherothrombotic Research in Tromsø, University of Tromsø, Tromsø, N
(3) Institute of Medical Biology, University of Tromsø, Tromsø, Norway

Introduction: Osteoprotegerin (OPG) is a cytokine that regulate bone metabolism and may be involved in atherosclerotic calcification. OPG-deficient mice develop severe osteoporosis and arterial calcification. In contrast, elevated serum OPG levels in humans have been reported to be associated with the presence and severity of coronary artery disease. Atherosclerosis of the carotid arteries can be assessed by ultrasound examination of plaque echogenicity, where echogenic plaques typically have a high content of calcified and dense fibrous tissue, while echolucent plaques contain relatively more lipid deposits. **Aims:** To investigate the relation between serum OPG and atherosclerotic carotid plaque morphology. **Material and methods:** Serum OPG was measured in 24 subjects with echolucent carotid plaques, 33 with echogenic carotid plaques, and 38 controls, recruited from a population health survey. Information on cardiovascular risk factors was obtained by interview and measurements of blood pressure, weight, height, and fasting blood samples were made. **Results:** Subjects with echogenic plaques had significantly lower mean levels of se-OPG (1.60 ng/ml, 95% CI 1.29-2.58 ng/ml) than controls (2.20 ng/ml, 95% CI 1.82-2.58 ng/ml, p=0.02) and non-significantly lower levels than subjects with echolucent plaques (1.82 ng/ml, 95% CI 1.36-2.28 ng/ml, p=0.4). Log-transformed OPG-levels were significantly lower in subjects with echogenic plaques than in controls even after adjustments for age, sex, body mass index, total cholesterol, HDL cholesterol, systolic blood pressure, smoking, previous or present cardiovascular disease (p<0.03). **Conclusions**: Osteoprotegerin is independently associated with echogenic carotid plaques. This is a further indication of a role for OPG as a link between the skeletal and the vascular system.

OC038

Markers of endothelial damage and inflammation correlate with a point-based score for stroke risk in atrial fibrillation

*Roldan V (1), Marin F (2), Garcia A (2), Marco P (3), Sogorb F (2), Lip G (4)**

(1) Haematology Unit. Hospital de San Vicente, Alicante, Spain
(2) Cardiology Dpt. Hospital General de Alicante. Alicante, Spain
(3) Haematology Dpt. Hospital General de Alicante. Alicante, Spain
(4) Department of Medicine, City Hospital. Birmingham, UK

A new point-based risk score that estimates the absolute risk for stroke or death in patients with new-onset atrial fibrillation (AF) in a community-based cohort has recently been described (JAMA 2003;290:1049-1056), based on 5 clinical risk factors. This risk score allows the classification of AF patients into 'low' or 'high' risk, and may help decisions on thromboprophylaxis. Abnormalities of haemostasis, endothelium and platelets have been described in AF, which may modify the risk of thromboembolism. Additionally, an inflammatory state has been observed in AF, and could participate in its pathophysiology. We hypothesised that thrombogenesis (assessed by prothrombin fragment 1+2, F1+2), endothelial dysfunction (assessed by von Willebrand factor, vWf) and inflammation (assessed by interleukin-6, IL6) in AF could be related with this new clinical score risk. We studied 191 consecutive patients (98 male; 72.3±9.2 years) with chronic nonvalvular AF who were not on anticoagulant therapy, and analysed plasma levels of IL-6, vWf and F1+2 (ELISA). Research indices were compared to 74 matched controls in sinus rhythm. Clinical risk factors for thromboembolism were recorded, and we calculated the new point-based risk score as described above. Patients with AF showed elevated levels of F1+2 (p<0.001) and IL6 (p=0.045). The risk score was correlated to IL6 levels (r=0.21, p<0.01), and vWf (r=0.29, p<0.001), but not F1+2 (r=0.11, p=0.111). In a wide cohort of non-selected and consecutive AF patients, IL6 (an inflammatory marker), vWf (a marker of endothelial dysfunction), but not F1+2 levels (an index of thrombogenesis), correlated with the new point-based risk score for stroke.

OC039

Associations of plasma fibrinogen, viscosity, D-dimer and tPA with risk of recurrent strokes in the PROGRESS study

*Rumley A (1), Woodward M (2), Lowe G (1)**

(1) Department of Medicine, University of Glasgow, UK
(2) Institute for International Health, University of Sydney, Australia

Introduction. Several prospective studies have shown significant associations between plasma fibrinogen, viscosity, fibrin D-dimer or tissue plasminogen activator (t-PA) antigen and risk of cardiovascular events (coronary heart disease, CHD and/or stroke). However there is little published information on the associations of these haemostatic and rheological variables with recurrent stroke, in patients with previous stroke or transient ischaemic attack (TIA). **Aims**. To study the associations of fibrinogen, viscosity, D-dimer and tPA with ischaemic and haemorrhagic strokes. **Methods**. Nested case-control study of ischaemic (n=472) and haemorrhagic (n=83) strokes occurring during a randomised, placebo-controlled multicentre trial of perindopril + indapamide in 6105 hypertensive and non-hypertensive patients with a history of stroke or TIA (PROGRESS study). **Results**.On univariate logistic regression analysis, fibrinogen was associated with increased risk of ischaemic stroke (odds ratio (OR) 1.18; 95% CI 1.04 – 1.34; p = 0.009). On multivariate logistic regression analysis including other predictors of stroke (systolic blood pressure, smoking and C-reactive protein) the odds ratio remained significant (1.34; 95% CI 1.10 – 1.63; p = 0.03). There was a borderline significant (p=0.07) inverse association with haemorrhagic stroke. Ischaemic stroke was also significantly associated with t-PA antigen on multivariate analysis (OR 1.03, 95% CI 1.00 – 1.06; p = 0.035), but not with plasma viscosity or D-dimer. **Conclusions**. This, the largest study reported to date of haemostatic variables and risk of (recurrent) stroke, confirms previous reports from smaller studies that plasma fibrinogen is a risk predictor for stroke; clarifies that this increased risk applies only to ischaemic stroke (in contrast, fibrinogen may show an inverse association with risk of haemorrhagic stroke); and suggests that the association is independent of potential confounders. Further studies are suggested to determine the additive value of plasma fibrinogen to classical risk predictors in prediction of both first and recurrent stroke; and to determine whether or not chronic reduction in plasma fibrinogen reduces risk of stroke.

OC040

Plasma angiopoietins 1 and 2, and angiopoietin receptor TIE-2 in congestive heart failure

Blann AD, Chong AY, Freestone B, Lip G*

Dept of Medicine, City Hospital, Birmingham, UK

Introduction: Increased plasma vascular endothelial growth factor (VEGF) in congestive heart failure (CHF) is evidence of excess angiogenesis, possibly driven by tissue hypoxia, itself a consequence of a low ejection fraction. However, VEGF is only one of a family of growth factors of possible relevance to the pathophysiology of CHF: others include angiopoietin-1 (Ang-1) that exerts its activity via receptor tie-2, and angiopoietin-2 (Ang-2). We hypothesised raised levels of Ang-1, Ang-2 and tie-2 in the plasma of patients with acute and chronic CHF compared to healthy age and sex matched controls. **Methods**: We recruited 39 patients with acute CHF (mean age 67±10), 40 with chronic CHF (mean age 63±9) and 17 healthy controls (mean age 67±7), all in sinus rhythm. Plasma samples were taken within 24h of admission in the acute CHF cohort. Citrated plasma was analysed for Ang-1, Ang-2, tie-2 and VEGF by ELISA. **Results**: Ang-2 (p<0.001), tie-2 (p<0.05) and VEGF (p<0.05) were all significantly higher in acute CHF compared to controls, Ang-2 was higher in acute CHF compared to chronic CHF (p<0.001), but there was no significant difference in Ang-1 levels between groups. Levels of Ang-2 correlated inversely with ejection fraction in CHF (r=-0.24, p=0.043). **Conclusion**: Elevated Ang-2, but not Ang-1, is present in both acute and chronic CHF patients that may, along side VEGF, indicate a role for this molecule in dissecting possible angiogenesis in CHF.

OC041

Increased circulating endothelial cells as an index of endothelial damage in congestive heart failure

Blann AD, Chong AY, Freestone B, Lip G*

Dept of Medicine, City Hospital, Birmingham, UK

Background: Circulating endothelial cells (CECs) in the peripheral blood probably represent the most direct evidence of endothelial cell damage. CECs are increased in haematological diseases, myocardial infarction, unstable angina and critical limb ischaemia. As congestive heart failure (CHF) is associated with endothelial abnormalities, we hypothesised that CECs are raised in CHF, and that they would correlate with the more established plasma indices of endothelial perturbation, that is, von Willebrand factor (vWf) and soluble E-selectin. **Methods**: We studied 30 patients with acute CHF, 30 patients with chronic stable CHF (all in sinus rhythm with ejection fraction ≤40%) and 20 controls. Patients with acute CHF were venesected within 24 hours of hospital admission. CECs were quantified using epifluorescence microscopy after immunomagnetic separation. Citrated plasma was analysed for soluble E-selectin and vWf by ELISA. **Results**: Levels of CECs, vWf and soluble E-selectin were significantly higher (all p<0.01) in patients with CHF compared to controls, with no significant differences between acute and chronic CHF. CECs correlated with plasma vWf (p<0.0001) and soluble E-selectin (p=0.022) but not ejection fraction or NYHA class. In stepwise multiple regression analysis, CHF was the only independent predictor of raised CECs (p<0.0001). **Conclusion**: CECs may be used as a novel measure of endothelial damage in CHF, which may have implications for the thrombotic risk associated with CHF and prognosis in this condition.

OC042

Association between obesity, fatty liver and fibrinogen as related to coronary artery disease in sample of the middle-aged urban population

Bogdanov M, Virc-Bogdanov S*

Obesity increases the risk of atherosclerosis and coronary thrombosis. This study investigated the relationship of obesity and fatty liver with some cardiovascular risk markers. In 548 (244 male 44.5% and 304 female 55.5%) subjects (34-60 years) we evaluated anthropometric, laboratory, sonographic findings and exercise test. In the whole group we compared the BMI (31.01 kg/m^2±4.7 SD), WHR (0.9±0.08 SD), biochemical findings [s-AST, s-ALT, s-γ-GT, s-tot.bilirubin, s-tot.cholesterol (7.2 mmol/L±1.9 SD), s-HDL-cholesterol (1.2 mmol/L±0.3 SD), s-LDL-cholesterol (5.2mmol/L±0.9 SD), s-triglyceride 2.35mmol/L±1.7 SD), ac.uricum 346.2 μmol/L±106SD), p-fibrinogen 4.18 g/L±1.4SD)], sonographic appearance (fatty liver). In 59 (65.4%) sonographic liver finding was described as normal and 55 (34.6%) had noted changes. Bicycle ergometry test used for confirmation of coronary artery disease was positive in 61 subjects. WHR has been shown to be correlated with p-fibrinogen and the ultrasound measure of fatty liver and was a better predictor of central fat distribution than BMI. The level of s-triglyceride does not have to influence fatty liver distinction. Exercise test result has been shown to correlate with BMI, s-cholesterol and p-fibrinogen. Varimax rotated factor analysis resulted in a four factor accounting for 71,2% of the scale variance. Factors were defined as (1) regulation of fibrinogen biosynthesis by steatohepatitis inflammation, (2) influence of visceral obesity to vascular system, (3) metabolic disturbances of obesity (4) influence of some hormonal abnormalities on some pro-thrombotic factors and (5) fat topography and hormonal abnormalities. Obese patients have higher plasma concentration of pro-thrombotic factors with a positive association with central fat. Ultrasound description of fatty liver in a group of subjects with coronary artery disease is in relation with the s-fibrinogen level. The relation between fat liver and fibrinogen level depends not only on the level of fatty liver, but also from the length of duration of changes in liver tissue.

OC043

Molecular defects in Tunisian families with Glanzmann thrombasthenia

Cheikh M (1), Mrad A (1), Gharbi Y (1), Derouich S (1), Kastally R (1), Rosa JP (2)*

(1) Hopital Habib Thameur, Tunis, Tunisie
(2) INSERM U348, Hopital Lariboisiere, Paris, France

Glanzmann thrombasthenia is a recessive autosomal bleeding disorder characterized by absence of platelet aggregation due to defective aIIbb3 integrin or GPIIbIIIa. Type I thrombasthenia is characterized by less than 5% aIIbb3 and no clot retraction. In type II thrombasthenia, aIIbb3 is 10 to30% and clot retraction is normal or subnormal. The rare variant type is essentially characterized by normal or subnormal levels of functionally defective aIIbb3. 43 families with Glanzmann Thrombasthenia were tested, the prevalence of type I was equal to that of type II. Two families carrying the variant type were identified. The molecular defects of the 43 families were characterized by PCR and sequencing. Different point mutations were identified and will be discussed.

OC044

Activation of platelets exposed to shear stress with smoke extracts of high-nicotine and zero-nicotine cigarettes: the protective effect of nicotine

Jesty J (1), Ramachandran J (2), Bluestein D (2)*

(1) Division of Hematology, Stony Brook University, Stony Brook, NY 11794, USA
(2) Dept Biomedical Engineering, Stony Brook University, Stony Brook, NY 11794, USA

Introduction. Tobacco smoke is a major risk factor in the development of cardiovascular disease and thrombosis. We have shown that cigarette smoke extracts not only activate platelets in a static situation, but sensitise them to activation by shear stress. However, pure nicotine partially protects platelets against shear-induced activation. **Aims**. We hypothesized that the activating effects of cigarette smoke on platelets may be reduced by the nicotine in the smoke. The availability of nicotine-free cigarettes in U.S. markets (Quest, from Vector Tobacco) enabled discrimination between the nicotine-dependent and non-nicotine-dependent effects of smoke on platelets. **Materials and methods**. Mainstream smoke (drawn through the cigarette tip) was extracted into aqueous buffer from normal (high tar, high nicotine) and zero-nicotine cigarettes. Gel-filtered platelets were freshly prepared from volunteer adult nonsmokers. Platelets were treated with smoke extracts and/or nicotine for 15 min in the presence of 3 mM Ca^{2+} before loading into a circulation loop for exposure to intermittent shear of 12 dyne/cm2 for 21 min (mimicking typical nonpathologic shear in the vasculature). Samples were removed every 3 min for assay of platelet activation state (PAS), using a modified prothrombinase-based assay (Jesty et al., Platelets 14:143-149, 2003), and were normalized to the maximum activity attainable by treatment with calcium ionophore. Platelet activation rates are the rates of increase in PAS with time. Pair comparisons were run individually, and each comparison derives from 6 runs under each of the pair conditions. **Results**. Mean platelet activation rates (summed over all pair comparisons) were: high nicotine extract, 0.0084 min–1; zero nicotine extract, 0.0159 min–1; zero nicotine extract + 50 nM nicotine, 0.0039 min–1. Probabilities of identity for the two key comparisons, derived from strict pairwise data (n = 2x6) by Student's t test, were: high nicotine vs zero nicotine, P = 0.005; zero nicotine vs zero nicotine + 50 nM nicotine, P = 0.007. **Conclusion**. Nicotine in tobacco smoke extracts significantly protects platelets against activation by non-nicotine smoke components.

OC045

Platelets express surface CD40L upon interaction with damaged vessel wall in vivo in humans: effects of aspirin intake

Giannini S (1), Rossi R (1), Guzzetta M (2), Falcinelli E (1), Ongini E (2), Gresele P (1)*

(1) Department of Internal Medicine, Section of Internal and Cardiovascular Medicine, University of Perugia, Italy
(2) NicOx Research Institute, Milano, Italy.

Introduction: The CD40-CD40L system has a key role in the immune response, inflammation, atherosclerosis and thrombosis, mediating cell-cell interactions. *In vitro* activated platelets express surface CD40L and release the soluble fragment sCD40L. The CD40-CD40L interaction is involved in platelet-induced endothelial cell activation and it has been claimed as an important mechanism in platelet-dependent atherothrombosis. However, no studies have directly demonstrated an increased expression of CD40L on platelets in conditions of *in vivo* platelet activation in humans. **Aims**: Aim of our study was to evaluate if platelets activated *in vivo* at a localized site of vascular injury express membrane bound CD40L and if this expression is inhibited by aspirin in humans. **Materials and methods**: Standardized bleeding time tests were performed with a simplate II device. Blood emerging from the bleeding time wound was collected at one minute intervals until the bleeding stopped, immediately anticoagulated in sodium citrate, fixed in 1% formaldehyde and labeled with FITC conjugated CD61 and PE conjugated CD40L monoclonal antibodies for subsequent flow cytometric analysis. In some experiments shed blood was analised before and one hour after the ingestion of 500mg aspirin. Platelet-induced endothelial cell activation was assessed determining IL-8 secretion by HUVEC (ELISA) after incubation with resting or thrombin activated platelets. **Results**: Platelets in the bleeding time blood expose membrane bound CD40L; the expression increases in a time dependent way ($p<0.01$ vs basal starting from the second minute) compatible with ongoing platelet activation. Although *in vivo* platelet CD40L expression (349% increase over basal) was lower than that obtained after *in vitro* stimulation with Thrombin Receptor Activating Peptide (TRAP) (603% over basal) it was sufficient to induce HUVEC activation. In fact *in vitro* activated platelet expressing amounts of CD40L similar to that reached in shed blood, were able to induce HUVEC IL-8 secretion. Aspirin intake did not reduce *in vivo* platelet CD40L expression while it inhibited *in vivo* P-selectin expression (-59%, $p<0.05$). **Conclusions**: Platelets activated at a localized site of vessel wall damage express surface CD40L *in vivo* in humans; the degree of CD40L expression is sufficient to provoke inflammatory reactions on endothelium; aspirin administration does not inhibit platelet CD40L expression. Platelet CD40L expression may play an important role in atherothrombosis and may represent one mechanism of aspirin resistance.

OC046

Ongoing prothrombotic state in patients with hypercholesterolemia: role for soluble CD40 ligand and oxidative stress

Sanguigni V (1), Pignatelli P (2), Ferro D (2), Del Ben M (2), Saliola M (2), Di Santo S (2), Alessandrro G (2), Mancini A (2), Sivo F (2), Violi F (2)*

(1) University of Rome Tor Vergata, Italy
(2) University of Rome La Sapienza, Italy

Introduction: Previous studies showed in hypercholesterolemic patients elevated circulating levels of sCD40L, a soluble form of a transmembrane protein, mainly expressed by activated platelets, with proinflammatory and prothrombotic activity. We performed in vivo and in vitro studies to explore the mechanism accounting for the interaction between CD40L and clotting system activation in patients with hypercholesterolemia. In particular, we evaluated whether oxidative stress could represent a link between CD40L and the clotting system. **Methods**: We studied 40 subjects (22 males, 18 females, age 41-68 years) affected by type IIa hypercholesterolemia and 20 healthy subjects matched for age and sex. In each subject we evaluated sCD40L (Quantikine CD40 ligand, R&D Systems, Minneapolis, USA), 8-hydroxy-2?-deoxyguanosine (8-OHdG) (Bioxytech 8-OHdG-EIATM Kit), a marker of oxidant stress and the plasma levels of prothrombin fragment 1+2 (F1+2) (Enzygnost F1+2, Behringwerke, Marburg, Germany), a marker of thrombin generation. In the in vitro study monocyte-mediated thrombin generation was evaluated in presence or not of the antioxidant vitamin C. **Results**: In hypercholesterolemic patients we found significantly higher sCD40L(4.2±0.3

vs.2.2 ±0.3 ng/ml; $p<0.009$), 8-OHdG (3.5±0.5 vs. 1.1?0.5 ng/ml; $p < 0.05$) and F1+2 (1.82?0.8 vs. 1.02?0.6 nM; $p<0.003$) compared to controls. A significant correlation between sCD40L and 8-OHdG (R:0.87; $p<0.0001$) and between 8-OHdG and F1+2 (R:0.68; p<0,0001) was demonstrated in all subjects studied. The in vitro study showed that CD40L, coincubated with monocytes, enhanced thrombin generation that was inhibited dose-dependently by vitamin C. **Conclusions**: The study demonstrates the existence of a relationship among sCD40L levels, oxidant status and thrombin generation and suggests that in hypercholesterolemic patients CD40L elicits clotting activation by enhancing oxidative stress.

OC047

Aspirin resistance and prognosis in the setting of non ST elevation acute coronary syndromes

Perdiou A (1), Zairis M (2), Tsiribis V (2), Patsourakos N (2), Lyras A (2), Foussas S (2), Tsoukanas K (2)*

(1) Hematology Department Tzanio Hospital Piraeus Greece
(2) Cardiology Department Tzanio Hospital Piraeus Greece

Background-There are limited data concerning to the impact of aspirin resistance (AR) on the long-term prognosis following acute coronary syndromes without ST segment elevation (NSTACS). **Methods**-Clotting time (CT) was estimated in 342 consecutive patients who admitted in our institute because of NSTACS. Determination of CT was made by PFA-100.Measurements were made upon admission for those who receive aspirin before the current event and 6 hours after aspirin administration in those who did not receive such therapy. The composite of death and myocardial infarction during the first year of follow-up was the primary study endpoint. **Results**-One hundred and two out of 342 (29.8%) patients was found to have AR (CT<300 sec). There were not significant differences in baseline characteristics between patients with or without AR. By the first year of follow-up the incidence of the composite endpoint was significantly higher in patients with AR than those without (11.3% vs. 19.4; $p=0.003$). **Conclusions**-AR is a common phenomenon among the patients with NSTACS and is associated with ominous long-term prognosis. More intensive antiplatelet therapy may be appropriate in these patients.

OC048

Application of the cone and plate(let) analyzer for testing the response to aspirin treatment

Spectre G (1), Brill A (1), Gural A (1), Turetzky N (1), Mosseri E (1), Savion D (2), Varon D (1)*

(1) Department of Hematology, Hadassah University hospital, Jerusalem Israel.
(2) Institute of Thrombosis and Haemostasis, Sheba Medical Centre, Tel-Hashomer, Israel.

Introduction. Pathological platelet activation underlies thrombotic complications of a variety of life-threatening conditions, such as coronary artery disease and cerebrovascular disease. Anti-platelet therapy is crucial in the treatment of such disorders. Recently, a correlation has been found between clinical outcome and pharmacological response to anti-platelet drugs. However, evaluation of the response to these drugs is problematic due to the lack of a rapid, inexpensive and reliable method. The Cone and Plate(let) Analyzer (CPA) was recently described as a functional test of platelet adhesion under flow condition. **Aims**. To evaluate the utility of a modified CPA test (using preincubation with an aggregation agonist) to monitor the effect of aspirin on platelet function, as compared to PRP aggregometry. **Materials and methods**. Citrated whole blood was obtained from 20 healthy volunteers under different doses of aspirin (0, 100, 300 and 500 mg/day). Platelet aggregation in response to arachidonic acid (AA) and ADP was compared to the CPA with and without preincubation of the samples with AA and ADP. **Results**. Preliminary *in vitro* studies showed that aspirin does not affect platelet adhesion, as measured by the CPA test. However, upon preincubation of the sample with AA (2.75 μM) or ADP (1.25 μM), a sharp decreased adhesion is observed with both agonists, reflecting the fact that activated platelets as well as small aggregates do not adhere to the surface. Addition of aspirin to the tested sample induced a significant recovery of platelet adhesion, in the case of pretreatment with AA but not with ADP. Based on these results, we studied the *in vivo* response to aspirin in healthy volunteers. Aspirin strongly inhibited AA-induced platelet aggregation in a dose-independent fashion (88±8% without aspirin and 13±4.8%, 11.6±5.3% and 12.4±7% for 100, 300 and 500 mg/day of aspirin, respectively). Similar to the *in vitro* findings, platelet adhesion measured by standard CPA was unaffected by aspirin.. The response to pre-incubation with AA, but not with ADP, was significantly ($p<0.001$) modified under aspirin treatment (0.6±0.3% before aspirin and 3.5±1.2, 4.4±1.7 and 4.1±2 under 100, 300 and 500 mg/day of aspirin, respectively). **Conclusions**. The modified CPA test was found to be a reliable method for testing the effect of aspirin on platelet function.

OC049

Regulation of NF-kB Activation in the anti-phospholipid syndrome: Involvement of ERK1/2 and p38 MAP kinase pathways

Buendia P (1), Lopez-Pedrera C (1), Barbarroja N (1), Montiel-Duarte C (2), Siendones E (1), Dorado G (3), Aguirre MA (1), Cuadrado M (1), Torres A (1), Velasco F (1)*

(1) Unidad de Investigacion, Hospital Reina Sofia, Cordoba, Spain
(2) Servicio de Hematologia, Clinica Universitaria de Navarra, Spain
(3) Departamento de Bioquimica y Biologia Molecular, Universidad de Cordoba, Spain

Introduction: The signal transduction mechanisms leading to the increased expression of tissue factor (TF) in monocytes of patients with antiphospholipid syndrome (APS) are largely unknown. Recent data indicate the involvement of activation of NF-kappaB and of p38/MEK-1 in aPL-mediated up-regulation of TF in endothelial cells (EC). Moreover, p38 and ERK1/2 MAP kinases are two essential mediators of VEGF-induced endothelial TF. NF-kB is activated by many of same stimuli that activate p38 and recent evidence indicates that p38 plays a role in the ability of certain stimuli to activate NF-kB transcriptional activity. **Aim**: We have evaluated the activation of these kinases in monocytes from APS patients and its association with NF-kB activation. **Materials and Methods**: Forty-four patients with primary APS (30 with thrombosis and 14 without thrombotic events) and 10 healthy controls were analysed. Monocytes were isolated from peripheral blood mononuclear cells by magnetic depletion of non-monocytes. Phosphorylated and non-phosphorylated forms of p38 and ERK1/2 MAP kinases and IkBalpha were studied in cytosolic extracts by Western blot. NF-kB binding activity was determined in nuclear extracts by EMSA. **Results**: Monocytes from 26 of 44 APS patients showed increased proteolysis of the cytoplasmic inhibitory protein IkBalpha and activation of nuclear NF-kB proteins p65 and p50. Mean levels of phosphorylated forms of p38 and ERK1/2 MAP kinases, as measured by densitometry, were significantly higher in APS patients compared to controls. In addition Pearson's relational statistic indicated significant inverse correlation between levels of pp38 MAP kinase and IkBalpha ($p=0.018$). Thus, increased levels of pp38 correlated with diminished levels of cytosolic IkBalpha expression. **Conclusions**: Our data suggest a direct implication of p38 in NF-kB activation in monocytes of APS patients. On the other hand, elevated ERK activity, which did not seem to be involved in NF-kB activity, might play a different role, (ie., as a mediator of TF-induced expression by VEGF in the APS monocytes), as suggested for endothelial cells. Additional studies are required to evaluate this hypothesis. Supported by FIS 01/0715 and JA 171/03

OC050

Platelet deposition under flow condition is increased in patients with antiphospholipid syndrome who experient thrombotic events

Shenkman B (1), Levi Y (2), Tamarin I (1), Savion N (3), Shoenfeld Y (2), Varon D (4)

(1) Inst. Thrombosis & Hemostasis, Sheba Med. Centre, Tel-Hashomer
(2) Med. Department B, Sheba Med. Centre, Tel-Hashomer
(3) Eye Res. Inst., Tel-Aviv University, Tel-Aviv
(4) Coagul. Unit, Hadassah Med. Centre, Jerusalem, Israel

Introduction: The inclination of patients with antiphospholipid syndrome (APS) to develop thrombosis is well established, whereas the mechanism of these thrombotic events is still obscure. It has been shown that coagulation system, platelets and endothelial cells are involved in the pathogenesis of thrombotic complications in APS. **Aim:** The aim of this study was to assess platelet function under defined flow conditions in APS patients and to correlate the results with thrombotic complications and the presence of lupus anticoagulant (LA) and/or anticardiolipin (aCL) antibodies. **Materials and Methods:** Platelet deposition on extracellular matrix under flow (200 and 1300 s^{-1}) was assayed by the Cone and Plate(let) Analyzer (CPA). The results obtained by the CPA were compared with platelet response to different concentrations of ADP in conventional aggregometry. In this study 87 APS patients were studied and 26 healthy volunteers served as a control group. **Results:** Under high shear, 1300 s^{-1} (but not under low shear, 200 s^{-1}) an increased platelet adhesion (surface coverage 26.1 ± 2.6 vs. 18.3 ± 2.1%) and platelet aggregation (average size 63.2 ± 11.0 vs. 44.5 ± 2.5 μm^2) (n = 17) were observed in the APS patients with thrombotic events as compared to healthy persons. This increase was associated with higher levels of von Willebrand factor (VWF) antigen (230 ± 51%) and ristocetin cofactor activity (181 ± 36%) in this group of patients. The high CPA parameters were not found in asymptomatic patients exhibiting positive test for APS. The CPA parameters were not dependent of the presence of either LA, aCL or both antibodies in all patient cohort. Furthermore, the CPA results were similarly increased in patients receiving or not receiving aspirin. Platelet deposition under flow did not correlate with platelet response to ADP in conventional aggregometry. **Conclusions:** The results of this study suggest that no interrelation exists between two mechanisms of platelet hyper-function in APS patients: one presumably is mediated by high level and activity of VWF while the other may be associated with direct platelet activation by APS antibodies. Further studies are needed to explore the differential role of each one of these mechanisms. The CPA test was found sensitive in differentiating APS patients with thrombotic complications from those without such events.

OC051

Laboratory diagnosis of antiphospholipid syndrome: difficulties and possibilities

Makatsaria A, Khizroeva D, Bitsadze VO, Baimuradova SM*

Chart of Obstetrics and Gynecology of Moscow Medical Academy

Antiphospholipid antibodies (APA) are frequently found in plasma of patients with pregnancy losses, arterial and venous thrombosis, small vessels thrombosis or thrombocytopenia, and are associated with antiphospholipid syndrome (APS). Obstetric complications of APS include placental infarction, miscarriage, preeclampsia, intrauterine growth retardation, intrauterine death and premature birth. The diagnosis of APS requires both clinical events and positive tests for APA or lupus anticoagulant (LA). Positive APA tests without clinical symptoms don't confirm the diagnosis of APS. Traditionally two basic tests for APA are used over the years to diagnose APS: one is for LA and another is for anticardiolipin antibodies (ACA). APA (ACA and LA) is heterogeneous family of immunoglobulins, which was many years considered to react with negatively charged phospholipids. Now it is well known that APA recognize not anionic phospholipids, but plasma proteins bound to suitable anionic surfaces. Some of the antigenic targets of these antibodies include beta-2-glycoprotein I (β2-GPI), prothrombin, protein C, protein S and annexin V. Patients with typical manifestations of APS in the absence of ACA and LA should be tested for antibodies to these proteins and to subgroups of APA (e.g. phosphatidylserine, phosphatidylethanolamine). This differential diagnosis is sometimes difficult even for expert laboratories because multiple tests are required. None of them combine optimal sensitivity and high specificity. Over a 2-year period (2001-2003) 52 women with recurrent pregnancy losses were tested for thrombophilic markers: LA, subgroups of APA, ACA, and antibodies against β2-GPI, prothrombin and annexin V. LA and/or elevated ACA were found in 10 patients (19,2%). Women with negative tests for LA and IgG, IgM ACA were tested for antibodies to other phospholipids. 9 patients had positive tests. Other seronegative patients were tested for β2-GPI, prothrombin and annexin V antibodies (IgG, IgM). The presence of these antibodies were demonstrated in 7 patients (13,5%), among them 1 had antiprothrombin antibodies, 3 - anti- β2-GPI antibodies and 3 - antiannexin V antibodies. These results prove that measuring of IgG, IgM antibodies against β2-GPI and other cofactors helps in serologic evaluation of APS in comparison with the commonly used tests. After diagnosis of APS all these women were treated with low doses of low molecular weight heparin (LMWH) (Fraxiparine) and 100 mg of aspirin once a day. Pregnant women with APS should begin LMWH treatment as soon as pregnancy is documented. There were no bleeding complications and no neonatal abnormalities. This therapy was effective in prevention of preclinical, embryonic and fetal loss in women with recurrent pregnancy losses and APS. The treatment with prednisone is out of date and should be avoided.

OC052

Elevated levels of prothrombin fragment 1+2 in patients with antiphospholipid antibodies but without clinical signs of antiphospholipid syndrome

Ambrožič A, Božič B, Rozman B*

University Medical Centre, Department of Rheumatology, Ljubljana, Slovenia

Introduction: Studies of specific markers for in vivo activation of coagulation in patients with antiphospholipid antibodies (aPL) are very rare. Increased levels of prothrombin fragment 1+2 (F1+2) in patients with APS were reported. **Aims**: To ascertain the relationship of F1+2 plasma levels with positive anticardiolipin antibodies (aCL) and antibodies against ß2-glycoprotein I (anti-ß2GPI) in patients without confirmed APS and to evaluate the effect of treatment on F1+2 values in patients with APS. **Methods**: 205 samples from 177 patients with suspected or confirmed connective tissue disease without APS and 15 samples from 9 patients with APS receiving anticoagulant (8) or antiplatelet (1) therapy were tested for plasma F1 + 2 values (test kit Enzygnost® F 1+2 micro, Behring, Germany), aCL (IgG, IgM) and anti-ß2GPI (IgG, IgM, IgA), both by in-house ELISAs. **Results**: Elevated levels of F1+2 were statistically significant associated with medium/high positive results for at least one isotype of aCL (p=0.027), anti-ß2GPI (p=0.019) and aCL and/or anti-ß2GPI (p=0.014) in the group of patients without confirmed APS. In aCL and ß2GPI negative/low positive patients 128/159 (81%) had normal F1+2 and 31/159 (19%) had elevated F1+2. In aCL and/or ß2GPI medium/high positive patients 29/46 (63%) had normal F1+2 and 17/46 (37%) had elevated F1+2. Furthermore, the mean level of F1+2 was significantly higher in patients with medium/high aCL or anti-ß2GPI than in those with negative/low positive aCL and anti-ß2GPI (p=0.035). In all 15 plasma samples from treated APS patients normal levels of F1+2 were measured during the treatment. **Conclusions**: Our study showed a significant association of elevated levels of F1+2 with medium or high positive aCL and/or anti-ß2GPI in patients with suspected or confirmed connective tissue disease but without clinical signs of APS in the past. aPL are believed to be one of the important causes for hypercoagulable state in those patients. Further, plasma values of F1+2 in all treated APS patients were within normal range and could therefore be a very useful indicator of the effectively suppressed coagulation activation in APS patients.

OC053

Detection of antiphospholipid antibodies (APAs) in patients with autoimmune and thrombotic diseases

Nagy E, Sallai K, Gergely P, Bodó I*

Central Laboratory of Immunology, Semmelweis Medical University, Budapest, Hungary

Introduction: Lupus anticoagulant (LA) and anticardiolipin (aCL) are antibodies seen either in patients with systemic autoimmune disorders, such as systemic lupus erythematosus (SLE), or detected as a primary condition resulting in thromboembolism and/or recurrent fetal loss. Proper detection of APAs requires both solid-phase immunoassays and coagulation tests. Coagulation testing itself is a complex procedure, including several screening and confirmatory tests, the optimal use of which remains controversial. **Aim**: was to set up an algorhythm for the use of the coagulation tests available so that both sensitivity and specificity are kept optimal. This was attempted in the setting of a diagnostic laboratory, which receives samples from autoimmune, coagulation and gynecology clinics. **Methods**: Plasma samples from 300 patients were tested both for LA and APLs. All sampels were screened for aCL and β_2-GP-I. Positive samples were also tested for anti-prothrombin and anti-phosphatidyil serine antibodies, and further typed for aCL Ig class (IgG or IgM). Three independent tests were used to screen for the presence of LA: the diluted Innovin time (dPT, 1:200) a lupus-sensitive aPTT (Actin-LA), and the diluted Russel viper venom time (dRVVT). Samples with normal results were reported as LA negative. Samples with prolonged or borderline clotting times were further analysed. A 1:1 mixing study was performed to demonstrate the presence of an anticoagulant. Samples with clear factor deficiencies (e.g. coumarin use) were reported as LA negative. Samples with partial or no correction were tested for phospholipid neutralization of the anticoagulant. For this purpose the following tests were performed: an LA insensitive aPTT, (Actin FS), a lupus sensitive aPTT in the presence of hexagonal phospholipids (Staclot LA), dRVVT in the presence of concentrated phospholipids (dRVVT Confirm). If phospholipid neutralization could be demonstrated in any of the above tests, samples were reported as LA positive. **Conclusion**: No single assay is specific and sensitive enough for LA, therefore multiple tests are required.

OC054

A survey on diagnosis of lupus anticoagulant among laboratories of the Italian Federation Of Anticoagulation Clinics (FCSA)

Biasiolo A (1), Tripodi A (2), Chantarangkul V (2), Gresele P (3), Marongiu F (4), Barcellona D (4), Erba N (5), Veschi F (6), Ghirarduzzi A (7), Pengo V (1)*

(1) Clinical Cardiology, University of Padova
(2) Angelo Bianchi Bonomi Hemophilia and Thrombosis Center, University of Milano
(3) Thrombosis Center, University of Perugia
(4) Institute of Internal Medicine, University of Cagliari
(5) Blood Tranfusion Center, Merate
(6) Coagulation Laboratory, Massa
(7) Thrombosis Center, Reggio Emilia

Search for Lupus Anticoagulants (LA) is frequently asked to clinical laboratories as part of the screening procedures for thrombophilia. As tests for LA are non-specific and lack standardization, laboratories follow guidelines as recommended by Scientific and Standardization Committee of International Society on Thrombosis and Haemostasis. Numerous surveys have been performed to assess the state of the art for LA diagnosis. We report here data on a survey carried out in Italy within the frame of activity of the Italian Federation of Anticoagulant Clinics (FCSA). The survey involved the 30 clinical laboratories, which were asked to collect plasma of patients positive for LA and to send samples to our laboratory to confirm the diagnosis. One hundred-eighty-five plasma samples were centrally tested by using dilute Russell Viper Venom Time (dRVVT) and Kaolin Clotting Time (KCT), mixing and confirmatory studies. Preliminary results confirmed LA activity in 125 plasma samples (67%) and showed a possible LA in 16 plasma samples (9%). In contrast, the remaining 44 plasma samples (24%) were fully negative. These preliminary data raise some concern as in 44 patients a false-positive diagnosis of LA was made. Moreover, positivity in this test may determine important clinical decisions as the prolongation in the use of antithrombotic drugs with consequent exposure of patients to undue risk of bleeding.

OC055

Objective assessment of deep vein thrombosis and pulmonary embolism can be deferred without increased risk of thrombosis

Siragusa S (1), Anastasio R (1), Porta C (2), Falaschi F (3), Pirrelli S (4), Malato A (1), Bonifacio G (1), Palmieri P (4), Bressan MA (3), Mariani G (1)*

(1) Thrombosis and Haemostasis Unit, Division of Hematology, University of Palermo, Italy
(2) Internal Medicine, IRCCS Policlinico San Matteo, Pavia, Italy
(3) Emergency Department, IRCCS Policlinico San Matteo, Pavia, Italy
(4) Division of Vascular Surgery, IRCCS Policlinico San Matteo, Pavia, Italy

Management of patients with suspected Deep Vein Thrombosis (DVT) or Pulmonary Embolism (PE) can be problematic if diagnostic imaging is not available (after normal working hours or in poorly equipped institutions). Pretest Clinical Probability (PCP) and D-dimer (D-d) assessment can be used to identify those patients for whom empirical, protective anticoagulation is indicated. To evaluate whether PCP and D-d assessment, together with the use of low molecular weight heparins (LMWHs), allow objective appraisal of DVT and PE to be deferred for up to 72 hours, 409 consecutive patients with suspected DVT and 124 with suspected PE were prospectively investigated. Patients identified as having a high PCP or a moderate PCP with positive D-d received a protective full-dose treatment of LMWH; the remaining patients were discharged without anticoagulant administration. However, all patients were scheduled to undergo objective tests for DVT or PE within 72 hours. Standard antithrombotic therapy was administered only when deferred diagnostic tests confirmed Venous ThromboEmbolism (VTE). In total, 23.8% (95% CI 20.3-27.3) of patients had confirmed VTE. At the short-term follow-up (72 hours), only a single thromboembolic event (0.53%, 95% CI 1.17–1.23) had occurred, while at the 3-month follow-up five events (0.9%, 95% CI 0.6–1.8) had occurred in patients in whom diagnosis of DVT or PE had been previously ruled out. Ninety per cent of subjects were managed as outpatients. Our study demonstrates that this approach allows the safe deferral of diagnostic procedures for DVT and PE for up to 72 hours, thus simplifying patient care.

OC056

Value of D-dimer, for the exclusion of deep venous thrombosis, in the low-moderate and high pre-test probability groups

El Kheir D, Gerdes V, Büller HR*

Amsterdam Medical Centre (AMC), Amsterdam, the Netherlands.

Introduction: Objective testing is required to adequately exclude or confirm clinically suspected deep vein thrombosis (DVT) of the lower limbs. However, non-selective use of objective tests, such as compression ultrasonography (CUS), is both expensive and time consuming, particularly when performed serially. To avoid this, the use of simple DVT exclusionary tools, such as D-dimer (DD) testing and/or standardised pre-test probability (PTP) scores, have been the focus of many clinical management studies. These studies were able to confirm that a normal DD test adequately excluded DVT in the low PTP group, but the same remained uncertain for the moderate and high PTP categories. **Aim**: To quantify the yield and safety of a normal DD result, for excluding DVT, in the low-moderate and high PTP groups, respectively. **Materials and methods**: We analysed the results of a prospective management study aimed at excluding DVT in outpatients referred with clinical suspicion of the disease. At presentation, DD testing, PTP assessment and CUS of the proximal (affected) leg veins were performed in all study patients. Clinical management decisions were based on DD and CUS test results, while PTP results were only utilised for the present analyses. Patients with a normal initial CUS underwent repeat testing 1 week later, unless they had a normal DD result. Anticoagulant therapy was withheld in all patients with negative test results. These patients were followed up, for 3 months, for the development of signs or symptoms of venous thromboembolism (VTE), which was then confirmed/refuted by objective testing. An independent, blinded, adjudication committee reviewed all deaths and suspected VTE complications. **Results**: A total of 1710 patients were included in our analysis, with 1393 (81.5%) in the low-moderate PTP group. DD was normal in 782 (56.1%) patients with low-moderate PTP, and in 53 (16.7%) patients with high PTP at presentation. The rate of VTE complications during follow up was 2.3% (upper 95% CI, 3.6%) and 9.4% (upper 95% CI, 20.7%) in the low-moderate and high PTP groups, respectively. **Conclusions**: A normal DD test, at presentation, safely excludes DVT in outpatients with a low-moderate PTP, while it is unreliable in those with a high PTP score. The latter should, directly, undergo objective testing for DVT.

OC057

Residual post treatment ultrasound detected thrombosis is associated with an increased risk of recurrence

Young L, Ockelford P, Rolfe-Vyson V, McKelvie S, Harper P*

Department of Haematology, Auckland City Hospital, Auckland, New Zealand

Introduction: Annual recurrence rates after initial anticoagulant therapy for deep vein thrombosis (DVT) vary between 5 and 15%. Selection of those patients at highest risk of a recurrent event may be useful so that prolonged secondary prophylaxis can be targeted on an individual basis. Residual thrombus on follow up compression ultrasound scan (CUS) at completion of oral anticoagulant therapy has been reported to be a potential risk factor for recurrent events. **Aims**: To determine if residual ultrasound detected venous thrombosis is predictive of recurrence risk in patients receiving initial LMW heparin (enoxaparin) and six months of secondary prophylaxis. **Results**: 316 patients with objectively confirmed DVT were recruited following referral to our hospital inpatient/outpatient Thrombosis Unit. All patients prospectively underwent full leg CUS on completion of anticoagulant therapy and were followed off treatment for a median follow up period of 29 months. Seventy three percent (73%) of patients had a proximal DVT. One-third had a spontaneous event, 18% had known malignancy, and 44% had a transient risk factor at presentation. CUS results were divided into those with minimal or no disease on ultrasound (67%) and those with significant residual thrombus (33%). There were 44 recurrences (14%) in the study population. Recurrence rates were significantly higher in the group with residual thrombus ($p=0.005$). The increase in risk remained significant following multivariate analysis to adjust for initial risk factors. Hereditary thrombophilia was not associated with increased recurrence risk. There were 46 deaths in the study cohort; significantly more occurred in the group with residual thrombus. This difference remained significant after adjustment for malignancy ($p<0.001$). **Conclusions**: The presence of residual thrombus detected at follow up by compression ultrasound scan is a risk factor for recurrent venous thromboembolic events. The increased risk of death in this group was an unexpected finding. The precise causes of death are currently being reviewed.

OC058

The long-term clinical course of acute deep vein thrombosis of upper extremities. A prospective cohort study

Prandoni P (1), Bernardi E (1), Marchiori A (1), Lensing A (2), Prins M (3), Sartor D (1), Piccioli A (1), Simioni P (1), Pagnan A (1), Girolami A (1)*

(1) Clinica Medica II, University of Padua, Italy
(2) Center for Vascular Medicine, University of Amsterdam, The Netherlands
(3) Department of Clinical Epidemiology, University of Maastricht, The Netherlands

Introduction. In contrast with the extensive documentation on the long-term incidence of recurrent venous thromboembolism (VTE) and post-thrombotic syndrome (PTS) after deep-vein thrombosis (DVT) of the lower extremity, the long-term clinical course of patients with upper extremity DVT is poorly defined. **Aims.** To assess the long-term incidence of recurrent venous thromboembolism (VTE) and that of the post-thrombotic syndrome (PTS) in patients with the first episode of DVT of the upper extremity. **Materials and Methods**. 53 consecutive patients with upper extremity DVT received an initial treatment with full-dose heparin followed by at least three months of oral anticoagulation. Follow-up assessments were scheduled at three and six months, and then every six months up to five years. Diagnosis of recurrent VTE was adjudicated according to standard methods, and the PTS was assessed using a standardized scale. **Results.** Of the 53 patients, 3 developed a recurrent thrombotic event. The cumulative incidence of recurrent VTE after one, two and five years was 2.0% (95% CI, 0.0 to 5.9), 4.2% (0.0 to 9.9), and 7.7% (0.0 to 16.5), respectively. The PTS developed in 13 patients (severe in 1). The cumulative incidence of the PTS was 20.8% (95% CI, 9.3 to 32.3) at six months, 25.1% (12.8 to 37.4) at one year, 27.3% (14.6 to 40.0) at two years, and remained stable afterwards. **Conclusions**. Symptomatic upper extremity DVT carries a low risk of recurrent VTE. Post-thrombotic sequelae occur in almost one fourth of patients within the first two years.

OC059

Chronic renal failure: Thrombotic events and relation with the levels of thrombomodulin, TFPI and von Willebrand factor

Sioulis A (2), Grekas D (2), Boutou A (1), Girtovitis F (1), Tasiopoulou K (2), Avdelidou A (2), Makris P (1)

(1) Haemostasis and Thrombosis Unit, A' Propedeutic Clinic, AHEPA, Aristotle University of Thessaloniki,
(2) Nephrologic Unit, A' Pathologic Clinic, AHEPA, Aristotle University of Thessaloniki, Greece

Introduction: Patients who go under haemodialysis often present with thrombosis of the arterial-venous anastomosis (fistula). In the past we had studied the changes in the levels of the normal inhibitors of coagulation, as well as in the levels of factors VII, VIII and V, coming to quite interesting conclusions. However, an important number of cases still remained unexplained. **Aim:** To study the levels of three haemostatic parameters, that is Tissue Factor Pathway Inhibitor (TFPI), Thrombomodoulin (TM) and von Willebrand factor (vWF), as indicators of the function of endothelium and to investigate any potential relation between their plasma levels and the presence of thrombotic events in patients that go under haemodialysis. **Material-Methods:** We studied 64 patients who undergo periodic haemodialysis for many years, because they suffer from chronic renal failure (CHF) of final stage. 40 of these patients are men (with a mean age of 57.6±13.8 years) and the rest 24 are women (with a mean age of 57.8±13.4 years). From these patients, 20(11 men and 9 women) manifested ≥1 thrombotic events (in the fistula or other sites), 3 (2 men and 1 woman) presented haemorrhagic complications and the rest 41 did not suffer from any thrombotic or haemorrhagic disorders. We studied the changes in the levels of TFPI, TM and vWF using the immunoenzymatic method (ELISA) before and after the haemodialysis. The same haemostatic parameters were also determined in 20 normal subjects (control group). **Results:** Our results are presented in Table I:

Table I

	TFPI	TM	vWF	
before	54.54	33.32	228.23	pts
	9.99	3.72	119.55	Control group
after	67.73	24.25	225.11	

Conclusions: 1) There is a significant difference in the levels of TM, TFPI and vWF before and after the haemodialysis and it is more pronounced in the 20 patients who presented the thrombotic events. 2) However, the levels of TM, vWF and TFPI are always a lot higher than the ones of controls, even after haemodialysis, without ever becoming normal.

OC060

Venous thromboembolism and spinal surgery

Fletcher J (1,2), Hitos K (1), Dexter M (3), Cree A (4), Dandie G (3), Saker K (2), Butler G (2)*

(1) University of Sydney Department of Surgery
(2) Westmead Vascular Laboratory
(3) Westmead Hospital Department of Neurosurgery
(4) Westmead Hospital Department of Orthopaedic Surgery

Background. The incidence of post-operative venous thromboembolism (VTE) in patients undergoing hip and knee surgery is well established as being high if prophylactic measures are not used and prophylaxis with low molecular weight heparin (LMWH) is recommended in these patients. There is less evidence on the incidence of deep vein thrombosis (DVT) in patients undergoing spinal surgery, with there being greater concern at the risk of post-operative bleeding in such patients with LMWH. **Aim.** To assess the incidence of VTE in spinal surgery patients. **Methods.** Bilateral lower extremity venous duplex scans were performed by experienced vascular technologists using a Toshiba Aplio ultrasound scanner in 170 consecutive patients, 89 males and 81 females, mean age 54.3±16.2 years. Scans were performed pre-operatively, within one week post-operatively and at 4-6 weeks. All patients received mechanical prophylaxis with graduated compression stockings, intermittent pneumatic compression and early post-operative ambulation. Heparin was used in 60.5% of patients, commencing pre-operatively in 16.3% and post-operatively in 44.2%; unfractionated heparin was used in 85.7% of patients when pre-operative heparin was given and LMWH in 94.4% of patients with post-operative heparin. **Results.** The incidence of abnormalities on the pre-operative scan was 36.3%, most frequently superficial thrombophlebitis (33.3%) in the small saphenous system with unsuspected pre-operative DVT in 3%. DVT occurred postoperatively in 3.6% with 2.4% identified within one week of surgery. Major DVT (iliofemoral and femoral) occurred in 1.2% with peroneal DVT in 1.2%. Another 1.2% of patients with no previous evidence of DVT were identified with posterior tibial and soleal vein DVT at 5-6 weeks post-operatively. Two-thirds of the DVTs occurred in patients who did not receive heparin. Blood transfusion (mean 2 units) was required in 12% of patients. Mean length of hospital stay was 7.0±2.8 days. There were no deaths and no cases of pulmonary embolism (PE). **Conclusion.** The incidence of DVT following spinal surgery in this prospective study where vigorous mechanical prophylaxis was applied with selective use of heparin was 3.6%. There was a surprisingly high incidence of pre-operative abnormality on venous scanning, possibly reflecting patient immobility prior to surgery, indicating the need for caution in interpretation of findings of DVT if only post-operative scanning is utilised.

OC061

Efficacy and safety of ximelagatran for prevention of thromboembolism using the EXPRESS regimen across different orthopaedic surgery patient groups

Eriksson BI (1), Agnelli G (2), Cohen AT (3), Dahl OE (4), Lassen M (5), Mouret P (6), Rosencher N (7), Kälebo P (1), Panfilov S (8), Andersson M (8)*

(1) Sahlgrenska University Hospital/Östra, Göteborg, Sweden
(2) University of Perugia, Perugia, Italy
(3) Guy's, King's and St Thomas' School of Medicine and Dentistry, London, UK
(4) Buskerud Central Hospital, Drammen, Norway
(5) University Hospital of Copenhagen, Hillerød, Denmark
(6) Frankfurt-Höchst Clinic, Frankfurt, Germany
(7) Cochin University Hospital, Paris, France
(8) AstraZeneca R&D Mölndal, Mölndal, Sweden

Introduction: Ximelagatran (Exanta™, AstraZeneca) is an oral direct thrombin inhibitor for prevention and treatment of venous thromboembolic (VTE) events. In the EXPRESS study, subcutaneous (sc) melagatran 2 mg, (at the time of operation) followed postoperatively by 3 mg sc melagatran and then oral ximelagatran 24 mg bid was significantly more effective than preoperative sc enoxaparin 40 mg od in reducing the risk of total VTE and proximal deep vein thrombosis (DVT)/pulmonary embolism (PE) in patients undergoing total hip (THR) or knee replacement (TKR).(1) **Aims**: A subgroup analysis was conducted on the EXPRESS intention-to-treat population to evaluate the efficacy and safety of the drug regimen in patients with different risk of either VTE or bleeding complications (type of surgery, gender, age, obesity, reduced creatinine clearance, use of general anaesthesia). **Methods**: The incidence of each binary outcome variable (VTE, proximal DVT/PE, severe bleeding, blood transfusion) was assessed by the above factors of potential prognostic significance in a logistic regression model, controlling for treatment, factor, and interaction between these. **Results**: No statistically significant interactions were found between treatment and differing risk factors for any efficacy or safety variables. The risk of VTE and proximal DVT/PE was significantly lower with ximelagatran than enoxaparin in both THR (12.9% vs 18.2%; $P = 0.0043$ and 1.8% vs 5.5%; $P < 0.001$) and TKR patients (35.1% vs 44.1%; $P = 0.0117$ and 8.2% vs 3.3%; $P = 0.0058$). However, the risk of severe bleeding was higher with ximelagatran (3.9%) than with enoxaparin (1.1%) in THR patients ($P < 0.0001$) and in patients $\geq$ 75 years old (6.9% vs 1.1%; $P = 0.0004$). Transfusion requirements and blood loss were generally higher with ximelagatran than with enoxaparin, regardless of potential prognostic factor. **Conclusions**: The efficacy and safety of sc melagatran followed by oral ximelagatran using the EXPRESS regimen was consistent across different groups of orthopaedic surgery patients, suggesting that ximelagatran is effective and well tolerated in a wide range of patients. The bleeding profile was less favourable in THR patients and compared to postoperatively initiated therapy, however, it should be noted that rates of fatal bleeding, critical site bleeding and bleeding requiring reoperation did not differ between ximelagatran and enoxaparin in the EXPRESS study.(1) 1. Eriksson BI et al. J Thromb Haemost. 2003;1:2490-6.

OC062

Dabigatran etexilate, new oral direct thrombin inhibitor, in the prevention of thromboembolic events after total hip/knee replacement: BISTRO-2 Study

Eriksson BI (1), Dahl OE (2), Büller HR (3), Hettiarachchi R (4), Rosencher N (5), Bravo ML (4), Ahnfelt L (6), Piovella F (7), Stangier J (4), Kälebo P (1)*

(1) Sahlgrenska Univesity Hospital/Östra, Göteborg, Sweden
(2) Buskerud Central Hospital, Drammen, Norway
(3) Academic Medical Center, Amsterdam, the Netherlands
(4) Boehringer Ingelheim
(5) Cochin (AP-HP) University-hospital, Paris, France
(6) Falköping Hospital, Sweden
(7) Thromboembolic Disease Unit - IRCCS Policlinico San Matteo, Pavia, Italy

Introduction: Dabigatran etexilate is an oral direct thrombin inhibitor undergoing evaluation for the prevention of venous thromboembolism (VTE) in patients with total hip (THR) or knee replacement (TKR). Following oral administration, dabigatran etexilate is rapidly converted to its active form, dabigatran. **Aims:** The primary objective was to establish a dose-response relationship with regard to efficacy and safety of Dabigatran in the prevention of VTE in patients undergoing THR/TKR. As a secondary objective, the dose effect of dabigatran was compared with the efficacy and safety of Enoxaparin 40 mg s.c. once a day. **Materials:** In a multicenter, parallel-group, double-blind study, 1973 patients undergoing total hip or knee replacement were randomized to oral doses of dabigatran etexilate (50 and 150 mg twice daily, 300 mg once daily, and 225 mg twice daily), with the first dose administered 1-4 hours after surgery, or enoxaparin (40 mg once daily) with the first dose administered subcutaneously prior to surgery, for a total of 6-10 days. The primary efficacy outcome was the incidence of VTE including deep vein thrombosis (DVT) detected by bilateral venography or symptomatic DVT and pulmonary embolism during the treatment period. The primary safety outcome was major bleeding episodes. **Results:** Of the 1949 treated patients, 1464 patients (75%) were evaluable for the primary outcome. VTE occurred in 28.5%, 17.4%, 16.6%, 13.1%, and 24% of patients assigned to dabigatran etexilate 50, 150 mg twice daily, 300 mg once daily, 225 mg twice daily and enoxaparin respectively. A significant dose dependent decrease in the frequency of VTE was seen with increasing doses of dabigatran etexilate. When compared with enoxaparin, significantly lower VTE rates were seen in patients receiving dabigatran etexilate 150 mg twice daily (odds ratio 0.65, $p = 0.04$), 225 mg twice daily (0.47, $p = 0.0007$) and 300 mg once daily (0.61, $p = 0.02$). Major bleeding rates were significantly lower than enoxaparin with 50 mg twice daily ($p=0.047$) but increased compared to enoxaparin with all higher doses of dabigatran etexilate, reaching statistical significance with the dabigatran etexilate 300 mg once daily dose (absolute increase +2.6%, 95% CI 0.1-5.2). **Conclusion:** In patients undergoing total hip or knee replacement, oral administration of dabigatran etexilate, commenced early in the postoperative period demonstrates good clinical benefit in comparison to preoperatively administered enoxaparin.

OC063

Influence of time of first dose on the efficacy and safety of postoperative ximelagatran for prevention of thromboembolism after orthopaedic surgery

Dahl OE (1), Eriksson BI (2), Agnelli G (3), Cohen AT (4), Mouret P (5), Rosencher N (6), Panfilov S (7), Andersson M (7)*

(1) Department of Orthopaedics, Section for Joint Implants and Medical Science, Buskerud Central Hospita
(2) Sahlgrenska University Hospital/Östra, Göteborg, Sweden
(3) University of Perugia, Perugia, Italy
(4) Guy's, King's and St Thomas' School of Medicine and Dentistry, London, UK
(5) Frankfurt-Höchst Clinic, Frankfurt, Germany
(6) Cochin University Hospital, Paris, France
(7) AstraZeneca R&D Mölndal, Mölndal, Sweden

Introduction: Ximelagatran (Exanta™, AstraZeneca) is an oral direct thrombin inhibitor for the prevention and treatment of thromboembolic events. Its active form, melagatran, may be administered subcutaneously (sc). In the METHRO III study, sc melagatran 3 mg, administered 4 to 12 hours post-surgery, followed by oral ximelagatran 24 mg bid, showed comparable efficacy to sc enoxaparin 40 mg od, started preoperatively, at reducing total venous thromboembolism (VTE), proximal deep vein thrombosis and/or pulmonary embolism (DVT/PE), and symptomatic DVT/PE in patients undergoing total hip (THR) or total knee replacement (TKR) surgery.(1) **Aims**: A subgroup analysis was conducted on the METHRO III intention-to-treat population to determine the effect of timing of the first postoperative melagatran dose on efficacy and safety. Methods: Logistic regression analysis was used to evaluate the effect of early (< 8 hours post-surgery) or late ($\geq$ 8 hours post-surgery) initiation of melagatran on risk of VTE, proximal DVT/PE, severe bleeding, and the need for blood transfusion. **Results**: Overall, the incidence of total VTE (including proximal DVT/PE) with early melagatran dosing (27.2%) was significantly lower than with late dosing (35.3%; $P = 0.0034$) and similar to preoperative enoxaparin (27.3%). Early postoperative melagatran was associated with a significantly lower incidence of VTE than late administration in both THR (22.1% vs 29.0%; $P = 0.0255$) and TKR (38.3% vs 51.7%; $P = 0.0143$) patients. The risk of proximal DVT/PE or severe bleeding was unaffected by timing of melagatran dose. However, compared with enoxaparin, the overall risk of blood transfusion was significantly lower with early melagatran dosing (OR 0.82; 95% CI 0.68-0.99; $P = 0.0349$), while following TKR, the risk was significantly lower with either early (OR 0.70; 95% CI 0.51-0.96; $P = 0.0285$) or late (OR 0.62; 95% CI 0.44-0.87; $P = 0.0062$) melagatran dosing. **Conclusions**: Commencement of sc melagatran < 8 hours post-surgery is significantly more effective at reducing the risk of postoperative VTE than late ($\geq$ 8 hours post-surgery) administration for patients undergoing THR or TKR surgery, providing a similar level of thromboprophylaxis to preoperative enoxaparin without compromising safety. Postoperative ximelagatran is associated with fewer blood transfusion requirements than preoperative enoxaparin. 1. Eriksson BI, Agnelli G, Cohen AT, Dahl OE, et al. Thromb Haemost. 2003;89:288-96.

OC064

Timing of initiation of thromboembolism prophylaxis in total hip/knee replacement with dabigatran etexilate, a new oral direct thrombin inhibitor

Dahl OE (1), Eriksson BI (2), Büller HR (3), Hettiarachchi R (4), Rosencher N (5), Bravo ML (4), Ahnfelt L (6), Piovella F (7), Stangier J (4), Kälebo P (1)*

(1) Department of Orthoaedics, Buskerud Central Hospital, Drammen, Norway
(2) Sahlgrenska Univesity Hospital/Östra, Göteborg, Sweden
(3) Academic Medical Center, Amsterdam, the Netherlands
(4) Boehringer Ingelheim
(5) Cochin (AP-HP) University-hospital, Paris, France
(6) Falköping Hospital, Sweden
(7) Thromboembolic Disease Unit - IRCCS Policlinico San Matteo, Pavia, Italy

Introduction: The timing of initiation of venous thromboembolism (VTE) prophylaxis in patients undergoing orthopedic surgery is a subject of ongoing debate. In Europe prophylaxis is routinely initiated 12 hours preoperatively. On the other hand, due to concerns about perioperative bleeding, North American surgeons generally start prophylaxis 12 to 24 hours postoperatively. **Aims:** To investigate the effect of timing of the first dose of dabigatran etexilate with regard to efficacy and safety. **Materials:** In a phase II parallel-group dose-finding study patients undergoing total hip or knee replacement (THR/TKR) were randomized in a double-blind manner to oral doses of dabigatran etexilate (50 and 150 mg twice daily, 300 mg once daily, and 225 mg twice daily), with the first dose administered 1-4 hours after completing surgery, or enoxaparin (40 mg once daily) with the first dose administered subcutaneously prior to surgery, for a total of 6-10 days. If the first oral dose could not be administered within 4 hours of completion of surgery, the oral study medication was given as early as possible thereafter. Sixty centers in 11 European countries and 2 centers in the Republic of South Africa participated in the study. The primary efficacy outcome was the incidence of VTE during the treatment period, that is, symptomatic or venographically detected DVT and/or Pulmonary Embolism (PE). Bilateral venography was performed within 12 hours of the last oral dose. The primary safety outcome was the rate of major bleeding during the treatment period. In a post hoc analysis, we examined the effect of timing of the first dose of dabigatran. **Results:** For all dose groups of dabigatran etexilate, the incidence of DVT was lower among patients who were administered their first oral dose within 2 hours postoperatively compared with administration more than 2 hours after surgery. In contrast, there were no time-dependent differences in the incidence of major bleeding. **Conclusion:** In patients undergoing total hip or knee replacement, oral administration of dabigatran etexilate started early in the postoperative period appears to be more efficacious than delayed administration, without compromising safety.

OC065

Ximelagatran/melagatran versus LMWH in major orthopedic surgery: relationship between efficacy and safety and timing of initial administration

*Zufferey P (1,2), Laporte S (2), Quenet S (2), Molliex S (1), Auboyer C (1), Decousus H (2), Mismetti P (2)**

(1) Anesthesiology and Intensive Care Department, Thrombosis Research Group, University Hospital of Sain
(2) Clinical Pharmacology Unit, Thrombosis Research Group, University Hospital of Saint-Etienne, France.

Introduction Ximelagatran, a new orally administered antithrombotic, is a prodrug of the subcutaneous form melagatran acting through direct inhibition of thrombin. There are conflicting data concerning its benefit-risk ratio compared to low molecular-weight heparins (LMWH). **Aims** To clearly assess the benefit-risk ratio of melagatran/ximelagatran in the prevention of venous thromboembolism (VTE) in orthopedic surgery. **Materials and methods** We performed a meta-analysis of randomized studies comparing short-term ($\leq$ 2 weeks) melagatran/ximelagatran with LMWH for preventing venous thromboembolic events after major orthopedic surgery. Relative risks (RR) were calculated for total DVT (deep-vein thrombosis), proximal DVT, VTE, pulmonary embolism (PE), transfusion and severe bleeding. Subgroup analyses were carried out to determine any influence of surgery type (total hip replacement, total knee replacement), the daily LMWH dose ($\leq$4000 *versus* >4000 anti-Xa IU) and the timing of initiation of melagatran/ximelagatran treatment. **Results** The literature search identified six studies (three phase 3 and three phase 2 studies) with a total of 8450 patients. With LMWH therapy, rate of venographically detected thrombosis was 27±2% for total DVT and 6.1±0.9% for proximal DVT. Melagatran/ximelagatran and LMWH were equivalent for all endpoints. Compared with post-operative administration, 'knife-to-skin' administration of melagatran / ximelagatran was more effective (total DVT: RR=0.68 [0.51-0.89] *vs* RR=1.14 [0.77-1.69]; proximal DVT: RR=0.37 [0.25-0.55] *vs* RR=1.28 [0.59-2.77]) but had a higher bleeding risk (number of transfused patients: RR=1.08 [1.04-1.14] *vs* RR=0.95 [0.90-0.99]; severe bleeding: RR=2.51 [1.60-3.92] *vs* RR=0.85 [0.52-1.40]). This timing effect was not affected by type of surgery. **Conclusions** These results support the existence of an effect of timing of initiation on benefit-risk ratio of thromboprophylactic drugs; the 'optimal' melagatran/ximelagatran schedule would therefore appear to depend on whether safety or efficacy is favored.

OC066

LMWH or ximelagatran versus VKA in the prevention of VTE after major knee surgery: a meta-analysis of randomized controlled trials

Iorio A, Ferrante F, Nenci G*

Sezione di Medicina Interna e Cardiovascolare - Università di Perugia - Italy

Introduction: Low molecular weight heparins (LMWH) have progressively shown over time and trials a more favourable efficacy and safety profile than unfractionated heparin and are probably the most commonly used prophylactic agent in Europe after hip and knee surgery. On the contrary, vitamin K antagonists (VKA) still have the preference of about 60% of the prescribing surgeons in North America for knee replacement. This is likely to be due to the higher rate of bleeding at the surgical site for LMWH than for VKA, particularly if heparin is started soon after surgery or even before, and this in spite of the higher rate of VTE occurring with the use of VKA as prophylactic agent. **Aims**: To perform a meta-analysis of the randomized controlled trials evaluating safety and efficacy of VKA in comparison to LMWH or ximelagatran in the prevention of venous thromboembolism after major knee surgery. **Materials and methods**: Computerized searches of MEDLINE and EMBASE were performed. The analysis was performed on venographically evaluated patients for the period of randomized treatment and for at least two further days of follow up for safety end points. The analysis was performed with the logarithm of the risk reduction method with EasyMA®. Cochran Q was used to evaluate heterogeneity between studies and treatments. **Results**: Nine studies (6 with LMWH and 3 with ximelagatran) were included in the analysis for a total of 10291 patients (5033 for LMWH and 5258 for ximelagatran). No statistical heterogeneity was found between the comparator treatments (LMWH or Ximelagatran), except that for symptomatic PE. For total DVT, VKA resulted less effective than LMWH (RR of 1.32 [1.18 – 1.47], P < 0.001) or oral ximelagatran (RR=1.33 [1.20 – 1.48], P < 0.001). For proximal DVT VKA tended to be less effective than LMWH (RR=1.27 [0.99 – 1.63], P=0.060) or ximelagatran (RR=1.35 [0.98 – 1.56], P=0.065). As far as safety end points are concerned, no difference was found between the treatments, but major haemorrhage was significantly lower for warfarin at cumulative analysis (0.72 [0.53 - 0.99]). No bleeding was fatal. **Conclusions:** Our meta-analysis offers a cumulative evidence of higher efficacy at the price of a higher bleeding rate of the new oral direct thrombin inhibitor ximelagatran as compared to vitamin K inhibitors in major knee surgery, similarly to what happens with LMWH.

OC067

A familial multi-vitamin K-dependent syndrom associated with compound heterozygosity in the gamma-glutamyl carboxylase gene

Darghouth D (1), LeRicousse S (2), Mrad A (2), Gharbi Y (2), Maherzi A (3), Kastally R (2), Rosa J (1)*

(1) U348 INSERM-IFR6, Hopital Lariboisiere, PARIS France
(2) Laboratoire d'Hematologie, Hopital Habib Thameur, TUNIS 1008 Tunisie
(3) Service de Pediatrie, Hopital Mongi Slim, La Marsa, Tunisie

Introduction The gamma glutamyl carboxylase (gGC), an endoplasmic reticulum membrane enzyme, catalyzes the post-translational conversion of glutamic acid (Glu) to gamma-glutamic acid (Gla), in vitamin K-dependent proteins such as blood coagulation factors (II,VII,IX,X,Protein S, Protein C), the bone proteins osteocalcine and matrix gla protein, or the growth arrest protein Gas 6. Defects in gGC lead to a severe congenital bleeding disorder, associated with alterations in bone development. **Aims** We wished to define the defect of a 2-year-old girl who presented with a life-threatening bleeding disorder associated with skeleton alterations. All vitamin K-dependent procoagulant and anticoagulant factors were found defective, while serum vitamin K level was normal. Both parents and one sister were clinically and biologically normal, while one brother appeared affected, consistent with an autosomal recessive inheritance. Altogether these data suggested a genetic defect in gGC. Materials and methods Genomic DNA PCR amplification and sequence of the 13 kb-long gGC gene of the propositus, her parents, her sister, and her brother. **Results** Two heterozygous base substitutions were detected in the propositus: a G1235:A transition and a C11134:A transversion, within exons 2 and 13, respectively (G177:A and C1858:A in the mRNA), and a G7408:T heterozygous transition within intron 6-7. Putative protein translation predicted the significant missense codon substitutions D31:N, located within the intracytoplasmic N-terminal domain, and T591:K within the C-terminal ER lumenal domain of gGC, both unreported to date. Family members analysis showed that the mother, clinically unaffected, was a compound heterozygote for D31:N and T591:K, and normal for the intron 6-7 G7408:T transition. The father was normal at D31 and T591, and heterozygous for the intron 6-7 G7408:T transition. Conclusions We thus conclude that the propositus is a compound heterozygote, D31:N and T591:K being coallelic and of maternal origin, while intron 6-7 G7408:T transition belongs to the paternal allele. Consistent with this conclusion, the unaffected sister was normal for both alleles, while the affected brother was identical to his sister, carrying both the D31:N / T591:K maternal, and intron 6-7 G7408:T paternal alleles. Further studies will be required to assess the exact impact of the D31:N/T591:K mutations on the structure and/or function of gGC, and of intron 6-7 on gGC mRNA maturation process.

OC068

Hemophilic arthropathy: A comparison between the findings of magnetic tomography and of simple X-rays

Makris P (1), Haritanti A (2), Fotiadis N (2), Girtovitis F (1), Dimitriadis A (2)*

(1) Haemostasis Unit of A' Prop. Pathological Clinic AUTH
(2) Radiological Laboratory AUTH- Greece

Introduction: Haemophilic arthropathy, as the result of repeated intraarticular bleedings, constitutes not only the most frequent and serious complication of hemophilia in the myoskeletic system, but also a factor of major morbidity and important disability of haemophilic patients. **Aim**: The aim of this study is 1) to appreciate, using the magnetic tomography (MRI) as the most accurate method of imaging, the localization and extent of alterations in the affected articulations, 2) to compare these findings with the ones of simple X-rays and 3) to determine the role of MRI in the diagnostic investigation and follow-up of hemophilic arthropathy. **Material and method:** With the MRI, we examined 37 articulations in 14 hemophilic patients aged 5-57 years, whom they all had a history of at least one episode of haemarthrus clinically confirmed. More precisely, we examined 21 knee articulations, 10 elbows and 6 ankle joints. The examinations were conducted in magnet 1,5 Tesla and each one articulation was examined in three levels, using the sequences T1 SE, T2 FSE and T2*GRE. Wherever it was necessary, techniques of fat elimination (STIR) as well as paramagnetic substance (T1 SE+Gd) were also applied. The examination took place with the articulation in neutral position (not in the period when haemarthrus was present), while simple X-rays were taken in the same time posterioanteriorly and laterally. **Results:** The MRI revealed: 1) hypertrophy of articular membrane, 2) diffuse depositions of haemosiderin in 22 articulations (damages that are not shown in the simple X-rays and play a very important role in the pathogenicity and development of the illness) and 3) destruction of articular cartilage that was found to be present in all its extent only with the MRI, while in 8 cases with focal damages in the cartilage there were not any discoveries in the simple radiographs. Moreover, the MRI revealed 21 cases of hydrarthrus, 12 degenerations of meniscuses, 9 osseocartilaginous damages and 4 ligament injuries, lesions that could not be diagnosed with the classic X-rays. However, in the advanced cases of arthropathy, where severe osteoarthritis had already grown, MRI did not offer more important clinical information than X-rays. **Conclusion:** The magnetic tomography constitutes the method of selection in order to detect any articulate lesions due to haemophilic arthropathy, particularly in the early stages.

OC069

Successful treatment of spontaneous intracerebral haemorrhage in a patient with prosthetic mechanical heart valves

Iorio A (1), La Torre D (2), Conti S (1), Gambelunghe G (2)*

(1) Sezione di Medicina Interna e Cardiovascolare - Università di Perugia - Italy
(2) Sezione di Medicina Interna e Scienze Endocrino-Metaboliche - Università di Perugia - Italy

Introduction. Intracerebral haemorrhage (ICH) is the deadliest event in patient under oral anticoagulant therapy. Moreover in these patients neurosurgical treatment is often unsuitable or, at best, delayed until normalisation of haemostatic function, which requires slow-acting or risky treatments, such as vitamin K, fresh frozen plasma, activated prothrombin complex. Recombinant FVIIa (Novoseven®) has proven useful in reducing the severity of ICH in patients with haemophilia and platelet disorders and is currently under study in non coagulopathyc ICH patients. To our knowledge, there are no previous reports of use of rFVIIa in patients with prosthetic heart valves treated with oral anticoagulants. **Results and Conclusions.** RG, 53 years old female, underwent mitral and aortic replacement with mechanical valves (respectively Sorin n°29 and Carbomedics n°16) when she was 41; thereafter she was on acenocumarol (target INR: 3 to 4.5), digoxin and diuretics. She has been admitted to our institution for a continuous headache started three days before and then associated with nausea and vomiting. At admission Glasgow coma scale was 15, neurologic examination was normal except for a slight eyelid ptosis and meningismus. Vital signs were normal. A CT scan showed a right parietal haemorrhage (1.5 cm) with ventricular invasion. INR was 3.22, hepatic and renal function normal. The patient received 10 mg of vitamin K and, after informed consent, a bolus of 80 μg/kg of rFVIIa, with normal INR 15 minutes later. Cerebral angiography, obtained immediately thereafter without adverse effects, ruled out vascular malformations or aneurysms and consequent surgical treatment. rFVIIa was repeated as a bolus three hours later and then infused for 12 hours at the dose of 15 μg/kg/h. Three hours after stopping the infusion the INR was and remained thereafter 1.0. The CT was repeated 24 hours later, showing reduction of the amount of blood in the parenchimal and ventricular locations and absence of hydrocephalus. Further reduction of the haematoma and normalized ventricular spaces were demonstrated on CT seven days later up to complete normalization at 14 days. Three and eight days after rFVIIa administration echocardiographic scans revealed normal hearth and prosthetic valves function; particularly, thrombi were not detected. Eighteen days after nadroparin 50U/Kg tid was started and continued for 20 days, when the patient was shifted to warfarin (target INR 2.5). Three months later the patient still enjoys good health.

OC070

Deficient platelet response to collagen: involvement of the glycoprotein VI mediated signaling pathway in two patients

Bellucci S (1), Huisse M (2), Boval B (1), Robert A (3), Fauvel-Lafeve F (4), Jandrot-Perrus M (2)

(1) AP-HP, Hôpital Lariboisière, Lab Hematology, 75010 Paris, France
(2) Faculté Xavier-Bichat, INSERM E348, Hématologie Hôpital Bichat, 75018 Paris, France
(3) AP-HP, Hôpital Saint-Antoine, Lab Hematology, 75012 Paris, France
(4) Hôpital Saint-Louis, INSERM U 553, 75010 Paris, France.

Background: Platelet glycoprotein VI (GPVI) is a main platelet receptor for collagen. Patients having either auto antibodies against GPVI or an inherited defect in GPVI present an abnormal bleeding tendency, and very decreased platelet reactivity to collagen. **Objectives and Results**: We have identified two cases of patients with an acquired deficiency in GPVI-mediated platelet responses. The first case, a 50-year old patient, presented a limb purpura related to the occurrence of a myelodysplasia and the second, a 77-year old patient, presented ecchymoses upon heparin treatment for pulmonary embolism in the context of a B lymphopathy. The patients' platelets failed to react with collagen and with the GPVI specific agonists: collagen related peptide (CRP) or convulxin. GPVI content was repeatedly normal and binding of specific ligands such as convulxin satisfactory. Nevertheless, specific activating MoAb and convulxin failed to induce any platelet secretion; collagen, CRP or convulxin were unable to provoke calcium mobilisation. Furthermore we showed, using a new model of perfusion chamber, that ex vivo collagen-induced thrombi formation was very impaired. **Conclusion**: Thus, for the first time, these data provide evidence for an acquired defective GPVI-mediated signalling pathway, straightly mimicking the data observed in constitutional GPVI deficiencies.

OC071

Reticulated platelets: a reliable parameter to reduce prophylactic platelet transfusion after autologous bone marrow transplantation

*Chaoui D (1), Robert F (2), Chakroun T (2), Rio B (1), Ramdane B (2), Lecrubier C (1), Casadevall N (1), Marie J (2), Elalamy I (1)**

(1) Service d'Onco-Hématologie Hôtel-Dieu Hospital Paris France
(2) Service d'Hématologie Biologique Hôtel-Dieu Hospital Paris France

Introduction: Reticulated platelets (RP) are the youngest circulating platelets. RP count is proposed as a surrogate for thrombopoiesis index. **Aims:** first, to determine the correlation between RP rate and platelet recovery and, second, to identify patients in whom platelet transfusion could be avoided. **Materials and methods:** 45 autologous bone marrow transplanted patients were included but only 38 were evaluable. Median age was 57 years old. Underlying diseases were myeloma (n=19), Non Hodgkin Lymphoma (n=15) and acute leukaemia (n=4). We prospectively monitored RP rate, platelet count and required platelet transfusions from autograft (day 0) to spontaneous platelet recovery. Three end points were retrospectively defined. Reticulated platelet nadir (RPN) is the lowest rate of RP after autograft (day 0). To predict platelet transfusion independence, we focused on the day of the first RP increase (RP > 7%) (Imminent platelet recovery: IPR). Platelet transfusion independence (PTI) was defined as the first day in which spontaneous platelet increase was observed. **Results:** Median time from BMT to RPN, IPR and PTI were: 6 [0-8], 8 [5-13] and 12 days [8-26], respectively. Mean of RP rate was significantly lower at RPN than at IPR and PTI phases: 3 [1-6], 13% [7-37] and 13% [6-32], respectively. 24 patients (63%) achieved platelet recovery within 4 days after the IPR. The others (27%), despite an RP increase had a delayed platelet recovery. PR level at day 8 predict a spontaneous PTI in the following 4 days with a 80% positive predictive value. All patients but 2 were severely thrombocytopenic (< 20 G/L) and required at least a platelet transfusion (1 to 9). Among the 24 patients with an early recovery after RP increase, 14 (58%) patients had a platelet transfusion. These transfusions may be avoided. **Conclusion:** In our pilot study, RP rate increase seems a reliable parameter to predict imminent platelet recovery and transfusion independence in almost 2/3 of patients in the following 4 days. Regarding platelet count evolution, transfusion could be avoided in about half of cases in patients with RP increase. These encouraging results may allow us to reduce the prophylactic platelet transfusion in transplanted patients according to their RP determination.

OC072

Recombinant FVIIa (rFVIIa) administration, as salvage treatment in patients with uncontrollable surgical or post surgical bleeding

Katsarou O, Kotsi P, Kouramba A, Anastasopoulou I, Gavalaki M, Markakis K, Karafoulidou A*

Introduction: Uncontrollable bleeding with coagulopathy, hypothermia, metabolic acidosis and shock, is a frequent cause of mortality, in patients undergoing surgery. Control of bleeding remains difficult, even after intensive transfusion of blood and blood products. Case reports present rFVIIa to be successful after administration in moribund trauma patients. Aim: We present our experience or rFVIIa use to control massive surgical or post surgical bleeding in patients who failed to respond to standard procedures. Patients: rFVIIa was used in 10 patients, mean age 58 years (22-80), 4 with disseminated malignancies, 2 with ruptured aortic aneurysms, 1 car accident with multiorganic injuries including liver, 1 emergency surgery with coagulopathy and 1 post surgical bleeding in patient with chronic renal failure under haemodialysis. Median transfusion requirements before rFVIIa use were: RBC 13 units (2-27), FFP 12 units (4-22), PLT 3 units (0-10). All patients had abnormal coagulation parameters. PT range: 18 sec – undetectable, APTT range: 58 sec – undetectable, FIB range: 40- 180 mg/dl. Two different doses of rFVIIa were used: high dose: 86-108 (median 90) μg/kg bw in 5 patients and low dose: 15-30 (median 20) μg/kg bw in the rest. Results: rFVIIa administration has successfully stopped or reduced bleeding in all patients. 50% of the patients required one single dose, while in the rest of the patients a second dose was administrated after 2 h in order to stabilize the results. All patients presented improvement in the values of coagulation parameters and reduction in transfusion requirements. The two different doses used, had similar results. No side effects were observed. Conclusions: rFVIIa appears safe and successful as salvage treatment in surgical patients with uncontrollable bleeding. Larger studies are needed in order to establish the optimal treatment schedule.

OC073

Prothrombotic risk in hypertensives with metabolic syndrome

Theodossiades G (1), Vyssoulis G (2), Karpanou E (3), Zervoudaki A (2), Betsas JA (2), Tsevrenis V (1), Kokkinos D (3), Stefanadis C (2)*

(1) 1st Regional Transfusion and Haemophilia Centre, Hippokration Hospital, Athens, Greece
(2) 1st Cardiology Department of Athens University, Athens, Greece
(3) 1st Cardiology Department of Onassis Cardiac Surgery Centre, Athens, Greece.

Introduction: The components of the metabolic syndrome (MS) include increased blood pressure, hyperglycemia, hypertriglyceridemia, abdominal obesity and low HDL cholesterol (NCEP ATPIII). All these criteria are common in hypertensive patients, conferring increased cardiovascular risk. Prothrombotic state is common as well in hypertensives, resulting to added risk. **Aim**: To assess thrombogenesis in patients with essential hypertension. Patients and Methods: We studied 10494 consecutive non-diabetic patients with uncomplicated essential hypertension of which 3098 with MS. After a 15-day wash-out period, total fibrinogen (TF) and plasminogen activator inhibitor 1(PAI-1) were measured following overnight fast. **Results:** Hypertensives with MS had higher TF and PAI-1 values (318 vs 291 mg/dL and 2.87 vs 2.29 IU/ml, p<.00001). These findings held true for all age decades of the hypertensive population. Both TF and PAI-1 increased with advancing age (r=.25 and .15, p<.0001) in hypertensives without MS, and significantly less in patients with MS (r=.19, p<.0001 and r=.05, p<.004), differentiating between groups (p<.001 and p<.00001, respectively). **Conclusion**: MS is common in arterial hypertension (29.5%), conferring added prothrombotic risk, almost independent of the age-related increase.

OC074

Prognostic role of fibrinogen and D-dimers in diabetic polyvascular disease?

Bosevski M, Kostoska S, Tosev S, Meskoska S, Borozanov V, Georgievska L, Peovska I*

Subject: Diabetes mellitus has been recognized as hypercoagulable state. We made hypothesis that hemostatic parameters could predict prognosis of diabetic vascular disease. **Patients and methods:** 82 patients with Insulin Dependent Diabetes mellitus and coexistent peripheral arterial disease and coronary artery disease were included in 36 months study (from March 1st 2000 to March 1st 2003). 62 men and 20 women with age 63,6±6,9 were evaluated for the following parameters: current smoking, ankle-brachial index, claudicating distance, ejection fraction, number of involved arteries, triglycerides, cholesterol, LDL, fibrinogen, D-dimers, antithrombin III, protein S and C, creatinin, glycaemia, histories of myocardial infarction, stroke, diabetes, arterial hypertension and previous revascularization, as well as number of other concurrent diseases. We developed Cox-proportional model for identification of variables, associated with cardiovascular events, and multivariate regression model to define the predictors of mortality. **Results:** We registered 126 cardiovascular events during three years follow-up (incidence of 0,05% for fatal and 0,57% for non-fatal events). Hazard ratios for cardiovascular events onset were: 1,07 for plasma level of fibrinogen (4,92±1,22 g/L), 2,55 for plasma value of D-dimers (983±315 μg/L) and 1,01 for protein S activity (61,2%±33,9%). Mortality of 6,67% was found in patients with diabetic polyvascular disease. The variables independently associated with mortality found by multivariate analysis were fibrinogen (r= 0,21, p 0,02, score 2,78), D-dimers (r=0,94, p 0,01, score 17,24) and ankle-brachial index (r=0,40, p 0,03, score 4,84). **Conclusions**: The reported data demonstrated that plasma levels of fibrinogen and D-dimers are independent predictors of a significant higher mortality risk in patients with diabetic polyvascular disease.

OC075

Do plasma levels of angiogenic factors reflect vitreous levels in patients with proliferative diabetic retinopathy?

*Ghosh Y (1), Reginald A (1), Banerjee S (1), Dhingra S (1), Tyagi A (1), Lip G (2)**

(1) Birmingham & Midland Eye Centre, Dudley Road, Birmingham B18 7QH
(2) Haemostasis Thrombosis & Vascular Biology Unit, City Hospital, Dudley Road, Birmingham B18 7QH, UK

Introduction: It has been established previously that proliferative diabetic retinopathy is associated with elevated plasma levels of angiogenic markers. **Aims**: To establish whether there is a statistically significant difference in plasma and vitreous levels of angiogenic factors [Vascular Endothelial Growth Factor (VEGF), soluble VEGF receptor (sFlt-1), Angiopoietin 1 & 2 (Ang-1, Ang-2) and soluble angiopoietin receptor TIE 2 (tie-2)] in patients with proliferative diabetic retinopathy undergoing vitrectomy. **Materials & methods**: Twenty-three patients (18 male), mean age 51 years (range 25 to 72) with proliferative retinopathy secondary to diabetes and with no previous vitreo-retinal surgery, were studied. All the patients underwent vitrectomy to clear persistent vitreous haemorrhage. Plasma and undiluted vitreous samples were obtained on the day of surgery. Plasma and vitreous levels of VEGF, sFLT-1, Ang 1 and 2 and tie 2 were assayed using ELISA. **Results**: Median VEGF levels were 120(pg/ml) in plasma versus 150(pg/ml) in vitreous (1-sample Wilcoxon test, p=0.887), sFLT was 1.0 ng/ml in both (p=0.26), Angiopoeitin 1 was 1.5 ng/ml (vs 1.0 ng/ml; p=0.134), Angiopoeitin 2 was 1500 pg/ml (vs 600 pg/ml; p=0.948) and tie 2 was 1.5 ng/ml (vs 1.0 ng/ml; p=0.673). All median levels based on Inter Quartile Ranges. **Conclusions**: There were no statistically significant differences between peripheral blood and vitreal markers of angiogenesis in patients with proliferative diabetic retinopathy. As previous studies have shown significantly raised levels of angiogenic markers in proliferative diabetic retinopathy, hence measuring plasma levels of these indices might be useful in determining patients at risk of developing proliferative retinopathy and provide an indicator for early treatment.

OC076

Plasma vascular endothelial growth factor and angiopoietins in diabetes is related to endothelial damage/dysfunction and atherosclerosis

Lim S (1), Blann AD (1), Lip G (1)*

(1) Haemostasis, Thrombosis and Vascular Biology Unit, City Hospital, Dudley Road, Birmingham, UK

Background*:* Microvascular complications, characterised by abnormal neovascularisation has been linked to endothelial damage/dysfunction and atherogenesis, and identifies patients with diabetes (DM) at high risk of cardiovascular complications. We hypothesised that plasma levels of vascular endothelial growth factor (VEGF) and angiopoietin-2 (Ang-2) are raised in patients with diabetes mellitus and that this is related to endothelial damage/dysfunction and atherosclerosis. **Methods and Patients***:* We measured plasma VEGF, Ang-1 and –2 in 97 patients with DM (41 with and 56 without overt cardiovascular disease, OCVD) and 35 age- and sex-comparable healthy controls. Common carotid intima-media thickness (CIMT) and plasma von Willebrand factor (vWf) and urine albumin: creatinine ratio (UACr) were measured as indices of atherosclerosis and endothelial damage/dysfunction respectively. **Results** [Data as mean (SD) or median (IQR]: Plasma levels of vWf (155 (72) vs 109 (37) IU/dL), VEGF (180 (125-550) vs 90 (10-230)pg/ml) and Ang-2 (6.0 (3.7-8.5) vs 4.0 (2.5-5.0)ng/ml) and CIMT (1.1 (0.2) vs 0.8 (0.1)mm) were higher in patients with DM compared to controls ($p<0.01$), with no significant difference between patients with and without OCVD. Plasma Ang-1 was not significantly raised in DM. Plasma Ang-2 correlated with vWf (r=0.405, p=0.002) and UACr (r=0.278, p=0.042) in all patients with DM but plasma VEGF correlated significantly with CIMT (r=0.322, p=0.019) in patients without OCVD only. Overall, HbA1c was the only significant predictor of CIMT on multivariate analysis (p=0.006). **Conclusion***:* Plasma VEGF and Ang-2 are selectively raised in patients with DM and may be associated with endothelial damage/dysfunction and atherosclerosis, particularly in patients free of OCVD.

OC077

Soluble CD40 ligand, interleukin-6 and tissue factor in diabetes and the effect of intensive multi-factorial intervention

Lim S, Blann AD , Lip G*

Haemostasis, Thrombosis and Vacsular Biology Unit, City Hospital, Dudley Road, Birmingham, UK

Background*:* The interaction between CD40L and CD40 has been linked to the pathogenesis of atherothrombotic complications in cardiovascular disease. Raised soluble CD40 ligand (sCD40L) levels have been shown in diabetes (DM) but the link with indices of vascular inflammation and thrombogenesis in vitro is unclear. We hypothesised that plasma sCD40L is related to circulating interleukin-6 (IL-6, a proinflammatory cytokine) and tissue factor (TF, an initiator of coagulation) in patients with DM with or without clinically overt cardiovascular disease (OCVD) and sought to determine if intensified multi-factorial cardiovascular risk intervention could reduce these indices, and if patients with OCVD would derive similar benefit as compared to those without. **Patients and Methods***:* We measured plasma sCD40L, IL-6, TF in 97 patients with DM (41 with, and 56 without, OCVD) and 39 age- and sex-comparable healthy controls. Of these, 36 patients with, and 32 without, OCVD participated in a 'package of care' of cardiovascular risk intervention over one year, including angiotensin-converting enzyme inhibitor-based anti-hypertensive and statin-based lipid lowering therapy. **Results***:* As expected, plasma levels of sCD40L (600 (193-1475) vs 30 (10-175) pg/ml, $p<0.001$), IL-6 (1.5 (1.0-10.0) vs 1.0 (1.0-1.5) pg/ml, p=0.001) and TF (850 (360-1900) vs 300 (11-925) pg/ml, $p<0.001$) were higher in patients with DM compared to controls. TF levels were highest in patients with OCVD. Total cholesterol (by 14%) and HbA1c (by 13%) were reduced (both $p<0.001$) by intensive intervention and this was associated with reductions in sCD40L in both patient groups (both $p<0.001$). Reduction in TF was seen only in patients free of OCVD. There was no significant change in IL-6 levels in both patient groups. The reduction in sCD40L and TF did not correlate with reductions in total cholesterol and HbA1c. **Conclusion***:* Intensive cardiovascular risk management can reduce high sCD40L levels, but can only partially correct abnormal vascular inflammation and coagulation in DM, particularly in patients with OCVD. These data suggest the need for earlier and more aggressive cardiovascular risk interventions in DM.

OC078

Increased intima-media thickness of carotid arteries in women with previous gestational diabetes mellitus

*Janša K**

Splošna bolnišnica Jesenice, Slovenia

Introduction: Gestational diabetes mellitus (GDM) is defined as any degree of glucose intolerance with onset or first recognition during pregnancy. Women with GDM are at increase risk for the development of diabetes mellitus (usually type 2) later in life. Diabetes mellitus type 2 is important risk factor for the development of atherosclerosis. There are 30 to 40% of cardiovascular complications at the onset of diabetes mellitus type 2. Early subclinical manifestation of atherosclerosis can be recognized by measuring the intima-media thickness. **Aims:** I wanted to prove if the women with previous GDM and so with a high risk for diabetes mellitus type 2 already had early signs of atherosclerosis. **Materials and methods**: I have compared the intima-media thickness of 15 women with previous GDM and 9 post gestational women with normal glucose tolerance. High-resolution ultrasonography for the noninvasive measurement of the intima- media thickness has been used. The IMT has been expressed as the mean of the three measurements of the far wall at three different sites of carotid arteries tree left and right (common carotid artery, carotid bifurcation and internal carotid artery). Lipid profile, resting blood pressure, smoking status, body mass index (BMI), fasting blood glucose and HbA1c have also been evaluated. **Results:** The women with GDM (age 30,8±6,0 years) compared to control group- the women with normal glucose tolerance (age 29,7±2,9 years) have significantly increased IMT of all measured part of carotid tree (mean left and right sites of common carotid artery: 0,61±0,08 mm in GDM vs. 0,53±0,03 mm in control, p=<0,05; carotid bifurcation: 0,85±0,24 mm in GDM vs. 0,62±0,1 mm in control, p=<0,05; internal carotid artery: 0,66±0,1 mm in GDM vs. 0,53±0,1 mm in control, p=<0,01). The two groups significantly differ in the body mass index, fasting blood glucose and level of triglyceride, but there are no differences between the groups in the whole cholesterol, LDL cholesterol, systolic and diastolic blood pressure, HbA1c and smoking status. **Conclusions:** The significantly increased intima-media thickness of carotid arteries in women with previous gestational diabetes mellitus vs. women with normal glucose tolerance demonstrates the women with previous GDM have early signs of atherosclerosis some years before onset of diabetes mellitus type 2.

OC079

Determination of platelet derived microparticles in patients with autoimmune trombocytopenia

Hlusi A, Slavik L, Krcova V, Pikalova Z*

Departement of Hemato-oncology, University hospital Olomouc, Czech Republic

Platelet derived microparticles (PMP) are fragments released from the plasma membrane of platelet in course of their rise, activation and destruction. PMP are parts of platelets with surfactant immunoglobulins and small amount of cytoplasm. PMP present some functions of platelets. Through surfactant immunoglobulins PMP activate coagulation cascade, especially external pathway of coagulation and in this way they supply the function of platelets. PMP was detected by flow cytometry using monoclonal antibody CD 51 (this marker is expressed on all platelets). Our protocol separates PMP and other microparticles (as endothelial microparticles) with the help of monoclonal antibody, which is, expressed only on platelets and PMP, but this protocol also very well separates PMP and platelets on basis of different particle size. For determination of normal distribution, we determined PMP in 35 healthy volunteers (age 20 - 37 years). Mean of normal value was determined as 1101 particles/l'l. Absolute value of PMP was calibrated by using Flow-Count as calibrator. Normal distribution is not significantly different among men and women. The aim of our study was to determine levels of PMP in-group of patients with autoimmune trombocytopenia and the correlation among episodes of haemorrhage and survival time of platelets. Our group consisted of 20 patients with autoimmune trombocytopenia. All patients had shortened survival time of platelets and bleeding episodes. The level of PMP in our group was significantly higher than in control group of healthy volunteers and it correlates with shortened survival time of platelet. We presume that determination of PMP becomes a good marker of bleeding episode risk in patients with autoimmune trombocytopenia.

OC080

The new mutation in the GP IIIa gene associated with high platelet aggregation is found in Russia

Sirotkina O (1), Sheydina A (1), Vavilova T (2), Schwarzman A (1)*

(1) Petersburg Nuclear Physics Institute RAS, Russia
(2) Saint-Petrsburg Pavlov State Medical University, Russia

Introduction. The normal function activity of platelets is dependent on the presence of platelet-membrane glycoproteins that have an important role in platelet adhesion and aggregation. One of these platelet receptors is the fibrinogen receptor IIb-IIIa. The IIb-IIIa complex consists on two subunits which is coding genes GP IIb and GP IIIa located on 17 chromosome. Nowadays only two mutations in these genes responsible of arterial thrombosis development are known – Leu33Pro (T1565C) GP IIIa and Ile843Ser (T2622G) GP IIb. The 33Pro GPIIIa isoform is associated with increased platelet aggregability in vitro and more efficient signaling then 33Leu GPIIIa. **Aims.** The aim of our study was to determine the frequency of molecular abnormalities in GPIIb/IIIa in Russian population and estimate their association with platelet hyperaggregability. **Materials and Methods.** We investigated 170 healthy individuals (49 males and 121 females) before age 45. The Leu33Pro GP IIIa mutation was analyzed by PCR and RFLP. **Results.** 112 individuals had wild genotype of GP IIIa gene (66%), 46 individuals were the heterozygous carriers of Leu33Pro mutation GP IIIa (27%) and 5 individuals were homozygous carriers of this mutation (3%). In this group we found the new unknown previously mutation in GP IIIa gene. This mutation consisted of the substitution T/G in 1585 position of the GP IIIa gene and the replacement Leu40Arg in protein (sequenced on ABI 373 using Thermo Sequenase II terminator cycle sequencing premix kit (Amersham Pharmacia)). The Leu40Arg polymorphism coupled with Leu33Pro was detected in 7 subjects. The Leu33Pro/Leu40Arg haplotype was associated with the higher maximal platelet aggregation in response to ADP and with absence of tendency to desaggregation compared with carriers of Leu33Pro mutation only. **Conclusion.** We had described the new genetics determinant that might be responsible for increased platelet aggregation. This finding may help to obtain the molecular mechanism of the predisposition to arterial thrombosis.

OC081

17 beta-oestradiol potentiates thrombin and tromboxane-dependent platelet aggregation and exposition of fibrinogen binding sites on platelet surface

Pietrapiana D (1), Moro L (1), Reineri S (1), Piranda D (1), Bordone R (1), Bertoni A (1), Torti M (2), Sinigaglia F (1)*

(1) Department of Medical Sciences, §DISCAFF, University ?A. Avogadro?, Novara, Italy
(2) Department of Biochemistry, University of Pavia, Italy

Introduction: The impact of oestrogens on the viability of cardiovascular system and mostly on platelet function is still an open and debated question. In particular at present oestrogen-dependent signaling in platelets is still unknown. **Aim**: The aim of this study was to investigate the ERbeta-mediated signal transduction pathways in human platelets in order to clarify how oestrogen can influence platelet function. **Materials and methods**: Gel-filtered platelets were incubated with oestrogen for different times and then eventually stimulated with different doses of thrombin or U46619, the thromboxane A2 analog. Platelet aggregation was measured by Born technique. Secretion was evaluated as ATP release by luminometric technique. Activation of integrin alphaIIb-beta3, the fibrinogen-binding site, was evaluated by using PAC-1 antibody in flow cytometry experiments. Sub-cellular fractionation and co-immunoprecipitation experiments were also performed. **Results**: Oestrogen caused rapid Src tyrosine-phosphorylation in human platelets, dependent on ERbeta engagement, which resulted in the formation of Src-dependent Src/PI-3K/Pyk2 complex associated with ERbeta. The complex assembly resulted in Pyk2 but not PI-3K activation but neither Akt nor MAPK activation could be observed. Moreover, ERbeta localized in platelet membranes, and 17beta-oestradiol caused either membrane-associated Src activation and Pyk2-translocation to platelet membranes. The effect of oestrogen on platelet function was also investigated. Whilst 17b-oestradiol alone did not induce any effect on human platelets, it significantly enhanced both aggregation and exposition of active alphaIIb-beta3 in low thrombin- or U46619-treated platelets. This effect was probably mediated by Src kinase that was activated by thrombin and oestrogen with synergic mechanisms. **Conclusion**: Taken together these results indicate that oestrogen can play a pro-aggregating role in platelet function by interfering with the mechanisms of inside-out signal transduction in human platelets. Influence of other thromboembolic risk factors on oestrogen-dependent pro-aggregating effect is under investigation.

OC082

gp91phox-dependent expression of platelet CD40 ligand

Pignatelli P (1), Sanguigni V (2), Lenti L (1), Lo Coco M (1), Carnevale R (1), Timi N (1), Finocchi A (2), Rossi P (2), Violi F (1)*

(1) University of Rome "La Sapienza"
(2) University of Rome "Tor Vergata"

Background CD40 ligand (CD40L) plays a key role in the pathogenesis of atherothrombosis. CD40L expression on platelets is mediated by agonists but the underlying mechanism is still unclear. **Methods** CD40L expression was measured both in platelets from healthy volunteers - with and without the addition of antioxidants, aspirin or a phospholipase A2 (PLA2) inhibitor - and in platelets from two patients with an inherited deficiency of gp91phox, the central core of NADPH oxidase. Immunoprecipitation analysis was also performed to determine whether normal platelets showed gp91phox expression. **Results** Unlike catalase and mannitol, superoxide dismutase (SOD) significantly inhibited collagen- and thrombin-induced platelet CD40L expression in platelets from healthy subjects. Immunoprecipitation analysis also showed that platelets from healthy subjects expressed gp91phox. In two male patients with inherited gp91phox deficiency, collagen- and thrombin-stimulated platelets showed an almost complete suppression of O2- and CD40L expression; a similar suppression was seen with arachidonic acid, thus suggesting a role for this pathway in agonist-induced platelet NADPH oxidase activation and CD40L expression. Likewise, incubation of platelets from healthy subjects with a PLA2 inhibitor almost completely prevented agonist-induced O2- and CD40L expression. **Discussion** These data provide the first evidence that platelet CD40L expression occurs via arachidonic acid-mediated gp91phox activation.

OC083

Participation of ADP and TXA2 receptors in the signal transduction that regulate platelet recruitment. Effects of erythrocytes

Moscardo A (1), Santos M (1), Valles J (1), Aznar J (2), Dasi MA (3), Piñon M (1)*

(1) Research Center, University Hospital La Fe, Valencia, Spain
(2) Department of Clinical Pathology,University Hospital La Fe, Valencia, Spain
(3) Pediatric Hematology,University Hospital La Fe, Valencia, Spain

Introduction. Platelet recruitment is a key process in thrombus growth. This is mediated by the release of granule contents (ADP, 5HT, adhesive proteins, etc.) and metabolic products (TXA_2) from activated platelets. The agonistic potency of this releasate is strongly increased by cell-cell interactions with metabolically active erythrocytes (RBCs) (1,2). **Aim**. To study the participation of receptors for some components of the platelet and platelet-RBC releasate in the signal transduction mechanisms involved in platelet recruitment, particularly those related to protein phosphorylation. **Methods.** Washed platelets (WP) or WP+RBCs (Htc. 40%) were stimulated with collagen and rapidly centrifuged to obtain a cell-free releasate within 1 min (1,2). Aliquots of this releasate were used as platelet agonist, and the biochemical effects and proaggregatory action were monitored (recruitment). Tyrosine phosphorylation (TP), cytoskeletal reorganization and cytoskeletal-associated tyrosine phosphorylated proteins were evaluated (3). When appropriate, receptors on recruiting platelets were specifically blocked. **Results.** Inhibition of tyrosine kinase activity down-regulated platelet recruitment, while PKC inhibition had no effect. In addition, releasates from WP+RBCs induced high TP levels, cytoskeleton reorganization and translocation of proteins to the cytoskeleton of recruiting platelets. These responses were of comparable final intensity, but even quicker than those induced by 1 U/mL thrombin. Interestingly, RBCs promote a significant translocation of FAK kinase and $\alpha_{IIb\beta 3}$ to the platelet cytoskeleton, an effect thought to play a role in $\alpha_{IIb\beta 3}$ clustering and focal adhesion formation. Individual blockade of ADP, TXA_2 or serotonin receptors reduced recruitment, TP and cytoskeletal reorganization on recruiting platelets. These reductions were markedly stronger if the ADP receptor P2Y12 or the TXA_2 receptor were blocked. **Conclusion.** Platelet recruitment constitutes simultaneous signaling events through different receptors that specifically regulate TP and cytoskeletal reorganization. (Grants FIS 01/1208/ FIS 03/0270). 1- J. Clin Invest 1991; 87: 571

OC084

Influence of oxidatively modified fibrinogen on platelet function

Dyr JE, Vanickova M, Suttnar J*

Institute of Hematology and Blood Transfusion, Prague, Czech Republic

Free radicals are inevitable by-products of biological redox reactions. Free-radical -protein interactions are now believed to be closely related to the physiology of aging and to pathologies such as atherosclerosis. Protein damage by free-radical exposure induces cross-linking and backbone fragmentation, as well as amino acid modification. The latter gives rise to carbonyl formation, protein-bound dopa (3,4-dihydroxyphenylalanine) and protein hydroperoxides. In addition, carbonyl groups may be introduced into proteins by reactions with aldehydes produced during lipid peroxidation. Among plasma proteins, fibrinogen is highly susceptible to oxidant attack. This adhesive plasma protein plays a central role in haemostasis. Both platelet adhesion and aggregation require recognition and binding of fibrinogen by the platelet integrin receptors GPIIbIIIa. In this study we have investigated the influence of fibrinogen oxidative modification on platelet adhesion, aggregation, and on thrombin kinetics of fibrinopeptides release. We modified fibrinogen molecule alternatively by three agents occuring in high local concentrations in oxidative stress conditions: malondialdehyde, Fe^{3+} / ascorbic acid, and hypochlorite. The total carbonyl content of fibrinogen was measured after derivatization with dinitrophenylhydrazine. The changes in fibrinogen chains size were detected using SDS-PAGE. The gel-filtrated platelets were reconstituted either in modified fibrinogen or in fibrinogen treated under the same conditions except for modification agents. The influence of fibrinogen oxidative modification on platelet ADP aggregation, platelet adhesion, and fibrinopeptides release by thrombin was studied. Exposure of fibrinogen to the hypochlorite, the Fe^{3+}/ascorbate, and to the malondialdehyde modification system resulted in structural modifications and altered functionality of the glycoprotein. The carbonyl content in modified fibrinogen was 0.5, 0.69, and 0.97 mols of carbonyls per mol of protein, respectively. The adhesion of platelets on modified fibrinogen was for all modifications an average of twenty percent lower as compared with control fibrinogen. The percentage of ADP-induced platelet aggregation decreased as a function of fibrinogen oxidative damage. Thrombin-catalyzed fibrinopeptides release was significantly slower in modified fibrinogen as compared with control fibrinogen. Our results suggest that oxidative treatment alters fibrinogen domains involved both in the recognition and the binding of the molecule to the platelets, and in fibrinopeptide release by thrombin. Acknowledgement: this work was supported by grant agency of Czech Republic GACR 303/03/0249, IGA NA/7616-3, and VZ UHKT 237360001.

OC085

Markers of haemostatic activation in pregnant women with deep-vein thrombosis

Božič M (1), Antolič B (1), Peternel P (1), Šajina-Stritar B (2), Stegnar M (1)*

(1) Department of Vascular Diseases, University Medical Centre, Ljubljana, Slovenia
(2) Department of Obstetrics and Gynaecology, University Medical Centre, Ljubljana, Slovenia

Background and aim: The effect of low-molecular weight heparin (LMWH) on the activity of the thrombotic process can be monitored with markers of haemostatic activation: prothrombin fragment 1+2 (F1+2), thrombin-antithrombin complex (TAT) and D-dimer. The aim was to investigate haemostatic activation in pregnant women with deep-vein thrombosis (DVT) on LMWH treatment and in healthy pregnant women. **Subjects and methods**: The patient group consisted of 11 women with objectively confirmed DVT prior to 32nd week of gestation. All patients were receiving 100 IU/ kg LMWH – dalteparin (FragminŇ, Pharmacia & Upjohn, Sweden) twice daily according to the body mass at the time of admittance. The LMWH daily dose remained constant throughout pregnancy regardless of the body mass gain. Nine healthy pregnant women were included as a control group. In patients and controls blood was drawn at 12th, 20th and 28th week of gestation and at least one month after delivery (baseline). F1+2 (Enzygnost F1+2 micro, Dade Behring), TAT (Enzygnost TAT micro, Dade Behring) and D-dimer (AsserachromŇ D-dimer, Diagnostica Stago) were determined with ELISA. In patients plasma levels of LMWH were measured with anti-factor Xa activity. **Results**: In the control group F1+2, TAT and D-dimer levels were similar at 12th week of gestation (median, 1st-3rd quartile, 0.6, 0.5-0.9 nmol/l, 2.2, 1.9-2.5 ug/l and 98, 68-165 ug/l, respectively) compared to baseline values (0.9, 0.5-0.9 nmol/l, 1.6, 1.4-2.3 ug/l and 67, 34-111 ug/l, respectively). A significant increase in all the markers was noted at 20th week of gestation (1.0, 0.9-1.1 nmol/l, 2.8, 2.5-3.2 ug/l and 259, 193-318 ug/l, respectively, all $p<0.05$) and a further significant increase at 28th week of gestation (1.4, 1.2-1.7 nmol/l, 3.5, 3.3-5.3 ug/l and 406, 298-446 ug/l, respectively, all $p<0.05$ compared to 20th week of gestation). In patients a similar trend in increasing of the markers throughout pregnancy was observed. At no point of sampling were levels of markers significantly higher in patients than controls. **Conclusion**: Since F1+2, TAT and D-dimer gradually increased throughout pregnancy in controls as well as in patients, and were comparable between both groups, it was presumed that a therapeutic dose of LMWH inhibits excess activation of systemic haemostasis in pregnant women with DVT.

OC086

Retrospective analysis of thrombophilic parameters in women with adverse pregnancy outcome

Kotsi P, Anastasopoulou I, Tsaousidou M, Katsarou O, Kanellopoulou G, Adraktas T, Tsoukala C, Karafoulidou A*

2nd Regional Blood Transfusion Center, Hemostasis Unit, Laikon General Hospital, Athens, Greece

Introduction Inherited or acquired thrombophilia is associated with pregnancy loss. Pregnancy loss is a common health problem. 20% of women will experience 1 abortion in their life and 5% two or more. In 40-55% of cases, causes remain obscure, despite obstetrical (10%), hormonological (28%) and chromosomal analysis (4%). **Aim** To evaluate the incidence of thrombophilia in women with gestational pathologies, in comparison with healthy women or with thromboembolic disease. **Materials and methods** 148 women, age 18-43 years old (mean 32 y), divided in 3 groups: 1)group A, 25 healthy women as controls,2) group B, 77 with gestational pathologies (54.5% 1or 2 abortions n=42, 18.92% 3 or more abortions n=15, 6.76% intrauterine fetal death n=5, 4.05% intrauterine growth retardation n=3, 6.76% with preeclampsia/eclampsia n=5, 5.41% with 2nd trimester miscarriages n=4, and 4.05% more than two of the previous categories n=3),3) group C, 46 with thromboembolic disease (52.1% with 1 DVT episode n=23, 20.2% with 1 PE episode n=9, 14.7% more than 1 episodes PE or/plus DVT n=8 and 13% with one episode PE plus DVT n=6). A medical and family history was taken and subjects were studied with the following laboratory parameters: TBC, PT, APTT, fibrinogen, d-dimers, antithrombin, protein C, protein S, factor VIII, factor IX, lupus anticoagulant, APC resistance, factor XII, plasminogen and factor V Leiden, factor II mutation G20210A, and MTHFR C677T. All subjects were at least 3 months away from the episode and free from medication. **Results and conclusions** No differences occurred between groups in TBC, PT, APTT, fibrinogen, antithrombin, protein C, factor IX, nAPCR after exclusion of factor V Leiden. Between groups different values obtained in d-dimers levels (p=0.086), protein S levels (p=0.072), and factor VIII levels which was statistically significant (p=0.002). Factor XII was evaluated in a minority of cases. 8 subjects had FXII < 60%, 7 of them from group B (9%). Incidence of thrombophilia in groups was: group A 11.1% (factor V Leiden 7.4%, G20210A 3.7%), group B 24.7% (factor V Leiden 9.2%, G20210A 3.9%, protein S deficiency 4.2%, factorVIII>175IU 7.8%, lupus anticoagulant 3.9%), group C 49.2% (factor V Leiden 28.5%, G20210A 14.3%, protein S deficiency 2.9%, factorVIII>175IU 11.5%). Combined thrombophilia was found in 7,8% of group B and 13% of group C. In conclusion women with pregnancy pathologies have increased incidence of thrombophilia, and should tested in that direction. Factor VIII levels were higher in this group in comparison with age matched healthy controls, factor XII may play a role in pregnancy loss.

OC087

Venous thromboembolism after elective cesarean section

Jacobsen A, Drolsum A, Kløw N, Dahl G, Qvigstad E, Sandset P*

Introduction: Pregnancy is associated with an overall 5-10 fold increased risk of venous thromboembolism (VTE). The absolute risk is highest during and shortly after delivery. Although operative delivery further increases the risk of VTE, there is no consensus on thromboprophylaxis after an elective cesarean. Aim: The aim of the study was to investigate the frequency of symptomatic and asymptomatic deep venous thrombosis (DVT), after low risk cesarean section. **Materials and methods**: Sixty-four women undergoing low risk elective cesarean section were screened for asymptomactic DVT using triplex Doppler sonography 3-5 days after delivery. Markers of activated coagulation were also followed and all women were screened for thrombophilia. Postoperative thromboprophylaxis was not given. **Results**: No DVT was detected by ultrasonography and no women developed symptomatic VTE during the six weeks follow-up period after delivery. Six women had thrombophilia. Five women were excluded because of infection, bleeding, or on patients own request, but none of these developed symptomatic VTE. During the same period, the department had 5364 deliveries. A cesarean section was performed in 1067 (20%) of the cases. In this cohort, we diagnosed objectively five (0.47%) cases of symptomatic postoperative pulmonary embolism (PE). No cases of symptomatic DVT were seen. All cases of PE had additional risk factors like obesity, severe preeclampsia, twin pregnancy, reoperation, immobilization, and placenta previa. **Conclusion**: The risk of DVT after low-risk, elective cesarean section is low, and general medical thromboprophylaxis is probably not justified.

OC088

Placental vascular abnormalities in neonatal alloimmune thrombocytopenia (NAIT)

Weir E, Althaus J, Blakemore K, Askin F, Kickler T**

The Johns Hopkins Medical Institutions, Baltimore, Maryland, USA

Introduction: NAIT is associated with fetal and neonatal thrombocytopenia and potential hemorrhagic complications. While maternal alloantibodies cause platelet destruction and abnormal hemostasis in NAIT, they may also cause disruption of the fetoplacental vasculature due to reactivity with paternally-derived endothelial cell antigens. **Aim:** To study the hypothesis that anti-HPA antibodies affect placental function in NAIT. **Materials & Methods:** We reviewed H&E-stained placental histology from 14 consecutive cases of pregnancies that were complicated by NAIT due to anti-HPA1a, HPA3b and HPA5b antibodies. Immunoperoxidase (IPOX) analyses were performed in 10/14 cases to assess for the presence of placental vascular disruption. The staining patterns of PECAM, VEGF, von Willebrand factor (vWF) and Tissue Factor (TF) were studied and compared to those of gestational age-matched controls. These results were then correlated with the early administration of IVIg and clinical outcome. **Results:** Nine placentas demonstrated variable histologic findings compatible with hypoxic/ischemic changes (HIC) including infarction, thrombi, villous dysmaturity, villous necrosis and increased syncytial knots. Six placentas showed evidence of chronic villitis and 5 showed no pathologic changes. The IPOX expression of PECAM was limited to the vascular endothelium and highlighted villous dysmaturity in 4/6 cases. Relative to controls, vWF expression was increased in the endothelial cells in 8 cases and in villous stromal cells in 8 cases, and TF expression was increased in endothelial cells, trophoblasts, and/or stromal cells in all cases. Increased expression of vWF and TF showed no significant correlation with HIC or villitis. Stains for VEGF showed no increased expression in any of the cellular compartments of the placenta. Chronic villitis was observed in 5/6 cases without IVIg therapy, and in one case in which IVIg was initiated late in pregnancy. Three fetuses died in utero, 2 suffered intracranial hemorrhages, and 3 developed intrauterine growth retardation. Poor fetal outcome correlated strongly with the absence of IVIg therapy but not with placental pathology. **Conclusion:** NAIT is associated with placental pathology that is characteristic of hypoxic or ischemic insults. Moreover, the results of IPOX analyses are typical of those found in endothelial cell damage. In addition, IVIg therapy appears to be associated with the absence of chronic villitis and a favorable clinical outcome, though the mechanisms underlying these relationships remains unclear.

OC089

Diagnosing pulmonary embolism in pregnancy: rationalising fetal radiation exposure in radiological procedures

Nijkeuter M (1), Geleijns J (2), de Roos A (2), Ginsberg J (3), Scherjon S (4), Meinders A (1), Huisman M (1)*

(1) Department of Internal Medicine, University Medical Center, Leiden, the Netherlands

(2) Department of Radiology, University Medical Center, Leiden, the Netherlands

(3) Department of Medicine, Hamilton Health Sciences, Hamilton, Ontario, Canada

(4) Department of Gynaecology and Obstetrics, University Medical Center, Leiden, the Netherlands

Introduction In pregnancy, the diagnosis of pulmonary embolism is problematic. First, there is doubt as to whether objective diagnostic tests are needed. Second, there is no consensus as to what objective test is the safest with respect to fetal radiation exposure. Helical CT has become a useful diagnostic test in ruling out pulmonary embolism in non-pregnant patients. However, a lot of physicians are reluctant to perform a helical CT in pregnancy because of assumed elevated radiation exposure and fear of radiation effects to the fetus. Perfusion scintigraphy is often assumed to be safer with respect to radiation exposure than helical CT. **Aims** To resolve this diagnostic dilemma, we calculated fetal radiation exposure in single- and multi-detector row helical CT and perfusion(ventilation)-scintigraphy in diagnosing pulmonary embolism according to our local hospital protocols. Further, we compared our data with data of the literature. **Methods** Since there are no generic dosimetric methods available for establishing fetal doses, a pragmatic approach was used, i.e. fetal dose was assumed to be equal to the uterus dose of a non-pregnant woman. Organ dose to the patient from CT can be estimated by multiplying the measured computed tomography dose index with organ dose conversion factors that are available for a mathematical model of a standard patient. **Results** The calculated doses to the fetus for single-detector row helical CT was 0.0026 mSv and 0.013 mSv for multi-detector row helical CT. In comparison, perfusion scintigraphy as performed in our institution with an activity of 40 MBq in a pregnant patient, exposed the fetus to 0.11- 0.20 mSv. Ventilation scintigraphy with 600 MBq of Krypton, added 0,0001 mSv of radiation to the fetus. **Conclusion** Performing helical CT, either single- or multi-detector row, exposes the fetus to less radiation than with perfusion scintigraphy. These findings are important when deciding on a diagnostic algorithm in pregnant patients presenting with a clinical suspicion of pulmonary embolism.

OC090

Increased titer of antiphospholipid antibodies in women with high risk pregnancy

Hoppensteadt D, Cunanan J, Oplatek A, Fareed J*

Loyola University Medical Center, Maywood, IL 60153, USA

Introduction: Antiphospholipid syndrome (APLS) is an autoimmune disorder in which vascular thrombosis and recurrent pregnancy loss occur in patients with elevated levels of antibodies directed against negatively charged phospholipids. Antiphospholipid antibodies (APL) have been associated with repeated miscarriages and fetal loss. Other high-risk pregnancy complications such as preeclampsia, placental insufficiency, and preterm labor have also been studied previously and are classified as antiphospholipid syndrome-associated diseases. **Aims:** The aim of this study was to determine the titer and specific isotype of the APL antibodies since these are important determinants of the APLS-associated clinical outcomes and the choice of prophylactic treatment. **Materials and Methods:** We studied a population of high-risk pregnancy patients (n=300) in order to determine the level of APL IgG and APL IgM. The APL antibody titer was determined with a commercially available ELISA assay (American Diagnostica, Stamford, CT). In addition the dilute Russells viper venom time (DRVV Test, American Diagnostica) was also measured in the patients and the control population (n=70). The following groups of patients were included: preterm labor, pre-eclampsia, fetus small for gestational age and normal pregnancy. The control group was compromised of a group of healthy non-pregnant females. **Results:** Among the patients with high risk pregnancy, the IgM titers were elevated in 25-35% (>6.0 MPL U) of this group, whereas only 8 % of the normal population (including normal pregnancy) exhibited elevated IgM titers (>6.0 MPL U). Almost 10% of the high risk patients had elevated IgG titers (>6.0 GPL U), however only 4% of the normal population exhibited higher titers of this subtype. There was a correlation between elevated APL antibody IgM and IgG levels and progression of pregnancy associated complications when compared to nonpregnant females or females with normal pregnancy. The APL IgM isotype titers were higher than the APL IgG isotype. In the DRVVT assay, 90% of the normal volunteers and normal pregnant women had a clotting time of less than 35 seconds (20±7 s). In the high risk patients, the DRVVT was prolonged in 35% of the plasma samples (42±9 s). **Conclusions:** These results suggest the APL IgM titers maybe a better predictor of pregnancy associated complications in comparison to APL IgG and DRVV. These studies warrant further clinical validation in a larger patient population.

OC091

Inherited protein S deficiency type I, but not type III is a risk factor for venous, but not arterial thrombosis; a study in 81 families

Brouwer JLP (1), Veeger N (2), van der Schaaf W (1), Kluin-Nelemans H (1), van der Meer J (1)*

(1) Division of Hemostasis and Thrombosis, Department of Hematology, University Hospital Groningen, The

(2) Trial Coordination Centre, University Hospital Groningen, The Netherlands

Background. Free protein S (PS) is commonly measured to detect inherited PS deficiency. It is assumed that type I and III deficiencies are comparable thrombotic risk factors, though this still needs to be established. **Aim**. To assess the absolute risk of venous (VTE) and arterial thromboembolism (ATE) in families with inherited PS deficiencies, type I and type III, respectively. **Methods**. First degree relatives (age >15 year) of probands with symptomatic PS deficiency type I or III were studied in our centre. Information about previous episodes of VTE and ATE was collected prior to blood sampling. PS was measured by ELISA, free protein S after PEG precipitation. PS deficiency was considered inherited if decreased levels were demonstrated at repeated measurements in at least 2 family members, excluding acquired conditions. **Results**. 134 relatives of 33 PS type I deficient probands and 212 relatives of 48 PS type III deficient probands were enrolled. VTE had occurred in 20/53 (38%) type I deficient and 4/81 (5%) non-deficient relatives, ATE in 3/53 (6%) vs 3/81 (4%). Annual incidences of VTE were 1.92 (deficient) vs 0.16 (non-deficient); relative risk (RR) 11.84 (4.05-34.65; 95% CI). For ATE, 0.23 vs 0.12; RR 1.95 (0.39-9.64). PS type III deficient and non-deficient relatives had experienced VTE in 8/86 (9%) vs 9/126 (7%) and ATE in 5/86 (6%) vs 9/126 (7%). Annual incidences of VTE were 0.32 vs 0.24; RR 1.32 (0.51-3.43). For ATE, these were 0.19 vs 0.24; RR 0.80 (0.26-2.35). **Conclusion**. Of inherited PS deficiency, only type I is associated with increased risk of venous thrombosis, while neither type I nor type III were risk factors for arterial thrombosis.

OC092

Markers of inflammation, D-dimer and recurrences after a first episode of venous thromboembolism

Cosmi B, Legnani C, Guazzaloca G, Coccheri S, Palareti G*

Division of Angiology and Blood Coagulation, Unitŕ Ricerca Clinica sulla Trombofilia "M. Golinelli", Italy

Introduction: D-Dimer (D-d) has been shown to have a high negative predictive value for recurrence after oral anticoagulant therapy (OAT) withdrawal for a first episode of venous thromboembolism (VTE). Elevated D-d may express a chronic hypercoagulable state induced by mediators of inflammation such as cytokines. **Aim** of the study: to determine whether markers of inflammation are increased in patients with recurrent VTE and whether they correlate with D-d after OAT withdrawal for a first episode of VTE. **Materials and methods**: Symptomatic outpatients with a first episode of venous thromboembolism (deep vein thrombosis of the lower limbs DVT and/ or pulmonary embolism-PE) were prospectively followed-up after withdrawal of OAT. Plasma concentrations of interleukin 6 (IL-6), interleukin 8 (IL-8), monocyte chemotactic protein 1 (MCP-1), C-reactive protein (C-RP) (Turbiquant, Dade Behring, Milan Italy) and D-d (Vidas D-Dimer, BioMerieux, Rome, Italy) were measured at the time of OAT withdrawal (T0) and 3 months afterwards (T3). IL-6, IL-8 and MCP-1 were measured with commercial ELISA methods. Recurrent events were diagnosed in case of symptoms of DVT or PE by objective methods during a 2-year follow-up. **Results**: 207 patients were included in the study (M/F 109/98; mean age:66; age range:23-93). Total follow-up was 240 patient/years. Recurrent events were recorded in 14 patients (7%). IL-8 and MCP-1 did not differ significantly either at T0 or T3 between patients with a recurrence and patients without recurrence. D-d, IL-6 and C-RP levels increased significantly at T3 when compared to T0 in patients with recurrences when compared to patients without recurrences. C-RP and IL-6 correlated significantly with D-D at T3 in patients who experienced a recurrent event (r = 0.50). **Conclusions**: Our data indicate that C-RP and IL-6 correlate with increased D-Dimer levels and may be a risk factors for recurrence after a first episode of VTE.

OC093

Success of initiatives to familiarize vascular physicians in Germany with outpatient treatment of deep venous thrombosis

Werner B, Jürgen D, Horst E G*

Background: We intended to familiarize vascular physicians in private practices with outpatient treatment of acute deep venous thrombosis (DVT). Teachings were set up with the help of the Professional Union of Phlebologists of Germany and Leo Pharma GmbH, Germany. Interested physicians were invited to include patients in a registry. The survey (study I) was concluded 12/2000 and the results were published. Participating centers were asked to report their experience a second time covering the period from 01/2002 to 06/2002 (study II). **Method**: Data were collected on the reasons for sending a patient to the hospital and on the results of outpatient treatment, respectively. Outpatients were anticoagulated with the low-molecular-weight heparin tinzaparin followed by phenprocoumon. Leg compression and deliberate ambulation were part of the treatment protocol. Follow-up covered the first 4 weeks after diagnosis. **Results**: 354 vascular physicians were instructed in a whole-day briefing session. 67 centres registered 827 patients in study I and 26 of the most active centres (providing 352 patients for study I) included 540 consecutive patients in study II. Outpatient treatment was performed in 76% of patients in the first and 92% in the second study. It increased from 93% to 97% for crural DVT, from 73% to 94% for popliteal, from 70% to 88% for femoral and from 38% to 65% for pelvic DVT. Medical reasons for hospital admissions decreased from 88% to 12% ($p<0.01$) while personal reasons remained the same. During follow-up no clinical suspicion of progression or recurrence was raised. In study I, compliance with tinzaparin was 96.3% and PT values were in the target range in 81% of assays (mean INR 2.2; 95%CI 2.0-2.3). No such data were collected in study II. Leg compression was performed in all but a few patients. The initial use of bandages decreased from 77% in study I to 23% in study II while the immediate application of stockings increased from 29% to 71% ($p<0.05$). **Conclusion**: Outpatient treatment of DVT by vascular physicians who received a specific instruction was effective. The experience led to the selection of more patients for this cost-efficient therapy.

OC094

Cost-effectiveness of bemiparin in the acute and long-term treatment of deep vein thrombosis

Rocha E (1), Gómez-Outes A (2), Martínez-González J (2)*, Kakkar V (3)*

(1) University Clinic of Navarra, Pamplona, Spain
(2) Laboratorios Farmacéuticos ROVI, S.A., Madrid, Spain
(3) Thrombosis Research Institute, London, UK

Introduction: The traditional treatment of patients with acute deep vein thrombosis (DVT) has been with unfractionated heparin (UFH) plus oral anticoagulants (OAC). **Aims:** To assess the cost-effectiveness of two regimens of bemiparin 115 IU/kg/d for 7-10 days (plus OAC or followed by long-term bemiparin 3,500 IU for three months) vs. dose-adjusted UFH for 7 days plus OAC for three months in the acute and long-term treatment of DVT. **Material and methods:** We performed a cost-effectiveness analysis by using a decision modelling approach. We expressed our results in terms of costs and incremental cost-effectiveness in euros (€). We considered for this analysis the treatment costs and costs derived from complications: recurrent DVT and/or pulmonary embolism, bleeding events, thrombocytopenia and deaths. The study perspective was the Spanish National Health System. The time horizon chosen was 3 months. **Results:** Total costs per patient (treatment costs and costs derived from complications) during a 3-month period were €4,128 for UFH plus OAC, €3,359 for bemiparin 115 IU/kg/d plus OAC and €3,220 for bemiparin 115 IU/kg/d followed by long-term bemiparin 3,500 IU/d. The use of bemiparin plus OAC or long-term bemiparin were associated with Euro cost savings of €769 and €908 respectively, compared to UFH plus OAC in the treatment of one patient with DVT during a 3-month period. Long-term treatment with bemiparin was associated with cost savings of €139 when compared to bemiparin plus OAC. Hospital stay was reduced in 2 and 3 days respectively in patients receiving bemiparin plus OAC or long-term bemiparin compared to patients who received UFH plus OAC. Bemiparin plus OAC or long-term bemiparin were more cost-effective than UFH plus OAC in all the ranges tested for complications and costs (sensitivity analysis). The reduction in hospital stay length and the effectiveness in preventing death and recurrent VTE were the most important factors on incremental cost-effectiveness ratio. **Conclusions:** Bemiparin plus OAC or long-term bemiparin were more cost-effective than UFH plus OAC in the initial and long-term treatment of DVT. Bemiparin offers the major benefit of convenient dosing, subcutaneous administration, no need of monitoring its anticoagulation effect in most patients and facilitation for treating patients at home. Long-term bemiparin is a cost-effective alternative to oral anticoagulants.

OC095

Outpatient tinzaparin therapy in 102 patients with pulmonary embolism - final results

Olsson (1), Bajc M (2), Bitzén U (2), Carlsson MS (3), Elf J (1), Jönsson K (3), Magnusson P (1), Olsson B (2), Jonson B (2)*

(1) Internal Medicine, University Hospital Lund, Sweden
(2) Clinical Physiology, University Hospital Lund, Sweden
(3) Internal Medicine, Central Hospital Växjö, Sweden

Introduction: Pulmonary embolism (PE) is usually treated in hospital. However, outpatient therapy is safe in deep vein thrombosis, although 32 % of such patients also have PE. Thus, it seems likely that outpatient therapy of small and medium-sized PE may also be safe. Aims: A) to identify patients suitable for therapy outside hospital wards, B) to evaluate tinzaparin for outpatient therapy, C) to follow long-term results of patients included. Patients and Methods: 100 patients were prospectively included. Initial symptoms were pain at breaths, cough, anxiety and insomnia. Mean age was 60.6 years. Echocardiography, lung X-ray, D-dimer and other blood specimens were taken. To select patients we measured extension of PE with quantitative planar or tomographic ventilation/perfusion scintigraphy (V/PSCINT or V/PSPECT). We scored 1 point for segmental Reduction of Ventilation (RoVent) or Reduction of Perfusion (RoPer) and 2 points for segmental absence. For inclusion at most 14 RoPer and 7 RoVent points were allowed. Daily s.c. injections of tinzaparin and oral anticoagulation were given in a patient hotel. Clinical follow up and V/P scan was repeated before discharge and at 6 months. Two reviewers blinded for the order of examination evaluated V/P scans. Results: The mean hotel stay was 4.6 days. Initial average mismatch score (RoPer – RoVent) was 5.7 and at follow up 5 days later only 3.3 No thromboembolic mortality was encountered. Three patients died from other diseases, within 2-4 months. Eleven patients reentered hospital due to pain, hyperglycemia or confusion. V/P scan improved in 78 %, unchanged in 13 % patients and worsened in 9 %. Conclusions: 1) Outpatient therapy was safe in small and medium-sized PE. 2) Some patients (11%) reentered hospital. 3) Interestingly, after tinzaparin for 5 days, reduction of perfusion defects by 42%, WBC by 40% and CRP by 51% was observed. 4) Quantitative V/P scan is ideal to measure extension of PE before and after therapy.

OC096

Analysis of predisposing factors and 6 month outcomes of DVT management in 668 patients treated with LMWH(tinzaparin) as outpatients

Rhodes S, Bond S, Green E*

Haematology Department, Great Western Hospital, Swindon, UK

In Swindon, eligible patients with a suspected or proven DVT are treated as outpatients using a once daily low molecular weight heparin (LMWH). Prospective audit using an electronic database has been ongoing since 1998. As a result of this data analysis we can identify patients at greater risk of recurrent thromboembolic disease and bleeding complications. As of August 2003 there was a total cohort of 717 patients: average age was 61 years, with 53% female patients. The major predisposing factors were recorded as immobility (32.5%), previous VTE (21.3%) and surgery (14.8%). 6-month follow-up data were available for 668 patients: 20 (3.0%) patients had confirmed thromboembolic complications, of which 18 (2.7%) occurred subsequent to the initial LMWH treatment phase (late). Bleeding complications occurred in 12 (1.8%), with 4 (0.6%) being classified as major- 3 gastrointestinal bleeds and 1 retroperitoneal haematoma. Of the 20 confirmed thromboembolic complications 2 (10%) had no predisposing factor at initial presentation. Other risk factors were malignancy (6 events), immobility (6 events), surgery/trauma (4 events), oral contraceptive/ HRT use (3 events), previous VTE (2 events), family history of VTE (2 events) and a long haul flight (1 event). 6 patients had more than 1 risk factor. 2 of the patients had 2 events and both of these patients had a malignancy. Incidence of thromboembolic and bleeding events at 6 months were low (comparable with clinical trial data and other UK audit data) in our centre. The most significant risk factors for recurrent thromboembolic complications were malignancy and immobilty. The database has allowed analysis of the data over different time periods enabling us to show that the service has been extended to more patients but with a reduction in complication rates. The service is now beginning to manage selected patients with a confirmed PE on an ambulatory basis.

OC097

Haplotypes of the EPCR gene, plasma sEPCR levels and the risk of deep venous thrombosis

Uitte de Willige S, van Marion V, Rosendaal F, Vos H, de Visser M, Bertina R*

Introduction The endothelial cell protein C receptor (EPCR) is an important component of the protein C (PC) pathway. Binding of PC to EPCR stimulates PC activation by increasing the affinity of PC for the thrombin-thrombomodulin complex. A soluble form of this receptor (sEPCR) circulates in plasma and inhibits both PC activation and APC anticoagulant activity. We hypothesized that variations in the EPCR gene and/or plasma sEPCR levels might influence the risk of deep venous thrombosis. **Aims** The aim of this study was to investigate whether variations in the EPCR gene and/or plasma sEPCR levels are risk factors for deep venous thrombosis. **Materials and methods** In a large population-based case-control study on risk factors for venous thrombosis, the Leiden Thrombophilia Study (LETS), plasma sEPCR levels were measured by ELISA (Asserachrom®, Diagnostica Stago). In addition, all subjects were genotyped with the TaqMan assay (Applied Biosystems) for 3 haplotype-tagging (ht) SNPs (H1: T3997C, H2: all common, H3: A4600G, H4: G3811A) in the EPCR gene. For the statistical analyses we excluded all users of oral anticoagulants (OAC), because of the significant influence of OAC on sEPCR levels. **Results** We found one haplotype (H4) to be associated with a 40% increased risk of venous thrombosis (OR=1.4, 95%CI: 1.0-2.2). H2 and H3 were not associated with an increased risk, whereas H1 showed a slightly decreased risk (OR=0.8, 95%CI: 0.6-1.1). High sEPCR levels (above 75th percentile, ≥137 ng/ml) are associated with a 40% increased risk of thrombosis (OR=1.4, 95%CI: 1.1-1.9). Low levels (below 25th percentile, ≤81 ng/ml) are associated with a decreased risk (OR=0.6, 95%CI: 0.4-0.8). The distribution of plasma sEPCR levels in the control population is trimodal. Individuals carrying two H3-specific 4600 G alleles have significantly higher sEPCR levels (439 ng/ml, 95%CI: 399-478) than GA heterozygotes (258 ng/ml, 95%CI: 248-269), which have again significantly higher levels than AA carriers (94 ng/ml, 95%CI: 91-96). 86.5% of the variation in sEPCR levels can be explained by the htSNP for H3 (see also Saposnik et al., Blood 2003; 103(4)). **Conclusions** The trimodal distribution of the sEPCR levels in the control group is genetically controlled by H3 of the EPCR gene. H4 of the EPCR gene is associated with a 40% increased risk of thrombosis. Also variations in sEPCR levels influence thrombosis risk.

OC098

Expression and characterization of a new factor V mutation (R1698W) found in combination with FV Leiden

*Lunghi B (1), Scanavini D (1), Ulazzi L (1), Busani C (1), Redaelli R (2), Tagariello G (3), Bernardi F (1)**

(1) Dipartimento di Biochimica e Biologia Molecolare, Università di Ferrara, Italia
(2) Divisione di Ematologia, Ospedale Niguarda, Milano, Italia
(3) Servizio Trasfusionale, Centro Regionale per le Malattie del Sangue e Servizio di assistenza agli Em

Introduction and aims Among the several acquired and genetic factors, which could modulate the APC resistance levels in carriers of the FV Leiden, and the associated thrombotic risk, we have investigated the intragenic determinants of FV levels. In particular we focused our research on the combination of FV Leiden with polymorphisms and mutations present in the FV counterpart gene. **Materials and methods** Selection of FV Leiden heterozygotes with low FV Levels (FVC<60%). Detection of FV mutations by sequencing of FV exons and splicing junctions. Expression into COS-7 cells of a mutagenized FV cDNA construct. Prothrombinase-based assay and ELISA of recombinant FV in conditioned media. **Results and Conclusions** We report the identification in a FV Leiden carrier (FVAg 46%, FVC 41%; APC res 0.64-0.67) of a novel FV gene mutation, predicting the substitution of Arg 1698 by a Trp in the exon 15. The R1698W change is located in the A3 domain in a contact loop with A2 domain. We also screened a group of 30 FV deficient subjects (FV:C range <1-58%) and found a subject (FV:C 29%) heterozygous for the R1698W FV mutation. This subject was doubly heterozygous for the H1299R mutation (HR2 haplotype), that has been previously found associated to slightly lower FV levels and could explain the FV levels well below 50%. In 7 independent transfections the mean antigen levels of the recombinant 1698W FV in conditioned media was indistinguishable from Wt, whereas the activity in a prothrombinase assay was significantly reduced (42%). The reduction in activity to half was maintained at 0.1-10 nM FXa. Moreover, in coagulation assay (PT assay in FV depleted plasma) the 1698W FV showed 50% activity as compared to Wt. In 4 time-course incubation experiments in FV depleted plasma at 37 C°, the decay in activity of the recombinant 1698W FV was found to be increased as compared with Wt (difference of slopes, p=0.007), which could provide an explanation for the reduced amount of 1698W FV molecules in plasma of subjects carrying this mutation. Although the expression data indicate the causative nature of the R1698W mutation, the interpretation of its relationships with APC resistance levels found in plasma of the FV Leiden carrier requires further investigation.

OC099

Genetic markers of inflammation and sensitivity to activated protein C (APC)

González-Ordóñ A (1), Macias D (2), Arias A (1), Fernández-Carreira JM (3), Morán M (1), Peliz M (4), Martín L (1)*

(1) Department of Hematology. Hospital S. Agustín. Avilés. SPAIN
(2) Department of Internal Medicine. Hospital S. Agustín. Avilés. SPAIN
(3) Research Unit. Hospital S. Agustín. Avilés. SPAIN
(4) Department of Emergencies. Hospital S. Agustín. Avilés. SPAIN

The phenotype of activated protein C (APC) resistance is involved in thrombosis independently of the factor V Leiden (FVL) status. The sensitivity to the anticoagulant activity of APC seems related with pregnancy, estrogens, lupus anticoagulant or increased FVIIIc also among FVL(-) individuals but the mechanisms responsible for this variability are not yet fully understood. Inflammation is a key component of vascular diseases and thrombosis. Therefore, the genes coding for cytokines could be theoretical candidates to explain some variability in FVIIIc and the related sensitivity to APC. **Population and methods.** From a randomly chosen population, we selected 108 FVL(-) subjects including 56 men and 52 women with a mean age of 60.7(12.9) years (range: 26-83 y) and a body mass index (BMI) of 27.5(4.1) Kg*m^{-2}. We genotyped (by PCR-RFLP) for three functional polymorphisms located in the genes encoding for cytokines: two in a promoter region [-174G>C of interleukin-6 (IL-6) and -2518 A>G of monocyte chemoattractant protein-1 (MCP-1)] and +3954 C>T in the exon 5 of the interleukin-1beta (IL-1b) gene. We analyzed the serum levels of IL-1b, IL-6 and MCP-1 by an ELISA method, the normalized APC sensitivity ratio (n-APC-SR) by a commercial APTT-based test and the procoagulant activity of the FVIII (FVIIIc). **Results.** In the overall series the n-APC-SR was 0.96(0.13) (range: 0.68-1.34) being similar in both gender. The n-APC-SR was independent of the BMI and probably inversely related with the age (r= -0.18, p= 0.06). The FVIIIc relates inversely with the sensitivity to the APC (r= -0.40, p <0.001). The n-APC-SR was related with the MCP-1 polymorphism (ANOVA, p<0.05) and marginally with the IL-1b polymorphism (p=0.05) but not with the serum levels of these cytokines. The 50 subjects with the G allele of MCP-1 (-2518 AG or GG genotypes) have a lower n-APC-SR than the homozygous carriers of the A allele [0.92(0.13) vs. 0.99(0.12), p< 0.01, student't test] although the activity for the FVIIIc was non-significantly higher [(151(50) vs. 139(37) U/dl, NS p]. Similarly, the rare subjects with the homozygous variant genotype of the IL-1b (+3954 TT) have a trend to a lower n-APC-SR than the rest [0.87(0.17) vs. 0.98(0.16), p= 0.06] although the activity for the FVIIIc was similar. **Conclusion.** We suggest the association between sensitivity to the APC and certain inflammatory mechanisms independently of the FVIIIc influence.

OC100

Frequency of cytochrome CYP2C9 polymorphism in Russian Population and it effects in 62 patients treated by warfarin

Vavilova T (1), Sirotkina O (2), Ulitina A (1), Kadinskaya M (1), Schwarzman A (2)*

(1) Saint-Petersburg Pavlov State Medical University, Saint-Petersburg, Russia
(2) Petersburg Nuclear Physics Institute RAS, Saint-Petersburg, Russia

The metabolism and elimination of warfarin are due to oxidation by cytochrome P450 family – CYP2C9. The enzymatic activity of this cytochrome is reduces in CYP 2C9*2 (Arg144Cys) and CYP 2C9*3 (Ile359Leu) variant alleles carriers. The presence of polymorphisms may associate with increased sensibility to warfarin and with risk of bleeding during treatment by oral anticoagulant (OAT). **Materials and methods.** The study included 297 persons, 44±2 years old from St.-Petersburg, Russia: 186 healthy men and 111 patients with documented thrombotic events or high thrombotic risk. Genotyping was done by PCR and RFLP with *KpnI*, *AvaII* и *Mph1103I*. 62 patients were on a long-term OAT because of primary or secondary thromboprophilaxis (the target level of INR from 2,0 up to 3,5). The mean maintenance warfarin dose and the duration of induction period from the beginning of treatment to target INR were studied. **Results.** Among the investigated persons 202 individuals (68%) had the wild-tipe CYP2C9*1/*1 genotype and 95 patients (32%) had at least 1 variant CYP2C9 -*2 or*3 allele with an allele distribution similar to that previously reported in Caucasians. The mean maintenance dose warfarin was lower and the induction period from the beginning of treatment to target INR was shorter in CYP2C9*2 or*3 carriers. The maintenance doses were 43.65±2.17, 31.87±2.27, 22.75±3.50 and 17,5 mg/week in subjects with CYP2C9*1/*1, CYP2C9*1/*2, CYP2C9*1/*3 and CYP2C9*2/*3 genotypes, respectively (p<0.05). The induction periods were 5.40±0.45, 4.22±0.64, 2.75±1.03 and 2 days in subjects with CYP2C9*1/*1, CYP2C9*1/*2, CYP2C9*1/*3 and CYP2C9*2/*3 genotypes, respectively (p<0.001). **Conclusion.** Cytochrome CYP2C9 gene polymorphisms investigation has the important clinical significance in selection and individualization of warfarin dosage and may prevent the over-coagulation in the initiation of therapy. The high frequency of*2 or*3 allele variants may be the reason to CYP2C9 genotype examination to optimize the OAT.

OC101

TNFR1 +36 G/G genotype and the metabolic syndrome both predispose obese women to higher levels of soluble TNFRs, PAI-1 and liver enzymes

Mavri A (1, 2), Bastelica D (1), Saut N (1), Verdier M (1), Renucci J (3), Juhan-Vague I (1), Alessi MC (1)

(1) Laboratory of Hematology, UMR 626, Faculty of Medicine, Marseille, France
(2) University Medical Centre, Dpt of Vascular disease, Ljubljana, Slovenia
(3) CDPA, CHU Timone, Marseille, France

Introduction: The metabolic syndrome (MS) includes obesity and several metabolic, hepatic, and fibrinolytic (mainly elevated levels of plasminogen activator inhibitor-1, PAI-1) abnormalities leading to an increased risk of diabetes and cardiovascular mortality. Inflammation may have an important role in the development of MS especially tumor necrosis factor (TNF), which actions are mediated by two receptors (TNFRs). **Aims**: We have examined whether polymorphisms in TNFRs genes may influence metabolic, inflammatory (IL6, CRP, TNF, TNFRs), PAI-1 and liver (ALT) levels in the MS. **Materials and Methods**: TNFR1 +36A/G and TNFR2 +587T/G polymorphisms were evaluated in 183 obese (BMI: 33.8±3.6 kg/m²) and 165 lean (21.9±2.1 kg/m²) women. Patients were grouped according to WHO criteria in those with (MS+; n=31) or without (MS-) the MS. Plasma levels of metabolic, inflammatory, liver parameters and PAI-1 were analyzed by routine biochemical methods or ELISA. **Results**: Obese subjects exhibit higher levels of all the studied parameters except TNF than lean subjects. MS+ and MS- groups differed significantly for all the studied parameters except for inflammatory markers. None of the metabolic parameters was associated with the two polymorphisms. Obese women TNFR1G/G had significantly higher concentrations of TNFR1 (879.9±223.4 vs 772.1±151.4 pg/ml, p<0.002), PAI-1 (65.39±52.75 vs 47.73±36.13 ng/ml, p<0.03) and liver enzymes (ALT: 24.8±32.1 vs 15.5±9.6 IU/l, p<0.005) than obese women carriers for A allele. These differences were not modified after adjustment for alcohol consumption. Differences in TNFR1 and PAI-1 levels were maintained in the MS+ (p<0.003 and p<0.01 respectively) but not in the MS- group. No differences were observed with the TNFR2 polymorphism. **Conclusions**: TNFR1 gene polymorphism is associated with plasma TNFR1, PAI-1, liver enzymes levels in obese women. These results provide evidence that TNFR1 GG genotype and the MS interact in the development of fibrinolytic and liver anomalies found in obesity.

OC102

Fibrinogen polymorphisms Taq I, Hae III and Bcl I are not major risk factors for deep-vein thrombosis

Božič M (1), Teran N (2), Peterlin B (2), Stegnar M (1)*

(1) Department of Vascular Diseases, University Medical Centre, Ljubljana, Slovenia
(2) Department of Gynaecology and Obstetrics, University Medical Centre, Ljubljana, Slovenia

Background and aim: It is not clear whether high plasma fibrinogen levels represent a risk factor for deep-vein thrombosis (DVT). It has been shown that certain polymorphisms in fibrinogen genes can influence the fibrinogen level. The aim was to determine if fibrinogen levels and polymorphisms Taq I (a-fibrinogen), Hae III (b-fibrinogen) and Bcl I (b-fibrinogen) increase risk for DVT. Subjects and methods: One hundred and fourteen patients with objectively confirmed DVT and 244 healthy subjects were included in the study. From all subjects blood was drawn on one occasion for the determination of fibrinogen level by the clotting method (Multifibren U, Dade Behring) and the presence of TaqI (common allele T1), HaeIII (common allele H1) or BclI (common allele B1) polymorphism. For the identification of the polymorphisms the relevant DNA regions were multiplied by PCR. TaqI polymorphism was detected regarding the amplicon size by GeneScan (Abi Prism 310, Applied Biosystems); the common allele (184 bp) was coded as T1 and the rare allele (212 bp) as T2. The Hae III polymorphism was detected by real-time PCR on a LightCycler (Roche) using the relevant hybridisation probes. The common allele was coded as H1 and the rare allele as H2. The Bcl I polymorphism was genotyped by digestion with the Bcl I endonuclease. The common allele was coded as B1 and the rare allele as B2. Results: Fibrinogen levels adjusted for age, gender and LDL-cholesterol were similar in patients and healthy subjects. However, in non-smokers fibrinogen levels above 5 g/l were associated with an increased risk of DVT (odds ratio 3.3, 95% CI 1.6-7.0). The frequencies of common alleles T1 (TaqI polymorphism), H1 (HaeIII polymorphism) and B1 (BclI polymorphism) were similar in patients (0.74, 0.66-0.82, 0.75, 0.67-0.83 and 0.78, 0.70-0.86, respectively) and controls (0.73, 0.67-0.79, 0.72, 0.66-0.78 and 0.77, 0.72-0.82). In controls T2 allele was associated with lower fibrinogen (2.88±0.84 g/l for T1T1, 2.80 ± 0.74 g/l for T1T2 and 2.42 ± 0.83 g/l for T2T2, ANOVA p=0.06). Alleles H2 and B2 were associated with higher fibrinogen only in non-smoking controls (2.70 ± 0.68 g/l for H1H1, 2.96 ± 0.79 g/l for H1H2 and 2.46 ± 0.42 g/l for H2H2, ANOVA p=0.04 and 2.68 ± 0.72 g/l for B1B1, 2.98 ± 0.75 g/l for B1B2 and 2.48 ± 0.30 g/l for B2B2, ANOVA p=0.07). On the contrary, either in all patients or in non-smoking patients no association was found between the polymorphisms and fibrinogen level. Conclusion: High fibrinogen increases the risk for DVT. The lack of an association between polymorphisms and DVT suggests that there is no major pathogenic role of these polymorphisms in DVT.

OC103

Inherited risk factors for ischemic stroke

Sirotkina O (1), Tcherkas Y (2), Elchaninov A (3), Merkulova A (4), Chukhlovina M (4), Denisenko A (2), Schwarzman A (1)*

(1) Petersburg Nuclear Physics Institute RAS, Russia
(2) Research Institute for Experimental Medicine, Saint-Petersburg, Russia
(3) Sokolov Central Hospital, Saint-Petersburg, Russia
(4) Saint-Petersburg State Pediatric Medical Academy, Russia

Introduction. Stroke and ischemic heart disease are the major causes of death and disability in industrial countries. Ischemic stroke is uncommon at young age and large proportions of stroke have undetermined etiology. **Aims.** The aim of our study was to determine the inherited risk factors for ischemic stroke. **Materials and Methods.** 148 relatively young individuals (83 males and 65 females, mean age 43.6±0.4) with ischemic stroke and 321 healthy control subjects (199 males and 122 females, mean age 40.8±0.4) were taken into analisys. Factor V Leiden mutation, 20210GA polymorphism in the prothrombin gene, G-455A in the β-fibrinogene gene, the 4G/5G PAI-1, C677T transition in the MTHFR gene, PlA1A2 GP III polymorphism and A1/A2 insertion promoter polymorphism in the factor VII gene were analyzed by PCR and RFLP. The total plasma homocysteine levels (tHcy) were estimated in patients group. **Results.** A significant increase in the prevalence of T677 MTHFR in patients with stroke compared to controls was found (allele frequency 33% and 27%, respectively, p=0.03, OR=1.47, CI 95% 1.08-2.0). The maximal tHcy level was observed in carriers TT genotype MTHFR - 17.5±2.2 μmol/l compared with 10.5±0.5 μmol/l and 12.0±0.8 μmol/l in carriers CC and CT genotype, respectively (p=0.002). A significant decrease in the prevalence of the protective A2 allele of the factor VII gene in patients with stroke compared to controls was also found (allele frequency 8.8% and 13.1%, respectively, p=0.04, OR=1.61, CI 95% 1.06-2.45). We observed gene-gene interaction between T677 allele of the MTHFR gene and A1A1 genotype of the factor VII gene (OR=1.9 CI 95% 1.39-2.59). **Conclusion.** The T677 allele of MTHFR gene associated with higher tHcy level and thrombophilic A1A1 genotype of the factor VII gene might play the important role in development of cerebrovascular decease and serve as the inherited risk factors for ischemic stroke.

OC104

Inherited prothrombotic risk factors (factor V G1691A, factor II G20210A, MTHFR C677T and platelet polymorphisms in pediatric ischemic stroke

Oliveira L (1), Ozelo M (2), Rossi F (2), Annichino-Bizzacchi JM (2), Moura-Ribeiro M (1), Castro V (2)*

(1) Neurology Department, Medical School, State University of Campinas - UNICAMP
(2) Hematology and Hemotherapy Center, State University of Campinas - UNICAMP

Pediatric stroke incidence is estimated at 2.5 cases in 100,000 per year, with about half of reported events being of ischemic origin. Risk factors include cardiac disease, vascular abnormalities or damage, infectious diseases and inherited or acquired coagulation prothrombotic abnormalities, such as anticardiolipin antibody, lupus anticoagulant, protein C, S and antithrombin deficiencies. Inherited prothrombotic risk factors include factor V G1691A, factor II G20210A, MTHFR C677T. Platelet polymorphisms such as HPA-1b, HPA-2b, HPA-5a, C807T and -5TC Kozak polymorphisms have been associated with stroke in adults but few reports are available in children, especially when associated to other inherited prothrombotic risk factors. Also, the impact of these risk factors may vary in different countries with distinct ethnic backgrounds. In these study, 23 children (13 female, 10 male, mean age 4 years, var.: 0-13y) presenting ischemic stroke confirmed by image methods were evaluated to protein C and S deficiency, presence of antiphospholipid, anticardiolipin antibodies (abs), and G1691A, G20210A, C677T mutations, as well as platelet HPA-1, -2 , -5/C807T haplotypes, and –5TC Kozak polymorphisms. Anticardiolipin ab was detected in 4 (17.4%) patients, protein C deficiency in 3 (13%), protein S deficiency in 1 (4.4%), anticardiolipin ab in 4 (17.4%) and antiphospholipid ab in 1(4.4%) patient. The evaluation of inherited prothrombotic risk factors showed a higher frequency of HPA-1b homozygous (8.7%) and HPA-2b homozygous (8.7%) than that previously described in our population (1.0% and 3.0%) but this difference failed to reach statistical significancy. No correlation was found in these patients with other platelet polymorphisms. G20210A mutation in heterozygozity was found in one patient (4.4%), G1691A mutation and C677T homozygous were not detected in any patients. This is the first report on pediatric stroke patients in which all these genetic risk factors were evaluated together. Our data suggest that platelet polymorphisms may have a role in pediatric stroke and reinforce the multifactorial characteristic of the disease.

OC105

Congenital thrombophilia in patients with cerebral ischemia and patent foramen ovalis (PFO)

Pengo V (1), Zanchetta M (2), Pedon L (2), Carrozza A (2), Bison E (1), Biasiolo A (1), Maiolino P (2), Iliceto S (1)*

(1) Clinical Cardiology, University of Padova, Italy
(2) Department of Cardiovascular Diseases, Cittadella(PD) Hospital, Italy

Causes of cerebral ischemia comprise atherothrombosis of arteries originating from the aortic arch and subsequent artery-to-artery embolism, thromboembolism from cardiac chambers, non-thrombotic occlusion of intracerebral penetrating arteries, other rare or unknown causes. Among cardiogenic cerebral ischemic events, those resulting from thrombi formed in right heart chambers or venous circulation migrating into the left part of the heart define the paradoxical embolism. In the same way of venous thromboembolism, thrombus formation in paradoxical embolism may be related to the presence of congenital thrombofilia. Aim of this study was to test for congenital thrombofilia subjects with cerebral ischemia undergoing cardiac intervention to close a Patent Foramen Ovalis (PFO) at the Cittadella hospital. Sixty consecutive patients, mean age 58 years, 32 males and 28 females, were studied for the presence of R506Q Factor V mutation (Factor V Leiden) and G20210A Factor II mutation (Prothrombin Variant). Five out of 60 studied patients (8.3%) compared to 4.2% in normal healthy subjects of Veneto Region area had Factor V Leiden (OR=1.8, 95% CI 0.8-3.2, p=0.3). Three patients were heterozygous and 1 patient was homozygous for this mutation. No difference in prothrombin variant was also detected among patients (2 out of 60, 3.3% as compared to normal subjects (4,2%, p=ns). In conclusion, the rate of congenital thrombophilia in these series is not significantly higher with respect to normal subjects. Thus, congenital thrombophilia does not explain these cases of paradoxical embolism. However, only a complete study of both inherited and acquired thrombophilia will make clear its role in the pathogenesis of cerebral ischemia in these patients.

OC106

Lipoprotein(a) and C-reactive protein in children with cerebrovascular events

Zrinski Topić R (1), Coen D (1), Fuček M (1), Miloš M (1), Leniček-Krleža J (2), Dodig S (3)*

(1) 1Clinical Institute of Laboratory Diagnosis, Zagreb University School of Medicine and Clinical Hospi
(2) 2Department of Laboratory Diagnosis and Neuropediatrics, Children˘s Hospital, Zagreb, Croatia
(3) Special Hospital for Respiratory Disease in Children and Adolescents, Zagreb, Croatia

Introduction: Cerebrovascular events in children, half of which are ischemic stroke, occur at an estimated incidence of about 2 per 100000 per year. The pathogenesis of atherosclerosis begins in childhood. Increased C-reactive protein (CRP) is a important predictor of cardiovascular events, independent of traditional risk factors. Elevated lipoprotein (a) (Lp(a)) has been identified as a genetically determined risk factor for stroke in young adults. Only preliminary data are available on theirs role as a risk factors for ischemic stroke in children. **Aim**: The aim of the study was to examine the prevalence of two atherosclerotic risk factors in children with cerebrovascular events. **Materials and methods**: Serum samples were obtained 3-6 months after acute phase of disease from 29 children (17 males and 12 females; age range 2-17 years) with a history of arterial ischemic stroke (AIS, n=14) and transient ischemic attack (TIA; n=15). The diagnosis were based on patient's history, clinical and neurological examination. Control group was 26 healthy children (15 males and 11 females; age range 2-15 years). CRP was measured by latex-enhanced nephelometry (N High Sensitivity CRP, Dade Behring). Lp(a) was quantified by immunoturbidimetric assay (Tina-quant, Roche Diagnostics). **Results**: By using cut-off value for CRP of 1,1 mg/L (90th percentile) we found a significantly higher frequency of elevated CRP values in children with a history of AIS (6 of 14; 43%) compared with control subjects (2 of 26; 8%). In addition, in this group of patients was higher frequency of Lp(a) values above 0.3 g/L (4 of 14; 29%) compared with control subjects (5 of 26; 19%). No difference in frequency of CRP and Lp(a) values were observed between children with a history of TIA and control group. **Conclusion**: Despite a low number of children in each group it seems that CRP and Lp(a) are important risk factor for arterial ischemic stroke in childhood.

OC107

Genetic determinants of hyperhomocysteinemia in ischemic stroke: the Role of MTHFR (C677T and A1298C), TSER and MTR A2756G

Kim N (1), Oh D (1), Park S (2)*

(1) Institute for Clinical Research, College of Medicine, Pochon CHA University, Seongnam 463-712, South Korea
(2) Department of Internal Medicine, College of Medicine, Seoul National University, Seoul 110-799, South Korea

Ischemic vascular disease is the leading cause of death in developed countries and is also emerging health problem. Hyperhomocysteinemia ia a risk factor for cerebrovascular and cardiovascular disease in general population. Although the mutations in homocysteine metabolism-related enzyme genes including methylenetetrahydrofolate reductase (MTHFR C677T and A1298C), thymidylate synthase enhancer region (TSER) and methionine synthase (MTR A2756G), possibly increase the risk of ischemic stroke, the data are still controversal. We aimed to study the role of these mutations in Korean population with 275 ischemic stroke patients and 223 healthy controls. (1) We found that adjusted odds ratio (AOR) of the 677TT genotype was not significantly higher in ischemic stroke patients than that in controls. (2) The odds ratio and 95% CI adjusted for the other risk factors were 2.13 (1.06 to 4.27) for the MTHFR 1298AC genotype. In addition, the adjusted OR for the 1298AC/CC genotype were significantly higher than in the controls (AOR, 2.35; 95% CI, 1.20 to 4.62). We found the MTHFR A1298C polymorphism is an independent risk factor for cerebral infarction. (3) Fasting homocysteine levels in plasma of ischemic stroke patients were significantly higher in TS 2R allele containing genotypes (2R2R, 2R3R) than without 2R allele containing genotypes (3R3R, 3R4R, 3R5R) (P=0.0229). Moreover, plasma homocysteine levels were significantly higher in 2R allele containing genotypes of ischemic stroke patients than that in controls (P=0.0398). However, these were not significant for patients in without 2R allele containing genotypes. (4) The prevalence of MTR 2756AG and GG genotypes alone did not differ between individuals with extremely high or extremely low tHcy levels. Combined MTR and MTHFR genotypes (MTR 2756AG and GG and MTHFR 677TT/AA and 677CT/ 1298AC) were found more often in the highest (n=4) compared with the lowest plasma tHcy decile (n=1). Our study shows that the 2756 A->G transition of MTR in combination with MTHFR 677TT/1298AA and 677CT/1298AC can be associated with extremely high tHcy plasma levels. In summary, our study shows that homocysteine metabolism-related gene (MTHFR, MTR and TS) mutations can be associated with elevated homocysteine level. And we found that the MTHFR A1298C polymorphism is an independent risk factor in ischemic stroke.

OC108

Is thrombin activatable fibrinolysis inhibitor a contributing factor for development of thrombotic complications in patients with ischemic stroke?

Antovic J (1), Rooth E (2), Wallen H (2), Kaponides G (3), von Arbin M (2), Wahlgren N (3), Stenmark J (1), Blombäck M (1)*

(1) Coagulation Research, Department of Surgical Sciences, Karolinska Institutet, Stockholm, Sweden
(2) Department of Medicine, Danderyd Hospital, Karolinska Institutet, Stockholm, Sweden
(3) Department of Neurology, Karolinska Hospital, Karolinska Institutet, Stockholm, Sweden

Background: Thrombin activatable fibrinolysis inhibitor (TAFI) is one of modulators of fibrinolysis activated by the thrombin/thrombomodulin complex into its active form – a carboxypeptidase B-like enzyme which down-regulates fibrinolysis. It has been shown that TAFI activity could be a risk factor for ischemic stroke, while TAFI antigen increases in acute phase of ischemic stroke. **Patients and methods**: We measured total TAFI antigen in peripheral blood, at admission, on day 1, 3 and 60 in 26 patients with ischemic (non - cardioembolic) stroke (IS) and we compared results with 13 healthy controls. **Results**: Statistically significant increase of total TAFI antigen compared to controls (98.8±10.4%) was noticed in patients with IS at admission (130.1±9.7%, p=0.05) and day 1 (137.5±11.1%, p=0.03). It tended to decrease (although without statistical significance) on day 3 (127.4%±12.8) and especially on day 60 (113.7±12.5%). **Interpretation**: The mechanism of total TAFI antigen increase is probably not unique. Total TAFI antigen comprises the proenzyme (pro-TAFI), the active form of the enzyme (TAFI) and the inactive form (TAFIi). The increase in total TAFI antigen could partly arise from an increase in the enzyme's active form (TAFI) caused by an increased generation of thrombin. On the other hand, pro-TAFI has been described as an acute phase protein and the increase in total TAFI antigen could be accounted for by an increase of the proenzyme as an acute-phase reactant. In spite of lack of clear explanations for the mechanism behind the TAFI antigen increase we believe that these findings may indicate that TAFI could be a contributing risk factor for development of thrombotic tendency in patients with ischemic stroke.

OC109

Bleeding complications of oral anticoagulation therapy: a prospective audit

Bond S (1), Rhodes S (1), Green E (1), James R (2), Taylor M (1), Rose P (2), Emmas C (3)*

(1) Haematology Department, Swindon and Marlborough NHS Trust, UK
(2) Haematology Department, University Hospitals of Coventry and Warwickshire NHS Trust, UK
(3) Astrazeneca, UK

Bleeding is the most serious complication of the use of oral anticoagulation in the prevention and treatment of thromboembolism. We designed a tool to prospectively audit the frequency and severity of over anticoagulation and bleeding in two anticoagulant services; a District hospital serving a population of 330,000 patients (3,400 anticoagulant patients) and a University hospital with a population of 300,000 (4,000 anticoagulant patients), both providing Anticoagulant Practitioner led inpatient and outpatient dosing. Data was collected over 10 months including INR at time of event, whether complications necessitated hospital attendence and/or admission, investigations carried out and treatment given. There were 347 events. 133 were asymptomatic high INRs (>8). The majority of these were treated with oral vitamin K as outpatients. There were 214 bleeding episodes, 54 major and 160 minor. The most common sites of bleeding were epistaxis (70/214), GI bleeding (45/214), haematoma (36/214) and haematuria (24/214). 106 patients were admitted to hospital, constituting 0.61% of the total emergency medical admissions over this period. Patients spent a total of 887 days in hospital. 14 patients died, 4 directly as a result of the bleeding episode. INR stability in the period prior to the event was measured by +/- 1 standard deviation from the mean. 52/347 of patients were new at the time of the event (receiving anticoagulant therapy for less than 4 weeks), 164/347 were unstable, 121/347 were stable and 10/347 were GP monitored patients with no INR data available. At the time of event 68% of patients had an INR above target range (major bleed 72%; minor 66%). The most common factors contributing to the event were concurrent illness (78/347), prescription of potentiating medication (65/347), increase in prescribed warfarin dose (21/347) or patients inadvertently exceeding their prescribed dose (15/347).

OC110

The relationship of D-dimer and residual vein thrombosis as risk factors for recurrent venous thromboembolism after anticoagulation withdrawal

Cosmi B, Legnani C, Cini M, Guazzaloca G, Palareti G*

Division of Angiology and Blood Coagulation, Unitŕ Ricerca Clinica sulla Trombofilia "M. Golinelli"; Bologna, Itlay

Introduction: After a first episode of venous thromboembolism (VTE), the disease tends to recur whatever the duration of oral anticoagulant therapy (OAT). D-dimer (D-d) and residual vein thrombosis (RVT) have been separately shown to be risk factors for recurrent VTE. **Aims**: to assess the relationship between D-d and RVT and the negative predictive value of their combination for recurrent VTE. **Materials and methods**: 703 consecutive symptomatic patients with a first episode of proximal deep vein thrombosis (DVT) of the lower limbs were prospectively followed-up after the day of OAT wihdrawal. After 90 + 10 days, D-d levels were measured (cut-off value: 500 ng/mL) and RVT was determined by compression ultrasonography of common femoral and popliteal veins. Recurrences were diagnosed in case of symptoms of VTE by objective methods during a 2-year period. **Results**: Abnormal D-d was present in 47.3% and RVT in 49.4% of patients. The proportion of subjects with RVT was similar among patients with normal (174/366: 47.5%) and with abnormal D-d (169/329:51.3%). The hazard ratio for recurrence was 4.9 (95% CI: 1.8-13.4) for patients with abnormal D-d and RVT versus those with normal D-d and absent RVT after adjustment for sex, age, duration of OAT, thrombophilia, type of index event and cancer. The negative predictive values of D-d, RVT and their combination for recurrence were 93.7%, 92.6% and 97.9% (95% CI: 95-99%), respectively. **Conclusions**: RVT and D-d are independent risk factors and in combination have a high negative predictive value for recurrent VTE.

OC111

Drug interactions and risk of acute bleeding leading to hospitalisation or death in patients with chronic atrial fibrillation treated with warfarin

Gasse C (1), Hollowell J (2), Meier C (3), Troost J (1), Schneider V (1), Haefeli W (1)*

(1) Department of Internal Medicine VI, Clinical Pharmacology and Pharmacoepidemiology, University of He
(2) AstraZeneca, Mölndal, Sweden
(3) University Hospital Basel, Department of Clinical Pharmacology and Toxicology, Basel Pharmacoepidemi

Introduction: Drug interactions with warfarin are a major cause of excessive anticoagulation, which may lead to serious bleeding. **Aims**: To investigate the relationship between drugs known to potentiate the effect of warfarin and the risk of bleeding in patients with nonvalvular atrial fibrillation (AF) undergoing long-term warfarin therapy (> 3 months) for stroke prevention. **Methods**: Nested case control analysis in patients aged 40 to 84 years from the UK General Practice Research Database, January 1991 to April 2001. Cases consisted of incident idiopathic bleeds occurring during current warfarin exposure and resulting in hospitalisation within 30 days or death within 7 days. Cases were matched with warfarin-exposed controls on age, gender, practice, and index date. Patients with a history of major bleedings or known bleeding risk factors were excluded. Interacting drugs were defined according to the British National Formulary (BNF 3/2001). **Results**: Among 4152 eligible patients, we identified 67 cases and 317 matched controls. More cases received at least 1 interacting drug within 30 days prior to the index date (48% [95% confidence interval, CI 35-60%] vs 28% [95% CI 23-33%]), and more cases used more than 4 drugs (polypharmacy) within 90 days prior to the index date (75% [95% CI 63-85%] vs 63% [95% CI 58-68%]). The most frequently prescribed interacting drug within 30 days prior to the index date was acetaminophen (cases vs controls: 23.9% [95% CI 14.3-35.8%] vs 10.2% [95% CI 7.0-14.0%]). Conditional logistic regression analysis yielded a crude odds ratio (OR) of 2.66 (95% CI 1.50-4.72) for the risk of bleeding in patients treated with warfarin and at least 1 interacting drug vs warfarin alone. After adjusting for polypharmacy, diabetes, hypertension, heart failure, and thyroid disease, the OR was 2.57 (95% CI 1.38-4.80). Heart failure was identified as an independent risk factor (OR 2.30; 95% CI 1.26-4.20). **Conclusion**: Concurrent use of drugs that may potentiate the effect of warfarin is associated with a 2-fold increased risk of major bleeding in long-term warfarin users. Supported by a BMBF grant #01EC9902 from the German Ministry for Research and Education and AstraZeneca, Sweden.

OC112

The effect of vitamin K substitution on anticoagulant treatment

Rombouts E (1), Van der Meer F (1), Rosendaal F (1,2)*

(1) dpt. of Haematology, Leiden University Medical Centre, Leiden, the Netherlands
(2) dpt. of Clinical Epidemiology, Leiden University Medical Centre, Leiden, the Netherlands

Background: Coumarin derivatives create a state of vitamin K deficiency, resulting in a diminished synthesis of functional vitamin K dependent coagulation factors. To prevent instability of anticoagulant effect, patients are often advised to keep the vitamin K content of their diets constant. Little is known, however, about the changes in INR due to fluctuations in daily dietary vitamin K intake. We therefore examined the effect of substitution of a low daily dose of vitamin K on anticoagulant treatment with phenprocoumon. **Objective**: To determine the dose-adjustment of the anticoagulant drug phenprocoumon needed to counteract substitution with low daily doses of vitamin K. **Methods**: Patients of the Leiden Thrombosis Service using phenprocoumon who completed the training for self-management of anticoagulant treatment were asked to participate. The total study period was 9 weeks, in which the INR was measured at least 3 times a week using the CoaguCheck S coagulometer (Roche laboratories). Patients received vitamin K for 3 weeks. The first and last 3 weeks served as control periods. 5 Patients received 50 µg, 10 patients 100 µg of oil based vitamin K_1 (250 µg/g). Primary endpoint was the percentage change in phenprocoumon dose needed after starting and stopping vitamin K to keep the INR within therapeutic limits. **Results**: Substitution of 50 µg of vitamin K had little effect on the INR and therefore only slight dose-adjustments were made (mean dose increase after starting vitamin K 3% (95%BI: -6% - 13%). Substitution of 100 µg, however, resulted in a dose increase of 9% (95% BI: 0% - 19%). In the three weeks follow up after stopping vitamin K substitution phenprocoumon doses were lowered to pre-substitution values (mean change of –7% (95% BI: -15% - 0%). There was considerable inter-individual variability in response to vitamin K. In the group receiving 100 µg of vitamin K dose-adjustments ranged from 0% to 37%. **Conclusion**: Vitamin K substitution of 100 µg resulted in an mean dose-increase of 9%. Average daily vitamin K intake is about 100 µg but ranges from nearly nothing to 2000 µg. Since dose adjustments of 5 to 10% are often made to correct sub- or supratherapeutic INR values a dose adjustment of 10% is a clinically important finding. More research is needed to explain the inter-individual difference in anticoagulant response after vitamin K intake.

OC113

Telemedicine for managing patients on oral anticoagulant therapy

Testa S (1), Alatri A (1), Morstabilini G (1), Denti N (1), Martellenghi E (1), Mazzei G (2), Negri D (3), Pani A (4), Camaiora A (5), Lari B (6)*

(1) Centro Emostasi e Trombosi AO Istituti Ospitalieri Cremona
(2) Laboratorio Analisi Ospedale di Sospiro, Cremona
(3) Laboratorio Analisi Ospedale Oglio PO-AO Cremona
(4) Centro Geriatrico"A. Soldi" Cremona
(5) GTO MMG Casalmaggiore, Cremona
(6) GTO MMG Piadena, Cremona

Introduction. In the last decade the indications of oral anticoagulant therapy have increased significantly. Several studies have shown that anticoagulation management by an Anticoagulation Clinic (AC) results in better clinical control compared with routine medical care. As a consequence we observed a substantial increase in the number of patients followed up at our AC. The patients, coming from the whole province were 150 in 1991 and 2525 in 2003. We identified 3 problems in the organization: 1. reduction of patient comfort at AC, due to overcrowding; 2. difficulty in reaching the AC for a substantial number of patient; 3. inadequate increase of health care staff. It was therefore necessary to reorganize the activity, maintaing the clinical quality level reached. **Aims** 1. Decentralize the activity in the health territorial care units of the Cremona area, through a telemedicine system. 2. Improve the quality of life of the patients living far from the AC site. 3. Reduce by 30% the number of patients seen daily at the AC. 4. Maintain the same clinical quality levels. **Materials and methods**: We installed a centralized net supported program (intra- and internet), *TAOnet*®, to collect and elaborate clinical data, connected with peripheral districts. PT-INR is performed on Coaguchek® portable monitors. Clinical data are obtained from the nourse and sent in real time to the AC. The AC sends within minutes the appropriate dose adjustment and the clinical suggestions to the district. All the process is under quality assessement as based upon ISO 9001-VISION 2000 standards. **Results** The project started in 1-2002. Six districts are available to the public and 310 patients, 12% of the total, are now on treatment. Patients expressed their overall satisfaction, as evaluated through an open questionnaire. We observed an increase of the time spent in the therapeutic range as compared to the previous six months (AC= 61%, health territorial care units= 68%; $p<0.05$). No difference in major complications was observed. **Conclusive remarks:** This new organization provides the following advantages: 1) direct communication between districts and AC, 2) improvement in time spent in the therapeutic range, 3) improvement in patient's satisfaction and in their quality of life, 4) continuing medical record update, 5) time gained by staff, 6) possibility to manage other antithrombotic drugs.

OC114

OAT with POC devices and remote computer monitoring in the setting of the Italian NHS: a controlled clinical trial

*Paccamiccio E (1), Ferrante F (1), Trottini S (1), Rosafalco M (2), Duca E (3), Maria V (3), Nenci G (1), Alfonso I (1)**

(1) Sezione di Medicina Interna e Cardiovascolare - Università di Perugia
(2) Instrumentation Laboratory, IL, Milan, Italy
(3) Distretto del Perugino ASL2, Perugia, Italy

Introduction. The number of patients chronically taking oral anticoagulant therapy (OAT) is progressively growing due to aging of the population and widening of the indications to treatment, and it often overcomes the capability of the dedicated specialised centres. **Aims**. To test the effectiveness and feasibility of specialised OAT monitoring with a remote computer modality in the setting of the Italian National Health System (INHS). **Materials and methods**. Three outpatient peripheral units from the INHS were identified. One-hundred-fifty unselected patients referring to the Thrombosis Centre (TC) of Perugia were enrolled on a first come basis after obtaining informed consent. As a control group, we studied a series of matched patients of the TC. The Point-of-care (POC) device for the capillary determination of INR was the Protime Microcoagulation System (IL, Milan), while the softwares used to manage OAT were P.A.R.M.A. 5 (IL, Milan, Italy) and Easy Tao (E-Medical Monitor, Barcelona, Spain). The project was planned and conducted with a research grant given by Region Umbria. **Results**. Patients recruitment started on October 2002 and fifty patients were assigned to each unit. The mean number of monthly accesses was 1.5 per patient. The analysis of the INR values showed that 62.1% of controls were in the therapeutic range and that 72.0% of time was spent into the therapeutic range. Neither major bleedings nor thromboembolic complications were documented. **Conclusions**. These figures were not different from those measured in the control group and in the historical analysis of the study group confirming the feasibility of this type of management of OAT.

OC115

Below-knee elastic compression stockings for prevention of the post-thrombotic syndrome. A randomized study

Prandoni P (1), Lensing A (2), Prins M (3), Frulla M (1), Marchiori A (1), Bernardi E (1), Tormene D (1), Mosena L (1), Pagnan A (1), Girolami A (1)*

(1) Clinica Medica II, University of Padua, Italy
(2) Center for Vascular Medicine, University of Amsterdam, The Netherlands
(3) Department of Clinical Epidemiology, University of Maastricht, The Netherlands

Introduction. Evidence that elastic compression stockings (ECS) prevent the post-thrombotic syndrome (PTS) in patients with symptomatic deep-vein thrombosis (DVT) is limited. Consequently, they are not widely employed. **Aims.** To evaluate the efficacy of ECS for prevention of PTS in patients with proximal DVT. **Materials and Methods.** 180 consecutive patients at their first episode of symptomatic proximal DVT who had a conventional anticoagulant treatment were randomized before discharge to wear or not below-knee ECS

(30-40 mm Hg at the ankle) for two years. Follow-up was performed up to five years. The presence and severity of PTS was scored using a standardized scale. **Results**. PTS developed in 44 of the 90 control patients (severe in 10), and in 23 of the 90 patients wearing ECS (severe in 3). All events but one developed in the first two years. The cumulative incidence of PTS in the control group was 40.0% (95 CI, 29.9 to 50.1) after six months, 46.7% (36.4 to 57.0) after one year, and 49.1% (38.7 to 59.4) after two years. The corresponding figures in the ECS group were 21.1% (12.7 to 29.5), 22.2% (13.8 to 30.7), and 24.5% (15.6 to 33.4), respectively. The hazard ratio for PTS in the study group as compared to control patients was 0.49 (0.29 to 0.84). **Conclusions**. Post-thrombotic sequelae develop in almost half of patients with a proximal DVT. Below-knee ECS reduce this rate by about 50%.

OC116

Do vena cava filters increase the incidence of post-thrombotic syndrome? Results from the eight-year follow-up of the randomised PREPIC trial

Quenet S, Rivron-Guillot K, Decousus H*

Introduction In a randomised trial involving 400 patients with proximal DVT [1], the insertion of a permanent vena cava filter led to a significant reduction in the occurrence of pulmonary embolism (PE) at 8 years, and a significant increase in the recurrence of DVT [2]. **Aim** As the post-thrombotic syndrome (PTS) is a chronic complication of DVT, our objective was to determine whether filter placement influences the long-term development of PTS. **Methods** From September 1991 to February 1995, 400 patients with acute proximal DVT were randomly assigned to receive a filter (n=200) or not (n=200). Patients were then clinically examined at three months and one year. At two years and then once a year thereafter, they received a telephone call from the coordinating centre, which was not aware of the treatment assignments. Objective signs of the PTS were assessed (oedema, varicose veins, trophic disorders and ulcers). PTS was considered present if at least one objective sign appeared or worsened compared with the last assessment. Kaplan-Meier analysis of the cumulative rate of events was performed. **Results** At eight years, the cumulative risk of PTS was 70.3% in the filter group and 69.7% in the no filter group. Half of these patients experienced their first sign of PTS within the first three years. At eight years, the most common signs of PTS were oedema and varicose veins which occurred respectively in 60% and 33% of patients in the filter group and in 53% and 38% of patients in the no filter group. **Conclusions** The development of PTS did not appear to be related to filter placement. (1. Decousus et al. *N Engl J Med* 1998; 338: 409-15. 2. Decousus et al. *J Thromb Haemost* 2003, suppl: OC440)

OC117

Postoperative asymptomatic deep vein thrombosis and the development of postthrombotic syndrome: a systematic review

Wille-Jørgens P, Jorgensen L*

Department of Surgical Gastroenterology K, Bispebjerg Hospital, University of Copenhagen, Denmark

Background: Several randomised trials have demonstrated a reduction of postoperative deep venous thrombosis (DVT) after administration of various antithrombotic regimens. However, the outcome in these trials is habitually asymptomatic DVT as assessed by systematic screening with sensitive methods. This article reviews the clinical significance of asymptomatic postoperative DVT with regard to the development of postthrombotic syndrome (PTS). **Methods:** A literature search was performed to locate articles or abstracts on the occurrence of PTS in patients formerly assessed for postoperative DVT by means of systematic sensitive objective measures. Meta-analyses were applied to detect an over-all trend towards an association between postoperative DVT and PTS after stratification according to individual study features. **Results:** The over-all relative risk of developing PTS was 63% (95% c.i: 50% – 81%) in patients without documentation of DVT as compared to patients with DVT, p < 0.0005. A uniform trend of the results was observed regardless of the methodological stratification conditions despite a certain heterogeneity among the included trials. **Conclusion:** Asymptomatic postoperative DVT is associated with an increased risk of late PTS. The finding emphasizes that DVT, detected after surgery by means of objective sensitive methods, is a clinically sound scientific endpoint in trials evaluating the efficacy of antithrombotic measures.

OC118

Inter-observer variables in results of compression ultrasonography performed in acutely ill medical patients

Malek G (1), Tomkowski W (2), Wisniewska J (2), Kuca P (2), Kober J (2), Burakowska B (1), Oniszh K (1)*

(1) Department of Radiology, National TB and Lung Diseases Research Institute, Warszaw, Poland
(2) Intensive Care Unit, National TB and Lung Diseases Research Institute, Warszaw, Poland

Background: Utility of vein ultrasonography in diagnostic procedure of deep vein thrombosis (DVT) is widely accepted. Comparison of vein ultrasonography results assessed by two independent radiologists with venography in asymptomatic medical patients at risk of thrombosis are available is poorly investigated. Study objective: To evaluate sensitivity and specificity of compression ultrasound (CUS) examinations (assessed by two observers) in diagnosis of proximal and distal deep venous thrombosis in acutely ill medical patients with exposure on risk of venous thromboembolism (VTE): congestive heart failure (NYHA class III and IV), respiratory infectious, inflammatory diseases - considered to be at moderate risk of VTE. Mainly asymptomatic course of DVT in acutely ill medical patients was expected. **Design**: CUS examination (equipment: Sequoia C 256, linear probe with pulse and color Doppler) was performed just before venography, scheduled on Day 6-15 of hospital stay. Extensive CUS was performed (simultaneously with recording on video-tape of all examination) and analyzed by observer one (OI). Whole length of common femoral veins, femoral veins, popliteal veins and calf veins: tibial anterior plus posterior and peroneal were investigated. CUS was compared with ascending venography, which was evaluated by two radiologists. Videotape recording was re-analyzed by second observer (OII), who was blinded for the results of venography and CUS assessed by OI. **Results**: Technically satisfactory venography was obtained in 160 patients. In 12 out of 160 patients (7.5%, 95% CI = [4.0%-12.7%]) venography confirmed presence of DVT. In all 12 cases course of DVT was asymptomatic. Among them proximal DVT was detected in 5 patients (3.1%, 95% CI = [1.0 %-7.1%]) and distal DVT in 7 patients (4.4%, 95% CI = [1.8% - 8.8%]). In all 160 patients CUS of proximal veins was technically satisfactory. Results assessed by OI: in 3 out of 5 patients with proven by venography proximal DVT, diagnosis was confirmed by CUS (sensitivity 60%), in one case result of CUS was false positive (specificity 99.4%). In 10 out of 160 patients calf CUS was technically insufficient. In 2 out of 7 patients with proven by venography calf thrombosis diagnosis was confirmed by CUS (sensitivity 28.6%) and in two cases result of CUS was false positive (specificity 98.6%). Results assessed by O II: in 3 out of 5 patients with proven by venography proximal DVT, diagnosis was confirmed by CUS (sensitivity 60%), in 29 cases result of CUS was false positive (specificity 81.3%). In 10 out of 160 patients calf CUS was technically insufficient. In 5 out of 7 patients with proven by venography calf thrombosis diagnosis was confirmed by CUS (sensitivity 71.4%) and in 14 cases result of CUS was false positive (specificity 90.7%). **Conclusion**: Due to huge differences between observers, compression ultrasound should not be used as reference screening method in diagnosis of DVT in asymptomatic medical patients.

OC119

Factors predicting long-term venous thrombotic complications after insertion of vena cava filters: results of the randomised PREPIC trial

Buchmuller-Cordier A, Laporte S, Decousus H*

Thrombosis Research Group, University Hospital of Saint-Etienne, France

Introduction In a randomised trial involving 400 patients with proximal deep vein thrombosis (DVT) [1], insertion of a permanent vena cava filter led to a significant reduction in the occurrence of pulmonary embolism (PE) at 8 years, and a significant increase in the recurrence of DVT [2]. There was no effect on overall mortality. **Aim** We performed a multivariate analysis of data from the PREPIC trial to identify, in addition to vena cava filter insertion, predictors of severe complications at 8 years. **Materials and methods** We analysed the predictive value of a number of baseline characteristics for two outcomes: PE and mortality at 8 years. Independent predictive factors were identified using univariate and multivariate Cox models. **Results** At 8 years, 9 patients in the filter group had experienced PE and 24 in the no filter group. PE was fatal for seven of these 33 patients. On multivariate analysis, insertion of filter (hazard ratio, HR=0.35; 95% CI [0.16-0.80]) was an independent predictor of PE; in addition, initial PE was associated with a significantly increased risk of PE at 8 years (HR=2.57 [1.18-5.62]). A trend to increasing risk of PE with increasing age was also found. Finally, 201 patients had died at 8 years (98 in the filter group and 103 in the no filter group). Three independent factors were found to be associated with an increased risk of death: cancer at inclusion (HR=2.08 [1.47-2.95]), cardiac or respiratory insufficiency (HR=1.79 [1.32-2.45]) and age (HR=1.64 [1.40-1.88] per 10 years). **Conclusions** These results confirm that in patients with proximal DVT, PE is more likely to occur in patients with a PE at inclusion than in those without a PE. (1. Decousus et al. N Engl J Med 1998; 338: 409-15. 2. Decousus et al. J Thromb Haemost 2003, suppl: OC440.)

OC120

Elastic stockings, hydroxyethylrutosides or both for the treatment of the post-thrombotic syndrome. A pilot randomized study

Frulla M, Marchiori A, Sartor D, Mosena L, Concolato A, Hartman L, Tormene D, Prandoni P*

Clinica Medica II, University of Padua, Italy

Introduction. In contrast with the extensive documentation on epidemiology, diagnosis, and prevention of the post-thrombotic syndrome (PTS), little is known about the treatment of this common and sometimes frustrating complication of deep vein thrombosis (DVT) of the lower extremities. **Aims.** To evaluate the efficacy of elastic compression stockings (ECS), hydroxyethylrutosides (HR), or both for the treatment of PTS. **Materials and Methods.** 120 consecutive patients with post-thrombotic manifestations, arising after one or more episodes of objectively documented DVT, were randomized to receive below-knee ECS (30-40 mm Hg at the ankle), the oral administration of HR (1000 mg b.i.d.), or both regimens for one year. Each group consisted of 40 patients. In all patients follow-up visits were planned after 3 and 6 months, and then after the completion of the scheduled 12 months. The presence and severity of PTS was scored using a standardized score (the Villalta scale). The efficacy of ECS and HR, alone and combined, was calculated using Cox regression models, and expressed as hazard ratio and its 95% confidence intervals (CI). **Results**. After adjustment for age, sex, modality of clinical presentation, location of the thrombotic episode, history of multiple ipsilateral thrombotic episodes, time elapsed between DVT episode and patient's recruitment, and PTS severity, hazard ratios for PTS recovery (defined as a PTS score lower than 5) for ECS versus HR, ECS alone versus the combined regimens, and HR alone versus the combined regimens were 1.48 (0.55 to 3.94), 1.46 (0.59 to 3.60), and 0.94 (0.37 to 2.40), respectively. The mean PTS score registered at each follow-up visit did not differ between the study groups. **Conclusions**. The combination of ECS with HR does not improve the results obtained by each strategy alone for the treatment of established PTS. ECS and HR are equally effective, and, therefore, interchangeable in patients with PTS. Larger studies are needed to confirm these findings.

OC121

Factor V Leiden, prothrombin G20210A and MTHFR C667T mutations in women with abruptio placentae

Procházka M (1), Slavík L (2), Procházková J (2), Hrachovec P (1), Krčová V (2)*

(1) Dept. of Obstetrics and Gynaecology, Medical Faculty, Palacký University, Czech republic
(2) Dpt. of Hematooncology, Medical Faculty, Palacký University, Czech republic

Objective: Abruptio placentae is a major cause of fetal and maternal mortality and morbidity, occuring in 0,4 - 1.3% of pregnancies. Recent studies suggest an increased risk of obstetric complications in women with hereditary or acquired thrombophilias. The aim of our study was to detect, wheteher carriership of the FV Leiden, G20210A and C667T mutations are associated with an increased risk of the premature separation of the placenta. **Design:** A retrospective case-control study. A cohort of 135 women with confirmed diagnosis of abruptio placentae was compared to prospectively obtained unselected control group of 198 pregnant women, who delivered between 2000 and 2003. Blood samples were taken in early postpartum period (24 – 72 hrs.). We investigated APC resistance - a modified functional APC resistance test using factor V deficient plasma. Individuals with APC ratio below 1.86 were tested with PCR-based analysis for the presence of the FV:Q506 allele. PCR methods for were used for the testing of the prothrombin gene G20210A mutation and mutation of methyletetrahydrofolatreductase (MTHFR) A/V 223. The study was performed on the Czech population; no other ethnic groups were included. **Results:** Women with abruptio placentae were carriers of factor V Leiden in 21 (15.5%) cases, prothrombin mutation G20210A was present 1 (0.74 %) and MTHFR +/- form in 63 (46.7%), +/+ form 5 (3.7%) cases. Women in control group were carriers of FV Leiden in 10 cases (5.05%), G20210A mutation 2 (1.01%) and MTHFR +/- 91 (45.95%), +/+ 7 (3.53%). **Conclusion:** Factor V Leiden presents a risk factor for premature placental separation (p= 0.0014) The frequency of prothrombin mutation G20210A is very low in our population and therefore difficult for statistical analysis. Mutation C667T are not associated with higher risk of abruptio placentae. (Supported by the grant from the Ministry of Health Czech Rep. IGA NH/6986 – 3, 2002)

OC122

Factor V Leiden, FII G20210A, MTHFR C677T mutations and first venous thrombosis during pregnancy and puerperium

Djordjevic V (1), Rakicevic L (1), Miljic P (2), Mikovic D (3), Kovac M (3), Radojkovic D (1), Savic A (1)*

(1) Institute of Molecular Genetics and Genetic Engineering, Belgrade, Serbia and Montenegro
(2) Institute of Hematology, University Clinical Center of Serbia, Belgrade, Serbia and Montenegro
(3) Hemostasis Department and Hemophilia Center, National Blood Transfusion Institute, Belgrade, Serbia

Venous thrombosis is an important cause of obstetric morbidity and mortality. Estimates of the incidence of pregnancy-associated venous thrombosis vary from 1 in 1000 to 1 in 2000 deliveries. The Factor V G1691A (FV Leiden), FII G20210A and MTHFR C677T mutations are most common genetic risk factors for thromboembolism. Purpose of our study was to establish the prevalence of these risk factors in group of 45 women (mean age:30 years) with a first episode of deep venous thrombosis during pregnancy or puerperium. Patients with antiphospholipid antibodies, an antithrombin III, protein C or protein S deficiency, were excluded from the study. Twenty heterozygous carriers of the FV Leiden mutation and one homozygous carrier were detected; which gives the frequencies of 44.4% and 2.2%, respectively. For the FII G20210A mutation, six heterozygous carriers were identified, giving the frequency of 13.3%. The MTHFR C677T mutation was observed in 31 patientes (22 heterozygous and 9 homozygous carriers) witch gives the frequencies of 48.9% and 20%, respectively . Our study suggests that testing for FV Leiden and FII G20210A mutations is strongly recommended in women with history of venous thrombosis during pregnancy and puerperium. We found a weak effect of MTHFR 667T allele, but it should be consider in association with other risk factors.

OC123

Safety and efficacy of nadroparin for the treatment or prophylaxis venous thromboembolism in pregnancy

Barillari G, Biffoni F, Springolo F, Marchsoni D*

Hemophilia and Thrombophilia Center, Department of Transfusion Medicine, General and University Hospital, Udine, Italy Thromboembolic disease is a rare but important complication of pregnancy and represents the leading non-obstetric cause of maternal morbidity or mortality. The need for the prevention and management of Venous Thromboembolism (VTE) in pregnant women, arise from the necessity of minimizing the risk of thromboembolic and obstetric (such as preeclampsia, intrauterine growth retardation, abruptio placentae, fetal death), post-partum and neonatal complications. Many studies have to now documented the efficacy and safety of LMWH in pregancy, however, only a few and small series of patients are reported to have been managed with Nadroparin. From June 2000 to December 2003, pregnant women carriers of thrombophilia or with acute VTE, who came to our observation, were managed with nadroparin as thromboprophylaxis (80 IU/Kg/d from the 28° week of gestation to delivery; 100 IU/Kg/d during puerperium), or therapy (at usual dosages). Platelet count was performed every second day, from the V to XXI day of heparin treatment to exclude type II HIT. Hemoglobin levels before and after the delivery (as estimate of delivery hemorrages) and transfusion requirements were recorded. A total of 64 pregnancies were managed with nadroparin administration. Eight pregnant women were treated with nadroparin because of DVT (N° = 6, occurring at 11°, 18°, 27°, 28°, 28° and 30° week of gestation) or pulmonary embolism (N° 2, at 27° and 28° w of gestation). Forty-six women for 56 pregnancies underwent thromboprophylaxis because of Leiden heterozigosity (N° 33 pregnancies), Leiden homozigosity (N° 2), Prothrombin heterozigosity

(N° 1), Protein C (N° 2) or Protein S (N° 2) deficiency, Antiphospholipid antibodies (N° 4), previous VTE during oral contracception, (N° 4), or during previous pregnancies (N° 4) or third trimester abortion (N° 2). Only in one case a minor hemorragic complication was observed (epystaxis during puerperium, requiring a lowering of nadro dosage to the pre-partum one). No major hemorrages nor HIT, neither neonatal abnormalities occurred. Post-partum Hb decrease was as expected in non anticoagulated women, and no transfusion with packed red cells were required. In conclusion: our data suggest that women with thrombophilia, previous VTE, and thromboembolism during pregnancy can be safely and effectively managed with nadroparin.

OC124

APC-NR and PC-NR as markers of prethrombotic changes in pregnancy

Vodnik T, Vukosavljević D, Ignjatović S, Majkić-SinghN*

Institute of Medical Biochemistry, Clinical Center of Serbia, Belgrade, Serbia and Montenegro

Introduction: The concentrations of plasma proteins involved in the process of coagulation change during regular pregnancy, what interferes with balance between procoagulant and anticoagulant systems. These changes include higher activity of coagulation factors, increasing the risk of thrombosis. Thrombosis of placental blood vessels gives rise to placental insufficiency, causing the repeated miscarriages, eclampsia and intrauterine death of fetus. The most frequent causes of venous thromboembolic complications are changes in Protein C system induced by Factor V Leiden mutation, where mutated factor V is less sensitive to APC (Activated Protein C). The condition characterized by poor anticoagulant response to APC is named APC resistance. Aim: The aim of this study was to test the functionality protein C system in normal and complicated pregnancy and APC resistance. Materials and methods: The testing was performed in 80 patients, e.g. pregnant women with regular and complicated pregnancy, 40 subjects in each group. The determination was carried out 3 times successively during the pregnancy. The following hemostatic parameters are determined: protein S, protein C, protein C Global and protein C APC sensitivity. Commercial "Dade Behring" tests were used to determine the parameters of hemostasis on automated BCT analyzer. **Results**: The values of protein C activity were within normal limits while protein S values were below lower limits. Significantly lower PC-NR and APC-NR values were found in all three gestation periods in pregnant women with repeated miscarriages in relation to pregnant women with regular pregnancy. In order to assess the diagnostic accuracy of investigated hemostatic parameters as markers of prethrombotic changes in pregnant women, the obtained values of investigated hemostatic parameters were evaluated by ROC analysis. **Conclusion**: PC-NR and APC-NR showed satisfactory diagnostic accuracy as markers of prethrombotic changes in pregnant women, more precisely, they were found to be good indicators of resistance to activated protein C in pregnancy.

OC125

Monitoring low molecular weight heparin in pregnancy: the timing of the peak measurement

Shiach C (1), Johnston T (2)*

(1) Haematology Department, Manchester Royal Infirmary, Oxford Road, Manchester England.
(2) Obstetrics Department,St Mary's Hospital, Hathersage Road, Manchester, England.

Background - The role of monitoring low molecular weight heparin (LMWH) by an anti-Xa assay remains disputed. Much confusion arises because different centres undertake this using different protocols. The timing of the peak measurement has been recommended at 2 hours, 3 hours and 4 hours in pregnant women. This study aimed to identify the true time of a peak LMWH level in pregnant women. **Patients and Methods** - 14 pregnant women took part in the study. Samples were taken at time 0 immediately prior to LMWH and then at 1, 2, 3, 4 and 6 hours after LMWH. LMWH concentration was measured using a one stage clotting anti-Xa assay. 37 separate studies were done. 6 women were studied only once. 8 women had studies 2-6 times during their pregnancy. **Results** - Data showed that the mean time of peak LMWH is 4.1 hours (95% CI 3.6 to 4.5). The median is 3.7 hours (95% CI 3.4 to 3.4 to 4.4). The interquartile range is 3.2 to 4.8 hours. Where a pregnant woman has no detectable LMWH at time 0 we change their dosing to a twice daily regime. Further analysis of the data showed that there is no significant difference in the time that women reach peak LMWH level between women having once daily and those having twice daily heparin (p=0.68) although those on once daily regimes have a wider scatter of results. This study shows that although pregnant women have increased rates of clearance of LMWH the time for LMWH to reach a peak is close to 4 hours which is very similar to results obtained in non pregnant individuals. Even where women need twice daily dosing there is no change in the time of the peak LMWH level.

OC126

Monitoring low molecular weight heparin in pregnancy

Shiach C (1), Johnston T (2)*

(1) Manchester Royal Infirmary, Manchester, England
(2) St Mary's Hospital, Manchester, England

Background - Prophylactic Low Molecular Weight Heparin (LMWH) is administered in pregnancy to prevent venous thromboembolism (VTE) and certain complications of pregnancy. LMWH metabolism is altered in pregnancy however the need for monitoring this drug is disputed. **Patients and Methods** - 43 pregnancies in 40 women were studied. 25 women had a previous VTE, 1 a CVA, 10 received treatment for previous complications in pregnancy. Clinical risk factors were identified in 14 pregnancies, 19 women had at least one thrombophilia risk factor. LMWH (Tinzaparin Leo) was monitored by an anti-Xa assay monthly. A pre-sample was taken prior to dosing and a post-sample at two hours. A therapeutic range was established of detectable LMWH in the pre-sample and levels of 0.15 – 0.35 iu/ml Heparin post-dosing. **Results** - 3/43 pregnancies had an unsuccessful outcome. 10/40 successful pregnancies were delivered by caesarean section. The median gestation at delivery was 38 weeks, median blood loss was 200 units. 2/40 live babies had reduced apgar scores at delivery. There was a significant increase in the proportion of small babies born. The mean dose required was 4,500iu in the first trimester, 7,000iu in the second and 9,000iu in the third. There was no correlation between weight and dose of LMWH. The frequency of twice daily dosing increased from 19% in the first trimester to 70% in the third. This study demonstrates that by monitoring LMWH levels appropriate and safe dose adjustment can be made during pregnancy. Most women require twice daily dosing in the third trimester.

OC127

Upper gastrointestinal hemorrhage, anticoagulant therapy and nonsteroidal antiinflammatory drugs–results of a prospective study

Skok P, Skok M*

Clinical Department of Internal Medicine Maribor, General Hospital Maribor and Health Centre Maribor, Slovenia

Introduction. Over the last years, the use of oral anticoagulant treatment has increased dramatically, principally for the prevention of venous thrombosis and thrombembolic events. **Aims and Methods**. To evaluate the safety of the management with oral antiocoagulants, nonsteroidal antiinflammatory drugs (NSAIDs) and antiaggregant agents in a prospective study. Included were patients who were admitted to our institution between 1 January 1994 and 30 April 2003 due to gastrointestinal hemorrhage. Emergency endoscopy was performed in all patients. **Results**. 6024 patients were investigated: 2290 women (38 %) and 3734 (62 %) men (av. age 59.1 years, SD 17.2). In 5209 patients (86.4 %) the source of bleeding was confirmed in the upper gastrointestinal tract. Among our patients 55 % were aged over 60 years, 26.7 % were older than 80 years. Sequelae of peptic ulcer disease were the most significant cause of upper gastrointestinal hemorrhage, in 48 % (2500/5209). In the last week prior to bleeding, 20.5 % (1068/5209) of patients were taking regularly NSAIDs, anticoagulant therapy, antiaggregant agents or corticosteroids at least in single daily dose. The majority, 94 %, were taking NSAIDs or antiaggregant agents, 8 % of them both preparations at the same time. 6 % (64/1068) of patients were using oral anticoagulant therapy, the majority of them had INR >5. 77 % of all patients were admitted to hospital due to hemorrhage which manifested at home, in 23 % of patients hemorrhage manifested during hospital stay. Only a minority of patients were receiving gastroprotective therapy. No significant difference in mortality of patients who were taking NSAIDs, corticosteroids, salycilates or anticoagulants compared to those who did not, was found, p=0.10. **Conclusions**. Upper gastrointestinal hemorrhage is a serious complication of different medication, particularly in elderly patients. Safe use of anticoagulant therapy, NSAIDs and antiaggregant agents is based on careful selection of patients and correct intake of the prescribed drug.

OC128

Patients on oral anticoagulant treatment: anticoagulation clinic vs assistant physician

Barreira R (1), Farinha M (2), Rodrigues I (3), Martins R (3), Mendes Z (4), Ribeiro J (2), Crespo F (1)*

(1) Serviço Patologia Clínica, Hospital Santa Cruz, Carnaxide, Portugal
(2) Serviço Patologia Clínica, Hospital S. Teotónio, Viseu, Portugal
(3) Serviço Patologia Clínica, Hospital Distrital Faro, Faro, Portugal
(4) Departamento Matemática, Universidade Lusíada

Introduction and Aims: In Portugal, patients on oral anticoagulant treatment are controlled mainly by specialized anticoagulation clinics or by assistant physicians, rather than by patient self-management. As the indications for long-term anticoagulant treatment are expanding, the number of patients on such a therapy has increased dramatically over the years. Patient monitoring by means of anticoagulation clinics, which provide not only monitoring of prothrombin time, but also patient education, and a more close clinical surveillance, may improve the overall quality of oral anticoagulation. Our aim was to compare 2 groups of warfarin anticoagulated patients, one attending a hospital based anticoagulation clinic and the other attending the assistant physician for anticoagulation control. The quality of anticoagulation control was assessed by comparing in both groups of patients the proportion of INRs within the therapeutic range, above 5.0 and below 1.5. **Materials and methods**: From August 2002 through March 2003 a total of 347 patients were selected, divided in two groups. One group consisted of 172 patients monitored by an anticoagulation clinic (AC group), and the other involved 175 patients monitored by the assistant physician (AP group). Patient characteristics being similar in both groups, all patients were on chronic oral anticoagulant therapy with warfarin for more than 3 months. Patients from AC group belonging to three different hospital based anticoagulation clinics, were randomly assigned to the study. Patients in the AP group were randomly enrolled when attending the routine consultation, and had their INR measured in the anticoagulation clinic laboratories. **Results and Conclusions**: In the AC group more patients had INRs within the therapeutic range than in the AP group, both among patients receiving lower-range (INR 2.0-3.0) anticoagulation therapy (71.6% vs 45.8%; p=0.0012) and in patients requiring higher-range (2.5-3.5) anticoagulation therapy (53.6% vs 30.1%; p=0.0016). In group AC fewer patients had INRs below 1.5 than in group AP (1.7% vs 14.9%; p<0.0001), but not significantly less INRs above 5.0 (1.7% vs 4.6%; p=0.2192). Patients treated at an anticoagulation clinic achieved better anticoagulation control, both among patients receiving lower-range anticoagulation therapy and in the patients requiring higher-range anticoagulation therapy. However, other aspects of assessing the quality of oral anticoagulation could and should be assessed, including the frequency of visits for INR estimation, the development of thrombotic or bleeding complications and the management of overanticoagulated patients.

OC129

Efficacy and risk of anticoagulant therapy in 102 patients with thrombosis and cancer

Ceresetto JM, Rabinovich O, Stemmelin G, Shanley C, Duboscq C, Gutierrez M, Mendizabal G, Carlos D, Vicente M, Bullorsky E*

Hospital Britanico de Buenos Aires, Argentina

Introduction: The management of acute venous thrombosis (AVT) in cancer patients has not been standardized. One of the main concerns about this treatment is a higher risk of thromboembolism and hemorrhage. **Objective**: To evaluate thrombotic and bleeding complications in patients with cancer and anticoagulation for a first episode of vein thrombosis. **Patients and methods**: Medical records of 102 patients with an active malignancy and AVT followed in our anticoagulation clinic between 1992 - 2002 were reviewed. Mean age: 62 years (range 30-87), M/F: 58-44. Neoplasm location: gynecologic 32, genitourinary 22, gastrointestinal 17, oncohaematologic 15, lung 10 and other location 4 patients; 74% of patients had disseminated disease. **Results**: The site of thrombosis was PE 32%, DVT 30%, Superficial Thrombophlebitis (ST) 19%, upper extremity 10%, inferior cava vein 5% and calf vein thrombosis 4%. Most of the episodes were considered spontaneous while 26% were related to surgery. 94 patients received full dose anticoagulation, 2 were not treated because of end stage malignancy and 6 received LMWH in prophylactic doses due to ST. 51% were initially treated with LMWH and 49% with unfractionated heparin followed by acenocoumarol (INR 2-3). 35 patients developed recurrent AVT during 2.2 years of follow-up. 69% recurrences occurred within adequate anticoagulation. All the patients (9 out of 9) that discontinued oral anticoagulation (OA) while the neoplasm was still active had a new thrombosis. Reasons for OA discontinuation were transitory bleeding (3), wrong oncologic evaluation (4) or patient's decision to discontinue therapy (2). Six of 7 patients with "only" ST and without OA had a recurrent and significant DVT, one of them bilateral. Major bleeding was also more frequent and occurred in 11% of patients; 3 were cerebral bleeding in patients without brain metastasis and INR < 3 (one fatal). **Conclusions**: 1) Cancer patients had a high rate of thrombotic complications with adequate OA therapy. 2) All patients that stopped anticoagulant treatment had a new thrombotic event, even patients with "innocent" ST had a severe new event. 3) Major bleeding was also frequent with 1/3 of these patients suffering a cerebral hemorrhage.

OC130

Vitamin K antagonists are less prescribed in outpatients with permanent lone atrial fibrillation: results of a large observational survey in France

Cohen A (1), Guenoun M (2), Le Heuzey J (3), Mismetti P (4), Leizorovicz A (5), for the FALSTAF Study Group*

(1) APHP Paris, France
(2) CHU Marseille, France
(3) APHP Paris, France
(4) CHU Saint-Etienne, France
(5) Faculté R.T.H. Laennec, Lyon, France

Introduction: Lone atrial fibrillation (LAF) has been associated with a lower risk of thromboembolism. However, controversial results have been recently reported, suggesting an increased risk of thromboembolism, particularly in elderly patients. Information regarding the current anticoagulant strategy in outpatients, usually based on a risk factor-based stratification, is lacking. **Aims**: The FALSTAF study was performed to describe the modalities of the prescription of antithrombotics in routine practice in ambulatory patients with permanent AF in France. The role of lone AF on antithrombotic prescriptions was particularly studied. **Materials and Methods**: We prospectively compared the prescription rate of antithrombotic drugs in patients with permanent (documented by two ECG at one month interval) lone AF and AF, with or without valvular disease, associated with at least one clinical or biological risk factor in a large survey of ambulatory AF patients in France. **Results**: From August to December 2002, 5893 patients with AF were included by 188 cardiologists and 582 general practitioners. Lone AF was present in 723 (12.3%) patients. Compared with other AF patients, in lone AF patients, the mean age was lower (72±12 years *vs* 76±9 years, p<0.001) and a history of stroke less frequent (6.8% *vs* 10.6%, p=0.002). Seventy percent of lone AF patients were men compared with 56% of men among other AF patients (p<0.001). Overall, 95.5% of patients were being prescribed an antithrombotic, including vitamin K antagonists (VKA) in 76.4% of patients and aspirin in 16.6% of patients. Compared with other AF patients, VKA were being significantly less prescribed in lone AF patients than in other AF patients (71% *vs* 77%, p<0.001), despite a younger age. On multivariate analysis, lone AF was significantly associated with non-prescription of VKA (Odds Ratio: 0.56, 95% CI: 0.43-0.73; p <0.0001). **Conclusions**: In 2002 in France, VKA were being prescribed in more than 75% of ambulatory patients with permanent AF. The prescription of VKA was lower in patients with lone AF.

OC131

Residual vein thrombosis assessment establishes the optimal duration of anticoagulants in patients with idiopathic or provoked deep vein thrombosis

Siragusa S (1), Milio G (2), Cormaci O (3), Anastasio R (1), Malato A (1), Bonifacio G (1), Amato C (2), Pellegrino M (4), Mariani G (1)*

(1) Thrombosis and Haemostasis Unit, Division of Hematology, University of Palermo
(2) Division of Angiology, University of Palermo
(3) Division of Vascular Surgery, Hospital "Garibaldi" of Catania
(4) Division of Surgery, Hospital of Trapani

The optimal intensity and duration of Oral Anticoagulant Therapy (OAT) after a first episode of Deep Vein Thrombosis (DVT) is still matter of debated. Patients with unprovoked DVT are currently treated for up to 12 months while patients with provoked DVT are usually treated for shorter periods of time. The persistence of vein clots, Residual Vein Thrombosis (RVT) was found to be associated with an incresead risk of recurrences. However, no prospective studies have been done using this parameter to select patients who could require prolonged OAT. The main advantage of this approach relates to the fact that patients can be treated on the basis of their individual risk of recurrence. In this study we prospectively investigated patients with a first episode of DVT and RVT was used to assess the duration of OAT. **Materials and methods**. During the period March 1999 - September 2002, 252 patients with DVT of the lower limbs (either idiopathic or provoked) were evaluated in a randomized controlled trial; patients with cancer or lupus anticoagulant were excluded. At the third months of OAT, RVT was assessed as previously described (Siragusa et al, Thromb Haemost 1993;538:1435); briefly, RVT was considered present when a clot occupying up to 60% of the vein lumen was detected by compression ultrasonography. Patients with RVT were randomly assigned to continue OAT for 1 year (group A1), or to stop it (group A2). In patients without evidence of RVT, OAT was discontinued (group B). Events, classified as recurrent DVT and/or Pulmonary Embolism (PE) or major and minor bleeding were evaluated; all patients were followed-up for additional 12 months after OAT discontinuation. **Results**. 218 patients completed the study; at the third months of OAT, RVT was still present in the 64.6% of patients. The rate of recurrent events at 12-months follow-up was 7.3%, 15.6% and 1.8% in group A1, A2 and B, respectively; these differences were statistically significant. The rate of major bleeding was 2.4%, 1.25 and 0% in group A1, A2 and B, respectively. Considering a time to event analysis (21 months), in patients without RVT the incidence of recurrent DVT remains low after OAT withdrawal while in patients with RVT the risk of recurrent VTE increased after the discontinuation of OAT. **Conclusions**. This is the first prospective, randomised trial assessing the optimal duration of OAT on the individual risk basis. This investigation shows that patients without RVT, after stopping OAT and no matter the type of DVT (either idiopathic or provoked), maintain a low risk of recurrences; therefore, in these patients OAT can be safely withheld after 3 months. In patients with persistent vein occlusion, OAT should be continued for more than 3 months although it is not clear for a long since prolonged OAT simply delay the risk of recurrence.

OC132

Comparative effects of antiplatelet, anticoagulant or combined therapy in patients with valvular and non-valvular atrial fibrillation

Narváez I (1), Iriarte J (1), Perez Gomez F (2), Caso R (1), Matinez B (1), Sagastagoitia J (3), Zumalde J (4), Molinero E (3)*

(1) FIDEC, Bilbao, Spain
(2) Hospital Universitario San Carlos, Madrid, Spain,
(3) Hospital de Basurto, Bilbao, Spain
(4) Hospital de Galdakano, Galdakano, Spain

Background. Anticoagulant therapy was more effective than aspirin in preventing stroke in patients with atrial fibrillation. In order to reduce both thromboembolic and bleeding events the combination of low dose warfarin and aspirin was investigated in three trials, concluding that this combination therapy with an INR below 1.5 was ineffective. In this trial the efficacy and safety of the combination of antiplatelets and moderate intensity anticoagulation has been evaluated. **Methods**. In a multi-centre, randomised trial we included 1209 patients with atrial fibrillation. Low risk patients were excluded. The intermediate risk group included patients with risk factors or>60 years: 242 received 600 mg/day of the cyclooxygenase inhibitor triflusal, 237 acenocoumarol (INR=2-3) and 235 the combination of both (INR=1.5-2). In the high risk group (patients with prior embolism or mitral stenosis), 259 received anticoagulants (INR=2-3) and 236 the combined therapy (INR=1.4-2.4). Median follow-up was 2.76 years. Primary outcome was a composite of vascular death, transient ischaemic attack and non-fatal stroke or systemic embolism. **Results**. Intermediate risk group: the primary outcome was lower in the combined than either the antiplatelet (HR 4.13, 95%CI 1.56-10.91; p=0.004) or the anticoagulant arms (HR 2.95, 95%CI 1.07-8.12; p=0.037). High risk group: the outcome was lower in the combined than in the anticoagulant arm (HR 1.97, 95% CI 1.06-3.96; p=0.03). Severe bleeding incidence was lower in the antiplatelet (2/235) than either the anticoagulant (23/479) or the combined arms (17/445); p=0.005 for both, without significant difference between anticoagulant and combined therapy. Non-valvular patients and those with mitral stenosis had similar event-rates during anticoagulant therapy. **Conclusions**. The combined antiplatelet therapy plus moderate intensity anticoagulation significantly decreased the vascular events compared with the anticoagulant alone and proved to be safe in atrial fibrillation patients.

OC133

Regression of severe atherosclerotic lesions after vitamin replacement in hyperhomocysteinemia with multiple heterozigous mutations

Gualdoni A (1), Arquati M (1), Porta B (1), Rossi E (2), Kluijtmans L (3), Cattaneo M (4), Cortellaro M (1)*

(1) Dipartimento Medicina Interna, Istituto Policlinico San Donato, Milan University, Italy
(2) Ospedale L. Sacco, Milan, Italy
(3) University Medical Center Nijmegen, The Netherlands
(4) Ospedale San Paolo, Milan University, Italy

Introduction: Hcy metabolism lies at the intersection of two metabolic pathways, remethylation and trans-sulfuration. The first is a reaction dependent on the activation of methylene tetrahydrofolate reductase (MTHFR), catalyzed by vitamin B12-dependent methionine synthase (MS). The second starts when there is an excess of methionine, or cysteine synthesis is required. In this pathway, the irreversible condensation of homocysteine and serine to cystathionine is catalyzed by the vitamin B6-dependent rate-limiting enzyme cystathionine β-synthase (CBS). Impaired enzyme function caused by genetic mutation or deficiency of the B vitamins pyridoxine and cyanocobalamin and folic acid can lead to hyperhomocysteinemia. **Case report**: A 31-yr-old male, non-smoker, presented marfanoid habitus, ectopia lentis and severe, symptomatic diffuse atherosclerosis (right renal arterial stenosis, arterial disease of the lower limbs and coronary vessel disease). Laboratory findings showed high homocysteine (364 mmol/L), low levels of vitamin B12 (103 pg/mL) and folic acid (3.7 mg/mL), MTHFR polymorphism (heterozygous for both the C677T and A1298C variants), and CBS heterozygous mutations G919A (i.e. the Celtic). The predominant CBS mutation in homocysteinuria (T833C) was absent. The patient had the wild-type T833T genotype; CBS activity in cultured fibroblasts, with and without pyridoxal-5-phosphate, was low-normal but not deficient. The patient received vitamin replacement (50 mg pyridoxine and 5 mg folic acid daily, plus 1000 mcg cyanocobalamin monthly). After three years the patient appears symptom-free, with normal levels of Hcy (mean 12 mmol/L). Coronary angiography and 2-D B-mode ultrasound scans of the legs showed complete regression of atherosclerotic lesions. On suspending vitamin B6 and B12 Hcy levels promptly rose again. The patient is now only taking pyridoxine and folic acid and his Hcy is normal. **Conclusions**: The severe clinical phenotype and the very high Hcy levels can be explained by the multiple heterozygous mutations of the enzymes involved in Hcy metabolism (MTHFR C677T and A1298C plus CBS G919A). Monomers of the CBS protein with the G919A mutation are degraded rapidly intracellularly and will therefore not be a major constituent of the active tetrameric protein. The drop in CBS activity justifies the clinical benefit of pyridoxine replacement to induce trans-sulfuration pathways.

OC134

Gene polymorphisms (C677T and A1298C MTHFR, A2756G MTR and 844ins68 CBS) in atrial fibrillation

Giusti B, Marcucci R, Gensini F, Cecchi E, Lapini I, Rossi L, Padeletti L, Pepe G, Prisco D, Gensini GF*

Department of Medical and Surgical Critical Care, Thrombosis Centre, University of Florence, Azienda

Atrial fibrillation (AF) is the most common sustained cardiac arrhythmia. AF is associated with the risk of developing stroke. Elevated plasma total homocysteine (tHcy) concentrations are a risk factor for cerebrovascular disease. Hyperhomocysteinemia may be associated with the presence of polymorphisms in genes codifying for enzymes involved in the Hcy metabolism. **Aims**: Aim of this study was to evaluate homocysteinemia and the prevalence of C677T and A1298C of 5,10-methylenetetrahydrofolate reductase (MTHFR), A2756G of methionine synthase (MTR) and 844ins68 of cystathionine β synthase (CBS) gene polymorphisms in patients affected by AF. We studied 245 patients with AF [mean age 73±8.84, 135 males and 110 females] and 245 matched healthy control subjects. tHcy plasma levels were determined by FPIA. For polymorphism detection, DNA was amplified by PCR and genotype was determined with microarray technology by using electronic chips (Nanogen technology). tHcy plasma levels were significantly higher in AF patients than in controls (14.8, 5.4-54.1 versus 11.5, 1.6-52.6 μmol/L, p=0.001). tHcy plasma levels were significantly higher iŋ AF patients with history of ischemic event(s) than in AF patients without history (15.4, 5.4-54.1 versus 13.9, 6.7-38.6 μmol/L, p<0.05). The prevalence of homozygous C677T genotype was not different in AF patients (17.7%) in comparison to controls (18.3%). The prevalence of homozygous C677T genotype was significantly ($p<0.05$) higher in patients with ischemic events (24.4%) than in those without events (9.9%). No difference in the prevalence of homozygotes for all the other polymorphisms investigated in AF patients and controls was observed. The risk of AF significantly increased in the higher quartile of Hcy (OR=4.50, 95% CI 2.73-7.44). The highest Hcy quartile and C677T homozygosity were associated with an increased risk of ischemic events (Hcy OR=2.62, 95% CI 1.40-4.92; C677T OR=2.95, 95% CI 1.53-5.67). In conclusion, our results demonstrate an association between elevated tHcy levels and the presence of AF. Moreover, tHcy is a risk factor for ischemic complications of AF. Our data stress the interest to extend the study to a larger number of subjects and the possible polymorphism interaction in order to better understand their possible role in AF.

OC135

Homocysteine, vitamins and C-reactive protein in the InCHIANTI Study

Gori A (1), Sofi F (1), Marcucci R (1), Giusti B (1), Fedi S (1), Sestini I (1), Rogolino A (1), Cesari F (1), Corsi AM (2), Ferrucci L (3)*

(1) Department of Medical and Surgical Critical Care, Thrombosis Centre, University of Florence, Azienda
(2) Laboratory of Clinical Epidemiology, Geriatric Department, National Institute of Research and Care
(3) Longitudinal Studies Section, Gerontology Research Center, National Institute on Aging

Several retrospective and prospective studies have demonstrated that increased total plasma homocysteine levels are associated with both arterial and venous disease. Elevated levels of homocysteine may reflect increasing age, male sex, renal failure, vitamin deficiencies (low folate vitamin B12 or vitamin B6), or inherited abnormalities of enzymes involved in the methionine metabolism, such as methylene tetrahydrofolate reductase (MTHFR). The aims of this study were to evaluate in the InCHIANTI Study, a prospective population-based Italian study of risk factors for disability in late life: 1- total homocysteine, vitamin B12 and B6 and C-Reactive Protein (CRP) levels and 2- the association between homocysteine levels and the genetic polymorphisms of methionine metabolism enzyme (MTHFR C677T and MTHFR A1298C). Therefore, we studied 460 men (78% aged, ≥ 65 years) and 560 women (81% aged, ≥ 65 years) randomly selected from the people living in two sites in the surrounding of Florence, Italy. Homocysteine plasma levels were significantly ($p<0.0001$) higher in men (median 14.8 μmol/L; range 7.1-95.9 μmol/L) than in women (median 12.8 μmol/L; range 5.4-54.8 μmol/L) and significantly correlated with increasing age ($r= 0.46$; $p<0.0001$). In the InCHIANTI population serum folic acid, vitamin B6 and B12 were 6.3 (0.7-45.3) nmol/L, 25.3 (0.4-689.2) nmol/L and 285 (25.2-1488.1) pmol/L respectively. Homocysteine showed a significant inverse correlation with folate, vitamin B6 and vitamin B12 ($r= -0.28$, $p<0.001$; $r=-0.31$, $p<0.001$ and $r=-0.29$, $p<0.001$ respectively). A statistically significant genotype-phenotype association ($p<0.01$) between homocysteine plasma levels and C677T MTR polymorphisms was observed, whereas no significant association with A1298C MTHFR polymorphism was found. Furthermore, in subjects with folic acid < 5nmol/L we observed a significant genotype-phenotype association ($p<0.001$) between homocysteine plasma levels and C677T MTHFR polymorphism, but not in those with folic acid ≥ 5nmol/L. CRP levels are significantly associated with advanced age ($p<0.05$). Vitamin B6 serum levels inversely correlated with age ($r=-0.42$, $p<0.001$) and with CRP serum levels ($r= -0.20$, $p<0.05$). In this study a relationship between inflammation, homocysteine and vitamin B6 status was found. Furthermore, these data demonstrate that in a large Italian population homocysteine levels were influenced by C677T MTHFR polymorphism in subjects with reduced folic acid levels.

OC136

Absolute risk of venous and arterial thromboembolism associated with mild hyperhomocysteinemia

van de Poel M (1), Libourel E (1), Bank I (2), Middeldorp S (2), Hamulyak K (3), Prins M (3), Büller HR (2), van der Meer J (1)*

(1) University Hospital Groningen, Netherlands
(2) Academic Medical Center Amsterdam, Netherlands
(3) University Hospitall Maastricht, Netherlands

Purpose: To assess the absolute and relative risk of venous and arterial thromboembolism associated with hyperhomocysteinemia (HH) in a family cohort study. **Methods**: Probands had had venous or arterial thromboembolism and revealed HH on oral methionine loading. Their first degree > 15 year old relatives were tested for HH as well as other thrombophilic disorders. Clinical data were collected prior to testing. Annual incidences were calculated from the number of events including venous thromboembolism (VTE), myocardial infarction (MI), transient ischemic attack (TIA), ischemic stroke (IS) and peripheral arterial disease (PAD), and observation years. Relative risks were calculated from annual incidences in relatives with and without HH. **Results**: Of 434 relatives, 147 (32%) had HH. The total follow up was 13360 patient years. Annual incidences (with 95% confidence intervals) of VTE in relatives with and without HH were 0.23 (0.12-0.41) vs 0.10 (0.05-0.20), relative risk of 2.2 (0.9-5.3). Annual incidences of MI were 0.17 (0.07-0.33) vs 0.16 (0.09-0.27), relative risk of 1.0 (0.43-2.45). Annual incidences of TIA were 0.13 (0.05-0.27) vs 0, relative risk of 108.1 (0.21-55969). Annual incidences of IS were 0.15 (0.06-0.30) vs 0.03 (0.007-0.10), relative risk 4.2 (1.09-16.3). Annual incidences of PAD were 0.15 (0.06-0.30) vs 0.06 (0.002-0.14), relative risk 2.5 (0.80-7.95). **Conclusion**: Although HH contributes to the risk of VTE the absolute risk hardly differs from the general population. Our data show differences in relative risks for various arterial diseases, however the absolute risks of MI, IS, TIA and PAD were similar.

OC137

Methionine loading test affects thrombin generation in high risk patients

Domagala TB, Undas A, Celińska-Lowenhoff M, Rybak M, Szczeklik A*

Department of Medicine, Jagiellonian University School of Medicine, Cracow, Poland

Introduction Homocysteine has been shown to predispose to thrombotic complications of atherosclerosis and venous thrombosis. There is very little data on the effect of methionine load on blood coagulation in patients with high cardiovascular risk. **Aim** We evaluated whether a methionine load could increase thrombin production in vivo. **Materials and methods** We studied 30 subjects with several risk factors for CAD, history of unstable angina or previous myocardial infarction (aged 53.9 ± 6.6 years). A standard oral methionine loading test (100 mg/kg of body weight) was performed in each individual and blood samples were taken prior to and 4 hours following the methionine ingestion to determine plasma total homocysteine levels using a HPLC method. We sampled the blood emerging from the bleeding-time skin incisions on a forearm every 30 seconds, and in the supernatants we determined thrombin-antithrombin complexes (TAT) by ELISA (Dade Behring). **Results** Plasma homocysteine levels increased from mean 13.8 ± 3.7 to 33.3 ± 7.36 μmol/L after 4 hours ($p<0.0001$). The estimated mean thrombin production at the sites of microvascular injury, as assessed by TAT levels, increased significantly by 30% following a methionine load ($p<0.0001$). A major difference in time-course of TAT generation was observed in the propagation phase at 3 minutes and later. **Conclusions** In patients with high cardiovascular risk a methionine load is associated with an increased thrombin formation with no correlation between this increase and the rise in plasma tHcy levels.

OC138

Hyperhomocysteinemia in cancer patients with thrombosis is independent of methylene tetrahydrofolate reductase gene mutation

Cunanan J (1), Tobu M (1), Iqbal O (1), Demir M (2), Fareed J (1), Deitcher S (3)*

(1) Loyola University Medical Center, Maywood, IL, USA
(2) Trakya University Medical School, Edirne, Turkey
(3) The Cleveland Clinic Foundation, Cleveland, OH, USA

Introduction: Plasma homocysteine level is considered to be an important surrogate marker of vasculopathy in thrombotic disorders. Methylene tetrahydrofolate reductase (MTHFR) gene mutations and nutritional factors (folic acid/ B_{12}) are primarily responsible for the observed increase in this surrogate marker. Cancer patients exhibit increased prevalence of thrombotic events. **Aims**: The aim of these studies was to show that an upregulation of homocysteine plays a role in cancer associated thrombosis. However, initial screening of cancer patients showed that the malignancy related thrombotic state was independent of molecular defects in Factor V Leiden, Prothrombin 20210 and MTHFR variants. **Materials and Methods**: In the same group of 102 patients who were diagnosed with cancer and in another group of cancer free patients with thrombosis enrolled in a treatment study with low molecular weight heparin (CORTES, n=50), blood levels of homocysteine were measured using a highly specific ELISA method (Diazyme Laboratories, San Diego, CA). **Results**: On a cumulative basis the cancer patients exhibited a relatively higher level of homocysteine (11.8±4.7 μM/L) in comparison to normal (n=140, 4.6±2.9 μM/L) and in contrast to cancer patients exhibiting homocysteine levels (7.8±3.1 μM/L). No difference in the MTHFR gene mutation profile was noted in the three groups. These results clearly suggest that, cancer patients with thrombosis exhibited a relatively higher level of circulating homocysteine levels, which are unrelated to a molecular defect in MTHFR. **Conclusions**: Cancer free patients with thrombosis do not exhibit this increase in circulating homocysteine levels. Thus, other relevant factors such as the use of chemotherapeutic agents like methotrexate and purine analogs may contribute to this apparently acquired upregulation of homocysteine. This observation warrants periodic monitoring of homocysteine in patients with thrombosis and cancer. Nutritional supplementation of folic acid and B_{12} may be helpful in the overall management of these patients.

OC139

Circulating tissue inhibitor of metalloproteinase-1 elevation correlates with impaired diastolic relaxation in patients with hypertension

Tayebjee M, Nadar S, MacFadyen R, Lip G*

University Department of Medicine, City Hospital, Birmingham, UK, B18 7QH

Background: Hypertension (HBP), hypertensive heart disease and left ventricular (LV) hypertrophy are integral to symptomatic diastolic heart failure. Tissue inhibitor of metalloproteinase 1 (TIMP-1) is linked to extracellular matrix fibrosis and is elevated in HBP. We explored the link between circulating TIMP-1, matrix metalloproteinase 9 (MMP-9) and resting echocardiographic LV filling. **Methods**: Circulating MMP-9 and TIMP-1 levels were measured in citrated plasma by ELISA in 74 patients with HBP (58 male, age 58 ± 11yrs) and 34 controls (23 male, mean age 53± 13years). Demography and standard resting echocardiographic indices of diastolic function were recorded. All had confirmed normal short axis systolic contractility. **Results**: Predictably there were significant differences in systolic and diastolic blood pressure, and baseline creatinine between the two groups. Although the hypertensive patients were unselected, there were significant differences in many of the parameters reflecting diastolic dysfunction (e,a, e', a', e'/a' and e/e'), and left ventricular mass (Table 1). Both MMP-9 and TIMP-1 were higher in the hypertensive group (Table 1). Within the hypertensive cohort, only TIMP-1 correlated with left ventricular mass (r=0.271,p=0.024), left ventricular mass index (r=0.323,p=0.007) and tissue Doppler parameters of diastolic dysfunction (e'(r= - 0.338,p=0.005), a' (r=-0.350, p=0.005) and e/e'(r=0.334,p=0.005). **Conclusion**: TIMP-1 is thought to increase tissue concentrations of collagen type I by preventing its breakdown by matrix metalloproteinases. Our findings therefore add weight to a hypothesis suggesting that TIMP-1 may be a key mediator of left ventricular diastolic dysfunction through definition of the ventricular matrix composition.

Table 1. Baseline Characteristics (data presented as Mean±SD or Median (IQR))

	Controls (n=34)	Hypertensives (n=74)	p
Age (yrs)	54±13	58±11	0.152*
Male (%)	68	78	0.232^
SBP (mmHg)	126±13	150±26	<0.0001*
DBP (mmHg)	79±8	88±14	<0.0001*
Cholesterol (mM)	5.7 (5.1-6.1)	5.2(4.8-6.1)	0.353
Creat (mM)	81±13	93±16	<0.0001*
LV mass (g)	172(130-229)	217(175-278)	0.0054**
LVMI	64(48-79)	80(63-98)	0.0055**
e (m/s)	0.71±0.15	0.81±0.15	0.004*
a (m/s)	0.66±0.12	0.81±0.16	<0.0001*
e/a	1.10(0.94-1.23)	1.00(0.85-1.16)	0.229**
e'	0.12(0.09-0.14)	0.09(0.07-0.10)	0.0017**
a'	0.09(0.05-0.10)	0.09(0.08-0.11)	0.123**
e'/a'	1.20(1.00-1.80)	0.88(0.71-1.05)	<0.0001**
e/e'	6.54(4.75-7.14)	8.89(7.55-10.75)	<0.0001**
IVRT (s)	111(99-130)	118(109-137)	0.435**
MMP-9 (ng/ml)	41(35-91)	70(49-120)	0.0039**
TIMP-1 (ng/ml)	305(238-380)	380(280-550)	0.0054**

(SBP, systolic blood pressure; DBP, diastolic blood pressure; Creat, serum creatinine; LV, left ventricle, LVMI, left ventricular mass index; IVRT, isovolumetric relaxation time; MMP, matrix metalloproteinase; TIMP, tissue inhibitor of metalloproteinase)

OC140

Circulating MMP-9, TIMP-1 and TIMP-2 in gestational hypertension

Tayebjee M, Karalis I, Nadar S, Beevers DG, MacFadyen R, Lip G*

University Department of Medicine, City Hospital, Birmingham, UK, B18 7QH

Background: Gestational hypertension (GH) is dangerous to both mother and child. Arterial invasiveness and growth are dependent on successful extracellular matrix (ECM) breakdown, which may be abnormal in GH. We hypothesised abnormalities in circulating Matrix metalloproteinase -9 (MMP-9) and tissue inhibitors of metalloproteinases -1 and -2 (TIMP-1 &2) in patients with GH, when compared to normotensive normal pregnancies and healthy non-pregnant controls. **Methods**: Plasma MMP-9, TIMP-1 and TIMP-2 were measured by ELISA in 23 women with GH, 30 normotensive pregnant women and 28 non-pregnant women, that were matched for age, gestational age and parity. **Results**: Levels of circulating MMP-9, TIMP-1&2 and the MMP-9/TIMP-1 & MMP-9/TIMP-2 ratios were significantly different between the three groups (p=0.026, p=0.006, p=0.007, p=0.001 and p=0.008 respectively). Post hoc Tukeys analysis (for p<0.05), demonstrated that the significant differences were as follows: for MMP-9 and TIMP-1 between the non pregnant and pregnant controls (153(61-218) vs. 210(119-281 and 197(173-228) vs. 180(145-196) respectively); for TIMP-2 between non pregnant controls and GH and normotensive pregnant and PIH (140(105-168) vs. 180(120-220) and 138(110-174) vs. 180(120-220) respectively) and for MMP-9/TIMP-1 and MMP-9/TIMP-2 between the non pregnant controls and pregnant controls (0.66(0.35-1.06) vs. 1.3(0.81-1.81) and 1.13(0.56-1.68) vs. 1.38(1,17-1.96) respectively) and the latter group and GH group (1.30(0.81-1.81) vs. 0.81(0.46-1.27) and 1.38(1.17-1.96) vs. 0.85(0.53-1.46) respectively). Within the GH group, MMP-9 and the MMP-9/TIMP-1 ratio correlated negatively with age (r= -0.581, p=0.004 and r= -0.563, p=0.005 respectively) and levels of diastolic blood pressure (r = -0.432, p=0.040 and r= -0.461, p=0.027 respectively). Using a multiple regression analysis, only age independently correlated with circulating levels of MMP-9 (p=0.010), however neither age nor levels of diastolic blood pressure had any effect on the MMP-9/TIMP-1 ratio. The MMP-9/TIMP-2 ratio correlated negatively with levels of diastolic blood pressure (r= -0.453, p=0.030). **Conclusion**: We have demonstrated altered MMP/TIMP ratios in maternal blood duringGH. These observations suggest pregnancy related changes in ECM breakdown and turnover. Given the importance of changes in ECM composition to vascular and cardiac structure in hypertension it is reasonable to suggest that these observations may be central to the pathophysiology of human GH.

OC141

Matrix metalloproteinase-9 and tissue inhibitor of metalloproteinase-1 in hypertension: Relationship to cardiovascular risk and treatment

Tayebjee M, Nadar S, Blann AD, Beevers DG, MacFadyen R, Lip G*

University Department of Medicine, City Hospital, Birmingham, UK, B18 7QH

Background: Hypertension results in structural changes to the cardiac and vascular extracellular matrix (ECM). Matrix metalloproteinases (MMP) and their inhibitors (TIMP) may play a central role in the modulation of this matrix. We hypothesized that both MMP-9 and TIMP-1 would be abnormal in hypertension, reflecting alterations in ECM turnover, and that their circulating levels should be linked to cardiovascular (CHD) and stroke (CVA) risk scores using the Framingham equation. Secondly, we hypothesized that treatment would result in changes in ECM indices. **Methods**: Plasma MMP-9 and TIMP-1 were measured pre and post treatment (median 3 years) from 96 hypertensive patients. Pre treatment values were compared to circulating MMP-9 and TIMP-1 levels in 45 age- and gender- matched healthy controls. **Results**: Circulating MMP-9 and TIMP-1 pre treatment were significantly higher in patients with hypertension than in the normotensive controls (p=0.0041 and p= 0.0166 respectively). Plasma MMP-9 levels fell, and TIMP-1 levels rose following treatment (p=0.035 and p=0.005 respectively). Levels of MMP-9 correlated with CHD risk (r= 0.317, p=0.007) and HDL cholesterol (r= -0.237, p=0.022), but not CVA risk. There were no significant correlations between TIMP-1 and CVA and CHD scores. **Conclusion**: Raised circulating MMP-9 and TIMP-1 at baseline in untreated patients with hypertension could reflect an increased deposition and retention of type I collagen at the expense of other components of ECM within the cardiac and vascular ECM. Following cardiovascular risk management, MMP-9 levels fell and TIMP-1 levels rose. Elevated levels of MMP-9 also appeared to be associated with higher Framingham cardiovascular risk scores. Our observations suggest a possible role for these surrogate markers of tissue ECM composition and the prognosis of cardiovascular events in hypertension.

OC142

Correlation of protein and mRNA expression of fibrinolytic and matrix metalloproteinase systems in endometriosis

*Ramón L (1), Gilabert-Estellés J (1), Castelló R (1), Gilabert J (2), España F (1), Chirivella M (1), Romeu A (1), Aznar J (1), Estellés A (1)**

(1) Hospital Universitario La Fe, Valencia, Spain.
(2) Hospital Arnau de Vilanova. Valencia, Spain.

Introduction: Endometriosis is a benign gynaecologic disease defined as the presence of endometrial tissue outside the uterus. This ectopic tissue has the ability to implant at ectopic sites, such as ovary and peritoneum, where a local extracellular proteolysis might take place. This process involves the plasminogen activator (PA) and matrix metalloproteinase (MMP) systems. **Aims**: The objective of this study was to analyse mRNA expression with quantitative real-time RT-PCR and protein levels of several components of PA and MMP systems in ovarian endometrioma and endometrium of women with and without endometriosis (control group). Material and methods: This study included 45 women with endometriosis and 28 women without the disease. **Results**: Eutopic endometrium of women with endometriosis showed higher mRNA expression of urokinase type-PA (uPA) and MMP-3. Ovarian endometrioma had higher mRNA and antigen levels of PA inhibitor type 1 (PAI-1) an MMP inhibitor type 1 (TIMP-1) than endometrium. In contrast, PAI-3 antigen levels and mRNA expression were reduced in endometriotic tissue in comparison to endometrium from women with and without the disease. **Conclusions**: The endometrium of women with endometriosis has an elevated proteolytic activator expression, which might contribute to the capability of implantation of endometrial cells at ectopic sites. The ovarian endometrioma has a high antigen and mRNA expression of protease inhibitors, which may limit the invasive capability of this tissue and explain the frequent clinical finding of an isolated ovarian endometriotic cyst. In conclusion, quantitative real-time RT-PCR can be a valuable tool for further investigations on plasminogen activator and MMP systems in endometriosis. (FIS PI020136 and PI020125, Fundación Investigación 2003 (H.U. La Fe. Valencia, Spain).

OC143

Popliteal arterial aneurysm – the role of proteolytic enzymes

Kozak M, Štalc J, Tominc U*

University Medical Center Ljubljana, Slovenia

Introduction: Most common arterial aneurysms are probably due to atherosclerosis. The pathogenesis of arterial aneurysm formation is not completely understood, however, involvement of proteolytic degradation of extracellular matrix components (collagen, elastin) due to matrix metalloproteinase (MMP) and fibrinolytic system activity could be important. **Aim**: The aim of our study was to assess the significance of matrix metalloproteinase and fibrinolytic system for popliteal artery aneurysm (PAA) formation. **Patients and methods**: In our study we included 22 patients with PAA (Group PAA: 20 males, 2 females, mean age 62,7 ± 10,3) and 17 age-, sex- and atherosclerosis risk factors-matched patients with peripheral atherosclerotic arterial disease (PAD) (Group PAD: 15 males, 2 females, mean age 67,1 ± 10,6). Concentrations of MMP-3, -9, -13, tissue-type plasminogen activator (t-PA), plasminogen activator inhibitor 1 antigen (PAI-1), D-dimer, fibrinogen, C-reactive protein, PAI activity, euglobulin clot lysis time (ECLT) and prothrombin time (PT/INR) were measured. Mann – Whitney U test was used for statistical comparison. **Results**: There was no difference in concentrations of observed parameters between groups. We found only significantly higher ($p = 0{,}04$) PAI activity in group PAA (median 9,3 IU/ml) compared to group PAD (median 5,5 IU/ml. **Conclusions**: We conclude that studied proteolytic enzymes (MMP-3, MMP-9, MMP-13 and enzymes of fibrinolytic system) are probably not involved in popliteal arterial aneurysm formation. PAI activity, higher in patients with aneurysm, could be explained with PAI released from intravascular thrombi in patients with aneurysm.

OC144

The roles of serum matrix metalloproteinases in patients with post myocardial infarction to heart failure

Jong G (1), Ma T (2), Kuo S (3)*

(1) Division of Cardiology, Armed Force Taichung General Hospital
(2) Department of the Health Service Management, China Medical University
(3) Department of Resourances Engineering, NCKU, Tainan and Department of Resources Engineering Dahan In

Introduction: Matrix metalloproteinases (MMPs) play a key role in the pathogenesis of atherosclerosis. MMP family consists of at least 20 numbers; MMPs are produced by the different cell types (vascular smooth cells, monocytes endothelial cells) involved in the atheromatous plaque formation and participate to extracellular matrix remolding and cell infiltration or migration. Myocardial infarction (MI) is thought to be involved in the destabilization and rupture of atherosclerotic lesions. The destruction of cardiac tissue due to myocardial ischemia could further result in heart failure. **Aims**: To investigate the possible mechanism of serum MMPs in patients with post MI to heart failure. **Materials and methods**: Twenty-eight myocardial infarction (MI) with heart failure (Killip FC II-III) patients (group A) and 27 normal subjects (MI with Killip I) (group B) were collected to evaluate the serum levels of MMP-2 and –9 by ELISA and Zymography. **Results**: It was observed that the serum levels of MMP-9 activity significantly increased ($p<0.01$) especially LAD lesion in the group A. There was no significant difference of MMP-2 activity between two groups ($p=0.36$). **Conclusions**: We concluded that increase of MMP-9 activity not only may be used as the marker of diagnosing the developing heart failure in patients of post MI, but also provide some explanation of the pathogenesis from post MI to heart failure.

OC145

Managed hemostasis "point-of-care" testing in a large hospital: a three-year experience and the assessment of clotting tests

Paniccia R (1), Costanzo M (1), Tronchin M (2), Messeri G (2), Gazzini A (1), Coviello S (1), Antonucci E (1), Abbate R (1), Gensini G (1), Prisco D (1)*

(1) Department of Medical and Surgical Critical Care, Thrombosis Centre, University of Florence, Azienda
(2) Laboratorio Analisi Biochimico-Cliniche, Azienda Ospedaliero-Universitaria Careggi, Florence, Italy

Point-of-care (POC) automated systems for coagulation evaluation are key tools in surgical and/or intensive health care units. Activated clotting time (ACT) is the most common hemostasis POC test to quickly monitor heparin anticoagulation during cardiopulmonary bypass, interventional cardiology and hemodialysis. Recently, these POC systems have been updated to rapidly perform aPTT and PT on whole blood, to obtain a shortening of time of results. To ensure safe and appropriate patient care, the clinical safety of POC tests in hemostasis is based on achievement of accurate and reliable results. This report was aimed to show the routine quality control (QC) testing and tracking, as a part of a comprehensive quality assurance program, for hemostasis POC devices, performed in Careggi Hospital (Firenze, Italy). Twenty-one Hemochron devices (International Technidyne Corp, USA) were located in 8 buildings. More than 18,500 analysis/year were performed in the different Units. A management staff for hemostasis POC was designed to control the use of these devices and specific and repeated training courses were held to hospital staff. QCs for each instrument and for each new lot of test cartridges were performed by the POC supervisor. Within-day CVs from normal and abnormal controls were respectively: for ACT <7% and <3%; for aPTT <8% and <4%; for PT <10% and <4%. Day-to-day CVs from normal and abnormal controls were respectively: for ACT <10% and <5%; for aPTT <9 % and <4 %; for PT <11 % and <4. %. In vivo duplicate testing values showed significant correlations: for ACT (n=90) $r=0.99$, $p<0.001$; for aPTT (n=45) $r=0.98$, $p<0.001$; for PT (n=60) $r=0.94$, $p<0.001$. Significant relationships were found between values obtained from POC tests and those from centralized laboratory: for aPTT (n=60) $r=0.98$, $p<0.001$; for PT (n=32) $r=0.88$, $p<0.001$. The sample collections and procedures of POC tests were found properly performed by the staff of each Unit. However, a logbook with registration of results was not set. Although the good performances of these hemostasis POC devices. The results of this survey show that the training of local personnel and logistic assistance is absolutely necessary. Supervision of POC systems by laboratory professional is mandatory and a continuous QC evaluation and reporting is only the first step. A more comprehensive supervision (QC results read on-line) will lead to greater improvements of POC tests management.

OC146

Once-daily LMWH versus UFH for the treatment of acute venous thromboembolism: a non-inferiority meta-analysis

Assante C (1), Cucherat M (2), Laporte S (1), Rivron-Guillot K (1), Decousus H (1), Mismetti P (1)*

(1) Thrombosis Research Group, University Hospital of Saint-Etienne, France
(2) Biostatistic Dept., Laennec University, Lyon Hospital, France.

Introduction LMWH are now considered to be the standard treatment for acute DVT and some of them can be administered either once or twice daily. Only one meta-analysis took into account these two different dose regimens by directly comparing once-daily LMWH with twice-daily LMWH. Furthermore, although there are several published meta-analyses that compared the efficacy of LMWH with that of UFH, none considered once-daily LMWH regimens separately. **Aim** We performed a meta-analysis of all available randomised trials directly comparing once-daily LMWH with UFH in the acute treatment of venous thromboembolism. This meta-analysis explicitly assessed the non-inferiority of once-daily LMWH against UFH. **Materials and methods** Relative risks (RR) and corresponding 95% confidence intervals (CI) were calculated. We chose to assess the efficacy non-inferiority and safety superiority of LMWH. Prior to the study, the non-inferiority threshold of LMWH was set at a level that conserved at least 75% of the efficacy of UFH compared with placebo (data from Brandjes's study [1]). Accordingly, the RR for the primary outcome (symptomatic recurrent thromboembolism) was 1.50. **Results** Eight studies, corresponding to 2759 patients, fulfilled the inclusion criteria for the meta-analysis (2 trials assessing tinzaparin, 3 dalteparin, 2 enoxaparin and 1 bemiparin). Compared with UFH, the risk of symptomatic recurrent thromboembolism observed is lower with once-daily LMWH (RR=0.79 [CI: 0.51-1.23]). The upper limit of the confidence interval is lower than the threshold of 1.50, allowing the conclusion of non-inferiority of once-daily LMWH against the reference treatment. For major bleeding, there was a trend in favour of once-daily LMWH (RR=0.62 [0.36-1.08]; p=0.09), likewise for death (RR=0.75 [0.50-1.13]; p=0.17). **Conclusion** We found that once-daily LMWH was as effective as UFH for the treatment of acute venous thromboembolism in terms of recurrent symptomatic venous thromboembolism, without an increase in safety complications. LMWH do not require laboratory monitoring of coagulation parameters so would be more convenient in the outpatient setting. A single daily injection would further simplify the treatment of venous thromboembolism, particularly in the outpatient setting. Brandjes DP *et al.* N Engl J Med 1992; 327: 1485-9.

OC147

Therapeutic implications of product individuality in commercially available low molecular weight heparins and their generic versions

Maddineni J, Walenga J, Jeske W, Hoppensteadt D, Fareed J, Messmore H*

Loyola University Chicago, Chicago, IL, USA 60153

Introduction: The currently available brand-name low molecular weight heparins (LMWHs) in the USA include dalteparin (Pfizer), enoxaparin (Aventis) and tinzaparin (Pharmion). Other products in Europe include certoparin (Novartis), reviparin (Abbott), nadroparin (Sanofi-Synthelabo) and parnaparin (Alpha-Wasserman). Each of these is characterized by their molecular weight profile and biologic activity in terms of an anti-FXa and anti-FIIa ratio. The molecular weight of these drugs ranges from 4 kD to 7 kD and the anti-FXa: anti-FIIa ratio ranges from 1.5 to 3.5. Furthermore, the component oligosaccharide chains exhibit product specific distribution profiles. It is now widely accepted that individual LMWHs are chemically unique agents and cannot be interchanged therapeutically (Merli G et al. J Thromb Thrombolysis 2001;11(3):247-59; Nightingale SL. JAMA 1993;270(14):1672). Recently, several generic LMWHs have become available in India (cutenox and markaparin) and South America. As the primary aim of a generic drug is to reduce cost without compromising patient care, a generic drug is required to be chemically and biologically equivalent to the branded drug. **Objective:** To determine the similarities and differences among the profiles of generic and commercial versions of different LMWHs. **Materials and Methods:** We have utilized a previously reported approach to systematically compare three generic versions of enoxaparin obtained from India and Brazil with the branded enoxaparin available in the USA. Testing included molecular and structural profiling, potency evaluation in clot-based and amidolytic anti-FXa and anti-FIIa assays, interactions with antithrombin III and heparin cofactor II and neutralization profiles. **Results:** While the molecular profiles (3.93 ± 1.4 kD) and anti-FXa potencies were comparable for all four agents, the generic products showed variations in the global anticoagulant assays USP, aPTT and Heptest. Two generic and the branded enoxaparin were readily digested by heparinase-I losing most of their anticoagulant activity, but one generic product resisted digestion possibly due to unique structural features. The protamine sulfate and platelet factor 4 neutralization profiles of all four agents were similar. **Conclusions:** These studies show that, while generic LMWHs may exhibit acceptable MW and anti-FXa profiles, they can exhibit assay-based differences and digestion profiles. In order to assure that the generic LMWHs are equivalent to branded LMWHs, there is a need to develop clear step-wise guidelines that will establish equivalency in physical, chemical, biochemical, pharmacokinetic, pharmacodynamic and drug interactions for these anticoagulant drugs.

OC148

Evaluation of the effectiveness and safety of bemiparin, a second-generation low-molecular-weight heparin, in several orthopaedic settings

Otero-Fernández R (1), Gómez-Outes A (2), Martínez-González J (2), Maeso R (2), Fontcuberta J (3)*

(1) Clinic Hospital San Carlos, Madrid, Spain
(2) Laboratorios Farmacéuticos ROVI, S.A., Madrid, Spain
(3) Hospital de la Santa Creu i Sant Pau, Barcelona, Spain

Introduction: Bemiparin has shown to be an effective and safe drug during clinical trials in orthopaedic patients. Reports on its use in wider populations during post-marketing authorisation have been encouraged. **Aims**: To evaluate the effectiveness, safety and tolerability of bemiparin in a wide population of orthopaedic patients in daily clinical practice. **Material and methods**: Prospective, open, multicenter, not randomized study. Patients from several orthopaedic settings were included. Symptomatic venous thromboembolism (VTE) [deep vein thrombosis (DVT) and pulmonary embolism (PE)], required further confirmation by objective methods (Doppler ultrasound, venography, gammagraphy or pulmonary arteriography). Major and minor bleeding, thrombocytopenia and deaths were also assessed. **Results**: A total of 7,959 patients were included and received bemiparin during 28 days (median). Bemiparin 3,500 IU/d was used in 84.9% of patients (high risk of VTE) whereas bemiparin 2,500 IU/d was used in 15.1% of patients (moderate risk of VTE). Reason for prophylaxis (number of cases) included: knee replacement (1,082), hip replacement (876), knee arthroscopy (769), hip fracture surgery (437), other lower limb surgery (1,569), spine surgery (231), other orthopaedic surgery (420), lower limb trauma (2,052) and other trauma requiring immobilisation (523). VTE was confirmed by objective methods in 80 (1.0%) of 7,959 patients (13 proximal DVTs, 65 distal DVTs and 4 non-fatal PEs). Two patients with PE had also distal DVT. There were 323 (4.1%) patients who developed bleeding events. Eleven (0.1%) of them were major because required treatment discontinuation. There were no cases of spinal haematoma, fatal bleeding or bleeding in critical organs. Mild to moderate thrombocytopenia that did not require treatment discontinuation was observed in 35 patients (0.4%). There were no cases of severe type II thrombocytopenia. A total of 27 patients (0.3%) developed mild to moderate non-serious allergic dermatitis around the injection site, and in 7 of them, treatment was discontinued. Twenty-five (0.3%) of 7,959 patients died during the study. The mean age of these patients was 85 years (range: 66 to 98). There were 3 deaths in which fatal PE could not be ruled out. **Conclusions**: Bemiparin is highly effective and safe in several orthopaedic settings in daily clinical practice. The incidence of complications does not differ from that specified in the Summary of Product Characteristics.

OC149

Bemiparin prospective observational study on the prevention of venous thromboembolism in medical patients

Gómez-Outes A (1), Martínez-González J (1), Maeso R (1), García-Hernández A (2)*

(1) Laboratorios Farmacéuticos ROVI, S.A., Madrid, Spain
(2) Logitest, S.L., Madrid, Spain

Introduction: Venous thromboembolism (VTE) is the cause of death in about 10-12% of all deaths occurring in hospitalised patients. The risk for deep vein thrombosis (DVT) of the lower limbs without prophylaxis in internal medicine is of about 19%. In a previous study, bemiparin suppressed markers of hypercoagulability in acutely ill medical patients with heart failure. **Aims**: To evaluate the effects of bemiparin on symptomatic confirmed VTE, bleeding events, thrombocytopenia and death in acutely ill medical patients in usual clinical practice conditions. **Material and methods**: Prospective, open, multicenter, not randomized, cohort study. Acutely ill patients hospitalised in medical departments were included and received either 2,500 IU or 3,500 IU/d of bemiparin, depending on the degree of VTE risk (moderate or high) assessed by the investigator. Main efficacy and safety endpoints were: symptomatic confirmed VTE [DVT and pulmonary embolism (PE)], major bleeding, thrombocytopenia and death. The observation period was 40 days. **Results**: A total of 297 medical patients were included from 13 centers in Spain due to several causes: lung disease 87 (29.3%), heart disease 80 (26.9%), gastrointestinal disease 18 (6.1%), hemiplegia and/or spinal disease 15 (5.1%), other neurological disease 10 (3.3%), rheumatic disorder 14 (4.7%), haematological disease 11 (3.7%), renal disease 8 (2.7%), other 54 (18.2%). The median age of patients included was 77 years (range: 31 to 98). Overall, 207 patients received bemiparin 2,500 IU/d and 91 patients received bemiparin 3,500 IU/d. In 11 cases, the patient was at high risk of VTE but received bemiparin 2,500 IU. Only one (0.3%) of 297 patients developed a confirmed VTE (non-fatal PE). This patient was at high risk of VTE but received bemiparin 2,500 IU/d. Overall, 4 (1.3%) of 297 patients experienced a major bleeding event. Major bleeding rates showed a trend to be lower in patients receiving bemiparin 2,500 IU vs. 3,500 IU (1% vs. 2.2%; Difference, -1.2%; P = 0.47). There were 2 cases of mild-moderate type I thrombocytopenia during the treatment period that did not require treatment discontinuation. There were no cases of severe type II thrombocytopenia. A total of 22 (7.4%) patients died during treatment period due to causes not related to VTE. **Conclusions**: Bemiparin appears to be highly effective and safe on the prevention of VTE in acutely ill medical patients. Further larger comparative studies are needed.

OC150

Low-molecular-weight heparin causes less heparin-induced antibodies than unfractionated heparin: A prospective study in neurologic patients

Harbrecht U (1), Andrea K (1), Britta B (1), Peter H (1), Thomas K (2), Christoph P (3)*

(1) Institute for Experimental Haematology and Transfusion Medicine, University of Bonn, Germany
(2) Department of Neurology, University of Bonn, Germany
(3) Schering AG, Germany

Background: Low-molecular-weight heparin (LMWH) is increasingly replacing unfractionated heparin (UFH) for thromboprophylaxis and treatment of thrombosis not least owing to less unwarranted side effects, probaply including heparin-induced thrombocytopenia (HIT). However, only few prospective studies have evaluated the frequency of heparin-induced antibodies (HI-Abs) and HIT in LMWH compared to UFH treated patients. **Objective**: We investigated prospectively the incidence of HI-Abs and HIT in neurologic patients treated with UFH or LMWH for prophylactic or therapeutic purpose. **Patients and Methods**: A total of 311 patients (44.4% neurovascular, 20.3% neuroinflammatory, 16.4% neurodegenerative/neoplastic, 19.0% miscellaneous) receiving i.v. UFH (n=96), s.c. UFH (n=104) or s.c. LMWH (n=111) were included in the study. The only inclusion cirterion was heparin treatment for at least five days. Blood for HI-Ab search was taken before/at the onset of heparin treatment and thereafter every five days. All HI-Ab determinations were done after end of heparin treatment from stored samples (-70°C) unless platelet count dropped > 50% or thrombocytopenia (< 120 G/L) developed. Heparin-platelet-factor-4-ELISA (Roche, Germany) and heparin-induced-platelet-activation-assay were used for detection of HI-Abs. Platelet counts were measured before and every 2-3 days during heparin treatment. **Results**: Mean duration of heparin therapy was 17.2. ą 9.0, 16.1 ą 12.6 and 12.6 ą 8.0 in i.v. UFH, s.c UFH and s.c. LMWH treated patients (total UFH vs. LMWH p<0.01). 31.3% of i.v. UFH , 11.8% of s.c. UFH and 1.8 % of LMWH treated patients developed HI-Abs during heparin therapy (i.v. UFH vs. s.c. UFH p< 0.001; total UFH vs. LMWH p < 0.0001). Peak of antibody formation occurred between day 8 and 10. The higher incidence of HI-Abs in patients receiving i.v. compared to s.c. UFH was dependant on total dose of administered heparin (p<0.01). 2.5% (5/200) of all UFH treated patients developed HIT, in contrast to none of the patients receiving LMWH (p=0.17). Incidence of thrombosis was much higher in HI-Ab positive compared to HI-Ab negative patients (11.6% vs. 1.9%; p<0.01). **Conclusions**: UFH in contrast to LMWH treated neurologic patients are at high risk to develop HI-Abs. HIT tended to be higher in UFH treated patients. Presence of heparin-induced antibodies is a risk factor for subsequent development of thrombotic complications.

OC151

Factors I, VII, VIII, IX, X and XI levels and the risk of deep venous thrombosis

*Mello T, Machado T, Ozello M, Annichino-Bizzacchi JM**

State University of Campinas, São Paulo, Brazil

Elevated levels of procoagulant proteins have been associated with an increased risk of venous thrombosis (VT). We investigated whether the increase of coagulation factors I, VII, VIII, IX, X and XI levels are a risk factor for VT. The correlation between ABO blood group and thrombotic risk was also evaluated. This study included 100 Brazilian patients with VT (71 females and 29 males, mean age, 36 years; range 16 to 63) without malignant or antiphospholipid disease and 100 age, race and sex-matched healthy controls. The coagulation factors were measured by a coagulometric method. Odds ratios were calculated as a measurement of relative risk. The mean factors VIII, IX, XI levels were higher in patients than in controls: 208IU/dl versus 146IU/dl (p<0.0001), 132IU/dl versus 117IU/dl (p=0.01), 142IU/dl versus 117IU/dl (p<0.0001) respectively. The 90th percentile of the factors VIII, IX and XI levels in the control group was: 220.4, 157.2 and 164 respectively Subjects with factors VIII, IX and XI levels above the 90th percentile had an increased risk of VT, as compared with those who had these factors levels at or below, that value : OR:6.8 CI:3.16-14.58; OR:2.4 CI:1.05-5.33; OR:2.8 CI:1.28-6.32 respectively. Patients of the non O blood group had a higher thrombosis risk than individuals of blood group O (OR:3.6 CI:1.96-6.56). We concluded that factors VIII, IX, XI levels and the non O blood group represent an increase in the risk of thrombosis. This is the first study to evaluate the factors IX and XI by the coagulometric method. This method may be better than the antigenic measurement since it demonstrates the real activity of these factors upon blood coagulation. If additional studies confirm these results, the determination of these factors should be included in routine thrombophilia screening.

OC152

High factor VIII (FVIII) levels in venous thromboembolism: role of the unbound component of FVIII

Schambeck C, Großmann R, Schwender S, Teuchert K, Walter U*

Institute of Clinical Biochemistry and Pathobiochemistry - Central Laboratory, University of Würzburg

Introduction: Theoretically, von Willebrand factor (VWF) could fully bind factor VIII (FVIII). However, there is even an unbound FVIII (uFVIII) plasma fraction. An altered uFVIII fraction might indicate a dysfunction of the FVIII regulation. This can be suggested in patients with a previous deep-vein thrombosis (DVT) and high FVIII levels. **Material and Methods**: 928 consecutive patients with a history of a DVT were referred to our outpatient department. 321 patients were considered to have high FVIII levels (i. e. levels exceeding the 98th percentile of levels of blood donors). 183 patients had to be excluded since a lot of clinical conditions cause high FVIII levels (acute phase reaction a.s.o.). Finally, plasma samples of 84 patients with unexplained high FVIII levels were available. Healthy blood donors were recruited as controls. To capture the FVIII-VWF-complex, superparamagnetic polystyrene beads with covalently attached streptavidin were coated with biotinylated anti-rabbit Ig and incubated with rabbit anti-human VWF-Ig. Plasma samples were slowly thawed at 4°C and added to the cooled beads. Finally, the beads were separated by a magnetic particle concentrator. The uFVIII fraction was calculated by deviding FVIII in the supernatant of the FVIII-VWF-complex-free sample from that present in the supernatant of the control sample. Additionally, the VWF residuum in the supernatant was determined. FVIII was measured by a chromogenic assay, VWF by an ELISA. **Results**: The thrombosis patients showed median plasma FVIII/VWF ratio of 1.3. Compared to blood donors (median ratio of 1.0), the ratio was significantly higher (p<0.001). Due to the strong impact of VWF on FVIII level, the uFVIII fraction had to be adjusted for VWF residuum. After a stepwise forward procedure of logistic regression, uFVIII had an odds ratio of 0.48 (95%CI 0.35-0.65). The lower odds ratio indicates a reduced uFVIII fraction in thrombosis patients. Analysis of covariance confirmed these results: the estimated mean of the uFVIII fraction in thrombosis patients (6.34%; 95%CI 5.97-6.70) was significantly lower than that in blood donors (7.58%; 95%CI 7.22-7.94). **Conclusions**:_The FVIII-VWF complex predominates in thrombosis patients with high FVIII levels. This may be due to a reduced clearance of this complex by low-density lipoprotein receptor-related protein (LRP). Interestingly, an increased FVIII/VWF ratio was observed in our patients as well as in LRP-deficient mice.

OC153

The relationship between inherited thrombophilia and residual vein thrombosis as risk factors for recurrent venous thromboembolism

Cosmi B, Legnani C, Cini M, Guzzaloca G, Palareti G*

Division of Angiology and Blood Coagulation Disorders, Unitŕ Ricerca Clinica sulla Trombofilia "M. G

Introduction: Residual vein thrombosis (RVT) has been shown to be a risk factors for recurrent VTE after oral anticoagulant therapy (OAT) withdrawal, while the role of congenital thrombophilia is still uncertain. **Aims**: to assess the relationship between RVT and thrombophilia as risk factors for recurrent VTE. **Materials and Methods**: Patients with a first episode of proximal deep vein thrombosis (DVT) of the lower limbs were enrolled on the day of OAT withdrawal and prospectively followed-up for 24 months. On the day of OAT withdrawal, RVT was determined by compression ultrasonography of common femoral and popliteal veins, while blood sampling for inherited thrombophilia was performed on 30 + 10 days afterwards. Recurrences were diagnosed in case of symptoms of VTE by objective methods. **Results**: Among 703 patients, thrombophilia was diagnosed in 148 (21%), while RVT in (52.7%). The proportion of subjects with RVT was 60% among patients with thrombophilia (88 /148) and 50% in subjects without thrombophilia (239/475) (p=0.06). The hazard ratio for recurrence was 1.48 (95% confidence intervals: 0.9-2.45) for patients with thrombophilia when compared with patients without thrombophilia, while it was 1.76 (95% CI: 1.05-2.75) among patients with RVT when compared with patients without RVT, after adjustment for age, sex, duration of OAT, thrombophilia, and type of index event. When compared with patients without thrombophilia and absent RVT, subjects with thrombophilia and RVT had a hazard ratio for recurrence of 2.1 (95% CI: 1.1 -5.7), after adjustment for sex, age, duration of OAT, D-dimer, type of index event and cancer. **Interpretation**: RVT is independent from thrombophilia as a risk factor for recurrent VTE after OAT withdrawal.

OC154

Retinal vein thrombosis and thrombophilic risk factors

Barillari G, Roman D, Giacomello R, Dello Russo P, De Stasio G, Bandello F, Biffoni F*

Hemophilia and Thrombophilia Center, Department of Immunohematology and Transfusion Medicine, General and University Hospital, Udine, Italy

Venous thromboembolism affects approximatively 1 per 1000 persons per year. However, little is known about the real incidence of retinal vein thrombosis. Furthermore, the real role of hemostasis-related genetic and/or acquired risk factors (such as antiphospholipid antibodies, natural coagulation inhibitors, polymorphisms in Factor V, Factor II and MTHFR, fasting homocysteinemia) has not been accurately stated yet. In this observational prospective study 30 consecutive patients with central or branch retinal vein occlusion (RVO) were examined to investigate the role of potential inherited and acquired thrombophilic risk factors. Patients with glaucoma, diabetes mellitus and uncontrolled hypertension were excluded. Median age was 55 yrs (19-82) and male/female ratio about 1:1. Among all hemostatic parameters evaluated (Antithrombin, Protein C, Protein S, free Protein S, APC Resistance, G20210A Prothrombin mutation; Antiphospholipid Antibodies, TAFI, Homocysteinemia, C677T MTHFR polymorphism), only abnormal fasting Homocysteine levels resulted significantly associated with RVO. In fact, in 19/30 patients (accounting for a prevalence of 63%) HyperHomocysteinemia was documented (fasting Hcy > 15 ΓM), while homozigosity for C677T mutation of MTHFR gene was observed in 5/30 cases (prevalence of 17%, not statistically significant as compared to normal population) and Anti-ß2 GP-1 Ab of IgM class were positive in 2/30 patients (at a low titer and in presence of normal Anti CLP Ab, being thus unsignificant). All other investigated hemostatic risk factors resulted normal or absent. In our series, fasting Hyperhomocysteinemia resulted strongly associated with Retinal Vein Occlusion. Further investigations are now necessary to determine the origin (congenital or acquired) of Hyperhomocysteinemia. Moreover, an L-Metionine loading test will allow a more accurate evaluation of the true prevalence of HyperHomocysteinemia in the pathogenesis of Retinal Vein Occlusion.

OC155

Risk factors for CNS thrombosis in neonates and children

Pergantou H, Kapsimali Z, Adamtziki E, Platokouki H, Vranou M, Aronis S*

Aim of the study: To estimate the frequency of prothrombotic factors and their relation to the development of central nervous system thrombosis (CNS) in neonates and children. **Patients***:* A total of 123 neonates and children with CNS thrombosis, referred to our Unit January 1999 to February 2004, were prospectively studied for the presence of congenital or acquired thrombophilic factors. Patients were divided into 3 groups: Group I : children n=77 (sinus:1) , Group II: neonates n=25 (sinus:2) and Group III: patients with congenital hemiplegia and/or psychomotor retardation n=21 (sinus: 0). Screening factors for thrombophilia: Fibrinogen, FII, FVII, FVIII, AT, PC, PS, Plg, PAI-1, FVLeiden, FII20210A, MTHFR C677T, LA, ACA, anti-b2GPI. **Results**: Congenital or acquired prothrombotic factors were identified in 82.6% of patients in group I, 72% in group II and 81% in group III. More than one prothrombotic factors were observrd in 16.9%, 36% and 23.8% of patients respectively in the three groups. The incidence of FVLeiden, FII20210A, and homozygous MTHFR C677T was much the same (35% vs 28% vs 33%). An underlying disease was more common in children and sick neonates (31% vs 20% vs 0%), hence a triggering event was reported in the majority of sick neonates (76%). A triggering event (maternal accident or/and thrombophilic factors and intrauterine asphyxia) was reported in 33% of congenital CNS thrombosis whereas only in 0.06% of children with CNS thrombosis. Catheter related thrombosis was more frequent in sick neonates. **Conclusion**: The prospective study of 123 patients with CNS thrombosis revealed that congenital or /and acquired prothrombotic factors were found in the majority of patients in the studied groups. An underlying disease or a triggering event were not frequent as risk factors hence idiopathic CNS thrombosis was a rare entity in all three groups (11.4%).

OC156

Coagulation activation in patients with and without thrombophilia during anticoagulant treatment for venous thrombosis

Vižintin Cuderman T, Božič M, Peternel P, Stegnar M*

Department of Angiology, University Medical Centre, Ljubljana, Slovenia

Introduction and aim: Presence of thrombophilia is considered to yield lifelong hypercoagulability and increased risk of thrombosis. The aim was to evaluate coagulation activation in patients with and without thrombophilia during anticoagulant treatment for deep venous thrombosis (DVT). **Subjects and Methods**: 28 consecutive patients (16 women, 12 men, mean age 60 years) with the first episode of DVT were included. They were treated with dalteparin (200 antiXa IU/kg once daily subcutaneously, mean duration of treatment 7 days) and with adjusted warfarin (INR 2-3) for 6 months. Coagulation activation was determined by the level of prothrombin fragments 1+2 (F1+2) and thrombin-antithrombin complexes (TAT) on day 1 (before treatment), days 2, 3, 4, 6 (dalteparin and warfarin treatment), days 60, 120, 180 (warfarin treatment), and on day 210 (no anticoagulant treatment). Presence of thrombophilia (antithrombin, protein C and S deficiency, lupus anticoagulants, factor V Leiden and G20210A prothrombin mutation) was determined on the last occasion (day 210). **Results**: Thrombophilia was established in 14 patients (lupus anticoagulants: N = 6, factor V Leiden: N = 6, factor V Leiden plus prothrombin mutation: N = 1, protein C deficiency: N = 1). In all patients F1+2 and TAT decreased significantly from day 1 to day 2: in thrombophilic patients F1+2 decreased from 1.40 to 0.90 nmol/L (p<0.01) and TAT from 6.00 to 3.20 mg/L (p<0.005), while in non-thrombophilic patients F1+2 decreased from 1.10 to 0.55 nmol/L (p<0.005) and TAT from 4.40 to 2.40 mg/L (p<0.05). Coagulation activation markers remained low throughout treatment. After discontinuation of treatment concentrations of both markers increased significantly in thrombophilic patients (from 0.20 to 0.60 nmol/L for F1+2, p<0.001 and from 1.25 to 2.60 mg/L for TAT, p<0.005), while in non-thrombophilic patients the increase was significant for F1+2 (from 0.30 to 0.60 nmol/L, p<0.001) but not for TAT (from 1.70 to 2.20 mg/L, p=0.056, all values are medians). When levels of coagulation activation markers were compared between thrombophilic and non-thrombophilic patients at the same time points, slightly higher concentrations of both markers were found in the thrombophilic group before treatment (1.4 vs 1.1 nmol/L for F1+2, p=0.40, and 6.0 vs 4.4 mg/L for TAT, p=0.32, all values are medians) and on several further occasions (days 2, 3, 4, 6 for F1+2 and 2, 3, 4, 210 for TAT), but the differences did not reach statistical significance. **Conclusions**: Anticoagulant treatment suppresses coagulation activation similarly in thrombophilic and non-thrombophilic patients with DVT.

OC157

A new TAFI antigen assay independent of polymorphism 325Thr/Ile and147 Ala/Thr

*Cost H, Grimaux M, Grosley M, Woodhams B**

Serbio SAS (Diagnostica Stago), Gennevilliers, France.

Introduction: Thrombin-activatable fibrinolysis inhibitor (TAFI), after activation by thrombin or plasmin, cleaves the carboxy-terminal lysine from partially degraded fibrin. This cleavage reduces the fibrin cofactor function of t-PA mediated plasminogen activation, resulting in a decreased rate of plasmin generation, thus inhibition of fibrinolysis. The plasma levels of TAFI are strongly influenced by genetic factors. Several polymorphisms have been identified in the TAFI gene and two majors variants have been described in the coding sequence of TAFI: 147Ala/Thr and 325Thr/Ile. A recent study by (1) showed that commercial available TAFI antigen assays exhibited differential immunological reactivity's with these different TAFI isoforms. **Method**: The Asserachrom TAFI assay is a new sandwich enzyme immunoassay based on the use of 2 specially selected monoclonal antibodies: F(ab')2 of 1B1 for capture and HRP labelled P4C2 as tag. The assay is calibrated with purified human TAFI. A study performed with plasma from 40 presumed normal human subjects has shown that this assay is not influenced by the 325 Thr/Ile or the 147 Ala/Thr polymorphisms. This assay only poorly recognises TAFI after activation by thrombin/thrombomodulin. The P4C2 antibody added to normal plasma inhibit TAFI conversion to TAFIa by thrombin/thrombomodulin, so its epitope seems to be near the site of TAFI cleavage at Arg 92. EDTA in dilution buffer does not influence the reactivity of the assay. **Results**: The average intra and inter assay coefficients are <5% and <7 %, respectively. The detection limit is 0.1 µg/ml. No prozone effect was observed up to 80 µg/ml. After addition of purified TAFI to normal human plasma recoveries from 96 to 105 % were obtained. Normal values found in 30 males and 30 females were 9.14 ± 1.57 µg/ml. No major differences were observed between males and females. **Conclusion**: This new one step, easy to perform, ELISA assay for TAFI is specific for TAFI (not TAFIa) and functions independently from the 325 Thr/Ile and 147 Ala/Thr polymorphisms. As the first true assay for plasma TAFI levels it may be more useful than any other commercial assay for clinical evaluation of this parameter in different physiological and pathological states in human. Gils A. et al.Development of a Genotype 325-Specific proCPU/TAFI ELISA, Arterioscler Thromb. Vasc. Biol. **23**, 1122-27,

OC158

Influence of the Thrombin Activatable Fibrinolysis Inhibitor (TAFI) Thr325Ile polymorphism on TAFI levels determined with three new assays

*Frère C (1), Aillaud MF (1), Saut N (1), Grosley M (2), Beltran J (2), Juhan-Vague I (1), Alessi MC (1)**

(1) Laboratory of Haematology, INSERM UMR 626, Faculty of Medecine, Marseille, France
(2) Serbio (Diagnostica Stago), Gennevilliers, France

Introduction – Reports have shown that, in ELISA, variable antibody reactivity towards TAFI isoforms (Thr325Ile) led to erroneous TAFI levels, reflecting qualitative rather than quantitative TAFI modifications. **Aims** – To assess 3 new methods for TAFI quantification in plasma. **Materials and Methods** –TAFI levels were measured in 208 individuals using 3 ELISA (2 based on recently developed antibodies (*P1G7/5081, 1B1/P4C)* and a commercially one from Milan Analytica (MA)) and 2 functional assays (a new method (TAFI Act) based on an original principle and Actichrome® TAFI from American Diagnostica). Based on the litterature, functional methods were supposed to similarly recognize the TAFI 325 isoforms. TAFI genotype at position 325 (C1040T) was determined in each individual. **Results and conclusions** – Significant correlations, but of variable intensity, were found between the assays: TAFIAct/Actichrome® (r=0.78, p<0.001), TAFI Act/*1B1/P4C2* (r=0.76, p<0.001), TAFI Act/MA (r=0.54, p<0.001), TAFI Act/*P1G7/5081* (r=0.21, p<0.01). TAFI levels exhibited a large variability between individuals, except when measured with the TAFI Act, Actichrome® or *1B1/P4C2* (coefficient of variability: 40 to 53 % versus 15 to 18 %). The contribution of the TAFI 325 polymorphism to this variability was then investigated. An association between TAFI levels and genotypes at position 325 was found with each ELISA (p<0.001) and both functional assays, the ThrThr genotype having the highest levels. When considering TAFI specific activity (ratio TAFI Act/Ag), a high ratio was observed in the IleIle genotype only with the MA and the *P1G7/5081*, suggesting a lower antigenic recognition of the Ile isoform with these assays. A linear regression analysis confirmed this finding showing that the genotype affected the slope between TAFI Act and MA or P1G7/5081 but not between TAFI Act and *1B1/P4C2*. These results allow to distinguish two kinds of assays. TAFI Act, Actichrome®, *1B1/P4C2* followed the same evolution and similarly reacted with the Thr or Ile 325 isoforms. In contrast, MA and *P1G7/5081* were less reactive towards the Ile isoform. The association between TAFI levels and genotypes ascertained with the *1B1/P4C2* without modification of the ratio TAFIAct/*1B1/P4C2* might reflect the existence of a genotype-related quantitative variation of circulating TAFI levels. Thus, the *1B1/P4C2* ELISA as well as functional assays are trustworthy methods to detect quantitative variations of circulating TAFI.

OC159

TAFI levels in patients with acute myocardial infarction treated with thrombolysis

Frère C (1), Renard S (1), Grosley (2), Beltran J (2), Gils A (3), Declerck P (3), Chandler W (4), Van De Werf F (5), Juhan-Vague I (1), Alessi MC (1)*

(1) Laboratory of Haematology, INSERM UMR 626, Faculty of Medecine, Marseille, France
(2) Serbio (Diagnostica Stago), Gennevilliers, France
(3) Laboratory for Pharmaceutical Biology and Phytopharmacology, Pharmaceutical Sciences, Katholieke U
(4) Department of Laboratory Medicine, University of Washington, Seattle, Washington, USA
(5) Department of Cardiology, University Hospitals Leuven, Leuven, Belgium

Introduction – The Thrombin Activatable Fibrinolysis Inhibitor (TAFI) plays a role in the down regulation of endogenous thrombolysis. TAFI inhibition in animal models was previously found to accelerate thrombolysis. Till now, behaviour of TAFI in acute myocardial infarction (MI) and thrombolysis has not been reported in humans. **Aims** – To study TAFI levels in acute MI and following thrombolysis with rt-PA or staphylokinase. **Materials and Methods** – TAFI levels were measured in 29 patients who suffered from an acute ST-elevation MI using four ELISAs exhibiting distinct reactivities towards TAFI and a newly developed functional assay. Samples were taken prior to therapy and at 1, 6, 12, 24, and 48 hours. Results were compared to those of 85 controls and analysed according to TAFI Thr325Ile genotype. **Results and conclusions** – In vitro activation of plasma TAFI with plasmin or thrombin increased apparent TAFI using the *P1G7/5081* assay while decreasing TAFI using *T12D11/T28G6* whathever TAFI genotype, indicating opposite reactivities of these two assays towards activated TAFI. Before thrombolysis, patients compared with controls had significantly higher TAFI (p<0.01) using *P1G7/5081* but lower TAFI (p=0.0244) using *T12D11/T28G6*, suggesting TAFI activation during myocardial infarction. Thrombolysis with staphylokinase did not lead to TAFI activation as indicated by stable TAFI levels. In contrast, thrombolysis with rt-PA led to TAFI activation as indicated by increased TAFI (p<0.001) using *P1G7/5081* and decreased TAFI (p<0.001) using *T12D11/T28G6*, correlated with a drop in fibrinogen and a rise in tPA and D-dimer levels. TAFI levels measured with *1B1/P4C2* and *T32F6/T9G12* assays were unchanged. In conclusion, TAFI consumption in acute MI patients prior to thrombolysis and the absence of TAFI level variations during staphylokinase treatment suggest that thrombin may be the most relevant activator of TAFI in vivo. Molecular forms of TAFI generated during TAFI activation are an apparent source of variability in TAFI plasma levels. Therefore assay characteristics must be considered when interpreting TAFI levels in clinical studies.

OC160

Mediation of fibrinolytic deficit in cancer patients by plasminogen activator inhibitor-1 and thrombin activatable fibrinolytic inhibitor

Florian-Kujawski M (1), Hoppensteadt D (1), Iqbal O (1), Demir M (2), Tobu M (1), Fareed D (1), Fareed J (1)*

(1) Loyola University Medical Center, Maywood, IL, USA
(2) Trakya University Medical School, Edirne, Turkey

Introduction: Cancer associated thrombosis is known to have a multifactorial pathogenesis involving up regulation of coagulation factors, down regulation of inhibitors and endothelial dysfunction. Cancer patients have been shown to exhibit fibrinolytic deficit with impaired clot lysis. This has been mostly attributed to an increase in the circulating levels of plasminogen activator inhibitor (PAI-1). Thrombin activatable fibrinolytic inhibitor (TAFI) has recently been identified as an additional mediator of fibrinolytic deficit that transforms fibrin to a plamsin resistant variant. **Aims**: The aim of these studies is to elucidate the role of TAFI in cancer associated thrombosis. In addition, to determine its effect as a mediator of fibrinolytic deficit and its correlation to PAI-1. **Materials and Methods**: Plasma samples obtained from 170 cancer patients with symptomatic thrombosis were analyzed for PAI-1, TAFI functional (F) and TAFI immunologic (I). An ELISA method was used for PAI-1 (Stago Parsipany, NJ) and TAFI-I (American Diagnostic, Stamford, CT), while a functional method was used for TAFI-F (Pentapharm Inc., Basel, Switzerland). **Results**: Baseline samples exhibited a marked increase in PAI-1 levels (140 ± 21 ng/ml) compared to normal (94 ± 14 ng/ml). The TAFI-I levels ranged from 56 – 183 %NHP (123 ± 28 %NHP) which was higher than normal (85.1 ± 14 %NHP; n= 82). Interestingly, TAFI measured by functional levels were disproportionately lower (85 ± 26 %NHP) suggesting the consumption of this protease in cancer patients. In contrast to the TAFI I/F ratio (approximately 1) for normal individuals, this ratio for cancer patients was 1.6 ± 0.1 (5.6 – 0.7). When the PAI-1 levels were compared with F and I TAFI levels, no correlation was evident. This suggests independent regulation of these two proteins in cancer. The increased PAI-1 and TAFI-I was independent of the fibrinogen levels. **Conclusions:** The results clearly suggest that thrombotic complications in cancer patients may be partly due to the fibrinolytic deficit, which is modulated by an up regulation of both PAI-1 and TAFI. Furthermore, the two regulators of fibrinolysis mediate their effects independently. Since the TAFI-I levels are disproportionately high, this enzyme may complex with endogenous proteins modulating its functionality. Cancer patients with fibrinolytic deficit may be benefited by anticoagulant therapy such as low molecular weight heparins and antithrombin agents.

OC161

Modulation of thrombin activatable fibrinolytic inhibitor (TAFI) by heparins: Variation among normal and patient populations

Florian-Kujawski M (1), Maddineni J (1), Hoppensteadt D (1), Janssen M (2), Wilmer M (2), Bick R (3), Iqbal O (1), Tobu M (1), Fareed J (1)*

(1) Loyola University Medical Center, Maywood, IL, USA
(2) Pentapharm Inc., Basel, Switzerland
(3) University of Texas, SW Med School, Dallas, TX, USA

Introduction: Both the unfractionated (UF) and low molecular weight (LMW) heparins have been reported to produce a molecular weight and concentration dependent inhibition of TAFI to TAFIa activation. This effect is predominantly due to their interaction with antithrombin (AT) and heparin cofactor II (HC II) and the eventual inhibition of thrombin. The observed profibrinolytic effects of heparins may be partly mediated by the inhibition of TAFI functionality. **Aims**: The aims of this study were to determine the effect of heparin on TAFI levels in both the experimental and clinical studies. **Materials and Methods**: A simple chromogenic substrate based method (Pefakit® TAFI, Pentapharm Ltd., Basel, Switzerland) for the measurement of functional TAFI levels was employed. All results are expressed in terms of percent normal human pool plasma (NHP). **Results**: Supplementation of heparins resulted in a concentration dependent inhibition of TAFI with IC_{50} value for heparin (1.2 µg/ml), Tinzaparin (0.8 µg/ml) and enoxaparin (0.7 µg/ml). Samples collected from patients on therapeutic heparin (PTT: 60-80 s) exhibited varying degrees of TAFI levels ranging from 10-80% (45.5 ± 18.4%). This led to the hypothesis that beside the AT and HC II modulation of thrombin-thrombomodulin and its activation of TAFI, additional factors may be responsible for the observed variations in TAFI levels. To validate this observation, plasma samples were collected from 140 healthy volunteers with normal AT and HC II levels, coagulation profiles and who were edication free. TAFI levels were measured in each of the individual plasma samples prior to and after heparin (0.25 U/ml). The plasma TAFI levels prior to heparin ranged from 22.3-165.7 % (89.5 ± 20.6%). Post heparin, the functional TAFI levels were reduced and ranged from 2.9-113.8% (39.9 ± 15.4%). Subset analysis of these samples reveal that despite the prolongation of APTT to therapeutic level (> 60 s) 27 individuals plasma showed levels of functional TAFI >75%. **Conclusions:** This observation clearly suggests that additional endogenous factors modulating TAFI or a variant form of TAFI may exist in certain normal individuals. The possibility of TAFI polymorphism should be investigated in patients who do not achieve the expected decrease in TAFIa activity after heparinization. Finally, the observed variations in fibrinolytic states in heparinized patients may be related to the differential activation of this modulator of fibrinolysis.

OC162

Does thrombin activatable fibrinolysis inhibitor (TAFI) contribute to hemostatic complications in patients with different types of brain injury?

Antovic J (1), Rooth E (2), Wallen H (2), Hannerz J (3), Nekludov M (4), Kaponides G (3), von Arbin M (2), Wahlgren N (3), Antovic A (1), Blombäck M (1)*

(1) Coagulation Research, Department of Surgical Sciences, Karolinska Hospital, Karolinska Institutet,
(2) Department of Medicine, Danderyd Hospital, Karolinska Institutet, Stockholm, Sweden
(3) Department of Neurology, Karolinska Hospital, Karolinska Institutet, Stockholm, Sweden
(4) Department of Neurosurgery, Karolinska Hospital, Karolinska Institutet, Stockholm, Sweden

Background: Hemostatic abnormalities are common findings in different brain pathology. They are induced by releasing of tissue factor (TF) and increased thrombin generation after the brain damage. Thrombin activatable fibrinolysis inhibitor (TAFI) is one of modulators of fibrinolysis activated by the thrombin/thrombomodulin complex into its active form – a carboxypeptidase B-like enzyme which down-regulates fibrinolysis. TAFI could contribute to hemostatic abnormalities in patients with different types of brain injuries. **Patients and methods**: We measured total TAFI antigen in arterial and cerebrovenous blood, as well in cerebrospinal fluid (CSF) at admission, day 1, 2, and 3 in 10 patients with isolated head trauma (IHT) and at admission, day 1, 3 and 60 in 26 patients with ischemic (non – cardioembolic) stroke (IS) and compared results with 13 healthy controls. We also measured TAFI antigen, overall fibrinolysis and TAFI dependent fibrinolysis in 12 women with idiopathic intracranial hypertension (IIH) and compared them with 12 healthy women. **Results**: In patients with IHT increase of total TAFI antigen both in arterial and cerebrovenous blood compared to controls was noticed at admission. It tended to decrease on day 2 and 3. In patients with IS increase of TAFI antigen was noticed at admission in patients and day 1 and it also tended to decrease on day 3 and especially on day 60. Increase of TAFI antigen together with impaired overall fibrinolysis, as well as TAFI dependent fibrinolysis was noticed in women with IIH. There was a statistically significant correlation between the level of TAFI antigen and CRP. TAFI antigen was not found in CSF. **Interpretation**: Mechanism of total TAFI antigen increase is probably not unique. Total TAFI antigen comprises the proenzyme (pro-TAFI), the active form of the enzyme (TAFI) and the inactive form (TAFIi). The increase in total TAFI antigen could partly arise from an increase in the enzyme's active form (TAFI) caused by an increased generation of thrombin. On the other hand, pro-TAFI has been described as an acute phase protein and the increase in total TAFI antigen could be accounted for by an increase in the proenzyme as an acute-phase reactant. In spite of lack of clear explanations for the mechanism behind the TAFI antigen increase we believe that these findings may indicate that TAFI could be a contributing risk factor for development of hemostatic abnormalities in patients with different types of brain injury.

[redacted]

FEATURED POSTERS

FP01

Abnormal heart rate variability is associated with platelet activation in stable coronary disease during recovery from myocardial infarction

Hamaad A (1,2), Blann AD (1,2), Lip G (1,2), MacFadyen R (1,2)*

(1) University Department of Medicine
(2) City Hospital, Birmingham

Aims: Abnormal autonomic tone (assessed by heart rate variability, HRV) predicts adverse outcomes in stable coronary disease. We hypothesized that increased platelet activation (assessed by soluble P selectin, sPsel) is related to HRV. **Methods:** We measured (HRV) indices and sP-sel (ELISA) in 41 patients (31male; 62±11yrs) during the rehabilitation phase (3 months) following an acute coronary syndrome (Non-ST elevation infarction, NSTEMI n=21; ST-elevation infarction, STEMI n=20). All patients were receiving aspirin. Patients in the NSTEMI group had all been managed with adjunctive percutaneous coronary intervention (PCI), those in the STEMI group all received thrombolytic therapy. Basal HRV was recorded using time domain indices derived from one 20-minute supine record (>95% analysable). Patients were grouped according to mean RR interval duration as high (>mean) or low (<mean) HRV. **Results:** Groups did not differ by age, sex, STEMI/NSTEMI status, concomitant therapy and LV ejection fraction but those with low HRV had higher sP-sel (table). The correlation between HRV and sPsel was significant in STEMI (r=-0.77, p=0.01), but not in NSTEMI (r=-0.37, p=0.188). **Conclusion:** Platelet activation in the rehabilitation phase of acute coronary syndromes is linked to HRV as defined by abnormal mean RR interval duration. This association appears more pronounced in patients with STEMI. Table- data presented as median (interquartile range) or mean (SD)

	Low HRV (n=20)	High HRV (n=21)	P-value
Age	59.5(12.5)	65.4 (9.6)	0.206
Male/Female	14/6	17/4	0.414
SBP (mmHg)	124 (26.8)	131 (17.5)	0.449
DBP (mmHg)	76 (13.7)	75 (7.5)	0.851
STEMI/NSTEMI	8/12	10/11	0.623
Clopidogrel (%)	32	27	0.601
Ejection fraction	0.61 (0.19)	0.65 (0.10)	0.591
Mean heart rate	93.0 (15.0)	68.8 (6.8)	<0.001
Mean RR duration (ms)	791 (145)	1065 (106)	<0.001
SDNN (ms)	29.4 (15.1)	55.1 (16.5)	<0.001
Triangular index	7.4 (3.7)	11.6 (3.8)	0.007
sP-selectin (ng/ml)	75.0 (50.0-97.0)*	48.0 (41.5-65.0)*	0.03

FP02

Abnormalities in heart rate variability is associated with platelet activation in acute ST-elevation myocardial infarction

Hamaad A (1,2), Blann AD (1,2), Lip G (1,2), MacFadyen R (1,2)*

(1) University Department of Medicine
(2) City Hospital

Aims: Abnormal autonomic tone in the acute phase of acute coronary syndromes (ACS) is related to adverse outcome. We hypothesized that this is due to excess platelet activation (marked by soluble P selectin, sPsel) or endothelial damage (by von Willebrand factor, vWf), and is further influenced by STEMI/NSTEMI status. **Methods**: We recruited 90 patients (65male; 63±11yrs) with acute coronary syndromes taking blood within 24 hours of admission. All patients were receiving aspirin (those on clopidogrel and beta-blockers were excluded). HRV was defined by time domain indices from 20-minute supine records (>95% analysable). Patients were grouped according to mean RR interval duration as high (>mean) or low (<mean) HRV. sPsel and vWf were measured by ELISA. Data presents as median (interquartile range) analysed by Mann-Whitney, or mean (SD), by t test. **Results**: The two groups defined by HRV were matched for age, sex, SBP, DBP, CK rise and STEMI status. Patients with low HRV had higher sP-sel but there was no difference in vWf (table). The correlation between HRV and sPsel was significant in STEMI (r=-0.50, p=0.002), but not in NSTEMI (r=-0.18, p=0.274). **Conclusion**: Abnormal mean RR interval duration is associated with platelet activation in acute coronary syndromes suggestive of sympathetic over-activity. This association is stronger in STEMI than in NSTEMI.

	Low HRV (n=41)	High HRV (n=49)	P-value
Age	63.5 (12.0)	63.8 (11.4)	0.916
Male/Female	29/12	36/13	0.861
SBP (mmHg)	131 (17.9)	123 (18.4)	0.06
DBP (mmHg)	69 (11.8)	64 (9.1)	0.09
STEMI/NSTEMI	20/21	24/25	0.985
Peak CK rise (IU/ml)	550 (176-1356)	464 (222-1324)	0.908
Mean heart rate	93.0 (15.0)	68.8 (6.8)	<0.001
Mean RR duration (ms)	691 (102)	961 (86)	<0.001
SDNN (ms)	26.5 (19.5-41.8)	49.5 (34.5-77.8)	<0.001
Triangular index	7.0 (4.0-9.0)	11.0 (10.0-17.0)	<0.001
sP-selectin (ng/ml)	65 (50-90)	50 (38.5-65.0)	0.003
vWF (IU/ml)	151 (22.8)	158 (21.6)	0.270

FP03

EPCR 23 bp insertion in atherosclerosis and early MI

Ulu A (1), Akar R (2), Emiroglu O (2), Ucanok K (2), Akar E (1), Akar N (1)*

(1) Department of Pediatric Molecular Genetics, School of Science, Ankara University, Ankara, Turkey
(2) Department of Cardiovascular Surgery, School of Science, Ankara University, Ankara, Turkey

Introduction: Factor V Leiden (FVL) has been shown to be the most important genetic risk factor leading to thrombosis by causing activated protein C resistance. Endothelial damage is a factor initiating coagulation. After the damage is healed by the coagulation system, the Protein C anticoagulant pathway takes its role. An endothelial protein C receptor (EPCR) has been suggested to play a role in the regulation of blood coagulation via APC formation. A 23 bp insertion in exon 3 of the EPCR gene was claimed to have a role in thrombosis. **Aim**: We assessed if the 23 bp insertion of EPCR gene affects thrombosis when present with other genetic risk factors, especially FVL. Materials and methods: Our study group included 175 atherosclerosis and 38 early MI. EPCR 23 bp insertion analyses was performed according to previously described techniques. FV 1691A was anaysed using Real Time-PCR (Roche Diagnostics, Germany). **Results**: EPCR 23 bp insertion was present in 2 (5.2%) patients with early MI, 1 (0.8%) individual in controls and 4 (2.2%) patients with atherosclerosis. **Conclusions**: We found that EPCR 23 bp insertion could be a risk factor in atherosclerosis patients with Turkish origin. But due to the low number of patients studied, further research including a larger series of patients is needed. (This study is supported by Ankara University Research Fund)

FP04

Soluble tissue factor in plasma from patients with acute myocardial infarction is not microvesicle associated

Seljeflot I (1), Lyberg T (2), Arnesen H (1)*

(1) Center for Clinical Research, Ullevål university Hospital, Oslo, Norway
(2) Dept of Cardiology, Ullevål university Hospital, Oslo, Norway

Introduction: Atherosclerotic lesions have been shown to contain large amounts of tissue factor (TF), a dominant initiator of the coagulation cascade. TF expression can be induced in different cell types, like monocytes, macrophages, smooth muscle cells and possibly also platelets. Trace amounts of TF are present as soluble forms in plasma (sTF). Elevated levels of sTF have been found in patients with acute myocardial infarction (AMI), and recent data have shown elevated levels of sTF in patients shortly after an AMI to predict future clinical events. The origin of sTF is unclear. It has, however, been suggested that sTF measured in plasma partly exists in a membrane-bound form, shed as microvesicles from the surface of cells generating TF. **Aim, Material and methods**: Aiming at identifying whether the sTF measured in plasma is bound to microvesicles, we have exposed citrated plasma (Ci-plasma) obtained by centrifugation at 2000 x g for 15 min, from 13 patients 6 weeks after an AMI, to additional ultracentrifugation at 100.000 x g for 60 min. The supernatants were pipetted off and separated in an upper layer, a middle layer and a lower layer. The invisible bottom sediments were thereafter resuspended in assay buffer (original plasma volume) on a minishaker at 3000 rpm for 2 min. Similarly obtained pellets were further investigated by transmission electron microscopy. A commercial ELISA method (American Diagnostica Inc) was used for determination of sTF. **Results**: The mean value (SD) of sTF in Ci-plasma was 173 (52) pg/mL. In the upper layer the concentration was reduced to 97 (40) pg/mL (~50 % of Ci-plasma, p<0.0001), whereas in the middle and lower plasma layers the values were 182 (46) and 195 (75) pg/mL, respectively. In the dissolved sediments the sTF concentration was undetectable in all samples. This was verifyied by the electron microscopy where no vesicle-like or membranous material could be seen. **In Conclusion**, the amount of sTF obtained in citrated plasma from patients after an AMI seems to be real soluble and not associated with microvesicles. However, the different concentrations of sTF found in the variuos layers of the plasma supernatant, indicate sTF molecular weight heterogeneity.

FP05

The effects of home-based versus hospital-based cardiac rehabilitation on plasma haemostatic markers in patients with coronary heart disease

Lee W, Jolly K, Lip G*

Haemostasis, Thrombosis and Vascular Biology Unit, University Department of Medicine, City Hospital, Birmingham, UK

Background: Raised levels of plasma viscosity, fibrinogen, fibrin D-dimer (an index of thrombogenesis) and von Willebrand factor (vWf, an index of endothelial damage/dysfunction) are known predictors of cardiovascular outcome in patients with coronary heart disease (CHD). The effects of home-based (nurse facilitated, based on the Heart Manual) versus hospital-based cardiac rehabilitation (CR) programs on these plasma haemostatic indices in patients with CHD are unknown. **Methods:** 72 patients (58 male, 59 ± 11 yrs) with CHD (following myocardial infarction or coronary revascularisation) were randomized to either a comprehensive hospital- (n = 35) or home-based (n = 37) CR programme. Plasma levels of vWf, D-dimer, fibrinogen and plasma viscosity were measured at baseline and after 3 months of CR. Baseline values were compared with 35 matched healthy controls (23 male, 57 ± 6 yrs). **Results:** Patients with CHD had significantly elevated plasma viscosity ([mean ± sd] 1.7 ± 0.2 vs 1.6 ± 0.8 mpa.s), fibrinogen (3.3 ± 0.8 vs 2.6 ± 0.6 g/l), vWf (189 ± 58 vs 127 ± 32 iu/dl) and D-dimer (median (IQR) 0.28 (0.2 - 0.5) vs 0.18 (0.13 - 0.3) ng/ml) when compared with healthy controls at baseline [all ≤ 0.001]. The baseline values of these haemostatic markers were not significantly different between CHD patients of home- and hospital-based CR programmes. After 3 months of CR, plasma viscosity (to 1.6 ± 0.1 mpa.s), fibrinogen (to 2.9 ± 0.7g/l), vWf (to 172 ± 50 iu/dl) and D-dimer (to 0.2 (0.12 - 0.3) ng/ml) levels were reduced in the whole CHD patient cohort [all p<0.001]. The changes in these haemostatic markers were not significantly different between the hospital-based and home-based CR programmes. Conclusions: CR improves haemostatic markers in patients with CHD, with no significant differences between home- and hospital-based CR programmes. These effects may contribute to the beneficial effects of CR programmes on cardiovascular outcomes.

FP06

Hemostatic markers in patients with chronic atrial fibrillation – relationship to thromboembolic risk

Vene N, Mavri A, Košmelj K, Stegnar M*

Department of Angiology, University Medical Centre, Ljubljana, Slovenia

Background: Chronic atrial fibrillation (AF) is associated with hemostatic activation and increased risk of thrombotic events, which depends on coexistent risk factors. Oral anticoagulant treatment (OAT) suppresses hemostatic activation and decreases the number of thromboembolic events. The **aim** of our study was to assess the relationship between hemostatic changes and thromboembolic risk profile before and during OAT. Methods: 152 patients with chronic AF (63% men, 69.2 ± 6.6 years old) referred for OAT were included in the study. Clinical risk factors were determined and according to SPAF criteria patients were classified as high (44%), moderate (39%) and low (17%) risk patients. Levels of coagulation markers: prothrombin fragment 1+2 (F1+2), thrombin-antithrombin complexes (TAT), D-dimer and fibrinolytic markers: tissue plasminogen activator (t-PA) and plasminogen activator inhibitor type 1 (PAI-1) antigen and activity were determined before OAT and after 3.9 ± 0.7 months of OAT (INR 2.57 ± 0.57). **Results**: Coagulation markers were independently associated with age (F1+2: p=0.02; D-dimer: p<0.01), female gender (F1+2: p<0.01) and heart failure (D-dimer: p=0.08). Fibrinolytic markers were associated with female gender (t-PA activity, PAI-1 antigen and activity, all p<0.01), hypertension (t-PA antigen: p=0.07; PAI antigen and activity, pŁ0.01) and diabetes (t-PA activity: p=0.08, PAI activity: p=0.07). Levels of coagulation markers increased proportionally with perceived thromboembolic risk (F1+2, D-dimer: pŁ0.01), as well as levels of fibrinolytic markers (t-PA and PAI-1 activity: p= 0.05; t-PA antigen: p=0.06; PAI-1 antigen: p=0.07). OAT significantly suppressed levels of F1+2 by 67%, TAT by 30% and D-dimer by 48% (all p<0.01). Levels of F1+2 and of D-dimer before and during OAT were significantlly correlated (F 1+2: r=0.35, D-dimer: r=0.65; both p< 0,01) and their levels during OAT also increased proportionally with the perceived risk (F1+2: p=0.06; D-dimer: p<0.01). **Conclusions**: Increased hemostatic activity associated with chronic AF is partly explained by associated clinical conditions and is concordant with perceived thromboembolic risk before as well as during OAT.

FP07

Anticoagulation in conventional versus transesophageal echocardiography guided cardioversion of atrial fibrillation

Dokler Glavnik A, Žohar P*, Gunzek R*, Bervar M*, Marinšek M*, Škrabl Močnik F**

General Hospital, Celje, Slovenia

Introduction: Atrial fibrillation (AF) is the most common sustained cardiac arrhythmia and is associated with thrombembolic events and hemodynamic impairment that results in considerable morbidity, mortality and cost. Current guidelines recommend that patients receive anticoagulants for 3-4 weeks before and 4 weeks after cardioversion (CV). Transesophageal echocardiography (TEE) guided cardioversion with low-molecular-weight heparin (LMWH) may reduce the duration of anticoagulation. **Aim**: We compared duration of anticoagulation in conventional aproach to CV and TEE guided cardioversion with LMWH. **Methods and results**: From October 2001 to December 2003 179 patients admitted with AF of more than 48 hours duration were included in our study. 97 patients were treated with conventional aproach to CV and 82 patients with TEE guided cardioversion. Clinical characteristic of patients in both groups were the same, regarding underlying disease, age and sex. CV was cancelled in all patients with atrial thrombi (n=10). The duration of pericardioversion anticoagulation in conventional treated group was 22 weeks and in the group with TEE with LMWH 4 weeks. **Conclusions**: Administration of LMWH in conjunction with TEE reduces the duration of pericardioversion anticoagulation from 22 weeks to 4 weeks.

FP08

Low molecular weight heparin limits prothrombotic reactions and may shorten in-hospital stay of patients with heart failure

Wachnicka-Truty R, Birkholz-Gołaszewska A, Korzeniowski A, Flasiński J, Górski J*

Disturbances of haemostasis in patients with heart failure are common and may worsen their progenosis. **Aim** of our study was to define intensity of thrombin generation and activity of fibrinolysis in 47 patients with aggravated heart failure treated with standard therapy (diuretics, ACE - inhibitors, betablockers, nitrates); 27 of them additionaly were given low molecular weight heparin (clexane 40mg daily s.c.) to specify if the administration of it may shorten their in-hospital stay. We determinated: thrombin-antithrombin III complexes (TAT), prothrombin fragment 1+2 (F1+2), plasminogen activator (PA) and its inhibitor (PAI-1) with Elisa commercial tests, ejection fraction (EF) with echocardiograph - at hospital admission (A) and on 7th day of therapy (B). **Results** EF% TATng/L F1+2 nmol/L PA IU/ml PAI-1IU/ml in-hospital stay days

Standard therapy

A 33+/-5 9,3+/-5,0 5,0+/-2,9 2,4+/- 0,9 8,4+/-3,8 10,2

B 35+/-4 8,7+/-3,7 4,6+/-3,0 2,6+/- 1,1 8,77+/-4,0

Standard therapy+clexane

A 34+/-4 9,9+/-4,2 4,7+/-2,1 2,7+/-1,0 9,9+/-3,3 8,3

B 32+/-6 6,1+/-3,9 5,1+/-2,4 2/,3+/-0,9 7,1+/-3,0

p<005 for TAT, PAI-1 and hospital stay after treatment between both groups treated. **Conclusion**: reduction of thrombin generation and positive fibrinolytic effect is in patients with heart failure most likely attributed to clexane therapy; in hospital stay in these patients was visibly shortened.

FP09

Replacing acenocoumarol with the low molecular weight heparin Tinzaparin sodium in patients undergoing general surgery operations: a pilot study

Volteas S, Bossinakou I, Kotsopoulou M, Mattheou S, Kalatzopoulos D, Nicolakeas M, Sikiotis K*

Hippocration Hospital, Athens Greece

Introduction Patients under acenocoumarol scheduled for general surgery operations need to substitute this with a safer anticoagulant agent. In this "bridging" process both unfractionated and low-dose heparin have been used with high complication rate. **Aim** The aim of the present study was to present an efficient and safe bridging process using the low-molecular-weight heparin (LMWH) Tinzaparin sodium (Innohep®, Leo Pharma). **Material and Methods** Twenty-four unselected patients (16 men and 8 women, aged 33-85 years, mean 67.5 years) treated with acenocoumarol for several cardiovascular disorders entered the study. Patients underwent a total of 30 scheduled general surgery operations and interventions. Acenocoumarol administration was stopped 4-6 days pre-operatively and Tinzaparin was given subcutaneously at an adjusted daily dose of 175 anti-Xa IU per Kg of body weight. Patients were operated under Tinzaparin (not given on the operation day) while acenocoumarol restarted 2-4 days post-operatively co-administered with Tinzaparin for 2 days (or longer) to achieve therapeutic INR levels. Tinzaparin administration was then stopped. A complete venous duplex scan was performed on admittance, pre-operatively and on days 2, 4-6 and 15-20 post-operatively. Complete haemorrheology tests (including platelet count, PT, aPTT, INR, D-Dimer, tPA, TAT complex and anti-Xa activity) were also performed. **Results** a. Therapeutic anti-Xa levels were achieved pre-operatively in all cases b. No major bleeding complications occurred: two patients developed relatively large haematomas postoperatively at the site of operation c. No DVT occurred: only one patient (under acenocoumarol for more than 20 years due to repeated thromboembolism) developed long-saphenous-vein thrombosis **Conclusions** The results of our pilot study indicate that a. The bridging process should start at least 4 days pre-operatively and last for 3-6 days post-operatively, according to the type of operation or intervention b. The bridging process using the LMWH Tinzaparin sodium is both safe and effective c. In selected patients hospital stay can be limited to 1-2 pre-op days, as the bridging process may start on an outpatient basis. Patients could also be discharged earlier and seen as outpatients for acenocoumarol adjustment post-operatively; larger studies are needed, however, to fully support these suggestions.

FP10

Oral anticoagulant therapy management in patient self-testing

Testa S, Alatri A, Morstabilini G*

Centro Emostasi e Trombosi AO Istituti Ospitalieri Cremona

Introduction Recent studies demonstrated that INR portable monitors have good accuracy and are user friendly. Patients on PST have shown the major time spent in the therapeutic range, as compared with PSM, anticoagulation clinic (AC) and routine medical care (RMC). Since few data are available on major complications in patients on PSM, we connected our Anticoagulation Clinic with patients at home, using a new net supported program *TAOnet*®, already on line with general physicians, health territorial care units of the Cremona area. **Aims:** - to ensure effectiveness and security of oral anticoagulant treatment in patients using portable monitors; - to obtain good management of PST and PSM, objectively defined through the availability of laboratory and clinical parameters; - to demonstrate the efficiency of a bi-directional net supported system. **Materials and methods**: All patients attended courses on anticoagulation therapy, portable monitors self-testing and/or self-management and on computer utilization procedures. Twenty patients, mean age 54 years (29-81y), are connected with our AC from November 2002, after informed consent was obtained. The main reason for patient acceptance was to save time and generally to improve quality of life. In summary, they refer directly to the hospital sending:1) their own clinical data, 2) the quality control, and 3) the INR value, through the compilation of an electronic data-sheet. They can also send to the AC further informations regarding their clinical status, co-medication, etc. In the standard model the patient receive the adjusted dosage through the net system by e-mail. **Results:** All patients expressed their satisfaction, as evaluated through an open questionnaire. We observed an increase of the time spent in the therapeutic range as compared to the previous six months (AC= 58%, home patients= 72%; $p<0.001$). No patient experienced major complications untill now. On 18 patients only two are on self management, because the majority of them (16 pts) prefer the validation of treatment by AC. **Conclusion:** This organization provide the following advantages: 1) direct communication between home patients and AC, 2) improvement in time spent in the therapeutic range, 3) improvement in patient's satisfaction and in their quality of life, 5) continuing medical record update.

FP11

Anti-Xa activity monitoring of the synthetic pentasaccharide Fondaparinux

Van Dreden P, Fontaine S, Woodhams*

Serbio Sas (Diagnostica Stago), Gennevilliers (France)

Introduction: The laboratory monitoring of unfractionated heparin and low molecular weight heparin therapy is well established, but to date no standardized assay for pentasaccharide has been proposed. Fondaparinux, a new antithombotic agent, is a synthetic pentasaccharide which only exhibits factor Xa inhibitor activity via binding to antithrombin III and acts without initiating release of tissue factor pathway inhibitor. It is usually administered without monitoring, however accumulated experience with the conventional antithrombotic agents suggests the possible need for monitoring of Fondaparinux in certain patient groups (pregnant or obese patients, paediatric patients, elderly patients, or thrombotic events, or patients with renal insufficiency). Fondaparinux had no effect on the activated clotting time or the activated partial thromboplastin time so these commonly used screening clotting assays cannot be used. The therapeutic concentrations of Fondaparinux is within the range of 0.1 to 1µg/ml. Quoting levels in terms of anti Xa is not considered appropriate for this drug as dosage is in gravimetric units. The aim of the present study was to investigate the use of a commercially available chromogenic assay anti-Xa assays: STA-Rotachrom Heparin (Diagnostica Stago) and an anti-Xa clotting assay Heptest (Haemachem). **Methods:** Normal plasma was spiked with increased amounts of Fondaparinux (range 0 to 3µg/ml) and both assays were performed according to the manufacturers' instructions on the STA-R analyser (Diagnostica Stago). For the assay the results were expressed as change OD/min or clotting time of the Fondaparinux spiked plasmas per µg/ml Fondaparinux. **Results:** The results showed that STA-Rotachrom Heparin gave 12%, 62% and 88% of factor Xa inhibition respectively for 0.1µg/mL, 1.0µg/mL and 2.5µg/mL Fondaparinux plasma concentrations, and a delta clotting times of 43.7", 107.9", 149", 154" for respectively 0.1µg/mL, 1.0µg/mL, 2.0µg/ml and 2.5µg/mL in Heptest assay. With this one-step chromogenic anti-Xa assay (STA Rotachrom Heparin) linear standard curves were obtained in the 0.1-2.0 µg/ml range. The within-run and day to day variation of the assays obtained using frozen plasmas with in vitro added Fondaparinux (0.5 and 1.5µg/ml) were respectively 3.5% and 3.8% for STA Rotachrom Heparin, and 9.2% and 11.6% for Heptest assay. The Heptest show a bending of the curve observed for plasma concentration lower than 2µg/ml then, the curve reached a plateau at concentrations around 2µg/ml. **Conclusion**: The good dose/response linearity obtained with the STA Rotachrom heparin indicate that this chromogenic assay can be used for monitoring Fondaparinux anti-Xa activity for both prophylactic and therapeutic doses of Fondaparinux. Good calibration can be obtained using the drug spiked into Normal plasma and the results expressed in gravimetric units of Fondaparinux. It must be stressed that due to the different sensitivities of the different anti Xa assays commercially available that the use of anti Xa units may be misleading as results in anti Xa units may differ according to the assay used.

FP12

The Ecarin Chromogenic Assay (ECA) for quantitative determination of direct thrombin inhibitors-From a routine method to a point-of-care test

Lange U (1), Frische I (1), Olschewski A (1), Nowak G (2), Bucha E (1)*

(1) HaemoSys GmbH, Winzerlaer Str. 2, Jena, Germany

(2) Friedrich Schiller University Jena, Medical Faculty, Research Unit "Pharmacological Haemostaseology"

Introduction: The Ecarin Chromogenic Assay (ECA) for quantitative determination of hirudin (ECA-H) or synthetic direct thrombin inhibitors (ECA-T) in plasma has proved to be a very sensitive, precise, robust and specific test. The ECA possesses many advantages compared to other tests: There is a linear correlation between inhibitor concentration and ECA-reaction time over a broad concentration range, the inter-individual variations in ECA are very low because ECA is independent on variations of coagulation variables (e.g. fibrinogen or prothrombin). ECA can be carried out as routine diagnostic test in automated systems as well as in manual coagulation analysers provided with an option for optical measurement and adapted for ECA. **Aim**: To enable the customer to perform single ECA determinations in case of need, ready-to-use cuvettes for both ECA-H and ECA-T were developed. The suitability of ECA as point-of-care test was to be investigated. **Materials and methods**: Special cuvettes containing lyophilised ECA-reagents were prepared. The determinations were carried out in handy, transportable and easily manageable single- or two-channel coagulometers, adapted for ECA. Precision, repeatability, sensitivity and robustness of ECA in the ready-to-use cuvettes were determined using hirudin- as well as argatroban-spiked plasma samples. The results of ECA-H were compared with those of ECT and aPTT in plasma samples of hirudin-treated patients. **Results and conclusions**: It was demonstrated that ECA-H for quantitative determination of hirudin as well as ECA-T for quantitative determination of synthetic direct thrombin inhibitors (shown with argatroban) can be easily carried out as single determinations using the ready-to-use cuvettes. After dissolution of the cuvette content the reagents are stable for at least 1h. The sealed cuvettes are stable for several months. Although the precision of ECA in the ready-to-use cuvettes is lower than in the conventional assay it is still highly satisfactory. Repeatability, sensitivity and robustness of the conventional ECA are well preserved. In plasma samples of patients treated with hirudin, hirudin levels determined using the ECA-H ready-to-use cuvettes correlate well with those obtained by ECT. ECA-H as well as ECA-T can be excellently carried out as point-of-care test in easily manageable single- or two-channel coagulometers.

FP13

A novel assay for tissue factor pathway inhibitor (TFPI) anticoagulant activity in plasma

Dahm A, Andersen T, Rosendaal F, Sandset P*

Introduction. Several studies have shown that full-length free TFPI is a much stronger anticoagulant in diluted prothrombin time (dPT) assays than truncated and lipoprotein associated TFPI. Although it has been suggested that TFPI anticoagulant activity is of importance for the effect of TFPI in vivo, no assays have so far been standardized to assay TFPI anticoagulant activity in patient samples. **Aims.** To develop an assay measuring the anticoagulant properties of TFPI and study the relationship between the TFPI anticoagulant activity and TFPI free antigen and TFPI total antigen. **Materials and Methods.** *TFPI anticoagulant assay:* 32 µL of plasma was first incubated for 5 min with either 8 µL TBS or anti-TFPI immunoglobulin, which completely blocked TFPI activity. Then, 30 µL recombinant, relipidated tissue factor (Innovin®) at 1/200 fold dilution was added and incubated for 3 min. Clotting was initiated by the addition of 30 µL $CaCl_2$ (35 mM). Results were expressed as a ratio, with clotting times in the absence of anti-TFPI as the denominator (a value of 1.0 indicating no TFPI anticoagulant activity). This ratio was normalized against the ratio obtained with reference plasma within each run to minimize day-to-day variation in clotting times. After normalization, high ratios reflect little functional TFPI anticoagulant, whereas low ratios reflect high activity. *TFPI antigen assays:* TFPI free and total antigen were assayed with commercial kits from Stago, of which TFPI free antigen is specific for circulating full-length TFPI. *Study population:* Control subjects (n=436) of the Leiden Thrombophilia Study (LETS). **Results.** Mean TFPI anticoagulant ratio was 0.97 (SD 0.0062, range 0.82-1.15). The assay coefficient of variation was 2.8% between days and from 0.6% to 1.5% within days. The regression coefficient (B) for TFPI free antigen, with TFPI anticoagulant ratio as dependent variable, was $-100 \cdot 10^{-4}$ (95% confidence interval $-110 \cdot 10^{-4}$ to $-90 \cdot 10^{-4}$), which means that an increase in TFPI free antigen of 10 ng/mL is consistent with a decrease of TFPI anticoagulant ratio of 0.10. The correlation coefficient (r) was 0.67. B for TFPI total antigen was $-20 \cdot 10^{-4}$ ($-23 \cdot 10^{-4}$ to $-16 \cdot 10^{-4}$) with r=0.47. **Conclusions.** A novel and reproducible assay for detection of TFPI anticoagulant activity in plasma has been developed. TFPI anticoagulant ratio was much stronger associated with free antigen than with TFPI total antigen, which supports the hypothesis that free TFPI is biologically relevant in vivo.

FP14

A novel coagulation assay used to detect procoagulant phospholipid correlates with microparticle numbers in resting and collagen-stimulated samples

Connor D, Exner T, Ma D, Joseph J**

Department of Haematology Research, St Vincent's Hospital, Darlinghurst, Sydney, Australia, 2010.

Introduction Phosphatidylserine (PS) plays a central role in haemostasis and can be detected by several types of assays. Numbers of circulating microparticles (which are PS rich) are calculated using both flow cytometric and ELISA techniques, whilst functional phospholipid activity can be assayed using PS-dependent coagulation tests. We have recently described a novel, simplified method (termed XACT) that can measure functional PS in both whole blood and plasma samples. **Aims** The main aim of this study was to examine the relationship between procoagulant PS activity (as detected by XACT) and number of annexin V positive microparticles (as detected by flow cytometry) in resting and collagen-stimulated samples from normal donors. **Materials and Methods** Venous blood was collected into 4.5ml citrate tubes from 10 normal donors. Whole blood, platelet rich plasma (PRP) and collagen stimulated (20mg/mL) PRP samples were prepared. Procoagulant activity was measured using a dilute FX-activated coagulation assay (XACT), which utilises PL-free porcine plasma. A flow cytometric method was used to count the number of microparticles (defined as Annexin V positive events less than 1.09Гm in size) and concentration calculated using BD TRU-COUNT tubes. **Results** Median values (with 5th and 95th percentile) for XACT times were 41.3s (35.7, 44.6) for whole blood; 48.7s (45.8, 52.9) for PRP; and 26.8s (23.9, 36.7) for collagen-stimulated PRP. Median values (with 5th and 95th percentile) for microparticle (MP) counts were 589 MP/ГL (297-1348) in whole blood; 1330 MP/ГL (1048-1894) for PRP; and 4730 MP/ГL (3083-7184) for collagen-stimulated PRP. The difference in XACT times and MP counts between PRP and collagen-stimulated PRP was highly significant ($p<0.0001$). There was also a significant correlation between XACT times and MP counts in PRP and collagen-stimulated PRP samples ($p<0.0001$). **Conclusion** This work demonstrates that the novel XACT assay can detect procoagulant phospholipid in resting and stimulated samples and directly correlates with number of annexin V positive MP's which confirms that this surface PS is functional. It also demonstrates that the removal of larger cell types (i.e. erythrocytes and leukocytes) results in prolongation of the XACT time, suggesting that a proportion of procoagulant phospholipid is associated with these cell types.

FP15

Von Willebrand factor cleavage in vitro at room temperature occurs without the need for divalent ions

Perutelli P, Amato S, Molinari A*

Thrombosis and Haemo

Introduction. Human von Willebrand factor (VWF) plays a pivotal role in the mechanism of platelet thrombus formation under conditions of high shear stress. VWF is synthesized by endothelial cells in form of an extra large polymer. The size of VWF is physiologically down regulated to a series of multimers by the specific VWF-cleaving metalloprotease, ADAMTS-13. VWF cleavage *in vitro* requires prolonged dialysis in denaturing agents and low ionic strength buffer in order to alter the tertiary conformation of VWF, and the presence of divalent ions (Ba^{2+} or Ca^{2+}) to activate ADAMTS-13. However, cleavage *in vivo* of the newly released VWF polymers occurs within seconds or minutes, thus indicating that fluid shear stress modulates VWF proteolysis. However, **Aim.** We evaluated VWF proteolysis *in vitro* at 37°C and 22°C controlled temperatures, in order to acquire further information on VWF proteolysis mechanism. **Materials and methods**. Normal pooled plasma was incubated in the presence of 1.5 M urea, 5 mM Tris (final concentrations) for 24 h at 37°C or 22°C in thermostatic bath. Plasma aliquot was pre-incubated for 5 min. with 10 mM $BaCl_2$. Digestion was stopped by adding 10 mM EDTA. VWF proteolysis was assessed by agarose gel electrophoresis and gel immunostaining. **Results.** VWF proteolysis was observed when plasma was incubated at 37°C in the presence of $BaCl_2$, whereas only partial digestion occurred in the absence of $BaCl_2$. Moreover, complete proteolysis occurred when plasma was incubated at 22°C, either in the presence or in the absence of divalent ions. **Conclusions.** Cleavage of endogenous VWF at temperature lower than physiologic occurs in the presence of denaturant and low ionic strength, without the need of supplementary divalent ions. Further investigations are necessary to elucidate whether the finding of VWF proteolysis at room temperature is due to a less specific or alternative cleavage mechanism.

FP16

Dietary habits and their role on the occurrence of coronary artery disease: is the Italian a real Mediterranean-diet?

Sofi F, Giuliani G, Vecchio S, Martinelli F, Fedi S, Cellai A, Gori A, Ferrini S, Abbate R, Gensini GF*

Department of Surgical and Medical Critical Care, Thrombosis Centre, Azienda Ospedaliero-Universitar

Epidemiological studies have demonstrated that dietary patterns are important determinants of the risk of coronary artery disease (CAD). "Progetto Nutrizione per la Salute e la Prevenzione di Malattia" is an ongoing study performed in order to investigate the dietary habits in relation to some chronic diseases. In a sample of population from Florence area, Tuscany, Italy (102 subjects with CAD and 410 healthy subjects) we assessed, by a dietary interview, intakes of several nutrients and lipid profile together with plasma levels of total homocysteine (tHcy), folate, vitamin B6, B12 and lipoprotein(a) [Lp(a)]. Lipid profile was significantly different between the two groups. Lp(a) and tHcy plasma levels were found to be higher in patients compared to healthy subjects (median: 194 mg/L vs 114.5 mg/L; p=0.02, and 14.8 µmol/L vs 10.2 µmol/L p<0.0001 respectively). Both serum folate and vitamin B6 levels were higher in healthy subjects than in patients (5.4±2.6 ng/mL vs 4.4±3.3 ng/mL, p<0.0001; 12.6±9.2 µg/L vs 7.4±3.4 µg/L, p<0.0001 respectively), while there was no difference in vitamin B12 concentrations. A significant correlation between serum tHcy, folate, vitamin B6, B12 and vitamin B6 and folate intakes was found. Concerning dietary habits we observed that total lipid intake was not adherent to Italian guidelines (<35% of daily Kcal) in 24.5% of patients and in 36.3% of healthy subjects. Poly-unsaturated-fatty-acids (PUFA) intake was significantly higher (p<0.005) in healthy subjects respect to patients. However, all patients and over 97% of healthy subjects had lower PUFA intake respect to recommended levels. Alcohol consumption was below 1 Alcoholic Unit (A.U.) in a large part of the population and an amount able to give a cardiovascular benefit (2-3 A.U./die) was present only in 20% of healthy subjects and in 36.2% of patients. Low (<60 mg/die) vitamin C intake was present in less than 5% of healthy subjects and in 10% of patients, reaching a statistically significant difference (p=0.03). Folate intake was higher in healthy subjects than in patients (346.7±124.4 µg/die vs 309.6±112.7 µg/die; p=0.009) while vitamin B6 intake was similar in both groups with a great part of healthy subjects showing vitamin intakes (68.4% for folate and 85.6% for vitamin B6) below recommended levels. Regression analysis showed that high levels of Lp(a) (>300mg/L) and tHcy (>19 µmol/L in men and >14 µmol/L in women) (OR 2.6 and 3.4 respectively) and low serum folate (<2.7 ng/mL) and vitamin B6 (<5 µg/L) (OR 3.04 and 2.1 respectively) were independent risk factors for CAD. **In conclusion** these preliminary data show the gap between nutritional recommendations and food practices even in a typical Mediterranean-diet population and confirm the pathogenetic role of Lp(a) and tHcy on the occurrence of CAD.

FP17

Oxidative stress-a link between endothelial injury, coagulation activation and atherosclerosis in haemodialysis patients

Pawlak K (1), Naumnik B (1), Brzosko S (1), Pawlak D (2), Mysliwiec M (1)*

(1) Department of Nephrology and Transplantation, Medical University, Białystok, Poland
(2) Department of Pharmacodynamics, Medical University, Białystok, Poland

Introduction. Recently, oxidative stress (SOX) has been implicated as an important etiologic factor in atherosclerosis and vascular dysfunction both in general and uraemic populations. Accelerated atherosclerosis plays an important role in the development of cardiovascular disease (CVD) in haemodialyzed (HD) patients. Aims. In the present study we try to establish whether enhanced SOX, involving endothelial injury, activation of coagulation and inflammatory reaction, could be implicated in the atherosclerotic disease in haemodialysis (HD) patients. **Materials and methods**. Markers of SOX, endothelial injury, coagulation and cytokines were measured in the plasma of HD patients with and without CVD, and healthy controls by ELISA methods. Remodelling of the carotid arteries was assessed by measuring intima-media thickness (IMT) as a surrogate of atherosclerotic disease in all groups. **Results**. Markers of SOX, endothelial injury, extrinsic coagulation pathway and IMT values were significantly elevated in HD patients, especially those with CVD when compared to the control group. Von Willebrand antigen (vWF:Ag) levels were more increased in the subgroup with CVD than those without. Furthermore, plasma levels of tumor necrosis factor α (TNF-α), monocyte chemoattractant protein-1 (MCP-1) and macrophage inflammatory protein-1β (MIP-1β), were significantly higher only in the HD group with CVD when compared to the controls. IMT was strongly and directly correlated with Cu/Zn superoxide dismutase (Cu/Zn SOD). Both IMT and Cu/Zn SOD were positively correlated with age, thrombomodulin (TM), vWF:Ag, tissue factor (TF), tissue factor pathway inhibitor (TFPI), prothrombin fragment F1+2 (F1+2), MCP-1, MIP-1β and TNF-α levels. Multivariate analysis identified vWF:Ag as the only independent variable significantly associated with increased IMT ($\beta = 1.523$, $p = 0.00018$). **Conclusions**. The present study suggests that enhanced SOX, involved proatherogenic cytokine and chemokines levels, endothelial injury and coagulation activation, may constitute a pathway for accelerated atherosclerosis in HD patients. The significant, independent association between IMT and vWF:Ag should be assessed in future studies to determine whether vWF:Ag elevation is causative or a by-product of increased IMT.

FP18

NCX 6550, a nitric oxide (NO)-releasing derivative of pravastatin, exerts antiplatelet and antithrombotic activity

Momi S (1), Rossiello M (2), Caracchini R (1), Monopoli A (3), Ongini E (3), Gresele P (1), Colucci M (2)*

(1) Department of Internal Medicine, Sect. of Internal and Cardiovascular Medicine, University of Perugia, Italy
(2) Department of Biomedical Sciences, Sect. of General Pathology, University of Bari, Bari
(3) NicOx Research Institute, Milan, Italy.

Introduction. Statins decrease cardiovascular morbidity and mortality, in both hyper and normocholesterolemic patients. One shortcoming of statins is their slow onset of action that reduces their efficacy in acute ischemic conditions. Recently, novel antithrombotic molecules have been developed by the addition of a nitric oxide (NO)-adduct to a known drug in order to exploit the additional antithrombotic effect of NO. **Aims.** In this study we evaluated the effect of the novel NO-releasing statin NCX6550 (nitropravastatin) *in vitro* and *in vivo* on a number of cellular functions relevant to atherothrombosis. **Methods.** *In vitro* we assessed the effects of test compounds on human platelet aggregation induced by U46619 and on tissue factor (TF) activity and expression by human mononuclear cells stimulated with LPS (1 µg/ml) or PMA (10^{-9} M). *In vivo* we evaluated the effect of the compounds on U46619-induced pulmonary thromboembolism in mice and on pro-coagulant activity of spleen mononuclear cells and peritoneal macrophages after administration of LPS (100 µg/mouse). **Results.** *In vitro*, NCX6550 inhibited U46619-induced human platelet aggregation in both buffer (IC_{50} = 117±12µM) and plasma (IC_{50} = 97±9 µM) with a NO-dependent mechanism (sensitive to guanylyl cyclase inhibition, ODQ 10µM), while pravastatin was inactive. In human mononuclear cells NCX6550, but not pravastatin, inhibited dose-dependently LPS- and PMA-induced TF expression (> 85% inhibition at 50 µM; TF antigen after 3h incubation with LPS: 0.66±0.25 *vs* 5.0±2.5ng/mg in NCX6550 and control, respectively; p<0.01), an effect associated with a comparable reduction of both TF activity (16.5±12.8 vs 198±92 U/10^6 cells) and TF mRNA. *In vivo,* NCX6550 (24 mg/kg i.p.) given 1h before U46619 injection, in contrast to equimolar dose of pravastatin (20 mg/kg i.p.), significantly reduced mortality (controls=85%; pravastatin=85%; NCX6550=55%; p<0.05) and platelet consumption (platelet x 10^9/L: NCX6550 48mg/kg = 208±89.9; pravastatin 40 mg/kg =94±25; p<0.05). Plasmatic NO-degradation products after NCX6550 increased progressively with a peak at 3 h (from 27±6µM to 64±17 µM). NCX6550 (0.6 mg/mouse i.p.) given 15 min before LPS, attenuated the clot promoting activity of spleen mononuclear cells and peritoneal macrophages harvested 3 h after LPS challenge (spleen mononuclear cells- clotting time: 197±18s and 255±42s in vehicle and NCX6550 groups, respectively; p<0.001; peritoneal macrophages-clotting time: ±s and ±s in vehicle and NCX6550 groups, respectively; p<0.001), while pravastatin was ineffective. **Conclusions.** Our results show that a novel NO-donating statin exerts antiplatelet and anticoagulant effects both *in vitro* and *in vivo.* Thus, NCX6550 may represent an interesting new anti-atherothrombotic treatment for patients with acute coronary syndromes.

FP19

Inhibition of integrin activation and expression in vascular smooth muscle cells

Sohn Y (1), Pyun W (2), You W (3), Jang Y (1,2), Seung K (4), Chung KH (1,3)

(1) Cardiovascular Research Institute and BK21 Project for Medical Science, Yonsei University College o
(2) Cardiology Division, Department of Internal Medicine, Yonsei University College of Medicine, Korea
(3) National Research Lab for Cardiovascular Therapy, BioBud R&D Center, Seoul 120-110, Korea
(4) Department of Internal Medicine, Catholic University Medical College, Korea

Backgrounds: The restenosis of coronary artery is responsive process after percutaneous coronary intervention and initiated by endothelial denudation, which causes aggregation and adhesion of platelets and inflammatory cells such as monocytes and lymphocytes. After that, activation, migration and proliferation of vascular smooth muscle cell cause neointimal hyperplasia as main mechanism for restenosis. The purposes of this study were to know the effects and mechanisms of new elegant disintegrin, saxatilin from Korean snake venom and down regulation of integrin by RNA interference in vascular smooth muscle cells. **Methods and Results:** The recombinant saxatilin was highly expressed from Phichia pastoris and purified. We observed the saxatilin inhibited adhesion and proliferation of vascular smooth muscle cells. We investigated adhesion of vascular smooth muscle cell and COS7 cell after saxatilin gene transfection on the cells. The surface integrins α_v and α_5 of vascular smooth muscle cell were down regulated by RNA interference successfully, which was proved by RT-PCR and revealed morphologic changes, inhibition of adhesion, proliferation, and actin cytoskeletal activation. **Conclusions:** These results may provide new insights into role of integrins, $\alpha_v\beta_3$ and $\alpha_5\beta_1$, on smooth muscle cell as well as role of smooth muscle cell in the process of neointimal hyperplasia and have significant implications for inhibition and down regulation of integrin targeted to smooth muscle cell might be beneficial for the prevention of restenosis after percutaneous coronary intervention.

FP20

Fibrocytes in atherosclerosis

Fletcher J (1,2), Vasista A (1), Guiffre A (1,2), Mamo P (1), Medbury H (1,2)*

(1) University of Sydney Department of Surgery
(2) Westmead Hospital

Smooth muscle cells (SMCs) play a major role in atherosclerosis maintaining plaque stability through the formation of a fibrous cap. While SMCs have been thought to migrate from the media, this view has been questioned with bone marrow shown as a source of alpha-actin positive cells present in atherosclerotic plaque. We hypothese that these alpha-actin positive cells may be fibrocytes which are spindle shaped adherent cells producing SMC alpha-actin upon stimulation with TGF-beta. They have characteristic CD markers, the key one being CD34. They also secrete extracellular matrix proteins, such as collagen I and III, which are found in the fibrous cap. We examined 20 human carotid endarterectomy specimens for the presence of fibrocytes by staining of specimens for SMC alpha-actin and CD34. SMC alpha-actin positive cells were found in the media and fibrous cap region. Double staining of specimens for SMC alpha-actin in combination with CD34 revealed that many of the SMC alpha-actin spindle shaped cells also stained positive for CD34. We found in vitro that monoyctes could transform into spindle shaped cells in less than 24 hours with the loss of CD14 and neo-expression of CD34 within a week. Our findings show that monoyctes are a progenitor for fibrocytes and that fibrocytes are a source of SMC alpha-actin positive cells found in atherosclerosis. We suggest that during the development of atherosclerosis, circulating monocytes can transform into either a foam cell or fibrocyte depending on local chemical mediators present at the time. Understanding what factors commit the monocyte to either pathway will provide potential targets for atherosclerosis treatment.

FP21

Influence of antiplatelet therapy on platelet-mediated thrombin generation after carotid stenting

Piñon M (1), Valles J (1), Santos M (1), Lago A (2), Tembl J (2), Aznar J (3), Moscardo A (1)*

(1) Research Center. University Hospital La Fe. Valencia Spain
(2) Neurology Department.University Hospital La Fe. Valencia Spain
(3) Department of Clinical Pathology.University Hospital La Fe. Valencia Spain

Background: Thrombin plays a pivotal role in thrombus formation. Stent procedures are known to produce platelet activation, and platelets contribute to thrombin generation. No data are available on the effects of antiplatelet therapy in platelet-mediated thrombin generation after carotid stenting. In addition, platelet-erythrocyte (RBC) interactions increase platelet reactivity (*Blood 99:3978-84). **Objective**: To study the effect of aspirin (ASA) and ASA+clopidogrel as antithrombotic therapy on thrombin generation after carotid stenting and to establish the modulatory effect of RBCs in this process. **Methods**: Platelet-mediated thrombin generation was analyzed in 22 patients (19 men and 3 women, average age 68+/-15) after implantation of a carotid stent. Patients were initially treated with daily ASA (300 mg) + clopidogrel (75 mg) for 1 month, and afterwards with 300 mg ASA. Normal subjects without medication were also evaluated (control). Thrombin generation in response to tissue factor was measured according to Hemker (*Tromb Haemostas* 1994, 72:713-21) in platelets alone (PRP) or PRP+RBCs (Htc 40%). **Results**: RBCs significantly shortened the lag time and increased the peak of thrombin generation. In PRP, patient treatment with ASA+clopidogrel for 30 days resulted in a significant increase in the lag time and reduction of the peak of thrombin generation (43%) when compared to controls. Change of therapy to ASA alone did not enhance thrombin generation when compared to ASA+clopidogrel. In fact, the same prolongation of the lag time and reduction of thrombin peak (40%) was detected in the patients (n=8, so far) when compared to controls. In platelets+RBCs, ASA+clopidogrel and ASA alone significantly reduced peak thrombin generation by 24 and 22%, respectively, when compared to controls. **Conclusions:** After carotid stenting, ASA+clopidogrel and ASA down-regulate platelet-mediated thrombin generation, which is also inhibited, to a lower extent, in the presence of RBCs. This mechanism may contribute to the clinical benefit of antiplatelet treatment. (Grants FIS01/1208/ FIS03/0270/GRUPOS03/005).

FP22

Role of PECAM-1 in acutely formed platelet thrombi during human microvascular anastomosis

Olsson E, Sarlomo-Rikala M, Böhling T, Lassila R*

Introduction: Previous in vitro studies suggest a regulatory role for platelet-endothelial adhesion molecule (PECAM-1) in platelet aggregation and interaction with collagen. **Aims**: We subjected in vivo-formed microthrombi to immunohistochemical analysis to characterize the association of platelets and PECAM-1. **Materials and methods**: we assessed acutely failed microanastomoses during free tissue transplantation in 12 human vessel samples. All patients except one (unstable fracture) were subjected to immediate or late reconstructive cancer surgery. Thrombus formation and platelet-vessel wall interaction were studied with two platelet-associated immunohistochemical markers, i.e. antibodies against CD 42b (glycoprotein, GP Ib) and CD 31 (PECAM-1). CD 31 was also stained to detect endothelial cells. **Results**: The absence of endothelial cells colocalized with thrombosis, and the staining in tensity of the markers was associated with the extents of adherent and/or aggregated platelets. Within the same vessels the findings ranged from adhesion to local fully occlusive thrombi. Both of the markers consistently decorated large or occlusive platelet thrombi. In adjacent vessel areas - in contrast to this dual staining pattern of the mature local thrombi - the adhesive platelet (mono)layers expressed only GPIb, whereas the PECAM-1 staining was fully absent. **Conclusions**: The staining pattern between adherent platelet layers and grown thrombi is distinct in respect of PECAM-1. This finding could reflect either shedding or a conformational change in PECAM-1 (i.e. dimerization) following its ITIM-engaged activities. If this PECAM-1-exerted regulatory step upon adherent platelets fails, local thrombus growth is marked by preserved PECAM-1 expression.

FP23

Effects of CML drugs (taxol, rapamycin and glivec) on platelet aggregation and on fibrinogen binding to platelets

Tetik S (1), Eksioglu-Demiralp E (2), Yardimci T (1)*

(1) Maramara University, Faculty of Pharmacy, Department of Biochemistry, Istanbul-Turkey
(2) Marmara University, Faculty of Medicine, Department of Haemotology-Immunology, Istanbul-Turkey

Background: One of the important complications in CML treatment with taxol, rapamycin and glivec is thrombocytopenia. These anticancer drugs therefore might play important role in platelet functions. Taxol and rapamycin are also used in stent eluting systems. Previously we have shown antiaggregating effect of taxol on platelets. **Aim**: To enlighten the underlying effects of taxol, rapamycin and glivec on platelets leading to thrombocytophenia, their effects on platelet aggregation and on fibrinogen binding to purified GpIIb/IIIa coated microbeads and fibrinogen binding to platelets are studied. **Materials&Metods**: Different concentrations of commercial taxol, rapamycin and glivec effects were examined. Platelets were obtained by thrombopheresis from normal subject. Agonist induced platelet aggregation was followed on Chronolog aggregometer. FITC labelled Fibrinogen (Fg-FITC) binding to purified GpIIb/IIIa coated microbeads and to isolated platelets was followed with FACsan Becton-Dickinson flowcytometer. **Results**: Taxol, rapamycin and glivec caused inhibition of ADP and Adrenalin induced agregation, concentration dependently. Whereas, only glivec inhibited fibrinogen binding to platelets. Rapamycin and taxol had no effect on fibrinogen binding to isolated platelets. Taxol rapamycin, and glivec showed no effect on Fg-FITC binding to purified GpIIb/IIIa coated microbeads.

FP24

The release of matrix metalloproteinase-9 in human platelets: regulation of platelet activation in in vitro and in vivo studies

Sheu J, Shen M, Hsiao G*

Graduate Institute of Medical Sciences, Taipei Medical University, Taipei 110, Taiwan.

Introduction. Matrix metalloproteinases (MMPs) are a family of Zn^{+2}- and Ca^{+2}-dependent enzymes, which are important in the resorption of extracellular matrices (ECMs) in both normal physiological processes and pathological states. Aims. The aim of this study was to identify the presence of matrix metalloproteinase-9 (MMP-9) in human platelets and systematically examine its inhibitory mechanisms of platelet activation. Materials and methods. In this study, we report on an efficient method for the quantitative analysis of pro-MMP-9 in human platelets using capillary zone electrophoresis (CZE). To elucidate subcellular localization of MMP-9 in human platelets, we investigated intraplatelet MMP-9 by immunogold labeling and visualized it using electron microscopy. Results and conclusions. MMP-9-gold labeling was observed on the plasma membrane, α-granules, open canalicular system, and within the cytoplasma both in resting and activated platelets. Furthermore, activated MMP-9 concentration-dependently (15-90 ng/ml) inhibited platelet aggregation stimulated by agonists. Activated MMP-9 (21 and 90 ng/ml) inhibited phosphoinositide breakdown, intracellular Ca^{+2} mobilization, and thromboxane A_2 formation in human platelets stimulated by collagen (1 μg/ml). In addition, activated MMP-9 (21 and 90 ng/ml) significantly increased the formation of nitric oxide/cyclic GMP. Rapid phosphorylation of a platelet protein of *Mr* 47,000 (P47), a marker of protein kinase C activation, was triggered by phorbol-12, 13-dibutyrate (PDBu) (60 nmol/L). This phosphorylation was markedly inhibited by activated MMP-9 (21 and 90 ng/ml). In an *in vivo* thrombotic study, activated MMP-9 (1 μg/g) significantly prolonged the latency period of inducing platelet plug formation in mesenteric venules. These results indicate that the antiplatelet activity of activated MMP-9 may be involved in the following pathways. (1) Activated MMP-9 may inhibit the activation of phospholipase C, followed by inhibition of phosphoinositide breakdown, protein kinase C activation, and thromboxane A_2 formation, thereby leading to inhibition of intracellular Ca^{+2} mobilization. (2) Activated MMP-9 also activated the formation of nitric oxide/cyclic GMP, resulting in inhibition of platelet aggregation.

FP25

Is assay of fibrin gel permeability a precise way to determine the effects of acetylsalicylic acid on coagulation?

Antovic A (1), Perneby C (2), Jacobsson Ekman G (3), Wallen H (2), Hjemdahl P (2), Blombäck M (1), He S(1)*

(1) Coagulation Research Division / Dept. of Surgical Sciences, Karolinska Institutet, Karolinska Hospital
(2) Clinical Pharmacology, Karolinska Institutet, Karolinska Hospital, Sweden.
(3) Department of Medicine, Unit of Clinical Allergy Research, Karolinska Institutet, Karolinska Hospital

Background: It has been reported that acetylsalicylic acid (ASA) induces the acetylation of lysine residues in fibrinogen molecule in vitro. We have found greater increase in permeability of the fibrin gel derived from plasma samples with exogenous thrombin during treatment of 75 mg ASA daily than in that of 360 mg. This may imply that the presence of ASA, especially in a low dose, alters the clotting property of fibrinogen in vivo, rendering the structure of fibrin more porous. The present study was aimed to assess whether more decreased dose of ASA can show the similar influence on the fibrin gel structure. **Material and methods:** Fifteen male healthy volunteers, aged 22-39 years participated in the study. Baseline blood samples were taken 3 times during 24 hours. Afterwards, they received 37.5mg ASA daily for 10 days. Sampling was performed 1, 4 and 24 hours after the last dose. After 2 weeks of washout period the participants were treated with the dose of 320mg ASA daily and samples were taken 1 hour after the last dose. The volunteers were instructed to immediately take 640mg ASA as a single dose. Sampling was performed 4 and 24 hours after dose of 960mg. The permeability of fibrin gels was assayed with flow measurement and permeability coefficient (Ks) was calculated. Three-dimensional (3-D) structure of the fibrin gel, and fibrinogen concentration was also determined. **Results:** Ks levels did not differ among baseline samples. During the treatment with 37.5 mg ASA, Ks increased significantly compared to the baseline levels. A significant but lower increase of Ks was also observed after treatment with higher ASA doses. The treatment with ASA did not influence fibrinogen concentration compared to the baseline results. The presence of thicker fibrin fibers and larger pores of network with irregular structure can be observed under the examination by 3-D in samples obtained during treatment with ASA. The changes were more obvious in those obtained during treatment with the lower dose. **Interpretation:** Possible changes in charge distribution and conformation of the fibrinogen molecules due to acetylation may serve as an explanation for the alternations in clotting property, observed as the influence on the fibrin gel porosity. Since increases of the fibrin porosity were ASA dose-dependent, it may be proved that clinical practice in use of ASA therapy with a dose as low as around 30 mg daily is beneficial for preventing thrombotic complications.

FP26

Plasma levels of factor VIII, IX and XI and risk of recurrent venous thromboembolism

Marchiori A, Simioni P, Tormene D, Fadin M, Gavasso S, Perlati M, Prandoni P*

Clinica Medica II, University of Padua, Italy

Background. Although high levels of factor VIII, IX, and XI have been reported to increase the risk of recurrent venous thromboembolism (VTE), the problem remains controversial. **Aims.** To assess the association between plasma levels of factor VIII, IX and XI and recurrent VTE. **Methods**. 251 consecutive patients with the first episode of objectively proved deep-vein thrombosis (DVT) of the lower extremities, who had received at least three months of conventional anticoagulation, were followed-up prospectively up to 10 years. Patients with malignancy, antiphospholipid antibody syndrome, and defects of antithrombin, protein C and S were excluded from the evaluation. The development of recurrent VTE was objectively documented. The association between plasma levels of factor VIII, IX and XI and recurrent VTE was assessed using Cox regression models. **Results**. The hazard ratios (HR) of recurrent VTE for each increase of 10 IU per deciliter of factor VIII, IX and XI were 1.02 (95% CI, 0.95 to 1.10), 0.96 (0.87 to 1.08) and 0.95 (0.84 to 1.08), respectively. Results did not change after adjustment for age, sex, modality of clinical presentation, presence of factor V Leiden or G20210A prothrombin mutation, and duration of oral anticoagulation. When the analysis was confined to the 98 patients with idiopathic DVT who were not carriers of factor V Leiden or prothrombin mutation, a significant association with VTE recurrence was found for high levels of FVIII (HR=1.26; 95% CI, 1.08-1.48 for each increase of 10 IU per deciliter). **Conclusions**. Plasma levels of FIX and FXI are not associated with an increased risk of recurrent VTE. High levels of factor VIII predict the development of recurrent VTE in the only subgroup of patients with idiopathic presentation who are not carriers of other known thrombophilic conditions.

FP27

The value of compression ultrasound in diagnosis of asymptomatic deep venous thrombosis in acutely ill medical patients

Wisniewska J (1), Tomkowski W (1), Lensing A (3), Kober J (1), Małek G (2), Oniszh K (2), Burakowska B (2)*

(1) Intensive Care Unit, National TB and Lung Diseases Research Institute, Warsaw, Poland
(2) Department of Radiology, National TB and Lung Diseases Research Institute, Warsaw, Poland
(3) Academic Medical Center, Amsterdam, Holland

Background: Utility of vein ultrasonography in diagnostic procedure of deep vein thrombosis (DVT) is widely accepted. According to MEDENOX data, majority of patients with DVT confirmed by venography had not clinical signs and symptoms of DVT. Any data in literature comparing vein ultrasonography with venography in asymptomatic medical patients at risk of thrombosis are available. **Study objective**: To evaluate sensitivity and specificity of compression ultrasound (CUS) examinations in diagnosis of proximal and distal deep venous thrombosis in acutely ill medical patients with exposure on risk of venous thromboembolism (VTE): congestive heart failure (NYHA class III and IV), respiratory infectious, inflammatory diseases - considered to be at moderate risk of VTE. Mainly asymptomatic course of DVT in acutely ill medical patients was expected. Design: CUS examination (equipment: Sequoia C 256, linear probe with pulse and color Doppler) was performed just before venography, scheduled on Day 6-15 of hospital stay. Extensive CUS was performed. Whole length of common femoral veins, femoral veins, popliteal veins and calf veins: tibial anterior plus posterior and peroneal were investigated. CUS was compared with ascending venography, which was evaluated by two radiologists. **Results**: Technically satisfactory venography was obtained in 160 patients. In 12 out of 160 patients (7.5%, 95% CI = [4.0%-12.7%]), venography confirmed presence of DVT. In all 12 cases course of DVT was asymptomatic. Among them proximal DVT was detected in 5 patients (3.1%, 95% CI = [1.0 %-7.1%]) and distal DVT in 7 patients (4.4%, 95% CI = [1.8% - 8.8%]). In all 160 patients CUS of proximal veins was technically satisfactory. In 3 out of 5 patients with proven by venography proximal DVT, diagnosis was confirmed by CUS (sensitivity 60%), in one case result of CUS was false positive (specificity 99.4%). In 10 out of 160 patients calf CUS was technically insufficient. In 2 out of 7 patients with proven by venography calf thrombosis diagnosis was confirmed by CUS (sensitivity 28.6%) and in two cases result of CUS was false positive (specificity 98.6). **Conclusion**: Due to low sensitivity, compression ultrasound should not be used as reference screening method in diagnosis of DVT in asymptomatic medical patients.

FP28

High incidence of symptomatic chronic thromboembolic pulmonary hypertension after symptomatic pulmonary embolism

Pengo V (1), Lensing A (2), Prins M (3), Marchiori A (4), Davidson BL (5), Biasiolo A (1), Pegoraro C (1), Iliceto S (1), Prandoni P (4)*

(1) Department of Clinical and Experimental Medicine, University of Padua, Italy
(2) Center for Vascular Medicine, University of Amsterdam, The Netherlands
(3) Department of Clinical Epidemiology, University of Maastricht, The Netherlands
(4) Department of Medical and Surgical Sciences, University of Padua, Italy
(5) Division of Pulmonary and Critical Care Medicine, University of Washington, U.S.A.

Background. Chronic thromboembolic pulmonary hypertension (CTPH) is associated with considerable morbidity and mortality. Its incidence following pulmonary embolism (PE) and associated risk factors are not well documented. **Aims.** To assess the incidence of CTPH following an episode of PE and to identify parameters associated with its development. **Materials and Methods**. We assessed the incidence of symptomatic CTPH in 223 consecutive patients with an acute episode of PE but without prior venous thromboembolism. CTPH was considered in the presence of otherwise unexplained persisting dyspnea. These patients underwent transthoracic echocardiography and if supportive findings were present, had a ventilation/perfusion lung scan and pulmonary angiography. CTPH was considered present with a systolic and mean pulmonary artery pressure exceeding 40 and 25 mmHg, respectively, a normal pulmonary capillary wedge pressure, and consistent angiographic appearance. Risk factors for CTPH were evaluated in a case-control design, which also included patients with acute PE but confirmed prior venous thromboembolism. **Results**. 223 patients were included in the cohort. The cumulative incidence of symptomatic CTPH was 1.0% (95% CI, 0-2.4%) at 6 months, 3.1% (95% CI, 0.7-5.5%) at 1 year, and 3.8% (95% CI, 1.1-6.5) at 2 years. None of the 132 remaining patients with more than 2-year follow-up developed this complication afterwards. In the case-control analysis, previous PE, younger age, larger perfusion defects, and idiopathic presentation were independently associated with an increased risk of CTPH. **Conclusions**. CTPH is a serious complication of PE that occurs with surprisingly high frequency. Future evaluations of new diagnostic and therapeutic strategies for PE should address and strive to minimize its incidence.

FP29

Observational study of bemiparin, first dose administered 6 hours after surgery, in hip or knee replacement surgery

Abad JI (1), Gómez-Outes A (2), Martínez-González J (2), Maeso R (2), Rocha E (3)*

(1) Carlos Haya Hospital, Málaga, Spain
(2) Laboratorios Farmacéuticos ROVI, S.A., Madrid, Spain
(3) University Clinic of Navarra, Pamplona, Spain

Introduction: Postoperative start of prophylaxis with bemiparin showed to be at least as effective and safe as preoperative start of prophylaxis with enoxaparin. **Aims:** To evaluate the effectiveness, safety, and pharmacoeconomic impact of bemiparin 3,500 IU/d (first dose administered 6 hours after surgery) in patients undergoing total hip or knee replacement in daily clinical practice. **Material and methods:** Prospective, open, multicenter, not randomized study. Main efficacy and safety endpoints included symptomatic and objectively confirmed venous thromboembolism (VTE) [deep vein thrombosis (DVT) and pulmonary embolism (PE)], major bleeding, thrombocytopenia and death by any cause. **Results:** A total of 1,009 patients were included from 23 centers in Spain. Of these, 882 (87.4%) received neuraxial anaesthesia. The rate of confirmed VTE was 0.3% (3 of 1,009 patients): 2 proximal and 1 distal DVTs. No cases of confirmed PE were shown. There were 14 (1.39%) major bleeding events: 10 excessive surgical wound bleedings, 3 hemarthroses and 1 gastrointestinal bleeding that required treatment discontinuation. There were no cases of spinal haematoma, fatal bleeding or bleeding in critical organs. There were 4 (0.4%) cases of mild thrombocytopenia that did not required treatment discontinuation. No cases of severe type II thrombocytopenia were observed. There were no deaths during the treatment period. The median length of hospitalisation was 9 days. 92.5% of patients continued prophylaxis out-hospital for a median time of 30 days (1st and 3rd quartile: 26 and 36). Interestingly, postoperative start of prophylaxis with bemiparin permitted that 29.4% of patients scheduled to undergo hip or knee replacement could be admitted in hospital the very same day of the intervention, thus reducing hospital stay costs in about 89,000 euros per 1,000 patients treated when compared to preoperative start of prophylaxis the day before surgery. **Conclusions:** Bemiparin 3,500 IU/d, commenced 6 hours after total hip or knee replacement surgery, is highly effective and safe in daily clinical practice. Postoperative dosing allows approximately one third of the patients to be admitted in hospital the very same day of surgery, thus reducing hospital stay costs, and makes easier the practice of neuraxial anaesthesia.

FP30

Abstract withdrawn

FP31

Statin and fibrate treatment of combined hyperlipidemia: the effects on some novel risk factors

Šebeštjen M (1), Keber I (1), Žegura B (1), Simčič S (2), Božič M (1), Migaud Fressart M (3), Stegnar M (1)*

(1) Department of Vascular Diseases, University Medical Centre, Ljubljana, Slovenia
(2) Institute of Microbiology and Immunology, Medical Faculty, Ljubljana, Slovenia
(3) Diagnostica Stago, Asnieres, France

Objectives: The effect of cerivastatin and fenofibrate on proteins involved in haemostasis and markers of inflammation was investigated in otherwise healthy middle-aged males with combined hyperlipidemia. **Background**: Besides classical risk factors, other so-called novel risk factors for coronary artery disease are playing increasingly important role as markers for the development and progression of atherosclerosis. **Methods**: Thirty-eight males, aged 49 ± 5 years were randomised to 12 weeks treatment either with cerivastatin in a daily dose of 0.2 mg to 0.4 mg to achieve the LDL cholesterol goal of <3.0 mmol/l, or with fenofibrate 250 mg daily. Fasting serum lipids, homocysteine, total and free TFPI, PAI-1 and t-PA antigen and activity, CRP, IL-6 and TNF-α were measured before and after treatment. **Results**: No change in homocysteine level was observed in the cerivastatin group, while in the fenofibrate group it increased (p<0.0001). The decrease of total tissue factor pathway inhibitor (TFPI) was significant after cerivastatin (p=0.002), but not after fenofibrate. Free TFPI did not decrease after either drug. Neither drug affected tissue plasminogen activator (t-PA) antigen and activity while fenofibrate increased plasminogen activator inhibitor (PAI-1) antigen (p<0.05) and activity (p<0.05). In cerivastatin group serum CRP values decreased by 49.5% (p=0.001), while in fenofibrate group serum CRP levels decreased by 29.8% (p=0.03). The decreases of CRP in the two groups differed significantly (p=0.04). IL-6 levels decreased significantly in fenofibrate group (39%; p<0,0001), while the decrease was not significant in cerivastatin group (15%; p=0,24) No significant decreases were observed for TNF- α. The decrease of CRP in cerivastatin group did not correlate with the decrease in IL-6 (r=0,22; p=0,44) and TNF- α (r=0,08; p=0,75). On the other hand in fenofibrate group the magnitude of CRP decrease significantly correlated with the magnitude of IL-6 (r=0,66; p=0,002) TNF- α (r=0,45; p=0,05). **Conclusions**: Cerivastatin has neutral effects on fibrinolysis, homocysteine and coagulation measured with free TFPI. On the other hand, fenofibrate increased PAI-1 antigen and activity and homocysteine, and did not effect coagulation. Both cerivastatin and fenofibrate reduced CRP level, the decrease being significantly greater after cerivastatin. Fenofibrate also significantly decreased IL-6 and TNF-a, while cerivastatin had no influence on these parameters.

FP32

Maximal doses of Atorvastatin improve inflammation, thrombogenesis and matrix remodelling in high-risk ischaemic heart disease patients

*Marin F (1), Roldan V (2), Garcia-Herola A (2), Lorenzo S (3), de Teresa L (2), Sogorb F (1), Lip G (4)**

(1) Cardiology Dpt. Hospital General de Alicante, Alicante, Spain
(2) Haematology Unit. Hospital de San Vicente, Alicante, Spain
(3) Clinic Analysis Dpt. Hospital General de Alicante, Alicante, Spain
(4) Department of Medicine, City Hospital, Birmingham, UK

Higher doses of statins could improve clinical outcomes compared to conventional doses, but whether this benefit is due to "additional" pleiotropic effects is uncertain. We hypothesised that high risk patients show abnormal indices of inflammation (C-reative protein, CRP), thrombogenesis (prothrombin fragment 1+2, F1+2), and matrix remodelling (matrix metalloproteinase-1, MMP-1, and its tissue inhibitor, TIMP-1) in spite of being treated with a 'standard' dose of atorvastatin (40 mg/day), and that using the highest doses of atorvastatin (80 mg/day) would beneficially improve these research indices. Methods. We studied 27 "high-risk" patients (inclusion criteria: severe triple vessel but rejected for by-pass for extensive coronary disease, severe effort angina after coronary artery by-pass and premature coronary disease with □3 risk factors) with an abnormal lipid profile despite 40 mg atorvastatin/day, at baseline and at 3 months after increasing the dose to 80 mg/day. Baseline results in patients were compared to 22 healthy controls. Results. At baseline, patients showed a proinflammatory [0.30 (0.15-0.60) vs 0.10 (0.03-0.35)] and prothrombotic state [0.50 (0.42-0.63) vs 0.32 (0.27-0.42)], with decreased levels of MMP-1 and TIMP-1 [3.92 (3.07-4.75) vs 4.28 (3.91-5.28), and 649 (530-808) vs 551 (437-670) respectively], all p value<0.05. When atorvastatin was increased to 80 mg/day, significant reductions in LDL-cholesterol, CRP and F1+2 levels were observed, whereas MMP-1 and TIMP-1 levels increased. No adverse effects were observed in any patients. Conclusions. In spite of atorvastatin 40mg daily, 'high risk' patients still demonstrated a proinflammatory and prothrombotic state, with abnormal extracellular remodeling. Doubling the dose of atorvastatin resulted in significant improvements in these pathophysiological processes.

FP33

Short-term nonlipid effects of simvastatin and micronised fenofibrate in high risk patients

Celińska-Lowenhoff M, Undas A, Iwaniec T, Szczeklik A*

Department of Medicine, Jagiellonian University School of Medicine, Cracow, Poland

Introduction It has been well documented that statins show anticoagulant and anti-inflammatory effects within a few weeks of treatment, however, little is known regarding similar effects of fibrates. **Aims** The aim of this study was to evaluate the immediate antithrombotic and anti-inflammatory effects of simvastatin and micronised fenofibrate in patients with high cardiovascular risk. **Materials and methods** In a randomized, double blind study, 30 patients with cholesterol LDL > 3.4 mmol/L and 2 or 3 other coronary risk factors were assigned to a group treated either with simvastatin [Merck Sharp and Dohme] (40 mg/d) or micronised fenofibrate [Fournier Laboratoires] (160 mg/d). Before, at 3 and 28 days of treatment C-reactive protein (CRP), interleukin 6 (IL-6), and thrombin-antithrombin complexes (TAT) were measured in venous blood. TAT levels were also determined in blood collected from standardized skin incisions at the same 3 days. All subjects (aged 53.9 ± 6.6 years) did not differ in respect with demographic characteristics and risk factors. **Results** LDL cholesterol lowered significantly during the treatment with both drugs. Thrombin generation, as evidenced by plasma TAT concentrations, was significantly attenuated as early as after 3 days of treatment with simvastatin (from 5.2 to 3.5 μg/L) and fenofibrate (from 4.3 to 2.9 μg/L) and the difference was more pronounced after a month of therapy (3.0 ug/L with simvastatin and 2.0 μg/L with fenofibrate). A suppression of thrombin formation was also observed at the site of microvascular injury. A major difference in the time course of thrombin generation was seen in the propagation phase at 3 minutes and later. CRP levels were significantly lower at 3 and 28 days of therapy with simvastatin (from 2.1 to 1.3 and 0.99 mg/L) and only 28 days of treatment with fenofibrate (from 2.3 to 1.0 mg/L). IL-6 lowered significantly from 2.8 to 2.4 pg/mL after 3-days' treatment with simvastatin and from 2.3 to 1.7 pg/mL after 28-days' therapy with fenofibrate. None of these effects correlated with the changes in lipid profile. **Conclusions** Our results suggest that both simvastatin and fenofibrate have rapid antithrombotic and anti-inflammatory effects in high-risk patients. This might provide rationale for early initiation of hypolipemic drugs in acute vascular events.

FP34

Interactions between tissue factor pathway inhibitor (TFPI) and lipoprotein lipase (LPL) in the metabolism of triglyeride-rich lipoproteins

Brodin E (1), Iversen N (2), Hansen J (1)*

(1) Center for Atherothrombotic Research in tromsø (CART), Institute of Clinical Medicine, Univer
(2) Department of Medical Genetic, Ullevaal University Hospital, Oslo, Norway

Introduction: Clinical studies have demonstrated a positive association between serum triglyceride levels and risk for coronary thrombosis. TFPI is a potent inhibitor of tissue factor (TF)-induced blood coagulation synthesized by and associated with the endothelial surface (EC). LPL is the major lipase in the metabolism of triglycerides, synthesized by parenchymal cells and anchored to GAGs at EC surface. A strong positive relationship between Very Low Density Lipoproteins (VLDL) and TFPI has been reported, and suggested as a compensatory mechanism for increased susceptibility for thrombosis in patients with hypertriglyceridemia. In contrast, *in vitro* studies have shown that TFPI enhances LPL activity, thereby increasing triglyceride hydrolysis. **Aims:** To investigate how native VLDL and LDL influenced the synthesis and release of TFPI in endothelial cells, and how TFPI affected the LPL-induced hydrolysis of VLDL in vitro and at the endothelial surface. **Material and methods:** A spontaneously transformed immortal endothelial cell line (ECV304) was used, and VLDL and LDL were isolated from healthy volunteers by density gradient ultracentrifugation. Sequential FFA measurements were used to evaluate the kinetics of the LPL induced hydrolysis. The levels of TFPI m-RNAs in the stimulated cells were determined by quantitative PCR (qPCR) using the ABI PRISM 7700 Sequence Detection System. **Results:** Stimulation of ECV304 for 24 hrs with n-VLDL (0-100 μg/ml) and n-LDL (0-400 μg/ml) caused a dose-dependent increase in TFPI to the medium 6.7-19.8 ng/10^6 cells, p<0.001 vs 10.3-148.4 ng/10^6 cells, p<0.001 respectively, without affecting the cellular content of TFPI. A similar dose-dependent increase in the expression of TFPI mRNA was observed upon stimulation with nLDL. Cellular binding of both r-TFPI and LPL to the endothelium was demonstrated, but TFPI bound more effectively than LPL. Addition of increasing concentrations of rTFPI to ECV 304 cells, preincubated with LPL, did not affect the hydrolysis of VLDL triglycerides. The maximal reaction velocity (V_{max}) of LPL induced hydrolysis of nVLDL was not affected by the addition of increasing concentrations of rTFPI to the reaction mixture in vitro. **Conclusions:** The present experimental study indicates an upregulation of TFPI synthesis and release by VLDL and LDL. LPL induced hydrolysis of VLDL is not influenced by TFPI neither in an endothelial system nor in vitro.

FP35

Delayed postprandial clearance of chylomicrons and increased ApoC-I in plasma VLDL in patients with echolucent carotid plaques

Notø A, Mathiesen E, Bjôrkegren J, Hansen J*

(1) Center for Atherothrombotic Research in Tromsø, University of Tromsø, Tromsø, N
(2) Institute of Community Medicine, University of Tromsø, Tromsø, Norway.
(3) The Atherosclerosis Research Unit, King Gustav V Research Institute, Karolinska Institute, Stockholm
(4) Center for Atherothrombotic Research in Tromsø, University of Tromsø, Tromsø, N

Introduction: Patients with echolucent, lipid-rich atherosclerotic plaques have increased risk of ischemic cerebrovascular events independent of degree of carotid stenosis. HDL cholesterol has been identified as an independent predictor for plaque echolucency and enrichment of postprandial VLDL with apoC-I have been identified as a marker of early atherosclerosis. **Aims:** To determine the metabolism of postprandial triglycerides and the apoC-I content of VLDL particles in relation to carotid plaque morphology. **Material and methods:** A total of 57 subjects with carotid plaques (24 with echolucent and 33 with echogenic plaques) and 38 controls were recruited from a population health survey. Plaque morphology was assessed by B-mode carotid ultrasound. Information on risk factors and blood samples were collected before and at 2-hrs interval after a standard high fat meal. **Results**: Subjects with echolucent plaques had lower age- and sex-adjusted mean HDL cholesterol level (1.50±0.49 mmol/l) than subjects with echogenic plaques (1.82±0.54 mmol/l, p=0.02) and controls (1.79±0.43 mmol/l, p=0.02). Measurement of plasma concentrations of chylomicrons after intake of the standard fat meal, revealed a delayed clearance of chylomicrons from the circulation in subjects with echolucent plaques (p<0.01). In the fasting state, isolated VLDL from subjects with echolucent plaques were enriched with apoC-I (116.9±124.2 nmol/l) compared to VLDL particles from subjects with echogenic plaques (58.4±41.0mol/l, p=0.007) and controls (54.0±41.6mol/l, p=0.003). The apoC-I/apoB ratio in VLDL was also found to be higher in the echolucent group) compared to the echogenic (p=0.10) and the control (p=0.02) groups. The latter findings were weakened in VLDL isolated 4 hrs after the meal due to a more pronounced enrichment of apoC-I in subjects with echogenic plaques and controls. **Conclusions**: The present study suggests that HDL cholesterol as a predictor for plaque morphology is associated with altered VLDL composition and delayed chylomicron clearance. In the fasting state, the apoC-I content of VLDL particles was shown to be a marker for echolucent plaques in carotid stenosis.

FP36

No clinically significant interactions between the oral direct thrombin inhibitor ximelagatran and amiodarone, atorvastatin, or digoxin

Dorani H (1), Schützer K (1), Sarich T (2), Wollbratt M (1), Teng R (2), Ohlsson L (1), Kessler E (1), Wall U (1), Kalies I (1), Hamer J (2)*

(1) AstraZeneca R&D Mölndal, Mölndal, Sweden
(2) AstraZeneca LP, Wilmington, DE, USA
(3) AUTHOR 11: GF Carlson MD, Affiliation 2
(4) AUTHOR 12: UG Eriksson PhD, Affiliation 1

Introduction: The oral direct thrombin inhibitor ximelagatran at a fixed oral dose has shown clinical benefit in the prevention of stroke and other thromboembolic complications in atrial fibrillation. Although ximelagatran has a low risk of drug interactions via the cytochrome P-450 enzyme system, patients receiving oral ximelagatran are likely to be receiving multiple medications. Investigation of the potential interaction of ximelagatran and medications expected to be commonly coadministered is warranted. **Aim**: The potential for interaction of ximelagatran with amiodarone, atorvastatin, and digoxin was assessed in 3 randomized studies in healthy volunteers. **Methods**: Study 1 was a single-blind, placebo-controlled, parallel-group study (n=26) with ximelagatran 36mg or placebo BID for 8 days and amiodarone (single 600mg oral dose) on Day 4. Study 2 was an open-label, two-way crossover study (n=16) with atorvastatin as a single 40mg oral dose during one treatment period and ximelagatran 36mg BID for 5 days plus a single dose of atorvastatin 40mg on Day 4 during the other treatment period. Study 3 was a double-blind, placebo-controlled, crossover study (n=16) with ximelagatran 36mg or placebo BID for 8 days and digoxin as a single 0.5mg dose on Day 4. **Results**: For melagatran, the active form of ximelagatran, AUC and C_{max} geometric mean ratios (90% CI) for combined therapy relative to monotherapy with either drug were within or only slightly outside predefined bounds for no interaction. Similarly, the AUC and C_{max} of amiodarone, atorvastatin, and digoxin were within or only slightly outside predefined bounds for no interaction. None of the coadministered drugs affected the concentration–effect relationship of melagatran on activated partial thromboplastin time. All drugs and combinations were well tolerated. One subject withdrew from the digoxin study (digoxin+placebo group) after experiencing bradycardia and headache shortly after receiving digoxin. **Conclusions**: No clinically significant pharmacokinetic or pharmacodynamic interactions were observed when ximelagatran was administered with amiodarone, atorvastatin, or digoxin, a finding that provides evidence that no dose adjustments are required for either of the drugs in these combinations.

FP37

Influence of prognostic factors on the risk of recurrence or bleeding in long-term secondary prevention of venous thromboembolism with ximelagatran

Eriksson H (1), Lundström T (2), Wåhlander K (2), Billing Clason S (2), Schulman S (3), for the THRIVE III I*

(1) Department of Medicine, Sahlgrenska University Hospital/Östra, Göteborg, Sweden
(2) AstraZeneca R&D Mölndal, Mölndal, Sweden
(3) Coagulation Unit, Department of Medicine, Karolinska Hospital, Stockholm, Sweden

Introduction: Ximelagatran (Exanta™, AstraZeneca) is an oral direct thrombin inhibitor under investigation for prevention and treatment of venous thromboembolism (VTE). Ximelagatran has a rapid onset of action and predictable pharmacokinetics without food or alcohol interactions and a low potential for drug interactions. In a previously reported, international, randomized, multicentre, double-blind trial (THRIVE III), oral ximelagatran (24 mg bid), administered without coagulation monitoring or dose adjustment, reduced the incidence of recurrent VTE compared with placebo in moderate risk patients over 18 months, following 6 months' standard anticoagulation.(1) Incidences of major bleeding and all-cause mortality were low and not significantly different between groups. **Aims**: A subgroup analysis was conducted to evaluate the influence of potential prognostic factors on the risk of recurrent VTE or bleeding, and their impact on ximelagatran efficacy. **Methods**: The influence of potential prognostic factors—gender, age, body weight, renal function, malignancy, type of VTE event, and history of previous VTE events—was investigated in the intention-to-treat population using Cox proportionate hazard modelling. **Results**: Ximelagatran was administered to 612 patients and placebo to 611 patients. Multiple regression analysis including treatment and prognostic factors revealed no statistically significant subgroup differences within treatment groups, except for in the placebo group: a lower risk of recurrent VTE among females than among males (hazard ratio 0.32; 95% CI 0.18-0.57; $P < 0.0001$) and a higher risk of recurrent VTE in patients with more than one previous VTE event (hazard ratio 1.87; 95% CI 1.07-3.24; P = 0.0272). In addition, the risk of bleeding was higher among females than males receiving ximelagatran (hazard ratio 1.72; 95% CI 1.18-2.51; P = 0.0048). However, there were no significant interactions between any of the potential prognostic factors and treatment effect for the risk of recurrent VTE or bleeding. **Conclusion**: The favourable tolerability profile of ximelagatran and its superior treatment effect vs placebo observed in the overall patient population were maintained in all subgroups analyzed. This suggests that long-term use of oral ximelagatran, without coagulation monitoring or dose adjustment, should be possible in a wide cross-section of patients for the secondary prevention of VTE. 1. Schulman S et al. N Engl J Med. 2003;349:1713-21.

FP38

Phase I double blind, placebo controlled, ascending single intravenous dose study with a synthetic direct thrombin inhibitor, TGN255

Combe S (1), Allen G (2), Kennedy T (1)*

(1) Trigen
(2) Gamms Consultancy

Introduction: TGN255 is a potent (Ki = 7-22nM), reversible, low molecular weight, and highly selective synthetic direct thrombin inhibitor. **Aims**: The aim of study was to evaluate the pharmacokinetics, pharmacodynamics and safety of three dosage levels of TGN255, after single intravenous administration. **Materials and methods**: Eighteen healthy male subjects were enrolled. Each dosage level included six subjects, five of whom received active compound and one received placebo. Three dose regimen were tested: 7 mg intravenous bolus over 30 sec followed by an infusion of 25 mg/h for 3 h, 10 mg bolus followed by an infusion of 40 mg/h for 3 h, and an infusion of 40 mg/h for 3 h. Blood samples were taken into 3.8% tri-sodium citrate. Plasma concentrations of TGN255 were evaluated through an LCMS/MS method. The dynamic activity of TGN255 was assessed through measurement of the thrombin clotting time (TT) and activated Partial Thromboplastin Time (aPTT). **Results**: There were no adverse events of either a general or cardiovascular nature (including ECG changes, or liver function tests) during the study period. The pharmacokinetic profile of TGN255 was dose proportional. The bolus induced an almost immediate rise in plasma concentration (within 2 minutes) of the drug which increased further following the start of the continuous infusion., The disposition of TGN255 followed a pattern with a short distribution phase occurring within 30 minutes after the end of the infusion, and an overall effective systemic half-life *ca.* 2h. Intravenous infusion of TGN255 induced a rapid, dose-related increase in the TT, reaching a peak within 2 to 3h after the start of the infusion, with maximum mean values being approximately 4.7 to 7.5 fold higher than at pre-dose. The pattern and duration of this effect reflected the rapid, biphasic disposition of TGN255, with a fall in TT to 3 fold baseline values within 30 minutes after cessation of infusion, and below 2 fold baseline 3h after the end of the infusion. The effect of TGN255 on aPTT was less marked and of a shorter duration. The maximum mean values were 1.8 to 2 fold baseline, between 2 and 3 hours after the start of the infusion. Thereafter, mean values declined to pre-dose values by approximately 3 to 5h post-end of infusion. **Conclusion**: The above results indicate that TGN255 has the desired pharmacodynamic properties of an antithrombotic drug, namely that of dose-related marked potentiation of thrombin clotting time with minimal effects on aPTT and, hence, on the incidence of unwanted bleeding in a clinical situation.

FP39

Comparative anticoagulant and antiprotease actions of BAY 59-7939 – an oral, direct Factor Xa inhibitor – and enoxaparin and fondaparinux

Hoppensteadt D (1), Nevelle B (1), Maddenini J (1), Perzborn E (2), Misselwitz F (3), Fareed J (1)*

(1) Dep Pathology, Loyola University Medical Center, Maywood, Illinois, USA
(2) Cardiovascular Research, Bayer HealthCare AG, Wuppertal, Germany
(3) Global Medical Development, Bayer HealthCare AG, Wuppertal, Germany

Introduction: In contrast to the low molecular weight heparin enoxaparin (Aventis) and the heparin-derived pentasaccharide fondaparinux (Sanofi-Synthelabo), BAY 59-7939 is a novel, oral, direct Factor Xa inhibitor. Both enoxaparin and fondaparinux require endogenous antithrombin III (AT) as a cofactor, whereas BAY 59-7939 directly inhibits Factor Xa. **Aim:** Since all three drugs produce inhibitory effects on thrombogenesis via distinct mechanisms, this study was designed to compare their effects using various laboratory tests. **Results:** In biochemically defined systems, BAY 59-7939 exhibited a strong inhibitory action toward both human and bovine Factor Xa (0.7–1.4 μM), which was independent of AT levels. Neither fondaparinux nor enoxaparin produced any Factor Xa inhibitory effects in AT-depleted systems. While fondaparinux and enoxaparin showed relatively stronger Factor Xa inhibitory effects than BAY 59-7939, both exhibited much weaker effects compared with BAY 59-7939 in the global clotting tests and protease-generation assays. At concentrations <1.4 μM, BAY 59-7939 exhibited a profound increase in the PT, aPTT and HepTest assays (INR >2.5; 2–3-fold elevation in aPTT and HepTest), indicating the simultaneous inhibition of both intrinsic and extrinsic pathways. Similar results were obtained with BAY 59-7939 in AT-depleted plasma. Neither fondaparinux nor enoxaparin produced any elevation of aPTT or PT in both AT-depleted and normal plasma at concentrations of up to 2 or 6 μM, respectively. However, fondaparinux and enoxaparin produced strong prolongation of HepTest. BAY 59-7939 prolonged the Russell's viper venom clotting time in both AT-depleted and normal human plasma in a concentration-dependent manner, whereas neither fondaparinux nor enoxaparin produced any effect. Enoxaparin at concentrations up to 2 μM modestly increased thrombin time, whereas fondaparinux and BAY 59-7939 did not. None of the agents affected agonist-induced platelet aggregation. **Conclusion:** BAY 59-7939 interacts potently with both the intrinsic and extrinsic coagulation systems, which is independent of AT, and is associated with relatively stronger anticoagulant activity than both fondaparinux and enoxaparin.

FP40

Pharmacokinetics and pharmacodynamics of dabigatran in patients undergoing total hip or knee replacement in BISTRO-2

Stangier J (1), Bravo ML (2), Hettiarachchi R (3), Dahl OE (4), Büller H (5), Rosencher N (6), Ahnfelt L (7), Piovella F (8), Reilly P (9), Eriksson BI (10)*

(1) Boehringer Ingelheim Pharma GmbH Co. KG, Germany
(2) Boehringer Ingelheim, France
(3) Boehringer Ingelheim, The Netherlands
(4) Buskerud Central Hospital, Norway
(5) Academic Medical Center, Amsterdam, The Netherlands
(6) Cochin University Hospital, Paris, France
(7) Falköping Hospital, Sweden
(8) IRCCS Policlinico San Matteo, Pavia, Italy
(9) Boehringer Ingelheim Pharmaceuticals Inc., USA
(10) Sahlgrenska University Hospital Östra, Göteborg, Sweden

Introduction: Dabigatran etexilate, the pro-drug of the potent, orally active, selective and direct thrombin inhibitor dabigatran is under development for the prevention of deep vein thrombosis in patients at risk of thrombotic events. **Aims**: The primary objective was to investigate the PK and PD of dabigatran in patients undergoing total hip or knee replacement, and to establish the exposure – efficacy and safety relationships of dabigatran. **Materials**: In BISTRO-2, a multicenter, parallel-group, double blind study, 1973 patients undergoing total hip or knee replacement were randomised to oral doses of dabigatran etexilate (50 and 150 mg twice daily, 300 mg once daily, and 225 mg twice daily) or enoxaparin (40 mg once daily) for a total of 6-10 days. The primary efficacy outcome was the incidence of VTE and the primary safety outcome was major bleeding episodes. For pharmacokinetic analysis, plasma concentrations of dabigatran were determined pre-dose on the day before surgery and on days 2, 4, 5 and 6 after surgery. Blood samples were collected for determination of the prolongation of the ecarin clotting time. In a sub-group of 325 patients, full PK/PD profiles were obtained after administration of the first dose of dabigatran etexilate after operation and at day 5 of the treatment period. **Results**: PK and PD parameters of dabigatran increased in proportion with dose. At steady state, the mean (CV%) AUCs of 50, 150 and 225 mg BID and 300 mg dabigatran etexilate QD were 446 (64%), 1450 (62%), 2420 (93%) and 3160 (64%) ng*h/mL, respectively. The mean maximum plasma concentrations at steady state were 56.4 (56%), 193 (56%), 310 (87%) ng/mL after 50, 150 and 225 mg BID and 329 (57%) ng/mL after 300 mg QD. Dabigatran trough concentrations increased with BID dosing and reached steady state on day 3. The mean dabigatran trough concentrations were 25 (72%), 95 (81%) and 149 (83%) ng/mL after 50, 150 and 225 mg dabigatran etexilate BID and 55 ng/mL (102%) after 300 mg QD. There was a linear relationship between ecarin clotting time and dabigatran plasma concentrations. PK and PD parameters were related to the incidence of DVT and bleeding by logistic regression analysis. A clear relationship between PK/PD parameters and DVT and bleeding was observed. **Conclusions**: Adequate dabigatran plasma concentrations were observed after oral administration early after surgery. The PK/PD profile of dabigtran in patients was predictable. The correlation between PK/PD parameters and the probability of DVT and bleeding was used for selection of dabigatran etexilate doses in Phase III clinical trials.

FP41

Effect of combination antı-angiogenesis therapy on markers of coagulation, platelet activation and angiogenesis in patients with advanced cancer

Caine G (1), Harris A (2), Christodoulos K (2), Lip G (1), Blann AD (1)

(1) University Department of Medicine, City Hospital, Birmingham, UK
(2) Cancer Research UK Medical Oncology Unit, Churchill Hospital, Oxford, UK.

Background: Coagulation, platelet, and angiogenic abnormalities are common manifestations of cancer, and recent data suggest that these processes are significantly inter-related. To investigate this further, we tested the effects of combination anti-angiogenesis therapy (marimastat, captopril and fragmin) on plasma levels of coagulation initiator tissue factor (TF), platelet marker soluble P-selectin (sP-sel) and angiogenic growth factor vascular endothelial growth factor (VEGF). **Materials and Methods:** 25 patients with advanced cancer and 25 age and sex matched controls were studied. Plasma levels of TF, sP-sel and VEGF were assessed by enzyme-linked immunosorbent assay (ELISA) at baseline, and (in the patients) at 4-and 8-week intervals post-combination anti-angiogenesis therapy. **Results:** At baseline, patients with cancer had raised plasma sP-sel (P<0.001) and TF (P<0.001), but not VEGF (p=0.066), when compared to healthy controls. A significant positive correlation was observed between VEGF and TF (r=0.8, P<0.001) in cancer patients but not controls. There were no significant differences changes in levels of sP-sel, TF or VEGF at 4- and 8-weeks, post-combination anti-angiogenesis therapy. **Conclusions:** Our data provide further evidence for a link between coagulation and angiogenesis in human cancer. Combination anti-angiogenesis therapy with marimastat, captopril and fragmin did not influence plasma levels of sP-sel, TF or VEGF.

FP42

Intrinsic "tenase" and prothrombinase activity of t-lymphoblastoid cells is enhanced by lipid peroxidation

Pickering W (1), Gray E (1), Goodall A (2), Barrowcliffe T (1)*

(1) Division of Haematology, NIBSC, Potters Bar, UK.
(2) Department of Cardiovascular Sciences, University of Leicester, UK.

Procoagulant phospholipids (PL) are normally provided by platelets, but our previous studies have shown PL-like activity on malignant T-cells. Lipid peroxidation (LP) occurs in several pathological states and can affect PL composition and activity. This study examines the effect of LP on intrinsic "tenase" and "prothrombinase" activities generated on the cell-surface of malignant T-cells. Four T-cell lines, CEM-CCRF, Jurkat, Molt-4, and A3.01, were cultured in RPMI under standard conditions. $CuSO_4$ (40 µM) and H_2O_2 (4 mM) initiated LP, and conjugated dienes (CD), "tenase" and "prothrombinase" activities were monitored over 4 hours. To block the additive apoptotic effect of H_2O_2 50 µM bongkrekic acid (BA) was added to the cells 1 hour before oxidation. Oxidation (CD) measured at 234 nm showed peak values at 1 hour, with Jurkat and Molt-4 being the highest. FXa and prothrombinase generation were measured in purified chromogenic systems, and calibrated against FXa and IIa standards. The basal activities of the cells for Xa generation were 95±6.3, 128±2.6, 153±5.9, 176±7.9 (pM±95% CI)) for CEM-CCRF, Jurkat, Molt-4 and A3.01 respectively, achieving peak levels of 228±7.5, 629±22.4, 575±18, 323±3.3 after 1 hour. BA reduced this peak activity by 11, 10, 21 and 4% respectively. "Prothrombinase" basal levels were 227±12, 263±18, 319±8, 304±4 (mIU/mL±95% CI) respectively, reaching peak levels of 491± 20, 522±13, 420±8, 469±16 after 2 hours. BA reduced this peak activity by 17, 12, 24, and 13% respectively. α-tocopherol (25 µM) an antioxidant also ameliorated the effect of LP on the "tenase" activity of the cell lines after 1 hour of LP by 71, 69, 44 and 37%, whilst "prothrombinase" activity after 2 hours LP was reduced by 56, 42, 47 and 69% respectively. In conclusion, BA reduces peak activity of the cell lines suggesting that the majority of this procoagulant activity appears to be due to the effect of LP. Furthermore *in-vitro* oxidation of PL increases T-Lymphoblastoid procoagulant activity, and suggests that LP enhances phosphatidylserine catalytic activity, and/or allows other PL to provide a potent coagulation surface.

FP43

Upregulation of monocyte chemotactic protein-1 and CD40 ligand in cancer patients and their modulation by subcutaneous enoxaparin

Fareed J (1), Tobu M (1), Demir M (2), Hoppensteadt D (1), Deitcher S (3)*

(1) Loyola University Medical Center, Maywood, IL, USA
(2) Trakya University Medical School, Edirne, Turkey
(3) The Cleveland Clinic Foundation, Cleveland, OH, USA

Introduction: Malignant cells constitutively produce monocyte chemotactic protein-1 (MCP-1). CD40 ligand (CD40L), a member of TNF superfamily, is primarily expressed on CD40 positive T-cells and activated platelets. **Aims**: The aims of these studies were to determine if MCP-1 and CD40L are up-regulated in cancer patients and to see if anticoagulant treatment enoxaparin down-regulates these factors. **Materials and Methods**: Blood samples were collected prior to and 3-7 days after the initiation of enoxaparin from cancer patients with acute symptomatic DVT and/or PE. These patients were enrolled in a randomized, parallel design study and were allocated to an initial treatment with enoxaparin alone for 1 week (n=70-72). A separate group of cancer-free patients with symptomatic thrombosis from a DVT treatment trial (n=50) were also included in this study. Commercially available quantitative sandwich enzyme immunoassay techniques (R&D Systems, Minneapolis, MN, USA) were used. **Results**: The baseline levels of the CD40L in cancer patients with thrombosis were markedly elevated (1323.8±29.0 pg/ml) in comparison to the normal plasma (n=47, 62.8± 18 pg/ml) and cancer-free patients with thrombosis (615±236 pg/ml). The MCP-1 levels were also increased in cancer patients (564.3±59 pg/ml) in comparison to the normal plasma (n= 47, 119.9±23 pg/ml) and cancer-free patients with thrombosis (215±75.5 pg/ml). Thirty-nine patients out of 70 (55%) exhibited >1000 pg/ml of CD40L. 39 patients out of 69 (58%) exhibited > 500 pg/ml of MCP-1. There was a good correlation (r^2=0.83) between MCP-1 and CD40L expression. Plasma samples drawn after treatment with enoxaparin (n=32), exhibited marked reduction in the CD40L (589.3± 125.6 pg/ml) and MCP-1 (342± 81.6 pg/ml) levels. The circulating anti-Xa levels ranged from 0.3-0.7 AXa U/ml (mean 0.56± 0.21U/ml). **Conclusions**: The circulating anti-Xa levels did not correlate with the decreased level of either MCP-1 or CD40L. The observed up-regulation of both of these markers of inflammation/immunoactivation in the baseline samples were consistent with a similar increase in von Willebrand Factor elevated in 97% of patients and CRP (elevated in 60% of patients). However, the relative decrease in these markers after enoxaparin treatment was not as dramatic as the one observed for the MCP-1 and CD 40L. Cancer-free patients with thrombosis did not exhibit similar increases in MCP-1 and CD40L.

FP44

Platelet–derived vegf, flt-1, angiopoietın-1 and p-selectin in breast and prostate cancer

*Caine G, Lip G, Blann AD**

University Department of Medicine, City Hospital, Birmingham, UK.

Background: Cancer is a complex multi-factorial disorder that may commonly show abnormal angiogenesis in such patients. Recently, platelets have been postulated to have a major role in both this processes, suggesting that anti-platelet strategies may be useful in cancer treatment. **Materials and Methods**: To further investigate the role of platelets in angiogenesis, we used an established in-house platelet lysate assay to analyse platelet contents in breast cancer (n=30) and prostate cancer (n=30) patients and age- and sex-matched controls (n=60). Markers of angiogenesis (vascular endothelial growth factor-A [VEGF-A], angiopoietin-1 and –2 [Ang-1, -2], and their respective receptors [Flt-1 and Tie-2] plus a marker of platelet activation (P-selectin [P-sel]), were all measured in platelet lysate by ELISA. **Results**: Platelet lysate from breast cancer patients contained higher levels of VEGF (p<0.0001), Ang-1 (p=0.0186) and P-sel (p=0.0002), compared to healthy controls. Platelet lysate from prostate cancer patients had elevated VEGF (p=0.008) but not Ang-1 or P-sel. There were no significant differences between levels of Flt-1 between patients and controls, and both Ang-2 and Tie-2 were undetectable in both patient groups and control platelet lysate. **Conclusion**: Our study provides further evidence that platelets may influence angiogenic abnormalities in human cancer. The platelet may be a useful target in anti-cancer strategies.

FP45

Optimal dosing of bemiparin for the prevention of venous thromboembolism in surgery for cancer

Gómez-Outes A (1), Martínez-González J (1), del Campo J (2), Rocha E (3)**

(1) Laboratorios Farmacéuticos ROVI, S.A., Madrid, Spain
(2) Logitest, S.L., Madrid, Spain
(3) University Clinic of Navarra, Pamplona, Spain

Introduction: Cancer patients have an augmented risk of venous thromboembolism (VTE) and bleeding. Low-molecular-weight heparins are drugs of first choice for thromboprophylaxis in surgery for cancer. **Aims**: To evaluate the timing of first administration and dose of bemiparin in surgery for cancer. **Material and methods**: Retrospective, open, multicenter, not randomized, cohort study. The incidence of symptomatic and objectively confirmed VTE, bleeding events, thrombocytopenia, death and adverse events was assessed. We also compared the investigator's VTE risk assessment (moderate or high) with the criteria of current Consensus Guidelines for the management of VTE. **Results**: A total of 197 patients were included. Prophylaxis was started postoperatively in 45 (22.8%) of them. According to the investigators' criteria, 124 (63%) patients were at moderate risk of VTE and therefore received bemiparin 2,500 IU/d, whereas 73 (37.1%) patients were at high risk and received bemiparin 3,500 IU/d. However, according to the criteria of current Guidelines, 189 (95.9%) patients were at high risk of VTE, and all of them should have received bemiparin 3,500 IU/d. The heterogeneity between the investigators' risk assessment and the criteria from Guidelines was statistically significant ($P < 0.0001$). Three (1.5%) patients developed a symptomatic confirmed VTE, all of them with bemiparin 2,500 IU/d administered in patients at high risk of VTE. There were 9 (4.6%) bleeding events during bemiparin prophylaxis. Four of them were major. Bemiparin started postoperatively showed a lower incidence of VTE (0% vs. 2%; $P = 0.39$), bleeding (2.2% vs. 5.3%; $P = 0.48$) and adverse events (2.2% vs. 9.9%; $P = 0.11$) than bemiparin preoperative dosing. Bleeding rates did not significantly differ between low and high bemiparin prophylactic doses (4.0% vs. 5.5%; $P = 0.72$). There was one case of moderate thrombocytopenia that did not require treatment discontinuation. There were no cases of severe type II thrombocytopenia. Two patients died during the study due to cardiorespiratory failure and sepsis, respectively. **Conclusions**: The risk of VTE was underestimated, resulting in an underdosing in many patients. Bemiparin appears to be highly effective and safe on the prevention of VTE in surgery for cancer. Postoperative start of prophylaxis with bemiparin probably provides a better safety profile in these patients and makes easier the application of neuraxial anaesthesia/analgesia.

POSTERS

PO001

Ischaemic cardiopathy and associated risk factors in two elderly women groups of low socio-economic condition

Narváez I (1), Saez de Lafuente J (2), Sáez Y (1), Vacas M (1), Molinero E (3), Sagastagoitia J (3), Magro A (2), Santos M (4), Sabino E (2), Iriarte J (1)*

(1) FIDEC. Bilbao. Spain
(2) Basque Country University. Bilbao. Spain
(3) Basurto Hospital. Bilbao. Spain
(4) MEDIKOSTA. Bilbao. Spain

Introduction: It has been stablished in several studies that people with low socio-economic level has a higher prevalence of coronary heart disease and cardiovascular risk factors. Our aim was to compare two groups of elderly women of low socio-economic condition and see if there are any differences in Ischaemic Cardiopathy and associated risk factors between them. **Material and Method**: We studied two groups of women aged ³ 65 years. Both groups present a common characteristic, which is a low economic condition. Group A: 301 women who lived in their home and received an economic grant from the town council. Group B: 122 women who lived in a geriatric residence totally subsidized by the town council. To each of the attendants under study, the following parameters were carried out: ECG, weight and height, blood pressure following WHO normatives, blood sample to determine Total Cholesterol (TC), Triglycerides (TG), LDLcholesterol (LDLc), HDLcholesterol (HDLc), uric acid, urea and glucose. For sample description we have used mean value (X) with standard deviation (sd) and to compare the different groups we used varianze analysis (ANOVA). We used SPSS/V10.1 statistical package. **Results**: Group A presented a higher prevalence of Ischaemic Cardiopathy (14.6 % vs 5.74%). Respecting cardiovascular risk factors studied, this group presented a higher mean values statistically significant for TC (237,50±42,85 vs 224,09±39 mg/dl) $p<0,003$, LDLc (159,47±38,03 vs 145,82±34 mg/dl) $p<0,001$, Uric Acid (5,56±1,60 vs 5,01±1,74 mg/dl) $p<0,002$, Body Mass Index (27,85±5,26 vs 26,40±5,54 Kg/m2) $p<0,01$ and Diastolic Blood Pressure (83,01±12,79 vs 80,33±10,54 mm Hg) $p<0,04$. **Conclusions**: We can conclude, looking to our data, that the differences in both groups in Ischaemic Cardiopathy and associated risk factors are due in part by the different diethetic and sanitary conditions of these populations.

PO002

Factors that may influence in the adequate control of arterial hypertension

Narváez I (1), Caso R (1), Martinez B (1), Molinero E (2), Sagastagoitia J (2), Vacas M (1), Saez Y (1), Saez de Lafuente J (3), Iriarte J (1), Iriarte M (1)*

(1) FIDEC, Bilbao, Spain
(2) Hospital de Basurto. Bilbao, Spain
(3) UPV/EHU. Bilbao, Spain

Hypertension is one of the most important modifiable risk factor for cardiovascular diseases. In the daily practice, control of arterial hypertension presents grate difficulties, for that reason we must frequently associate two o more agents to achieve their target blood pressure levels. Our aim was to evaluate factors that may influence in the adequate control of arterial hypertension. **Material and method**: 40 patients with a mean age of 65.2±8.4 years (23 males and 17 females) that received pharmacological treatment were analysed. These patients were controlled with 24h Ambulatory blood pressure monitoring (ABPM) before and after treatment and were followed up during 24 months. Systolic blood pressure (SBP), Diastolic blood pressure (DBP), pulse pressure (PP) values were estimated at baseline and after treatment. Presence of smoking habit, hypercholesterolemia, diabetes and Body Mass Index was also studied. **Results**: Patients were divided in two groups. Group A (GA): 24 patients with controlled blood pressure levels and Group B (GB), 16 patients with persistent elevated blood pressure levels. Baseline office SBP was in GA 157.04±12.09 mm Hg and in GB 167.32 ±14.7 mm Hg ($p < 0.031$); office SBP after treatment in GA 133.54 ±7.6 mm Hg and in GB 150.69 ± 5.4 mm Hg ($p < 0.0001$); office PP after treatment in GA 53.26 ± 9.2 mm Hg and in GB 67.31 ± 12.5 mm Hg ($p < 0.001$); SBP (ABPM) after treatment in GA 123.83 ± 12 mm Hg and in GB 132.31 ±11.3 mm Hg ($p < 0.032$). Patients with monotherapy in GA 6.84 % and in GB 31.25% and with combined therapy in GA 37.16% and in GB 68.75 % ($p < 0.01$). We didn`t find statistical significant differences between DBP, age, sex, cardiac frequency and all risk factors in the studied situations. **Conclusions**: Therapeutic control is difficult in patients with higher baseline SBP. This group had SBP and PP significantly higher even with combined therapy. DBP is easily controlled even with monotherapy. These results are independent from age, sex and associated risk factors.

PO003

Coronary heart disease estimation in an elderly population

Vacas M (1), Martinez B (1), Caso R (1), Narváez I (1), Saez Y (1), Iriarte M (1), Iriarte J (1), Molinero E (2), Sagastagoitia J (2), Gandarias JM (1)*

(1) FIDEC, Bilbao, Spain
(2) Hospital de Basurto, Bilbao, Spain

Background: Evidence from epidemiologic studies indicates that the same factors that are associated with increased risk of coronary heart disease (CHD) in the middle-aged people are relevant in older adults (those aged ³ 65 years). The relative risk associated with some risk factors decreases with advancing age but this is offset by greater incidence of CHD among older adults. A growing body of evidence from clinical trials indicates that risk factors modification in older adults reduces CHD risk as effectively as it does in middle-aged adults. **Aim**: To estimate coronary risk in an elderly population using a calibrated Framingham function for Spanish population. **Material and Method**: 646 subjects (56% females and 44 % males) with a mean age of 73.4±6.48 years and representative of Biscay elderly population has been selected. To each of the selected the following were carried out: clinical history, two blood pressure measurements, and blood sample to determine glucose, total cholesterol and HDL-cholesterol. We used the Framingham calibrated function to evaluate the 10-year probability of developing coronary heart disease events, such as fatal or non-fatal myocardial infarction with or without symptoms and angina. The 10-year risk probability of developing CHD was divided in four groups. Low coronary risk < 5%; Moderately low risk beteween 5-9 %; Moderate risk between 10-19 %; High risk between 20-39 % and Very high risk > 39 %. **Results**: Mean coronary risk was 7.3 %. 13.31 % had low risk (19.8 % men and 79.1% women); 60.99 % moderately low risk (35.8% men and 64 % women); Moderate risk 23.52 % (76.6 % men and 22.4 % women); High risk 2.16 % (92.9 % men and 7.1 % women). **Conclusions**: Mean coronary risk in our sample was moderately low. Looking to our results we see a higher coronary risk (>10%) in men than in women. None of the subjects studied had very high coronary risk.

PO004

Prothrombotic risk in white coat hypertensives

Theodossiades G (1), Vyssoulis G (2), Karpanou E (3), Zervoudaki A (2), Tsevrenis V (1), Kokkinos D (3), Stefanadis C (2)*

(1) 1st Regional Transfusion and Haemophilia Centre, Hippokration Hospital, Athens, Greece

(2) 1st Cardiology Department of Athens University, Athens, Greece

(3) 1st Cardiology Department of Onassis Cardiac Surgery Centre, Athens, Greece

Introduction: Patients with white coat hypertension (WCH) are at increased cardiovascular risk compared to normotensives, but much less than hypertensives. Furthermore, increased blood pressure (BP) is usually accompanied with thrombotic tendency. **Aim**: To explore the prothrombotic risk in patients with WCH. **Patients and Methods**: We studied 5514 non-diabetic patients, 1414 with WCH and 4100 with uncomplicated, untreated essential hypertension. WCH was defined when daytime measurements in 24h ambulatory BP were < 130/85 mmHg. After a 12h fast, total fibrinogen (TF) and plasminogen activator inhibitor 1(PAI-1) were measured in all patients. **Results**: Overall, TF and PAI-1 were lower in patients with WCH (291 vs 302 mg/dL and 2.36 vs 2.54 IU/ml, p<.00001), with lower incidence of increased values respectively (17.2 vs 23.5%, p<.00001 and 18.2 vs 21.7%, p<.005). When grouping patients in age decades, these differences were not observed in the middle ages and were relatively small in younger (<40 year old) and older (>60 year old) patients. **Conclusion**: Patients with WCH are at increased prothrombotic risk, almost similar to established hypertensives. This may play a major role in their overall risk assessment

PO005

Pathogenetic role of nitric oxide in thomboembolic complications in patients with chronic hart failure

Mirsamatova G

Endothelial dysfunction in patients with ischaemic hart diseases evokes a proliferation of smoothmussels cells in to wall's vessels, increase lipid's passing. It promotes further progress of atheroscleroses and coronary thromboses that cause a persistence of myocardium ischaemia The aim is the study of in order to investigate the role of NO in pathogenesis of chronic hart failure (CHF). We examined 45 patients (from 44 to 64 year old) of II functional class on categorizations NYHA. In all of them was measured NO by spectrofotometric determination of its stable metabolites (NO_2 + NO_3) and aggregation activity of thrombocytis (AAT) and erythrocytes (AAE). The aggregation potency of platelets and NO matters has been characterized by high index. A direct correlation of stable metabolites NO with AAT and AAE confirmed the important role of NO in aggregation pathogenesis of CHF. In patient of CHF with expressed clinical syndromes high level of NO corresponded max figures AAT and AAE. AAT was higher than AAE and the difference between parameters AAT and AAE was 17% (p<0.01). Also these high levels of AAT had a negative correlation with hypokinetic type of blood circulation. Studies have demonstrated that the difference in formation of NO between AAT and AAE may be a reflection of different cell pathogenic mechanisms: in unfavourable conditions thrombocytis was changed more than erythrocytes.

PO006

A comparison of off-pump and on-pump coronary-artery bypass surgery by sonoclot analysis

Paniccia R (1), Caciolli S (3), Palmarini M (2), Costanzo M (1), Pretelli P (2), Stefano P (3), Attanasio M (1), Abbate R (1), Gensini GF (1), Prisco D (1)*

(1) Department of Medical and Surgical Critical Care, Thrombosis Centre, University of Florence, Azienda

(2) U.O. Anestesia e Rianimazione 1, Azienda Ospedaliero-Universitaria Careggi, Florence, Italy

(3) U.O. Cardiochirurgia, Azienda Ospedaliero-Universitaria Careggi, Florence, Italy

Aim of this study was to investigate whether a different hemostatic profile at Sonoclot analysis (SIENCO Inc, USA) exists in off-pump coronary artery bypass (OPCAB) patients compared with on-pump coronary artery bypass patients (cardiopulmonary bypass – CPB - patients). The Sonoclot analyzer measures changes in blood viscoelastic properties by recording these changes in the form of a graph. Sonoclot "signatures" show a lag period (SonACT), corresponding to ACT (sec), and a primary wave whose slope, expressed as Clot Rate (CR), reflects the rate of fibrin formation, and is considered as an index of clot formation. Then, an inflection is produced as platelets are incorporated into the fibrin mesh and a secondary upslope leads to peak, which occurs at completion of fibrin formation. Subsequent downslope is produced as platelets induce further clot retraction. The time to peak (minutes) (TP) reflects clot retraction, and is an indicator of platelet function (PF). Twelve OPCAB and 12 CPB patients were studied. Sonoclot analysis in OPCAB patients was performed pre and post-heparin bolus, 45 min and 75 min after heparin administration, post-protamine infusion and 24 hours after the surgery. In CPB patients the procedure was similar to those for OPCAB patients except for extracorporeal circulation (ECC) period in which Sonoclot analysis was performed 30 and 60 min after ECC beginning. At baseline, in OPCAB and CPB patients no difference was found for the parameters examined. After heparin, during surgery and 24 h after surgery SonACT was significantly higher (at least p<0.05) in CPB than in OPCAB patients. In CPB patients CR values were found significantly increased post-protamine infusion (p<0.01) and 24 hrs after surgery (p<0.05) compared both with baseline values and CR values of OPCAB patients. Also TP values were significantly prolonged in CPB patients post-protamine infusion and 24 hrs after surgery (p<0.05 for both). The results of this pilot study indicate that OPCAB patients show a different profile in Sonoclot analysis in comparison with CPB patients. The clinical significance of this finding is yet to be determined.

PO007

A comparison between inthima-media thickness and coronary artery disease

Liva S, Pegoraro C, Cucchini U, Andriani C, Pelliccioni S, Maiolino G, Napodano M, Ramondo A, Pengo V, Iliceto S

Clinica Cardiologica Università di Padova, Padova, Italy

Measurement of intima-media thickness (IMT) in common carotid artery is a non-invasive method to evaluate systemic atherosclerosis. Aim of this study was to ascertain whether the degree of IMT was associated with the severity of coronary atherosclerosis. Eighty-nine consecutive patients undergoing catheterization to evaluate coronary artery disease (CAD) were studied. Coronary angiography of each patient was reviewed by an independent observer who determined the percent of diameter stenosis. The severity of CAD was determined by the number of significantly stenosed coronary arteries. Patients were classified as follow: code 1, normal vessel; code 2, < 50% stenosis; code 3,4 and 5 stenosis ≥50% in 1,2,or 3 major coronary arteries, respectively. A Duke score was also calculated. Classical risk factors (smoke habit, diabetes, hypertension, hypercholesterolemia) were recorded in each patient. IMT was measured in the common carotid artery 1 cm proximal to carotid bulb, bilaterally. Data of coronary artery involvement were dichotomized in below and equal/over 50% (code 1,2 and code 3,4,5) and analyzed in multiple logistic regression analysis together with IMT and classical risk factors. Only smoke habit resulted a predictor of coronary involvement (p=0.02), while IMT was a weak predictor (p=0.06). In another model of linear regression considering IMT and classical risk factors, smoke habit and age were predictive of IMT severity. In conclusion, the relationship between IMT and coronary atherosclerosis is not fully evident in this series of patients, possibly due to the small sample size of studied population.

PO008

The effects of incremental shuttle walking on activation of haemostatic and haemorheologic markers in patients with coronary heart disease

Lee W, Ingram J, Jolly K, Lip G*

Haemostasis, Thrombosis and Vascular Biology Unit, University Department of Medicine, City Hospital

Background: Activation of the coagulation cascade after short-term physical exertion has been shown in patients with CHD. However, most previous studies have used either bicycle ergometer or treadmill exercise protocol, which is not widely available to most patients. Most CHD patients choose walking as a mean of exercise and therefore the **aim** of this study was to assess the effect of an incremental shuttle walk test (ISWT) on plasma haemostatic markers. **Methods:** Plasma viscosity (PV), fibrinogen (Fg), D-dimer (Dd), soluble P-selectin(sPsel) and von Willebrand factor (vWf) levels were measured before and immediately after ISWT in 52 clinically stable CHD patients (47 male, 58±10yrs) who had completed a 12 weeks course of cardiac rehabilitation and in 19 matched healthy controls (15 male, 59±7yrs). The ISWT is a standardised incremental field walking test that provokes maximal performance and has been shown to correlate strongly with maximum oxygen uptake. **Result:** Baseline Fg, vWf and sPsel levels were significantly higher in CHD patients than in controls (all $p<0.05$). Fg (mean±sd, from 2.9±0.7 to 3.2±0.7 g/l), vWf (163 ± 44 to 179 ± 49 iu/dl), Dd (0.23±0.1 to 0.26±0.2 ng/ml) and PV (1.6±0.1 to 1.7±0.1 mpa.s) (all $p=0.001$) but not sPsel (78±18 to 81±20 ng/ml, $p=0.112$) levels were significantly raised post ISWT. Increment of Fg was correlated with total walking distance and peak heart rate ($p=0.02$). **Conclusion**s: A single bout of shuttle walking in patients with CHD appears to elevate fibrinogen, vWf, Dd and PV compared with healthy individuals with intact endothelium and normal haemostasis.

PO009

Use of low-molecular-weight-heparin in early cardioversion

Dokler Glavnik A, Škrabl Močnik F, Žohar P, Bervar M, Marinšek M, Gunzek R*

General Hospital, Celje, Slovenia

Introduction In persistant atrial fibrillation (AF) cardioversion (CV) is delayed because of prolonged anticoagulation. This period of waiting can be shortened if thrombi within the heart are excluded by transesophageal echocardiography (TEE). Administration of low molecular-weight-heparin (LMWH) in conjugation with TEE offers several advantages over unfractionated heparin (UFH). Methods From January 1999 to 2003 we treated 73 patients with AF lasting more than 48 hours and less than 1 month. We excluded thrombi with TEE. 23 patients (group A) were initially anticoagulated with UFH and therapeutic APTT was reached. 50 patients (group B) were treated with LMWH in therapeutic dose. After 24 hours on UFH or LMWH and warfarin CV was performed. We followed up a time of hospital stay and embolic incidents one week and six months after the procedure. **Results** Mean age in group A was 68±11 years and in B group 66±11 years. Arterial hypertension was the prevalent cause of AF in both groups. We excluded 9 (12%) patients from the study, because we found thrombi in left atrium or left atrial appendage. Hospital stay was significantly longer in group A 7.4 ± 2.6 days versus group B 2.8 ± 1.9 days. There were no embolic incidents detected during six months follow up time after cardioversion. **Conclusion** Early cardioversion of AF is safe if thrombi are excluded with TEE and proper early anticoagulation therapy is introduced. The use of LMWH for cardioversion significantly reduces hospital length of stay.

PO010

Left ventricular diastolic dysfunction is associated with abnormal haemorheology, thrombogenesis and endothelial damage/dysfunction

Lee W, Lip G*

Haemostasis, Thrombosis and Vascular Biology Unit, University Department of Medicine, City Hospital

Background: Heart failure (HF) is associated with an increased risk of thromboembolic events. About 35% of patients with HF have normal left ventricular (LV) systolic function, with diastolic dysfunction as the underlying cause. We hypothesised that LV diastolic dysfunction is associated with an increased risk of haemostasis, which may be related to abnormal haemorheology (raised plasma fibrinogen levels and plasma viscosity [PV]), endothelial damage/dysfunction (raised von Willebrand factor, vWf) and thrombogenesis (raised fibrin D-dimer, Dd). **Methods**: 72 patients with CHD (58 male, 59 ± 11 yrs) who were in sinus rhythm and with preserved LV systolic function (LV ejection fraction 61 ± 10%) and 35 matched healthy controls (23 male, 57 ± 6 yrs) were studied. Conventional transmitral pulsed Doppler indices (early/atrial [E/A] velocity ratio, E-wave deceleration time [EDT], isovolumic relaxation time [IVRT]) and pulsed Doppler Tissue imaging indices (peak systolic [S'], early and late diastolic velocities [E', A']) obtained at the septal and lateral mitral annuli were measured and related to plasma haemostatic markers levels. **Results**: Patients with CHD have significant prolonged EDT (median 240 vs 204 ms) and IVRT (149 vs 125 ms), shortened S' (10 vs 12 cm/s), E' (12 vs 14 cm/s) and A' (12 vs 13 cm/s) velocities with higher E/E' ratio (6.2 vs 5.4) compared to controls (Mann-Whitney test, all $p<0.05$). PV (median 1.7 vs 1.6 mpa.s), fibrinogen (3.3 vs 2.5 g/l), Dd (0.28 vs 0.18 ng/ml) and vWf (182 vs 120 iu/dl) levels were significantly higher in CHD patients than in controls (all $p<0.01$). PV and fibrinogen levels were correlated with S', E' and E/E' ratio (Spearman's $r=0.3$, $p<0.01$). vWf levels were correlated with E/A ratio ($r=0.2$), EDT ($r=0.3$), IVRT ($r=0.3$), S' ($r=0.4$), and E' ($r=0.2$) (all $p<0.05$). Dd was correlated with EDT ($r=0.3$, $p=0.016$). On multivariate analysis, vWf was independently related to S' ($p=0.024$) and IVRT ($p=0.016$), whilst PV was independently related to E/E' ratio ($p=0.034$). **Conclusions:** Diastolic LV dysfunction in patients with CHD is significantly associated with abnormal haemorheology, thrombogenesis and endothelial damage/dysfunction. The activation of coagulation in combination with endothelial dysfunction may contribute to increased thromboembolic risk in these patients despite preserved systolic function.

PO011

Plasma vascular endothelial growth factor (VEGF) and the angiopoietin/Tie2 System in proliferative sickle retinopathy

Mohan J (1,3), Lip P (2), Bareford D (3), Blann AD (1), Lip G (1)*

(1) Haemostasis, Thrombosis and Vascular Biology Unit, University Department of Medicine, City Hospital
(2) Department of Ophthalmology, The Birmingham and Midland Eye Centre, City Hospital, Dudley Road, Birmingham, UK
(3) Department of Haematology, City Hospital, Dudley Road, Birmingham B18 7QH, England, UK.

Introduction Proliferative sickle retinopathy (PSR) is an important cause of ocular pathology in sickle cell disease (SCD). Angiogenic growth factors are upregulated in conditions with active retinal neovascularisationor with retinal ischaemia. Data on plasma markers of angiogenesis are limited in SCD; in particular, whether levels are related to severity of retinopathy are unknown. Aims To measure the levels of plasma vascular endothelial growth factor (VEGF), its soluble receptor (sFlt-1), angiopoietin-1 and –2 (Ang1, Ang2) and their soluble receptor Tie2, [as indices of angiogenesis] in SCD patients with proliferative sickle retinopathy (PSR), in SCD patients with non-proliferative retinopathy (NPR), and in SCD patients without retinopathy (NR). Materials and Methods We measured these indices (all in citrated venous plasma by ELISA) in 56 SCD patients and in 23 control subjects with normal haemoglobin (AA subjects) matched for age, gender & ethnic origin with the PSR patients. Comparison of data in the SCD patients and AA subjects was by the Student's unpaired t test and among the SCD subgroups was by one-way ANOVA. Results We found raised levels of the following indices in SCD compared with AA subjects: VEGF (median 120, [IQR; 72-780] vs 11, [10-110] pg/ml; $p<0.001$), Ang1 (2.2, [1.0-11.4] vs (0.5, [0.5-2.5] ng/ml; $p<0.001$), Ang2 (5.1, [2.3-7.7] vs (1.3, [1.0-2.0] ng/ml; $p<0.001$) but no difference in sFlt-1 or Tie2. Of the 56 SCD patients, 24 had PSR, 16 had NPR and 16 had NR. However, there was no difference in any of the indices among the three SCD subgroups (VEGF: $p=0.800$, sFlt-1: $p=0.864$, Ang1: $p=0.675$, Ang2: $p=0.377$, Tie2: $p=0.910$). Conclusions We conclude that raised plasma VEGF and angiopoietins reflect abnormal angiogenesis in SCD, but not differences in ocular proliferation in SCD.

PO012

Fluid shear stress, blood coagulation and epigenome topography of granulocytes nuclei at atherosclerosis: what is evident?

Teplyakov A

Research Institute for Ecopathology and Occupational Disease

A widespread, but incorrect, view of the neutrophils is the short-lived, terminally differentiated cells that have a highly condensed nucleus and hence is unable to induce gene expression. However, these cells upregulate genes involved in phagocytic function, respiratory burst activity and cytokine secretion. Most studies of neutrophil gene expression have examined cytokine stimulation and have focused on a few specific genes of known interest, rather than the global genetic research. At the same time, we cannot exclude the granulocytes participation in supporting of cell-cell communication balance, coordinated by endothelium. **Goal**. To estimate the epigenetic topography changes of neutrophil nuclei in response to fluid shear stress and blood coagulation at modeling of fluid shear stress and thrombosis using original research technique. **Object**: 29 patients, suffering from atherosclerosis. The chromatin of granulocyte nuclei was studied using Computer TV Morphodensitometry System "DiaMorph" (Russia) in the smears dyed especially for DNA. It is the method for reconstructing morphologic characteristics of biologic objects from a digital matrix of optical parameters using digital image processing and an automatic TV device for quantitative image analysis of complex structural biologic objects. The primary advantage of its method is the capacity to combine morphometric data (area and perimeter) with cytophotometric ones (optical and integral optical density), and analyze the microanatomy of individual chromatin blocks. Nearly 100 parameters can be measured. After fluid shear stress we have detected the changes of classical morphometrical and optical parameters nuclei in whole. The size of nuclei had significant decreased (area and perimeter nuclei in whole) whereas the hetero/euchromatin ratio had significantly increased in comparison to initial. As result of more detail analysis, we detected and intranuclear rebuilding also: the significant increase of q1 area and perimeter, q2 area and perimeter with increase of integral optical density as indicator of decreasing methabolic activity in both components. After fluid shear stress we have detected the changes of classical morphometrical and optical parameters nuclei in whole. The size of nuclei had significant decreased (area and perimeter nuclei in whole) whereas the hetero/euchromatin ratio had significantly increased in comparison to initial. As result of more detail analysis, we detected and intranuclear rebuilding also: the significant increase of q1 area and perimeter, q2 area and perimeter with increase of integral optical density as indicator of decreasing methabolic activity in both components. After blood coagulation the topography of granulocytes nuclei have taken the other manner. The classic morphometric parameters of nuclei had no significant changes, excluding the significant increase of hetero-euchromatin ratio, comparable to results, receiving after fluid shear stress. However, the optical density of nuclei in whole was strongly increased. There more, the inhibition of methabolic processes has detected. It has indicated on possible necrosis association, i.e. "dark nuclei" problem interpretation. The strong "darkness" has been observed as q1 and q2, well as q4 (!). More significant changes are detected at q1 and q2. **Evaluation**: the q1 and q2 significant enlargement, increase of integral optical density It has been known, that granulocytes released the most of proinflammatory cytokines under any stressed conditions as fast reactant. The other logical step of our research has included the comparative analysis of cytokines level changes after both tests. This analysis has shown the striking results: after fluid shear stress the detected cytokines level was increased at many time in comparison to blood coagulation. Thus, results of present paper have shown the general genetic and epigenetic changes have took place, that is evidence once more the active genetic control of main kinds of granulocytes response to different stimuli at atherogenesis. This postulate is counterbalanced to present viewpoints about unable to induce gene expression by granulocytes.

PO013

New polymorphism in the first intron of the ABCA1 transporter gene

Sheydina A, Pchelina S, Demina E, Schwarzman A*

Petersburg Nuclear Physics Institute, RAS, Russia

Introduction. The ATP-binding cassette transporter ABCA1 mediates cellular cholesterol efflux. As it is known now there are binding sites for the nuclear receptors particularly for liver X receptor (LXR) in the promoter region and first intron of the ABCA1 gene. **Aims**. The purpose of our research was to search for new SNPs in the first intron of ABCA1 gene, associating with low level of high density lipoproteins (HDL). **Materials and methods**. Three pairs of primer flanking the sites of transcription factors were designed as well as detailed PCR protocols. The single strand conformational polymorphisms analysis (SSCP) of those fragments was conducted in patients with low level HDL and high level of triglycerides. All patients were men, survived after myocardial infarction (MI) at the age under 45 (30 subjects). All probes with the modified mobility were sequenced on ABI 373 using Thermo Sequenase II terminator cycle sequencing premix kit (Amersham Pharmacia). **Results**. The nucleotide substitution G18200A (NCBI, GeneBank, AF275948) was found in one of the fragments. This substitution was located in the first intron of the ABCA1 gene 29 bp downstream of the site of transcription factor LXR. Studies of functional consequences of this substitution are in progress. **Conclusions**. The described polymorphism of the ABCA1 gene might be associated with the modified expression of the gene and, thus, might play the role in predisposition to MI in young men.

PO014

Enhanced level of tissue-type plasminogen activator antigen in hypertensive small deep infarcts

Ionova V, Suslina Z, Maximova M, Tanashian M, Klimovich L*

Institute of Neurology of Russian Academy of Medical Sciences, Moscow, Russia

A few studies on fibrinolytic system investigated patients with established essential hypertension have been published. The aim of the study was to investigate the state of endogenous fibrinolytic system in patients with hypertensive small deep infarcts (SDI). **Materials and methods**: 80 patients with SDI in the carotid system due to hypertension were under study, mean age 60.9 ± 8.9 years. The hypertensive SDI group had SBP equal to 147-175 mm Hg and/or DBP equal to or below than 109 mm Hg. The diagnosis was verified by MRI. Laboratory investigations of tissue-type plasminogen activator (t-PA) antigen and plasminogen activator inhibitor 1 (PAI-1) antigen were made on the 1st day of the lacunar stroke at rest and in response to «cuff»-test. All data were compared with those of 20 healthy persons. For determination of t-PA and PAI-1 antigen, the reagent kits TintElize t-PA and TintElize PAI-1 were used. Fibrinolytic reserve of the vascular wall was assessed with the help of «cuff»-test. **Results**: Hypertensive SDI patients had a higher plasma concentration of t-PA antigen at rest than control subjects ($p<0.01$). There were no significant differences in PAI-1 antigen levels between the two groups. «Cuff»-test caused significant increases in the plasma t-PA antigen as well as of PAI-1 antigen in hypertensive SDI patients and in normotensive control subjects. The increase in t-PA antigen in response to «cuff»-test was significant greater in hypertensive SDI patients than in normotensive control subjects ($p<0.01$). Thus, hypertensive SDI is associated with activation of endogenous fibrinolysis as compensatory reaction.

PO015

Hyperhomocysteinemia is significant risk factor for cerebral arterial occlusive diseases in North West Russia

Shmeleva V, Kapustin S, Papayan L*

Cerebral arterial occlusive diseases (CAOD) and their complications are an important cause of mortality and morbidity in our population. Hyperhomocysteinemia (HHcy) is an established independent risk factor for arterial thrombosis and atherosclerosis. The aim of this study was to evaluate the significance of HHcy in the development of early onset CAOD in our selected patients. 78 unrelated patients (40 men and 38 women, mean age 40.5+-10.3), with documented early onset CAOD were involved in this study. Fasting plasma levels of total homocysteine (tHcy) were determined by HPLC. Mean level of tHcy in our patient group was significantly higher ($p<0,005$) than in age and sex matched controls ($n=40$): 14.7+-1,3 µmol/l vs. 10.7+-0.6 µmol/l. The prevalence of ↑tHcy was significantly higher ($p<0,005$) among patients with recurrent arterial thrombosis. Our study indicated that ↑tHcy is associated with high risk of cerebral occlusive disease in our patients and play important role in the recurrence of thrombosis. Genetic and environmental factors act in concert to cause HHcy. Among the genetic factors underlying ↑tHcy MTHFR C677T substitution is the most frequent in the general population. MTHFR genotyping was performed by PCR and restriction digest. We found mean plasma tHcy levels significantly higher in homozygotes for MTHFR C677T substitution than in heterozygotes and wild type. We also conclude MTHFR TT genotype to be strong genetic determinant of ↑tHcy in our region.

PO016

Oral methionine load induces von Willebrand factor changes in women with peripheral occlusive disease

Peutelli P (1), Amato S (1), Bottini F (1), Minniti G (2), Cerone R (2), Molinari A (1)*

(1) Thrombosis and Haemostasis Unit, Department of Hematology and Oncology, Giannina Gaslini Children
(2) Department of Pediatrics I, University of Genoa, Italy

Introduction. Hyperhomocysteinemia induces endothelial dysfunction and injury followed by platelet activation and thrombus formation. Von Willebrand factor (VWF) is a large multimeric plasma protein that mediates adhesion at the site of vascular damage. Under high shear stress conditions, VWF acts as a bridge between the injured endothelium and platelet membrane receptors. **Aim**. We investigated quantitative, functional and structural changes of VWF, induced by oral methionine load, in healthy women and women with venous or arterial occlusive disease. **Materials and methods**. We investigated 37 healthy women (median 34.5 years) and 42 patients (median 36.5 years). Total homocysteine (tHcy), VWF antigen (VWF:Ag), VWF ristocetin cofactor activity (VWF:RiCof), VWF multimer composition, and VWF proteolysis fragments were assayed before and after oral methionine load (100 mg/kg body weight). **Results**. Methionine load induced mild hyperhomocysteinemia in 7 healthy women (28.7 to 34.6 μ M/L) and 10 patients (28.4 to 37.8 μ M/L). No significant difference was found between fasting and post load levels of VWF:Ag and VWF:RiCof in patients and controls, and no difference was found between the two populations. Fasting and post load levels of the larger VWF multimers were lower than in controls (12.9% vs. 15.6%, and 10.4% vs. 13.2%, $p<0.05$). The relative proportion of the larger VWF multimers inversely correlated with tHcy increments and the age of the patients ($p<0.05$). Patients showed increased proteolysis fragments after load (19.8% to 23.2%, $p<0.05$), whereas control did not. **Conclusions**. Oral methionine load increased tHcy levels in healthy women and patients, inducing mild hyperhomocysteinemia in some of them. As a consequence, patients significantly decreased the size of VWF, depending on tHcy increment and age. The proteolysis of the molecule did not affect levels and function of VWF.

PO017

Analysis of 5 SNPs of the ABCA1 gene in patients with ischemic stroke

Taraskina A (1), Sheydina A (1), Sirotkina O (1), Elchaninov A (2), Pchelina S (1)*

(1) Petersburg Nuclear Physics Institute, RAS, Russia
(2) Sokolov Central Hospital, St.Petersburg, Russia

Introduction. As it is known now ischemic stroke is the arterial disease. It was shown that cassette transporter ABCA1 mediates cellular cholesterol efflux that may determine the degree of atherosclerotic progression. At present time several SNPs in the promoter and 5'-untranslated region of the ABCA1 gene associated with increase and decrease in coronary events were described. The R219K polymorphism in the coding region of the ABCA1 gene is considered as a protective factor for premature CHD. **Aims**. We suppose that SNPs in the ABCA1 gene might be associated with ischemic stroke. **Materials and methods**. 138 relatively young individuals (77 males and 61 females, mean age 42.2±0.4) with ischemic stroke and 286 healthy control subjects (183 males and 103 females, mean age 41.8±0.4) have been analyzed. In order to determine genetic risk factors in the development of ischemic stroke we analyzed distributions of the G(-191)C, C69T, C(-17)G, R219K and 319insG polymorphisms of the ABCA1 gene. **Results**. No association was found between all studied polymorphisms and ischemic stroke. The following allele frequencies were T69-0.37 and 0.43, C (-191) – 0.44 and 0.51, G(-17) -0.26 and 0.27, K219 0.27 and 0.29, G319 -0.17 and 0.13 in patients and control groups, respectively. **Conclusions**. Other mechanisms may play role in the pathogenesis of ischemic stroke.

PO018

ASO titer and efficacy of streptokinase in acute myocardial infarction patients

Ostovan M, Hooshmand S*

Introduction: recent streptococcal infection and antibodies against streptococcal products may affect the efficacy of streptokinase as a thrombolytic agent in acute myocardial infarction. **Aims**: the aim of this study was to evaluate the relationship between ASO titer prior to administeration of streptokinase and its efficacy in acute myocardial infarction. **Materials and Methods**: 100 patients with diagnosis of acute myocardial infarction who received thrombolysis with streptokinase were allocated into two groups ; 50 patients who responded to streptokinase ,defined as 50% reduction in sum of ST elevation after 90 min,and 50 patients who didnt respond .ASO titer was measured prior to injection of SK in all patients. **Results**: all patients with effective thrombolysis had ASO titers of less than 200,but only 28% of patients with ineffective thrombolysis had ASO titers of less than 200.($P < 0.001$) .side effects like skin rash and hypotension also were more frequently seen in patients with ASO titers higher than 200.(P value : 0.01 and 0.01 respectively). **Conclusion**: effectiveness of streptokinase as a method of thrombolysis is lower in patients with high ASO titers.

PO019

Lymphocyte platelet adhesion in acute coronary syndrome

Solpov A, Govorin A, Gorbunov V, Vitkovsky Y*

Chita Medical Academi, Chita, Russia

Background. Leukocyte platelet aggregation plays important role in acute coronary syndrome (ACS) pathogenesis. However, role of lymphocyte platelet adhesion in ACS development is unknown. **Methods**. Patients with acute myocardial infarction (AMI) (Q-wave and non-Q-wave) were examined. All patients were received traditional therapy. Investigation was performed on first and tenth days after acute attack. The lymphocyte-platelet adhesion and trombocyte aggregation were determined. ADP, collagen and adrenaline agonists were used as platelet aggregation agonists. **Results**. We established that LPA count on the first day was different. The numbers of LPA were ranged 5 - 29%. On tenth day in patients who had decrease LPA the parameters of platelet aggregation increased. In contrast, patients who had increase LPA the platelet aggregation decreased. In some patients parameters of LPA and platelet aggregation did not change. **Conclusion**. Thus, dynamics of lymphocyte-platelet adhesion and platelet aggregation parameters in acute coronary syndrome are opposite.

PO020

Different molecules of endothelial origin - master of cytokines network balance: new evidence of lymphocytes functioning at atherosclerosis

*Teplyakov A**

Researh Institute for Ecopathology and Occupational Diseases

We hypothesized also, that the intra- and inter-cell communications, which are realized the cytokines network balance, coordinated by endothelium. The cytokines network imbalance has been participated in atherosclerosis development and complications via "long term endothelial injuries healing in response to any proinflammatory signals". We have estimated, that the proinflammatory cytokines releasing have fast reacted to as blood coagulation well as fluid shear stress. Goal: to analyze the endothelial origin molecules involving in cytokines network and adhesive cascades, presented by sP-, sE-selectins, sICAM-1 and sVCAM-1 in our study, and to analyze the chromatin topography of lymphocytes nuclei and described molecules level changes at atherosclerosis (i.e. to define its interested to cytokines network balance in our understanding the last). Object: 29 patients, suffering from atherosclerosis. 10 volunteers comprise a control group. The chromatin of lymphocyte nuclei was studied using Computer TV Morphodensitometry System "DiaMorph" (Russia) in the smears dyed especially for DNA. Initial data has shown, that the ET-1 level was close related to lymphocytes epigenetic chromatin changes. We detected that q1 and q2 quotes were close positive correlated to ET-1 level ($r=0.76$ and 0.86, $p<0.05$) as shown on fig.1, accompanied by decrease of its optical and integral optical density. ET-1 level was close negatively correlated to q4 quota ($r=-0.96$, $p<0.05$) also. As result, we detected the correlations, indicated on significant increase of hetero/euchromatin ratio. We postulate, that cell-cell communications coordinate the balance between different molecules of endothelial origin without presence of endothelium even. We detected elevation of ET-1 after both tests, the source of it is unknown. Observed reaction was based on receptor-ligand linkage for selectins, realized under fluid conditions, and the sE-selectin binding resulted to prevent the ET-1 negative (proapoptotic or just calm) consequences. We postulate logically, that other cell-cell communication mechanisms are switched on (shedding or reinternalization). Thus, the endothelium is needed to show from a new position as Master of cytokines network balance.

PO021

Haemorheological alterations in patients with previous myocardial infarction and angiographically normal coronary arteries (MINC)

Mannini L, Paniccia R, Cecchi E, Giuello A, Bruschettini A, Margheri M, Giglioli C, Comeglio M, Abbate R, Gensini GF*

Department of Medical and Surgical Critical Care, Thrombosis Centre, University of Florence, Azienda

Epidemiological studies have established the role of traditional cardiovascular risk factors in cardiovascular disease and different pathophysiological mechanisms involved in the formation and the progression of the atherosclerotic plaque have been identified. Among these factors, some reports suggest a role for haemorheological and fibrinolytic alterations, in patients with MINC. Aim of this study was to evaluate haemorheological pattern and fibrinolytic potential in MINC patients. We studied 12 subjects [8 M, 4 F; median age 45 yrs (range 35-63)] admitted to the Coronary Intensive Therapy Unit of University of Florence with diagnosis of MINC and 12 control subjects [6 M, 6 F; median age 42 yrs (range 25-56)] matched for age, sex and traditional cardiovascular risk factors. Haemorheological study was performed before and after venous stasis (sphygmomanometer cuff maintained at a pressure intermediate between systolic and diastolic for 10 minutes). Blood tests performed were: erythrocytes filtration test on washed red blood cells (with erythrocyte filtrometer Myrenne MF4, France); whole blood viscosity test (WBV) and plasma viscosity test (PLV) studied with viscosimeter Contraves LS 30 (Germany); euglobulin lysis time (ELT) and t-PA and PAI-1 plasma levels (ELISA method, Biopool, USA). In baseline samples no differences were observed in the haemorheological profile of patients respect to controls [WBV (shear rate 0.512 cP): 23.59 (range 20.11-23.79) and 24.40 (range 21.40-25.71) respectively], but after venous stasis, a marked alteration of haemorheological profile was observed, in patients with MINC compared with control subjects [WBV (shear rate 0.512 cP): 33.21 (range 28-96-51.00) and 25.50 (range 20.93-28.16) respectively] was found. As fibrinolytic activity is concerned, PAI-1 plasma levels, but not ELT and t-PA levels, were significantly higher in baseline conditions in patients with respect to controls (8.3 vs 20 ng/mL, $p<0.01$). After venous stasis a comparable activation of fibrinolytic activity was observed both in patients and controls. These preliminary results indicate that haemorheological and haemostatic alterations are detectable in MINC independently of the absence of relevant atherosclerotic coronary lesions.

PO022

Long-term clinical outcomes of a platelet glycoprotein IIb/IIIa receptor blocker (Abciximab: ReoPro®) coated stent in coronary artery disease

Jeong M, Kim W, Kim J, Ahn YK, Cho JG, Park J, Kang J*

Chonnam National University Hospital, Gwangju, Korea

Background: Previously we reported the inhibition of coronary restenosis with Abciximab (ReoPro®)-coated stent in a porcine model. ReoPro® inhibits platelet aggregation, the proliferation of vascular smooth muscle cells and inflammatory reaction. **Methods**: We performed a prospective randomized trial to compare two types of stents for the revascularization in native coronary artery. The primary effective end points were major adverse coronary events (MACE): cardiac death, acute myocardial infarction, target vessel revascularization (TVR), restenosis at 6-month clinical and angiographic follow-up. **Results**: One hundred fifty-five patients were enrolled between Aug, 2001 and Jun, 2003. Mean ages (56.0±10.0 vs. 56.9±10.8 years), baseline diameter stenosis and minimal luminal diameter were not different between the two groups. There was one myocardial infarction and revascularization during hospital stay in control stent group. During clinical follow-up, there were two myocardial infarctions in control group. Follow-up coronary angiogram was done 62.3% (48/77) in coated and 65.4% (51/78) in control groups. Diameter stenosis and late loss were significantly less in the ReoPro®-coated stent group compared with controls (16.4±5.8% vs. 34.3±6.1%, p=0.009; and 0.33±0.28 mm vs. 0.88±0.41 mm; p=0.002). The restenosis and TVR rates of ReoPro®-coated stent were relatively lower compared with control stent [14.6%(7/48) vs. 29.4%(15/51), p=0.062; and 9.2%(7/76) vs. 14.7%(11/75); p=0.327]. **Conclusion**: A ReoPro®-coated stent is safe and may be effective in the prevention of coronary restenosis. Final result will be presented at the meeting.

PO023

Protein C as diagnostic marker in early diagnosis severe intra-abdominal infections

Vukosavljević D, Vodnik T, Majkić-Singh N, Karamarković A*

Institute of Medical Biochemistry, Clinical Center of Serbia, Belgrade, Serbia and Montenegro

Center for Emergency Surgery, Clinical Center of Serbia, Belgrade, Serbia and Montenegro

Systemic response to infection is sepsis. The term sepsis in the abdominal surgery designates presence of the septic abdomen as the major trigger of a range of pathophysiological events. Sepsis is frequently associated with disturbances within the blood coagulation and fibrinolitic system. Protein C has a very important role in control of microvascular coagulation and inflammation and it is highly important in pathophysiology of sepsis. It is one of the basic regulatory system of homeostasis expressing potent antocoagulant and antiinflammatory properties. The aim of the study was to analyse hemostasis disturbances during the severe intra-abdominal infections (IAI) with sepsis syndrome. Protein C is determined by commercial tests Dade Behring on analyzer BCT- Behring Coagulation Timer, using spectrophotometric method with chromogenic substrate. The study group consisted 20 patients with severe IAI (mostly diffuse peritonitis) and control group 20 surgically treated (hernia repair) patients without of infection signs. The blood samples for determination protein C were obtained preoperatively, as well as on the postoperative days. In control group, protein C activity is permanently maintained within the normal range. Average preoperative protein C values among survived and deceased patients treated for IAI with sepsis syndrome were significantly different ($p<0,037$). Postoperative activity was changed and characterized by decreased values in the whole study group. Difference in average protein C value between the study and control groups was statistically significant over the whole studied period ($p<0,001$). We may be concluded that protein C represents an important biological marker in early diagnosis of coagulation disorders and inflammatory cascade in sepsis.

PO024

Is factor VII deficiency predisposing to foetal loss? (Study of a large family)

Lo Pinto G, Perroni L, Cusano R, Barbaresi M, Costa M, Malatesti V*

Ospedali Gallie, Thrombosis Center, Genetic Laboratory, In vitro fertilization unit (Genetic Department), General Analysis Laboratory

Introduction: factor VII is a vitamin-K dependent glycoprotein. It circulates in plasma in two forms: the majority as a single-chain inactive zymogen and a much smaller amount as the active two-chain form. Factor VII gene maps to the long arm of chromosome 13 at 13q34. Inherited factor VII deficiency has an estimated prevalence of between 1:300 000 and 1:500 000. The transmission is autosomal recessive. For unclear reasons, there is a relatively poor correlation between factor VII levels and the risk of bleeding. **Clinical case**: a woman aged 35 was studied because three early abortions occurred between the 6th and 8th week of pregnancy. In her family factor VII deficiency was reported; this defect was investigated in her father, in her mother, in two of her three sisters and in one of her two brothers. All of them are affected. The thrombophylic screening was normal, and the deficiency of Factor VII (15% - N.V. 70-120%) was confirmed. As the family history was suggestive for a genetic cause of the defect, also mutation analysis was performed. For mutation detection of coagulation factor VII, DNA of the subjects examined was obtained by phenol-clorophorm extraction; the exons and the intron-exon junctions of the gene were amplified and then sequenced on a 3100 Avant sequencer (Applied Biosystem). The propositus resulted compound heterozygous for the mutations 9729delgggt and E265K. Her mother is heterozygous 9729delgggt and her father heterozygous E265K. Two sisters, both mothers of two children, were examined for the two mutations; one of them is heterozygous for the deletion, the other is compound heterozygous. The other family members are to be examined. **Discussion**: it is already known that the fibrin clot formation is an important phase for blastocistys implantation in the endometrium. We think that, in this woman, factor VII deficiency may have contribute to hamper this process causing recurrent foetal loss. Other sister, with two children, is compound heterozygous as our patient; it means that other factors play a role in early poliabortivity.

PO025

The relationship between ABO blood subgroups, von Willebrand factor, factor VIII and ristocetin cofactor

Sousa N (1), Anicchino-Bizzacchi JM (1), Siqueira L (1), Leite E (2), Locatelli M (1), Barjas-Castro ML (1)*

(1) Hemocentro Unicamp - State University of Campinas - UNICAMP - Campinas - Brazil
(2) Faculdade de Ciências Farmacêuticas - UNESP - Araraquara - Brazil

Introduction: Von Willebrand factor (VWF) plays a key role in primary hemostasis. Various factors influence the FVW plasma level and ABO blood groups are considered the most important factor. Recent studies have demonstrated that individuals carrying one O allele have significantly lower plasma levels of VWF and FVIII than to those carrying no O allele. **Aims**: The objective of this study was to correlate the ABO gene polymorphisms with plasma levels of VWF, FVIII and ristocetin cofator. Material and methods: Blood donors of different blood groups defined by sorological and molecular tests were submitted to VWF:Ag (ELISA) and FVIII (coagulometric method) dosage and tested for ristocetin cofactor(RiCof). The blood groups genotyping were: 10(AA), 10(BB), 10(AB), 10(AO1), 10(BO1), 14(O1O1), 10(O1O1V), 20(A2O), 20(A2B), 4(A3O), 2(AXO), 1(B3O) and 1(BmO). The subgroups A3O, AXO, B3O and BmO were analysed as only one group. **Results**: Group O individuals and those carrying this allele demonstrated significantly lower levels of VWF:Ag, FVIII and RiCof than individuals of groups AA, AB and BB. When subgroup A2O was studied these factors presented lower levels (Median (Md):FVW=89%; FVIII=96%; RiCof=99%) than AA, AB and BB(Md:FVW=120%-p<0.001; FVIII=117%-p<0.001, RiCof=119%-p<0.001) and A2B(Md:FVW=169%-p<0.001; FVIII=112%-p<0.001; RiCof=132%-p=0.001) and higher levels than O1O1(Md:FVW=69%-p=0.018; FVIII=75%-p=0.048; RiCof= 65%-p<0.001). The same factors analysed in A3O1, AX01 and B3O1/BmO1 donors (Md:FVW=75%; FVIII:C=88%; RiCof=76%) were significantly lower compared with those in the groups AA, AB and BB(Md:FVW=120%-p<0.001; FVIII=117%-p=0.041; RiCof=119%-p<0.001) and A2B(Md:FVW=169%-p<0.001; FVIII=112%-p=0.001; RiCof=132%-p<0.001). However, no statistically significant differences were observed when this subgroup was compared with O1O1, AO1 and A2O1. **Conclusions**: We demonstrated a high correlation between the plasma levels of VWF and FVIII (R=0.77; p<0.001) and between VWF and RiCof (R=0.75; p<0.001). The results of this study clearly demonstrated the influence of ABO subgroups (H antigen) on the WVF:Ag plasma level and consequently on the FVIII plasmatic level and functional activity of FVW:Ag (ristocetin cofactor).

PO026

A proteomic approach for the resolution of vitamin K dependent proteins

Uras F (1), Salman Dilgimen A (1), Uras A (2)*

(1) University of Marmara, Faculty of Pharmacy, Department of Biochemistry Istanbul, Turkey
(2) Biochemistry Laboratory of Vakif Gureba Training Hospital, Istanbul, Turkey

Introduction: Different strategies have been developed for the isolation of each one of the vitamin K dependent plasma proteins (Gla-proteins). Based on time consuming chromatographic methods, not appropriate for clinical studies, highly purified proteins were isolated from high volume human plasma. Prothrombin, factor VII, factor IX, factor X, protein C, protein S, protein Z and osteocalcin are well-known plasma proteins. But some Gla-proteins have not been well characterized and their physiological function is not clear. **Aim:** It would be useful in clinical practice and research to perform a one step procedure for simultaneous isolation/quantification of Gla-proteins from the plasma of low volume. The purpose of this study is to resolve the human Gla-proteins by two-dimensional gel electrophoresis (2-D). **Materials and methods:** In this study Gla-proteins were isolated from normal human plasma by barium citrate adsorption and ammonium sulfate elution. Then the protein mixture, prothrombin complex, was subjected to 2-D with silver staining. **Results:** The protein pattern was obtained by 2-D which was carried out with an immobilized pH gradient in the first dimension and by sodium dodecyl sulfate-polyacrylamide gel electrophoresis in the second dimension. Over 20 major and minor protein spots were visualized by silver staining. **Conclusion:** When we compare the number of well known plasma Gla proteins with the number of the protein spots, we concluded that some of the protein spots might be artifacts of the Gla proteins but some of them might be due to unknown Gla-proteins. Further studies utilizing mass spectrophotometric evaluation of the 2-D pattern are required to prove the presence of new proteins. Quantitative analysis of the protein pattern by computer-assisted densitometry may be helpful in clinical studies for simultaneous quantification of Gla-proteins.

PO027

Factor XIII Val34Leu polymorphism as a modulator of resistance to fibrinolysis in subjects treated with aspirin

Undas A, Brożek J, Iwaniec T, Szczeklik A*

Department of Medicine, Jagiellonian University School of Medicine, Cracow, Poland

Introduction Factor (F)XIII Leu34 allele has been found in some studies to protect against myocardial infarction. Paradoxically, in vitro studies demonstrated that Leu34 is associated with faster FXIII activation and formation of tighter fibrin clots that might implicate less sensitivity of fibrin to plasmin. We have reported (Circulation 2003) that aspirin slows down the rate of FXIII activation in the Leu34 carriers to a greater extent than in the Leu34 non-carriers. This effect is likely attributable to modification of FXIII activation by acetylated fibrin. **Aims** To test the hypothesis that the Leu34 allele affects lysis of clots and aspirin enhances this modulation, we performed turbidimetry of plasma clots prior to and after aspirin ingestion in 3 healthy subjects homozygous for the FXIII Leu34 allele versus 3 subjects homozygous for FXIII Val34 allele. **Materials and methods** Tissue-type plasminogen activator (Hematologic Technologies) 1 μg/ml was added to 100 μl of plasma with human thrombin 1U/ml (Sigma) and calcium chloride 10 mmol/l (final). Absorbancy was read at 405 nm in a microplate reader (Dynex) for 15 minutes. **Results** Both genotype groups did not differ in regard to fibrinogen levels (range, 2-3 g/l). Turbidimetry revealed no differences in fibrinolysis rate depending on the presence or absence of the Leu34 allele before aspirin. In contrast, aspirin resulted in a significantly shorter fibrinolysis time, defined as the time in which absorbancy decreases by 50% comparing with the maximum value, in the Leu34-positive and –negative group (by 2.9 vs 1.4 minutes, respectively); the fastest lysis rate was observed in the Leu34Leu subjects on aspirin (mean, 6.6 minutes). **Conclusions** Our results suggest that in FXIII Leu34 carriers treated with aspirin, plasma clots are significantly less resistant to lysis than the Val34 homozygotes. It might be speculated that effectiveness of fibrinolysis in patients receiving aspirin depends in part from the FXIII Val34Leu polymorphism.

PO028

Factor VII activity and blood coagulation at the site of microvascular injury

Brzezinska B, Undas A, Padjas A, Iwaniec T, Musiał J*

Department of Medicine, Jagiellonian University School of Medicine, Cracow, Poland

Introduction: Duration of the initiation phase in thrombin generation depends on factor VII activity and tissue factor (TF) activity with a little effect on the propagation phase. The impact of factor VII activity on thrombin generation in vivo, when blood coagulation is triggered by vascular injury, has not been fully elucidated. **Aims**: The aim of our study was to evaluate the effects of factor VII activity on thrombin generation in a model of blood coagulation upon vascular injury. **Material and methods**: We assessed thrombin-antithrombin (TAT) complexes by ELISA (BCT- Berhing Coagulation Timer; Dade Behring) in blood samples taken every 30 seconds at the site of microvascular injury as described previously (Undas et al. Blood 2001) in patients receiving long-term treatment with coumadin (acenocoumarol). Factor II activity was measured by chromogenic method assay (BCT-Berhing Coagulation Timer; Dade Behring). We enrolled patients on anticoagulation (INR 2.0-3.0) for a mean of 15 months: 36 patients (mean age, 50 yrs), with a history of deep venous thrombosis (DVT) and 20 patients (mean age 60 yrs) with atrial fibrillation (AF). The control group included 29 sex- and age-matched healthy subjects.

Results: Factor VII activity is not associated with duration of the initiation phase in healthy subjects and patients on anticoagulation when thrombin formation is assessed at the site of microvascular injury. The propagation phase has not been affected by factor VII activity. It has been found that the initiation phase of thrombin generation is significantly longer (by 30 -60 seconds) in patients with AF than those with DVT, but then the rate of increase of TAT levels in the propagation phase measured in both patient groups is higher in case of AF as compared to DVT. **Conclusions**: Our results suggest that the initiation phase of thrombin generation induced by sudden TF expression upon vascular injury is not related to factor VII activity, which is in contrast to in vitro data. Individuals treated with acenocumarol form the heterogeneous groups in respect to the influence of factor VII on thrombin generation. It seems that in subjects with multiple thrombosis risk factors the effect of factor VII on thrombin formation may be blunted.

PO029

Role of fibrin in thrombin behavior

de Bosch N

Centro Nacional de Hemofila. Banco Metropolitano de Sangre

Thrombin binds to fibrin in two different sites distinct from thrombin catalytic site. One is a low-affinity site in the fibrin E domain. A high-affinity binding site is in the γ'414-427 of a hetero-dimeric Fibrinogen (Fbg) molecule containing one γ'/γA chain that can be separated by ion exchange chromatography (Fbg2) from the homodimeric γA/γA fibrinogen molecule (Fbg1). In afibrinogenemic patients factor 2 fragment I+II and TAT complex are increased. In our patients thrombin generation (TG) of 200 uL of PPP triggered by 50 uL of cephaline reagent in 200uL of 25mM Ca Cl_2, measured by chromogenic substrate, the rate and maximum level of thrombin generation were greater than in normal plasma. When Fbg1 was added to these plasmas the TG had a modest reduction, but the TG effect was marked when Fbg2 was added (60% reduction). Same down-regulating effect was observed in reptilase depleted normal plasma. Fbg1 and 2 concentrations were the same and ranged from 1.1 to 1.9 mg/ml in different experiments. We could demonstrate that the clot from each of these Fbgs had the same improvement of the lag time for thrombin burst in the afibrinogenemic PRP TG. When γ' peptide 408-427 was added to afibrinogenemic plasma or Fbg depleted normal plasma the burst of thrombin was 1 to 2 min delayed in the onset of thrombin generated, that was similar to the amount obtained without the peptide. In the same generation mixtures we determined TAT every minute over 6 minutes. TAT was lower in the generation mixture that contained the peptide. This last finding suggests that thrombin in the presence of the γ' high-affinity binding sequence becomes less sensitive to ATIII inactivation.

PO030

Factor XIII level and prevalence of FXIII-A Val34Leu polymorphism in patients with peripheral arterial disease and Raynaud's disease

Shemirani A (1), Csiki Z (2), Szomják E (2), Katona É (1), Bereczky Z (1), Muszbek L (1)*

(1) University of Debrecen, Medical and Health Science Center, Department of Clinical Biochemistry and Molecular Pathology, Debrecen, Hungary
(2) University of Debrecen, Medical and Health Science Center, 3rd Department of Medicine, Debrecen, Hungary

Introduction: Factor XIII (FXIII) is a tetrameric zymogen (A2B2) that is activated in the final stage of blood coagulation by the concerted action of thrombin and Ca2+. Its active form, FXIIIa cross-links fibrin chains and α2-plasmin inhibitor to fibrin and by this way protects newly formed fibrin from the prompt elimination by the fibrinolytic system. Excessive fibrin cross-linking by FXIII has been implicated in the development of atherosclerosis and thrombosis. A polymorphism of FXIII A subunit (FXIII-A) has been reported to provide protection against arterial thrombotic diseases. **Aims**: Determination of plasma FXIII activity and antigen levels and the prevalence of FXIII-A V34L polymorphism in patients with peripheral obstructive arterial disease and Raynaud's disease and their relationship with known risk factors of atherosclerosis. Materials and methods: The determination of plasma FXIII activity and complex FXIII A2B2 antigen was carried out with REA-chrom spectrophotometric activity assay (REANAL-Labexpert) and with commercial sandwich ELISA (R-ELIA FXIII, REANAL-Labexpert). A real-time PCR assay using fluorescence energy transfer detection and melting point analysis was developed for the determination of V34L genotypes. **Results**: FXIII activity and plasma FXIII concentration were significantly elevated in patients with peripheral arterial disease (114±22% versus 100±19% and 24.6±5.4 mg/L versus 21.4±3.4 mg/L, respectively). FXIII levels were also elevated in Raynaud's disease (114±19% and 24.3±4.8 mg/L). The specific activity of FXIII was unchanged in the disease groups. The prevalence of L34 allele in the patients' groups did not deviate significantly from that observed in the control group and the specific FXIII activity remained the same in the three groups of different V34L genotypes. A slight, but significant correlation of FXIII levels with fibrinogen and LDL cholesterol levels was observed. **Conclusions**: FXIII activity and antigen levels are elevated in peripheral vascular disease that might be due to the increased destruction of platelets. FXIII-A V34L polymorphism does not provide protection against these diseases.

PO031

Factor XIII subunit B: a protein A-binding protein

Kerényi A, Haramura G, Muszbek L*

University of Debrecen, Medical and Health Science Center, Department of Clinical Biochemistry and Molecular Pathology, Debrecen, Hungary

Introduction: Blood coagulation factor XIII (FXIII) is a tetrameric protein that consists of two potentially active A (FXIII-A) and two protective (carrier) B subunits (FXIII-B). FXIII-A is predominantly synthesized by cells of bone marrow origin and FXIII-B is synthesized by hepatocytes. The complex between the two types of subunits is formed in the plasma and FXIII-B prevents FXIII-A from the slow spontaneous activation that would otherwise occur in plasmatic conditions. In the plasma FXIII-B is present in excess and half of FXIII-B circulates as free protein. It has been proposed that FXIII-B in addition to its function in the clotting system might be involved in protective inflammatory processes. Protein A is a Staphylococcal protein is that characteristically binds to the Fc portion of IgG between the CH2 and CH3 domains. The protein is involved in defending the microorganism against the destructive potential of the Fc region of IgG. **Aims**: We attempted to study the interaction of staphylococcal protein A with the plasma FXIII complex and its individual subunits. Materials and Methods: Micro-plates coated with highly purified human FXIII-B were used for studying the binding to protein A and to antibodies against different human and animal immunglobulins. **Results**: A tight binding of protein A labeled with biotin or peroxidase to FXIII-B was demonstrated. The extent of protein A binding to FXIII-B was comparable to the binding to human IgG. Protein A also bound to FXIII-B when FXIII-B was part of the plasma FXIII complex, although to a lesser extent. No binding to FXIII-A could be observed. Anti-human IgG antibody produced in goat or rabbit also bound to FXIII-B and FXIII A2B2 complex, but not to FXIII-A. Anti-mouse IgG produced in rabbit or goat gave hardly any reaction with human FXIII-B and non-immune IgG did not show any binding. Reaction with anti-human IgM and with antibodies against isolated kappa and lambda chains was significantly less than the reaction with anti human IgG and there was no reaction with anti-human IgA and IgE. **Conclusions**: Protein A and anti-human IgG react with FXIII-B, perhaps to an epitope that is similar to an epitope on human IgG. The reaction of FXIII-B with protein A might interfere with the protective mechanism of Staphylococcus aureus and thus, FXIII-B might participate in the non-specific anti-microbial defense mechanism.

PO032

Effect of short wave frequency electromagnetic radiation on lymphocyte-platelet adhesion and tissue factor expression by leukocytes

Nardina I, Vitkovsky Y*

Chita Medical Academy, Chita, Russia

Recently a new method of short wave frequency electromagnetic radiation for treatment of different diseases associated with immune and haemostatic disorders has been successful. Our aim was to study influence of short wave frequency electromagnetic radiation on lymphocyte-platelet adhesion and tissue factor expression by leukocytes of peripheral blood in vitro. Healthy donors' and patients' blood was irradiated by apparatus "Amfit-0,2/10-01" in waveband 53,57-78,33 GHz. It was established that healthy donors had 13 – 15% lymphocyte-platelet aggregates and electromagnetic radiation did not change it. In patients who had low contents (5-6%) the lymphocyte-platelet aggregates increased 2-3-fold after irradiation. In patients with infection processes who had high level of that parameter (30-35%) the electromagnetic radiation promoted a decrease in lymphocyte-platelet aggregation. Electromagnetic radiation led a reduction of tissue factor expression, a main trigger of hypercoagulability, by leukocytes of peripheral blood. Thus, short wave frequency electromagnetic radiation can be a perspective method for treatment and rehabilitation of patients with disorders of immunity and haemostasis.

PO033

FVIII levels during attacks of familial Mediterranean fever

Akar N, Ekim M, Gürman C*

Departments of Pediatric Molecular Genetics and Nephrology of Ankara University, Ankara, Turkey

Introduction: Familial Mediterranean Fever primarily affects populations surrounding the Mediterranean basin. During the attacks of the disease, increasing levels of fibrinogen, erytrocyte sedimentation rate and high white blood cell count are used routinely for the diagnosis of FMF. Factor VIII is a well-known acute phase reactant and is increased during infection. Increasing levels of FVIII during the attacks and decreasing during the resolution of the attacks in FMF patients were reported. **Aim**: From this point, we hypothesized that increase and decrease of FVIII levels during the attacks of FMF may be another criteria for the diagnosis of FMF. Materials and methods: The patient group included 27 unrelated FMF Turkish patients who were compliant to colchicine therapy. Only patients with two mutations at MEFV gene were included. Mutation analysis was performed by DNA sequencing (Beckman Coulter, USA). FVIII levels were measured by one-stage clotting assay with FVIII-deficient plasma. **Results**: FVIII levels during the attacks were found to be 195.08 + 86.5 IU/dl. Of the 27 FMF patients, 20 had elevated levels of FVIII. Fibrinogen levels during the attacks were found to be 544.1 + 126.0. All of the 27 FMF patients had elevated levels of fibrinogen. There was a significant correlation with fibrinogen levels at the 0.01 level. Six patients were evaluated after the resolution of the acute attack. FVIII levels were 213.0 + 31.3 and 130.0 + 35.0 at the onset and following the attack respectively (p= 0.028). It was 603.5 + 174.9 and 529.0 + 94.9 for fibrinogen. The difference was not significant (0.17). **Conclusions**: Our data indicated that FVIII levels could be a good indicator during the attacks of FMF in some patients but cannot be used as a diagnostic criterion. However, it decreases prior to fibrinogen indicating that FVIII also cannot be used as a marker for the resolution of acute phase.

PO034

Successful use of recombinant activated factor VII (rFVIIa) in a patient with severe bleeding during transabdominal retropubic prostatectomy

Monteiro C, Jorreto M, Gonçalves L, Fraga M, Pereira R*

Center of Thrombosis, Haemostasis and Vascular Biology, Department of Transfusion Medicine, S. Jo&at

Introduction: Transabdominal retropubic prostatectomy is a common surgical procedure for patients with prostatic cancer or prostatic hypertrophy. Despite the improvements of surgical techniques, transabdominal retropubic prostatectomy is still frequently associated with severe bleeding, which may require blood transfusion. This is mainly due to the complicated anatomical localization of the prostate, in a densely vascularized area with increased fibrinolysis, which may compromise surgical haemostasis. Several studies indicate that systemic administration of recombinant activated factor VII (rFVIIa) induces short-term local haemotasis, even in patients without previous coagulopathy. rFVIIa has been considered as a universal agent, prompting its use in the management of severe uncontrolled surgical bleedings. **Aims**: We describe the case of a patient with uncontrolled surgical bleeding during a transabdominal prostatectomy, in whom rFVIIa has been successfully used. **Case Report**: Male, 66 years old, without previous bleeding disorder, submitted to a transabdominal retropubic prostatectomy. During the surgery, the patient had severe blood loss, with hypovolemic shock and severe coagulopathy. The patient was transfused with 11 units of red blood cells (RBCs), 8 units of fresh frozen plasma (FFP), 7 units of platelets concentrates (Plts) and 1 g of fibrinogen. He was transferred to the Intensive Care Unit, but the blood loss from the suprapubic tube was still significant (1200 ml). He returned to the operating room for revision of haemostasis, and was transfused with 4 units of FFP, 6 units of RBCs and 1 g of fibrinogen. The blood loss was detected in the haemorrhoidal plexus; due to the difficulty of establishing local haemostasis, a single bolus of rFVIIa, 90 µg/Kg, was given. After this administration, bleeding decreased immediately, and he only received more 3 units of FFP and 3 units of RBCs. He recovered completely. **Conclusion**: In this case, the administration of a single dose of rFVIIa proved to be safe and effective, in the management of uncontrolled surgical bleeding, decreasing the need for other blood components. In the PROSE study, it was demonstrated the reduction in perioperative blood loss and transfusion requirements in patients undergoing transabdominal prostatectomy, by the prophylactic use of a single dose of rFVIIa. In surgeries where significant blood losses are expected, should this haemostatic agent be used prophylatically?

PO035

Tensile strength of blood clot

*Savushkin A V**

Chita State Medical Academy, Chita, Russia

The aim of blood coagulation is to prevent the circulation system from the liquid loss. The clot is a hydraulic plug and its function is to opposite blood pressure. So hemostatic clot must be strong enough not to be destroyed under a pressure. Thrombi are also the result of coagulation process. Most of arterial and vein thrombi are nonocclusive during "silent" phase of diseases, which may be rather long. From mechanical viewpoint hydraulic action to such thrombi from liquid blood may be quite different than to a hemostatic clot. There are not only pressure forces but a significant tensile either. If the tensile force would increase to a critical level, thrombus destroys and thromboembolism develops. We studied the tensile strength of blood clot in our experiments. The blood samples were obtained from 47 volunteers and stabilized with sodium citrate. Cylindrical clot (diameter 6 mm, length 30 mm) was formed within the cell of special thermostat tensile equipment. The clot was stretched at 11 mm/min in 5 minutes after coagulation performed. The clot became longer and thinner during stretching. Then the sample was destroyed. The clot length equalled 67$\pm$4 mm and diameter 3.2$\pm$0.4 mm just before the gap. Destroying tensile force was 57.6$\pm$17.8 mN and critical stress equalled 2.0$\pm$0.6 mN/m ^{2}. Thus, we obtained some biomechanical characteristics of blood clots in stretching gap.

PO036

Blood clot: hydraulic resistance and its changing

*Savushkin A V**

Chita State Medical Academy, Chita, Russia

The problems of transport of matter, energy, and information are very important within complex organisms. The hydraulic way is widely spread and perfect. Moving of fluid inside vessel circuit is energetically profitable and has a great deal of "in" and "out" transport points. However, there is a significant danger of the lost of the transport matter - blood - and the death as a result of it, if the vessel would be damaged. The coagulation blood system had been formed during evolution to opposite it. Haemostatic blood clot plays a role of hydraulic plug and stops hemorrhage. It is obviously from this point of view that the hydraulic resistance is one of the main clot characteristics. Therefore we tried to examine it. Blood clots (diameter 11 mm and length 30 mm) formed within glass cylinder thermostated tube, which modeled a part of vessel. Thirty volunteers` blood samples were stabilized with sodium citrate and coagulated with calcium chloride within the tube. The leaking of isotonic sodium chloride solution started after coagulation had performed. The surplus pressure was not stable and increased with velocity 98 N/ m^2 min during thirty minutes. Volumes of leaked liquid were measured. Hydraulic resistance was calculated as R=P/Q (R - resistance, P - surplus pressure, Q - volume speed of liquid). The average minimal resistance equalled 307 $\pm$ 48 (nN sec/m ^{5}) and it was registered at the beginning of the measurement (pressure 98 N/m ^{2}). Then it reached maximal meaning (2943$\pm$196 nN sec/m ^{5}) under 1766 n/m^2 and after that decreased by mean 973$\pm$360 (nN sec/m ^{5}) at 3532 N/m ^{2}. It was surprising, but minute volumes leaked through clots did not increased in proportion to a hydraulic pressure augmentation as it could be prognosticated. Such a result was observed in every experiment. Minute volume speed did not increase in 50$\pm$4% and decreased in 16$\pm$2% of summarized results during the experiment. We suppose that fibrin net, as a strength base of clot, was not stable under the pressure and was modified by it. So, the hydraulic resistance of normal blood clots meaning was obtained and nonlinear relationship between pressure and volume rate of solution leaking through the clot was registered.

PO037

Erythrocyte desert out the blood clot phenomenon (filtration "back to front")

*Savushkin A V**

Chita State Medical Academy, Chita, Russia

The main result of coagulation is to transverse the liquid blood to another aggregate state - haemostatic clot or thrombus. There are some differences between them but clots and thrombi have common essence: the base of them is spatial fibrin net with blood cells within the loops. Near 50% of clot volume is erythrocytes capacity. The base characteristics of a clot and a thrombus are hydraulic resistance and hydraulic strength because a fibrin net must be able to opposite blood pressure without destruction to prevent hemorrhage. Fibrin gel is known to be able to leak a solution through itself and it is possible that erythrocytes of clot could be washed outside with oozing liquid too. RBC can vary form and dimension. They are able to change disc-like form to rod-like one and their dimension could be decreased from 5-7 mcm to 2-4 mcm while streaming inside a capillaries. Moreover, leaking of RBC through filters with a different pore size is a laboratory test to diagnose cell membrane state. The erythrocyte desertion of blood clot was studied. The blood samples were obtained from twenty volunteers. Then blood was located within special equipment, in cylinder vessel modeling the part of blood circuit and clotting performed there. The clot length was 30 and the diameter was near 7 mm. After coagulation had finished the clot was affected by constantly (98 N/m^2 min) increasing hydraulic pressure for 45 minutes. The volumes of isotonic sodium chloride solution leaked through the gel were measured in minute interval. They contained erythrocytes deserted the fibrin net. The clot volume decreased under the pressure in the experiments. Capacity of percolated solution, the clot volume and RBC number into oozed liquid were registered. The leaked capacity equalled 53.6 $\pm$ 36.3 ml that is 100-fold more than start clot volume. The final clot bulk was only 32$\pm$9% against the start one. 37.3$\pm$19.5 % of RBC deserted the gel with leaking solution, but the final erythrocyte concentration in the clot was 97$\pm$2% of the start one because of clot compression. So, we stated that about 40% of erythrocytes are able to desert out of the clot by leaking solution and the concentration of RBC into the deformed compressed clot can be the same as in undeformed one.

PO038

Warfarin is superior to Acenocoumarol in the management of patients requiring low doses of oral anticoagulants

Ceresetto JM, Rabinovich O, Stemmelin G, Shanley C, Duboscq C, Gutierrez M, Mendizabal G, Doti C, Vicente M, Bullorsky E*

Hospital Britanico de Buenos Aires, Argentina

Introduction: The main difference between Warfarin (W) and Acenocoumarol (AC) is their half-life of 36 and 9 hours respectively. Warfarin's longer half-life theoretically provides a more stable anticoagulation and avoids F VII fluctuations. Because of FII longer half-life AC is presumed to be as effective as W. **Objective**: We prospectively evaluated the coagulation parameters on the day following a scheduled withhold of vitamin K antagonists (VKA) in patients with chronic anticoagulation with low doses of either AC or W, who has been stable for at least the last 2 months. **Patients and methods**: All patients were tested for Prothrombin time, INR and Factors II, VII and X levels the day after a withhold of a dose, as planned in the regular schedule. We performed 143 assays in 67 patients to be considered for this study. This represent 11% of the whole anticoagulated patients in our anticoagulation clinic. Fifty-four assays were performed in patients receiving W and 89 AC. Most of the patients (n=49) were anticoagulated for atrial fibrillation, only one patient with AC and 9 with W were treated for mechanical heart valves (target INR 2.5-3.5). **Results**: 28% of the INR assays in patients receiving W and 55% in the AC group were unsatisfactory considering their targeted INR. Moreover only 29% of patients with AC and 59% with W had an adequate F II assay (less than 40%). There were no episodes of symptomatic embolism during the study.

	Acenocumarol	Warfarin	
Prothrombin Time	37%(± 13.8%, 1SD)	24%(±11.9%, 1SD)	p < 0.001
INR	1.95 (± 0.45%)	2.68 (± 0.88%)	p < 0.001
F. II	52% (± 18.7%)	38% (± 16.6%)	p < 0.001
F. VII	57% (± 20.3%)	37% (± 17.3%)	p < 0.001
F. X	33% (± 17.0%)	20% (± 10.5%)	p <0.001

Conclusions: 1) Patients under chronic VKA treatment that required low doses of anticoagulation were significantly better anticoagulated with W than with AC. 2) INR and F II dosages with AC were unsatisfactory in 55% and 71% of assays 3) Although we found no episodes of thromboembolism, patients requiring low doses of AC should probably be switched to Warfarin.

PO039

Validation of CoaguChek S on samples of patients on stable oral anticoagulation

*Laszlo P**

Department of Haemostaseology, University of Debrecen, Hungary

Introduction: Some years ago, portable equipment for prothrombin time determination (CoaguChek S, Hofmann La Roche, Indianapolis) has been developed for self-management of oral anticoagulation. The instrument estimates the PT and INR from capillary sample of whole blood. Before wide range spread of self-management of cumarin treatment in our country, we had possibility to validate the above mentioned equipment on samples of patients on stable oral anticoagulation. **Materials and Methods**: The reference values were determinated by a photo-optical coagulometer (Electra 900C, MLA) using a human recombinant thromboplastin (Innovin, Dade Behring, ISI=0.95). **Results**: Capillary and citrated samples of 34 patients on stable oral anticoagulant therapy were investigated parallel. 2 patients were excluded, because they showed extremely high deviation (>30%) from the reference values. In these cases the determination was repeated at latter. Due to paired t-test, the mean of differences was statistically significant (0.13; p= 0.0009), but not clinically important. The orthogonal regression line showed good correlation between the two methods, the slope, intercept and r square were 1.18; -0.26 and 0.95 respectively. **Conclusions**: Due to our experience, the CoaguChek S reliable, but give a little bit elevated INR result, what might be the consequence of the higher ISI of the applied thromboplastin in the test strip. However, the cases of excluded patients suggest the need of previous laboratory control between CoaguChek S and a coagulometer at each new patient. Lupus anticoagulant was not confirmed at the excluded patients.

PO040

Dental surgery in patients treated with oral anticoagulants

Dimova C (1), Kostovska S (2), Dejanova V (2), Kovacevska I (1), Andonovska B (1)*

(1) Clinic of oral surgery, Faculti of Dentistry, University St.Cyril and Methody, Skopje R. Macedonia

(2) Faculty of Medicine, University St.Cyril and Methody, Skopje, R. Macedonia

Introduction: Contraversial attitudes and studies mere found in the liteature concerning the oral anticoagulation therapy – OAT (reduction, complite cut or maintenance of the same therapy level) associated with the extraction therapeutic measure. The aforementioned provoked this research in the field of the oral surgical praxis. **Aim**: The aim of this work was defining a protocol for those patiens, as well as lowering the incidense of post extraction extended bleeding, and reducing the risk fir developing thromboembolism. **Material and methods**: Subjects for this research were 20 randomly slected patiens, who are under continueted OAT. Patiens of both genders with average age of 55± 8 years. All the relevant data were taken in a specially designed form during a previous survey. In addition to this detail anamnesis procedure, in wich the disease treatment with the anticoagulant therapy schemes was taken in note, extra and intra oral examinations were also made. X-ray was used as an additional diagnostic method, and for the close estimation of the kind of the indicated tooth extraction. Special attention in our research was paid to the thrombi-test, which was foloved foall the patients the value of 28 % ± nine was found for our group of study. **Results**: Spontaneus bleeding of more than 25 minutes duration occured in none of the 20 patients. No relationship seems to exist between bleedings and tooth mobility or complicated extraction. **Conclusion**: Reducing the therapeutic level or the complete cut of the oral anticoagulation therapy in collaboration with the specialists in transfuziology, a safe tooth extraction was provaded with a minimum risk of postextraction prolonged bleeding, and free from development of thromboembolism at all patients. The need of another study of tooth extraction without interruption of OAT is forced itself in future.

PO041

Evaluating the interaction of allopurinol with the oral anticoagulants

Rodrigues, Martins R, Viegas E*

Aim: Allopurinol is a medicine described in several articles as not interfering or increasing the influence of oral anticoagulants. The aim of this medical research was checking its interference on the values of INR in the patients who go and consult the oral anticoagulation service. **Methods**: Since September 1994, every patient was studied. The patients treated with allopurinol were checked the percentage in which INR raised or lowered. The patients who were taking other medication, or had intercurrence were out. The analysis of prothrombin time was made by il® a.c.l.1000 and futura plus and the result was given in INR. **Results**: Allopurinol was given to 33 patients from the 1864 patients registered. In 12 (36.4%) patients the INR raised (average=0,75; maximun value=2,87) and in 6 (18,2%) patients decreased this value (average=1,03; maximun value=1,91). 3 patients were excluded as they showed different response in several times and 12 patients were excluded as they had intercurrence. **Conclusion**: It was found the tendency referred by the scientific literature, that is, the allopurinol has an effect of increasing the influence of oral anticoagulants in most patients. However, 18.2% of the patients we studied, reduced the value of INR, and we did not find this effect described in any bibliography we consulted. Although changes we observed were not responsible for the thromboembolic or hemorrhagic complications, we think, that it is important to always watch the possibility of the interaction between the allopurinol and the oral anticoagulant therapy as well as fulfil other studies about this subject. References: Hoffbrand AV, Lewis SM, Tuddenham. Postgraduate Haematology; Beutler E, Lichtman MA, Coller BS, Kipps TJ, Seligsohn U. Williams Hematology; Jobin F. La Thrombose; Horton JD, Bushwick BM. Warfarin Therapy: Evolving Strategies in Anticoagulation, Clinical Pharmacology; AHFS Drug Information; Martindale The complete drug reference.

PO042

Recurrence of deep vein thrombosis in a patient with combined thrombophilic disorder, complicated by warfarin-induced liver damage

Hirmerová J (1), Mecová E (1), Chudáček Z (2)*

(1) 2nd Dpt. of Internal Medicine, University Hospital Pilsen, Czech Republic
(2) Dpt. of Radiology, University Hospital, Pilsen, Czech Republic

Optimal length of anticoagulation following venous thromboembolism is still a matter of debate. The goal of the therapy is to prevent recurrence but not to expose the patient to the risk of serious bleeding. Current recommendations suggest 3-6 months of warfarin therapy with target INR 2-3 after the first episode of venous thromboembolism in the case of reversible or time-limited risk factor. At least 6 months of oral anticoagulation is recommended after the first idiopathic event. In practice, however, not every patient is treated adequately. We present a case of a 25 year old patient with a history of popliteal deep vein thrombosis of the right leg 15 months ago, now admitted for ultrasound findings of deep vein thrombosis in popliteal and femoral location bilaterally, probably not acute. Later on, selective venography revealed even an occlusion of external iliac veins bilaterally, not acute as well. After his previous thrombotic episode, the intensity and duration of warfarin therapy had not been adequate and that had probably caused recurrence and extension of thrombotic process. He had been previously positively tested for factor V Leiden (heterozygous), now we revealed also protein C deficiency. We considered anticoagulation treatment indicated, at least to prevent further extension of thrombotic process. After a course of low-molecular-weight heparin we started warfarin therapy. That was complicated by hepatopathy, suspicious of warfarin-induced liver damage. The diagnosis was supported by improving following withdrawal of warfarin and confirmed by liver biopsy. This complication, which is described as extremely rare, was a contraindication to further coumarin therapy. We were forced to use low-molecular-weight heparin for long-term anticoagulation. The patient is followed on outpatient-basis and his family is currently being tested for thrombophilia.

PO043

Ambulatory programme of monitoring oral anticoagulant therapy in the Basque country: evaluation of the point of-care device ProTime

Vacas M (1), Santos M (2), Longa M (2), Martin S (1), Lafuente P (1), Iriarte J (1), Gandarias JM (1)*

(1) FIDEC. Bilbao.Spain.
(2) MEDIKOSTA. Bilbao. Spain.

Introduction: In recent years a high increase in oral anticoagulated patients due to the new indications has taken to the Department of Health of the Basque Government to initiate an ambulatory programme of monitoring oral anticoagulant treatment making use of a point-of-care (POC) device, ProTime (ITC, Technidyne Co). **Aim**: To evaluate the reproducibility as well as the therapeutic agreement of ProTime with the Prothrombin Time reference manual technique and a high sensitivity thromboplastin. **Patients and Method**: 60 anticoagulated patients stabilised over 3 months in a therapeutic INR range between 2-3.5. The capillary whole blood sample was obtained simultaneously to venous blood collection and capillary PT determination was performed on the ProTime monitor. PT plasma was tested with the manual PT reference technique (RT) using Thromboplastin Bilbao (TBi) an in-house high sensitivity rabbit thromboplastin (ISI=1.08) calibrated against International Reference Preparation (RBT/90) and recommended as reference reagent in the Spanish External Quality Assessment Oral Anticoagulant Control. The statistical methodology for comparing the INR results of the two systems included: determination of the mean, standard deviation, interval of confidence to 95%, regression analysis and the plot of the average value of a pair of measurements versus their difference. A test of simple concordance and the kappa index was also used in three INR ranks: <2.0, 2-3.5 and >3.5. Intra-assay reproducibility was analysed in 10 samples by triplicate. In the processing of the data the statistical package SPSS/v10.1 was used. **Results**: The coefficient of variation in reproducibility test ranged between 0-5.0%. The average value of INR was 2.80±0.76 (IC 95% 2.60¸ 3.00) for the ProTime and 2.95±0.87 (IC 95%: 2.73¸3.18) for the RT. The coefficient of correlation was 0.96. The degree of simple concordance was of a 95% and applying the Kappa Index was 81.9%. When studying the correlation in the INR results in the three studied ranks, we observed that the monitor underestimated the value of reference of INR from 4.5. **Conclusions**: The ProTime monitor presents a good correlation with the system of reference. The fact to include two internal controls in test cartridges gives a greater security in the test results. From our experience, we considered necessary to apply the demanded criteria of quality for oral anticoagulant monitoring in POC devices and developed an external quality programme.

PO044

Patient relationship to the oral anticoagulant therapy with regard to the age, level of education and duration of treatment

Vukelic-Damijani N (1), Caser L (1), Skalamera R (2), Vujaklija-Stipanovic K (1)*

(1) Institute of Transfusion Medicine, Clinical Hospital Centre, Rijeka, Croatia
(2) Department of Clinical Psychology, Clinical Hospital Centre, Rijeka, Croatia

Oral anticoagulant therapy (OAT) is more often, long-lasting and complex therapy, which requires continuous and qualitative education as well as active participation of patient under treatment. In our anticoagulant clinic, we tested 240 patients by anonymous 20-item questionnaire. The patients' replies were grouped and analysed due to different age, level of education and duration of treatment. The intention was to find out the patient's attitude and opinion in respect of OAT and respective affects on their everyday life. The patients' reply grouped and analysed in conformity of duration of treatment (14% 1-6 months, 16% 6-12 months, 41% 1-5 years, 29% >5 years) pointed out that fears and psychology pressure due to illness and specific treatment are present mainly in the rather new patient. The test affected on patients of different ages (12% <53 years, 19% 54-63 years, 50% 64-74 years, 19% >75years) produced different results too. The youngest patient are the one mostly obsessed by therapy. They are afraid of such treatment but also frustrated during everyday life and appear as most upset patient group. The selection of patients' answers recorded under educational level (24% primary education, 56% secondary education, 20% high school/university) have noticed minimal differences although graduated patients have got better approach with less fears and nervousness. The results obtained emphasized that patients on OAT are worried and afraid not only due to illness but also because of specific therapy, especially younger patients and those who just started the treatment. Therefore, OAT apart from regular coagulation monitoring requires permanent professional education and supervision in order to adapt patients soon as possible to the most valuable treatment.

PO045

Self-management of anticoagulation: a randomised trial (SMART)

Fitzmaurice D, Murray E, McCahon D, Jowett S, Sandhur H, Hobbs R*

Department of Primary Care and General Practice, the University of Birmingham, Edgbaston, Birmingham

Introduction: The increased demand for oral anticoagulation has led to a need for alternative models of care. Self-management (PSM), analogous to diabetic self-care has been proposed as one such alternative. **Aims**: This paper reports the first large-scale UK randomised trial of PSM compared to routine care. Outcome measures were in terms of both clinical and health economic measures. **Materials and methods**: All adult patients receiving warfarin for a long-term indication who had received warfarin for at least 6 months, from 50 primary care centres were invited to participate. Following consent patients were randomised to either control or intervention. Intervention patients were trained in 2x3hour sessions to measure their own INR using a point of care testing device (Coaguchek S, Roche Diagnostics, UK) and interpret their dose of warfarin using a hand-held algorithm. Patients completing training were followed up for 12 months. **Results**: 617 patients were randomised (337 intervention/280 control, from 2470 invited). Using intention to treat analysis, there was no significant difference in percent time in range (PSM 70% vs Control 68%). There were no significant differences in adverse events. Cost-effectiveness data will be available for presentation. **Conclusions**: Whilst PSM is a feasible alternative to routine UK management, only 25% of patients were willing to participate and of these only 57% were able to complete 12 months self-management.

PO046

Importance of continuous education in anticoagulated patients

Iriarte J (1), Longa M (2), Zorraquin A (2), Santos M (2), Vacas M (1), Narvaez I (1), Sabino E (3), Gandarias JM (1), Saez Y (1), Saez de Lafuente J (3)*

(1) FIDEC. Bilbao. Spain
(2) MEDIKOSTA. Bilbao. Spain
(3) UPV/EHU.Bilbao.Spain

Background: Studies have shown that continuous education performed by dedicated healthcare professionals is associated with less complications; we can reduce haemorrhagic and thromboembolic complications in five and ten times respectively among patients with more knowledge about its disease and treatment. **Aim**: Our main objective was to know the impact of grade of knowledge that frequent educative conferences have among oral anticoagulated patients. **Material and Methods**: To achieve this objective we have selected two groups. Group A: 50 patients who only received one educative conference and Group B, 80 patients that received continous education about its disease and treatment. A multiple-choice test was fullfilled by all of them. We included thirteen questions about oral anticoagulant treatment (OAT) including among others: the reason of takin OAT, problems linked to little or too much anticoagulation, the target INR, the interference with other drugs, what to do in case of an emergency or a complication and so on. **Results**: Only 12 % of patients of group A answered succesfully the questionnaire and in Group B, 81.44 % of patients answered correctly the questionnaire. **Conclusions**: Looking to our results, we see the importance of periodic educative conferences in order to increase patients' konwledge and therefore reduce the number of INR controls and thromboembolic and haemorrhagic complications.

PO047

A new approach to identify blood sample collected from hospitalized patients receiving anticoagulant therapy

Katz B, Kirgner I, Eidelman L , Zwang E, Vardimon H, Goncharov I, Mar-Zev F , Deutsch V*

Hematology Institution Tel- Aviv Souraski Medical Center Israel

Introduction: Two common laboratory tests are heavily utilized for the primary screening of coagulation disorders and monitoring of anticoagulation treatment. Activated Partial Thromboplastin Time (aPTT) is used to measure the intrinsic coagulation pathway and monitor heparin therapy. Prothrombin Time (PT) tests the extrinsic coagulation system and is used for monitoring oral anticoagulant treatment. Many clinical laboratories incorporate routine coagulopathy work-up on samples with extended PT/aPTT results. However, an aberrant PT/aPTT result is the consequence of either anticoagulant therapy or a coagulopathy that should be identified. **Aims:** Identify patients receiving anticoagulant therapy and to avoid coagulopathy work-up in this group of patients. Examine compliance of internal medicine departments for usage two types of coagulation samples. **Materials and methods:** Two types of coagulation sampling tubes, containing identical Na-citrate concentrations were introduced in Tel Aviv Sourasky Medical Center departments and clinics. The common blue cap coagulation tube (for patients not receiving anticoagulation), and a second type of coagulation tube with light blue cap (for patient treated with anticoagulation) was introduced for identifying patients receiving anticoagulant therapy. Following a period of education and use of this system, we examined compliance of internal medicine departments for performing coagulation tests sampling. **Results:** Screening of 152 routine coagulation samples of different internal medicine departments indicates 83.5% compliance with respect to proper coagulation sampling. The compliance ratios varied between 100% to 50% in different departments. Indicating reeducation of certain departments with further improve the compliance. Of the inappropriate coagulation tube sampling, 16.5% of all samples sent to the laboratory, 64.3% were of patients receiving anticoagulants collected in normal (blue cap) coagulation tubes and 37.5% were of patients receiving no anticoagulation that were collected in tubes designated for patients receiving anticoagulant therapy. **Conclusions:** Our data indicate good compliance ratios among internal medicine departments, which can be further improved. The usage of anticoagulant therapy designated tubes may increase the accuracy of coagulopathy diagnosis in hospitalized patients, and significantly improve the efficiency and cost-effectiveness in clinical laboratories by eliminating coagulation work-up of patients receiving anticoagulants.

PO048

Prolonged increase of plasma vitamin K_2 concentration by natto (*Bacillus subtilis natto*) ingestion

*Yatagai C, Yanagisawa Y, Ohsugi T, Sumi H**

Kurashiki University of Science and the Arts

Natto is the typical Japanese traditional fermented soy-food and has been used as a folk medicine for heart and vascular diseases. A novel strong fibrinolytic enzyme named nattokinase was reported previously (Sumi et al., Experientia, 43: 1110, 1987; Fibrinolysis, 6:86, 1992). In addition, natto is the only food known that naturally contains menaquinone type vitamin K (MK-7) (Sumi et al., Fibrinolysis, 2:67, 1988). Menaquinone type (vitamin K2) is know as the substance that is essential for composition of osteocalcine (bone Gla protein), which is specific protein combining calcium in a bone. In the present study, using healthy volunteers, prolonged increase of plasma menaquinone-7 concentration was observed by ingesting natto or natto bacillus (Bacillus subtilis natto). Isoelectric focusing was performed using LKB column (110 ml), as reported by Vesterberg & Svensson (Acta Chem. Scand., 20:820, 1966). Vitamin K was determined by HPLC method with a fluorescence monitor (Sumi et al., Food Sci. Technol. Res., 5:48, 1999). After shaking (100 rpm) of 2% soypeptone S-3% glycerol with natto bacillus for 2-10 days at 37°C, the main molecular forms of vitamin K2 produced were water-soluble with pIs 5.0-4.0 by isoelectric focusing. The molecular weights were 80,000-100,000 by gel flirtation on Sephacryl-S 200. Significantly, higher concentration of plasma MK-7 was observed in 7 healthy volunteers taking natto every day. Increase of MK-7 continued until 7 days after natto ingestion. Increase of plasma MK-7 concentration was also confirmed after ingestion of natto bacillus (1.8x1010 viable cells). After ingestion of 4 hrs, the maximum arise was about 6.3 times (7.5? 2.7 ng/ml plasma; $p<0.005$) than the control level. In any cases, these were no difference observed in phylloquinone (vitamin K1) concentration and in the blood coagulation system tested by PT and APTT.

PO049

How does age influence the prescribing of antithrombotic therapy for ambulatory patients with permanent atrial fibrillation?

Leizorovicz A (1), Guenoun M (2), Le Heuzey J (3), Jeandel C (4), Mismetti P (5), Cohen A (6)*

(1) Faculté R.T.H. Laennec, Lyon, France
(2) CHU Marseille, France
(3) APHP Paris, France
(4) CH Montpellier, France
(5) CHU Saint-Etienne, France
(6) APHP, Paris, France

Introduction: Prescription of antithrombotics in atrial fibrillation (AF) patients and its determinants in elderly patients are not well known. **Aims:** The FALSTAF study was performed to describe the modalities of the prescription of antithrombotics in routine practice in ambulatory patients with permanent AF in France. The effect of age on antithrombotic prescription was particularly studied. **Materials and Methods:** We prospectively surveyed consecutive outpatients with documented permanent AF with or without valvular disease, excluding those with valvular prostheses. Cardiologists or general practitioners were selected at random. **Results:** A total of 5893 patients were included by 188 cardiologists (2367 patients) and 582 general practitioners (3526 patients). Their mean age was 75.8 years, 58% were men, and 31.7% had valvular disease. Overall, 95.5% of patients were being prescribed an antithrombotic drug, including vitamin K antagonists (VKA) in 76.4% of patients and aspirin in 16.6% of patients. High age was a significant predictor (p=0.001) for the non-prescription of antithrombotics or VKA, even after multivariate adjustment for other factors that had a significant negative influence on prescribing, such as poor autonomy, history of severe haemorrhage and potentially haemorrhagic diseases. Above 80 years, 7.4% of patients were not receiving antithrombotic prophylaxis. Among patients receiving an antithrombotic therapy, the use of VKA decreased sharply after 75 years in favour of aspirin. **Conclusions:** In our study, a majority of ambulatory patients with permanent AF were receiving antithrombotic therapy. However, the use of VKA was not optimal in elderly patients and better prophylactic strategies may be warranted for them.

PO050

Surface-expressed mediators on activated platelets are required for pulmonary leukocyte recruitment in a murine model of allergic inflammation

Pitchford S, Giannini S, Momi S, Casali L, Gresele P*

Department of Internal Medicine, Section of Internal and Cardiovascular Medicine, University of Perugia, Italy

Introduction: A characteristic of murine models of allergic inflammation is the pulmonary recruitment of leukocytes, a process which is platelet dependent (Pitchford *et al* 2003*.J.Allergy.Clin.Immunol.*112 109-118) and has also been shown to be suppressed in animals congenitally lacking adhesion molecules (De Sanctis et al.1997.J.Appl. Physiol.83, 681-687). The mechanisms by which platelets are essential for leukocyte recruitment are unknown. **Aims**: The effects of re-infusion of pre-activated platelets on leukocyte recruitment were studied in a murine model of allergic inflammation. **Methods**: Male C57BL/6 mice (n=4-6) immunised on days 0 and 7 with ovalbumin (OVA. 10μg/mouse i.p. 0.4ml in 0.1M $Al_2(OH)_3$ or Alum alone), were exposed to aerosolised OVA (1%saline, 20 minutes. t.i.d.) on days 15,16,17. Groups were selectively depleted of platelets via busulfan (20mg/kg i.p.) on days -4,-2,1. Washed platelets_stimulated with thrombin (1U/ml), fixed with 1% paraformaldehyde (SFP), were resuspended in saline, and reinjected into platelet-depleted mice before aerosol challenge on days 15 &16 (2x108 platelets i.v.). Similar experiments were carried out with washed, unstimulated fixed platelets (FP). Broncho-alveolar lavages (BAL) were performed 24 hours after day 17, and cytospins prepared and stained (Diffquik) for leukocyte differentiation. Total cell counts were assessed using a Burker chamber. Data were expressed as means±SEM of 105 eosinophils/ml. **Results**: A significant increase in eosinophil recruitment was observed between sham and OVA immunised mice (Sham: 0.1±0.1 OVA: 80.9±21.7. P<0.001). Busulfan administration depleted platelets >90% without affecting peripheral blood leukocyte numbers, and significantly inhibited eosinophil recruitment (10.3±2.5 P<0.01). SFP injection significantly restored eosinophil recruitment compared to platelet depleted mice, whilst FP injection did not (SFP: 51.7±9.3 FP: 3.7±0.8 P<0.05). A significant increase in the percentage of cells positive for P-selectin and PSGL-1 was observed between SFP compared to FP (P-selectin SFP: 55.6±11.5 vs. FP: 25.9±7.6 P<0.01); (PSGL-1 SFP:24.8±4.7vs. FP: 7.8±1.8. P<0.01). **Conclusion**: This study demonstrates that surface bound mediators on activated platelets are necessary for pulmonary eosinophil recruitment in a murine model of allergic inflammation.

PO051

Activated platelets induce APC-resistance in vivo

*Leone M (1), Momi S (1), Colucci M (2), Gresele P (1)**

(1) Department of Internal Medicine, Sect. of Internal and Cardiovascular Medicine, University of Perugi
(2) Department of Biomedical Sciences, Sect. of General Pathology, University of Bari, Bari, Italy.

Introduction: Activated platelets have been shown to inhibit both the anticoagulant and profibrinolytic activity of activated protein C (APC) in vitro. **Aims:** We investigated the effect of platelets on the anticoagulant and antithrombotic activities of human APC in mice in ex vivo studies and in a model of thrombin-induced pulmonary thromboembolism. **Methods**: In vitro we assessed the effect of platelets on the APC resistance test using a clotting assay. To evaluate the role of platelets in APC-resistance in vivo we evaluated the direct effect of APC injection in normal and thrombocytopenic mice against thrombin-induced pulmonary thromboembolism in mice. **Results:** Control in vitro experiments indicated that collagen-stimulated murine platelets reduce the APC sensitivity ratio (APC-ratio) of mouse plasma from 2.15 ± 0.39 to 1.33 ± 0.10 (p<0.05). The platelet-dependent APC resistance was inhibited (≈50%) by preincubation in vitro with G4120, an antagonist of GPIIb/IIIa. The injection of collagen (250 mg/ml) plus adrenaline (1.5 mg/ml) in mice was accompanied by a reduction of the APC-ratio of platelet-poor-plasma collected 2 min after injection (1.52 ±0.16 as compared to 1.96 ±0.23 in plasma from vehicle-treated mice), suggesting that platelet activation caused the shedding of platelet-derived microparticles endowed with APC resistance. No change in plasma APC-ratio was observed when the platelet agonists were injected in mice made thrombocytopenic (<10 % of basal count) by an antiplatelet antiserum. In agreement with these data, the injection of lethal doses of thrombin caused markedly less mortality in thrombocytopenic that in normal mice (17 % versus 60% with 1000 U/kg thrombin), probably because of an unopposed APC anticoagulant-pathway activation in the former. Finally, to assess directly the role of platelets on APC-resistance in vivo, we evaluated the effect of APC injection (1 mg/kg) on thrombin-induced mortality in normal and thrombocytopenic mice. When the two groups of animals were treated with doses of thrombin causing a similar (≈80%) mortality rate (1000 U/kg in control and 2000 U/kg in thrombocytopenic animals), the injection of human APC was associated with a reduction in mortality of 50% in normal animals and of 80% in thrombocytopenic mice (p<0.01). **Conclusions**: These data suggest that in vivo platelet activation induces a relative APC resistance phenotype, and thus might increase thrombotic risk. In vivo platelet activation may decrease the response to antithrombotic drugs acting via the PC anticoagulant pathway. Drugs capable of reducing platelet-dependent APC resistance might be effective in facilitating APC-mediated anticoagulant effects.

PO052

The thrombolytic effect of longolytine in external application in rabbits

Tamara S (1), Lidia P (1), Tamara S (1), Rosa M (1), Leonid N (2), Galina A (1)

(1) Moscow State University, Moscow, Russia
(2) Institut of molecular genetics, Moscow, Russia

Introduction: Longolytin a mixture of proneolytic enzymes isolated from the cultural fluid of low saprophyte fungus arthrobotrys longa possesses fibrinjlynic, thrombolytic and PA activities in vitro and in vivo after intravenous injection to rats. However it is little known about external using jf thrombolytic preparations. The aim of investigation is to study the thrombolytic effect of longolytine used as external agent on model of thrombosis in rabbits. **Material and methods**: We have created the model of thrombosis on the ear border vein in rabbits. This model permits to obsverve the process of thrombus dissolving in vivo by thrombolytic preparations. In the first experience series the formed thrombi were applicated with solution of longolytine in glycerine.(21cases) .In the second series (33 cases) there were used longolytine mixed with heparin (5u/ml) for prophylaxis of thrombosis. Thrombi of control rabbits we applicated with only glycerine (first series) or glycerine mixed with heparin (second series).

We were watching for thrombus dissolving and determinating thrombus parameters every hour for experimental day. **Results**: Experimental data were estimated by value of speed of thrombi dissolving (mm^2/min). In first series the speed in experimental rabbits was 0.048 mm min that 6 times faster than in control rabbits 0.008 mm^2/min. Thrombus in animals of second series, that were applicated with complex longolytine and heparin dissolved at a speed 0,106 mm^2/min, compared to control – 0,025 mm^2/min. In above experimental and control groupe there were not observed dependence of thrombus dissolution on thrombus size. Dissappearance of inflammation reaction was also faster in experimental animals. **Conclusion**: External application of thrombolytic preparation longolytine and complex longolytine and heparin caused dissolving of thromb formed in border vein in rabbits. The complex longolytine and heparin accelerated the speed of thrombus solution compared to longolytine alone.

PO053

Antithrombotic effects of BAY 59-7939, an oral, direct Factor Xa inhibitor, in models of thrombosis and bleeding time in rats and rabbits

Perzborn E (1), Buetehorn U (2), Lampe T (3), Pernerstorfer J (3), Pohlmann J (3), Roehrig S (3), Schlemmer K (2), Straub A (3)*

(1) Cardiovascular Research, Bayer HealthCare AG, Wuppertal, Germany
(2) Preclinical Pharmacokinetics, Bayer HealthCare AG, Wuppertal, Germany
(3) Chemical Research, Bayer HealthCare AG, Wuppertal, Germany

Introduction: BAY 59-7939 is an oral, direct Factor Xa (FXa) inhibitor in development for the prevention and treatment of thromboembolic diseases. **Aim**: To evaluate the antithrombotic properties of BAY 59-7939 in models of venous and arterial thrombosis in rats and rabbits. **Results**: In a rat venous thrombosis model, thrombosis was induced by stasis and concomitant administration of tissue factor. Intravenous administration of BAY 59-7939 resulted in dose-dependent inhibition of thrombus development, with an ED50 of 0.098 mg/kg. Ex vivo, BAY 59-7939 increased PT and inhibited FXa dose dependently. However, at the ED50, PT was only slightly increased (1.8±0.3-fold), and FXa activity was inhibited by only 32±5%. In the rat arterio-venous shunt model, oral administration of BAY 59-7939 reduced thrombus mass dose dependently, with an ED50 of 5.0 mg/kg. Ex vivo, BAY 59-7939 affected clotting times and FXa activity dose dependently. At oral doses near the ED50 (3 and 6 mg/kg), FXa was inhibited by 61±2% and 78±2%, respectively, and PT was prolonged 2.4±0.2-fold and 3.7±0.4-fold, respectively; aPTT was increased 1.4±0.02-fold at 6 mg/kg. BAY 59-7939 reduced thrombus development dose dependently, with an ED50 of 4 mg/kg in the $FeCl_3$-induced carotid artery thrombosis model, and an ED50 of 2.0 mg/kg in the mechanical-damage-induced jugular vein thrombosis model after oral administration in rats. In the rabbit arterio-venous shunt thrombosis model, oral administration of BAY 59-7939 reduced the clot weight dose dependently, with an ED50 of 0.6 mg/kg. Ex vivo, clotting times and FXa activity were affected dose dependently. After an oral dose of 1.0 mg/kg, above the ED50 dose, FXa was inhibited by 91±9%, but PT and aPTT were only slightly increased, by 1.32±0.05-fold and 1.31±0.06-fold, respectively. Prolongation of PT (r = 0.98) and aPTT (r = 0.80) correlated strongly with the plasma levels of BAY 59-7939. In addition, the anti-hemostatic effects of BAY 59-7939 were investigated in models of bleeding time in rats and rabbits. Rat tail-bleeding time and rabbit ear-bleeding time were unaffected at an antithrombotic effective dose (3 mg/kg). **Conclusions**: These results show that BAY 59-7939 has a favourable antithrombotic activity: bleeding risk ratio in several well-characterized models of thrombosis. The findings suggest that direct inhibition of FXa with BAY 59-7939 may offer a safe and effective oral therapy for thromboembolic diseases.

PO054

Pharmacokinetics of BAY 59-7939 – an oral, direct Factor Xa inhibitor – in rats and dogs

Weinz C (1), Buetehorn U (2), Daehler H (2), Kohlsdorfer C (2), Pleiss U (1), Sandmann S (2), Schlemmer K (2), Schwarz T (2), Steinke W (2)*

(1) Drug Metabolism and Isotope Chemistry, Bayer HealthCare AG, Wuppertal, Germany
(2) Preclinical Pharmacokinetics, Bayer HealthCare AG, Wuppertal, Germany

Introduction: BAY 59-7939 is an oral, direct Factor Xa inhibitor in development for the prevention and treatment of thromboembolic diseases. **Aim:** To investigate the pharmacokinetics of BAY 59-7939 *in vivo* in Wistar rats and Beagle dogs. **Results:** The absorption of [^{14}C] BAY 59-7939 from the gastrointestinal tract was 67% in rats and 95% in dogs. The absolute bioavailability was high: 60% in rats and 60–86% in dogs. Plasma concentrations of the parent drug after oral and intravenous administration showed linear pharmacokinetics in both rats and dogs. Plasma clearance in rats (0.4 L/[kg·h]) and dogs (0.3 L/[kg·h]) was low. The volume of distribution was moderate: 0.3 L/kg in rats and 0.4 L/kg in dogs. In rats, the plasma elimination half-life of unchanged drug was 0.9 hour after intravenous administration and 1.2–2.3 hours after oral administration. In dogs, the elimination half-life was about 0.9 hour after both intravenous and oral administration. After administration of [^{14}C] BAY 59-7939, radioactivity was heterogeneously distributed to organs and tissues, with similar patterns after intravenous and oral administration. There was no evidence of irreversible binding or retention of radioactivity in organs and tissues of rats. The protein binding of the parent drug varied between the different species, with fractions unbound to plasma proteins (f_u) of 1.3% in rats, 10.4% in dogs, and 5.1% in humans, respectively. The excretion of radioactivity occurred rapidly in rats, >95% of the dose was excreted during the first day after administration. After oral administration, 67% of the dose was excreted in the faeces and 25% in the urine. Residues in the bodies of rats 7 days after administration were low: 0.2% of the dose. Both elimination pathways were of equal importance in dogs: following oral administration 52% of the dose was excreted in the urine and 43% in the faeces. **Conclusion:** These findings show that BAY 59-7939 has a favourable pharmacokinetic profile with high oral bioavailability and a dual mode of excretion without accumulation in the body.

PO055

The assessment of MDA and SOD after the administration of Allopurinol in the Ischemia-reperfusion syndrome of the small bowel

Sapalidis K (2), Makris P (1), Girtovitis F (1), Anestakis D (1), Deligiannnidis N (2), Gamvros O (2)*

(1) Haemostasis Unit, A' Medical Propedeutic Clinic, AUTH, GR
(2) 3rd Surgical Clinic, AUTH, GR

Aim: The aim of this study is to evaluate the ideal timing for the administration of allopurinol with respect to ischaemia-reperfusion syndrome of the small bowel. **Material and Methods:** 20 rabbits were divided in four groups of 5. Enteric ischaemia was caused for 50 minutes to all of the animals, followed by 50 minutes of reperfusion. Group A was the control group (no allopurinol administration). Group B had an allopurinol (30mg/Kg) administration 10minutes prior to ischaemia. Group C had an allopurinol (30mg/Kg) administration 2 minutes prior to reperfusion. Group D had an allopurinol administration (15mg/Kg) 10minutes prior to ischaemia and the same quantity was re-administrated 2 minutes prior to reperfusion. 3 blood samples were obtained: i) 15 minutes prior to ischaemia ii) 5 minutes prior to reperfusion iii) after the reperfusion had been completed. In all samples dismutase's (SOD) concentration was determined. All of the animals were sacrificed and tissue malonylaldehyde (MDA) was determined. ANOVA multivariate analysis was employed. **Results:** The comparison of the results showed that, application of allopurinol in groups B and C had only a small favourable effect. On the other hand, allopurinol's application in group D showed a maximal protective effect. **Conclusion:** Allopurinol has a protective effect, blocking the development of necrotic lesions in the intestinal mucosa. The optimal effect is achieved when allopurinol is administered both before the ischemia and before the reperfusion phase. The beneficial results are confirmed by determining the tissue levels of MDA and SOD.

PO056

The postoperative inflammatory reaction (IR) in dependence of using different surgical scalpels in experiment

Tatyana S, Ludmila L, Margarita K, Ospan M, Galina A

Moscow State University, Moscow, Russia

Introduction: The IR is one of important reasons of postoperative disturbances: thrombosis, hemophilia, adhesion formation. The inflammation depend from many factors, among them the characteristics of surgical instruments plays a great role. **Aim:** In present work has aimed to study specials of the IR and state of coagulation and fibrinolysis systems in postoperative time in dependence of using different scalpels. **Materials and methods:** The operation on Wistar line rats uterine horns carry out under hexanel narcosis. We had: ordinary scalpel (1-st group), mono- and bipolar electrosurgery scalpels (2-nd group), harmonic scalpel (3-st group), argono-scalpel (4-th group). Blood from v.jugularis were taken preoperatively, and on the 1, 7, 15, 21 and 45 day after surgery. In that time we made macroscopic and histology investigation of wound surface, and citomorphology search of peritoneal fluids (PF) cells. **Results:** In 1-st group in the PF was observed rough elevated contents off polymorphonuclear cells (PNC) from 1-st day, and the quantity of macrophages linear increased and fibrinogen level shortness augment only in plasma. It showed acute character of IR. We observed two periods depression of fibrinolitic activity, which suited elevation of amount monocytes in PF. Plasminogen activator activity (PAA) was decreased in 3-fold by the 15-th day after injury, after that it come back in norm. Plasmin activity was decreased in all period of experiment. The dates of macroscopic and histology researches indicated on prolonged IR with y 4-th groups. The augmentation of the PNC and diminution of macrophages cells in PF in 2-nd and 3-st groups were insignificant, and in 4-th - PNC rose only in the 1-st week of experiment. It was been shown that in all groups amount of monocytes raised by 7-21 day and wavy changes of quantity of eosinophils occurred. In all time of investigation the maintenance of fibrinogen in plasma was authentically higher of norm. In PF in 2-nd and 3-rd groups this protein has been found in 1-st week, and 4-th - only on 1-st day. In 2-4 groups fibrinolitic activity of plasma was reduced, but at that time PAA was increased. The titer of PAI activity rose from 1-st day and before ending of experiments in all (2-4) groups. **Conclusion:** Thus, using of an ordinary scalpel leads to the acute IR and short disturbances functions of haemostasis system. The application of surgical injury induces the chronic of IR, which makes slow wound healing, and prolonged disorders of the coagulation and fibrinolysis.

PO057

The formation of stable prethrombotic state is result in an action of different psychostimulators

Tamara S, Lidiya P, Kira N, Victoria S, Galina A*

Moscow State University, Moscow, Russia

Introduction. Modern humans experiencing large informational overloads, often use different pharmacological preparations (Opilong) for activation of mentality. But it is not always justified. **The aim** is to investigate the peculiarities of haemostasis and fibrinolysis in repeated influencing of Opilong=synthetic analog of dermorphine (Op) and a weak static MF (sMF). **Material and methods**. Different parameters of haemostasis were studied in 7 groups of Wistar rats: (1) control (n=60); (2) intact rats-learning without action of factors (n=20); (3 and 4) learned rats on natural MF (38.2 □T) and static MF (up to 300 □ T); (5 and 6) opilong-treated rats (n=40) without and with information load, (7) sMF+Op-induced rats (n=20). Opilong was used in dose of 40 □g/kg. Information load was the complicated task that rats were to solve in the maze. **Results**. It was found that the Op and sMF facilitated realization of cognitive processes. 90% of rats were able to solve the task instead of 40 % in the intact group. The most intensive effect was observed as a result of sMF+Op action. Biochemical analysis indicated that information load on the background of Op and sMF actions provoked to development of prethrombotic state. 62,3% of rats in 4, 6, and 7 groups had high nonenzymatic fibrinolysis (35,6 mm instead of 8,7 mm in control). The fibrinogen content in 60% of cases shifted to region of the higher values (from 240,5 to 742,2 mg%). Recalcification time was significantly decreased from 87,5 sec to 62,3 sec in 25,7 % of rats. The region of ATIII (94,3% +36,9%) values became a half of its original size (90,6% + 18,0%). The fibrinolytic activity (ELT) was reduced sharply (with 179,2 min up to 430,5 min) while the activator activity was increased from 12,5 mm up to 53,6 mm. Extreme values was observed in Op+sMF rats. **Conclusion**. The data obtained demonstrate that the attempts to facilitate a thought process by the psychostimulant actionsof different nature can result in stable prethrombotic state.

PO058

Determination of coagulation inhibitor activity and resistance to activated protein C in non-small cell lung cancer patients (NSCLC)

Dworakowska D (1), Lapinski M (2), Skibowska A (3), Mital A (4), Tomaszewski D (2), Dworakowski R (5), Kazimierska E (1), Skokowski J (2), Szutowicz A (3), Czestochowska E (1)*

(1) Department of Internal Medicine, Endocrinology and Haemostatic Disorders, Medical University of Gdan
(2) Department if Thoracic Surgery, Medical University of Gdansk, Poland
(3) Department of Clinical Biochemistry, Medical University of Gdansk, Poland
(4) Department of Pathophysiology, Medical University of Gdansk, Poland
(5) Department of Cardiology, Medical University of Gdansk, Poland

Introduction: Coagulopathies are frequently observed in patients with malignancy and in many cancer patients, the coagulation system is activated without clinical signs of thromboembolism. Non-small cell lung cancer (NSCLC) is the most common human malignancy and its treatment outcome is poor on overall. **Aim**: The aim of this study was to determine whether NSCLC patients (with no symptoms of thromboembolism) show any alteration in activity of coagulation inhibitors or in resistance to activated protein C (APCR). **Material and Methods**: The study group consisted of 20 consecutive NSCLC patients (18 men and 2 women), aged from 47 to 78 years (with a mean of 63 years), who underwent radical pulmonary resection. All patients were under IIIb stage of disease and remained active smokers. Control group consisted of 20 healthy donors, similar to patients group according to sex, age and smoking habit. In study group blood samples were collected preoperatively. The clotting system was assessed measuring antithrombin (AT), protein C and S activity, APCR, fibrinogen and d-dimer level. Additionally homocystein level was assessed. All parameters ware measured in blood serum using commercially available kits. **Results**: There were no statistically significant differences between NSCLC patients and control group in mean values of APCR (1.9±0.35 vs 2.1±0.28, respectively, p=0.16), AT activity (102%±10.4% vs 108%±9%, respectively, p=0.07) and protein C activity (117%±18% vs 120%±19%, respectively, p=0.66). Mean protein S activity in NSCLC patients was significantly lower than in control group (70.05%±24% vs 52.8%±25%, respectively, p=0.037). Mean fibrinogen and d-dimer levels were in NSCLC patients higher than in control group (6.26g/l±0.7g/l vs 3.6g/l±1.9g/l, respectively, p<0.001 for fibrinogen and 260ug/l±194ug/l vs 144ug/l±66ug/l, respectively, p=0.02 for d-dimer). There was no difference in mean homocystein level between patients and control group (13.2umol/l±2.2 umol/l vs 13.1umol/l ±3.5umol/l, respectively, p=0.98). **Conclusion**: Our results suggest that in spite of no symptoms of thromboembolism, there are same alterations of clotting system in NSCLC patients.

PO059

Angioplasty (ANG) and anticoagulation (ATC) in superior vena cava syndrome (SVCS)

Celebrin L, Carlevaro O, Bluguermann J, Mauro D, Bezares R, Antonio D, Parise F*

SVCS is caused frequently by extrinsic compression or invasion by tumors of the superior mediastinum and other causes, and rarely by in situ thrombosis (T) without compression. **Aims**: To analyze the results of ANG and ATC in SVCS. **Materials and Methods**: We report 6 patients (p) treated between 1997 and 2002 with SVCS. The mean age was 58 years (22-73), 1 female. The clinical presentation was upper chest and neck edema in 58%, dyspnea and cough in 25%, and upper limbs edema in 17%. Diagnosis were: 1 non Hodgkin Lymphoma, (p1); 2 lung neoplasms (p2, 3); 2 undeterminated neoplasms (p4,5) and 1 clinical Trousseau Syndrome (p6) with primary tumor undetected. The venous obstructions were located in 4 p in the vena cava and jugulosubclavian confluent, and in 2 p in the subclavian veins; in 4 cases there was compression and thrombosis and in 2 was observed in situ thrombosis (p5, 6). All p were treated with ANG with multiple stent implantation (mean 3,2 stents/p) and ATC, and in two cases was also given thrombolytic treatment (p 4 and 6). **Results**: Rapid relief of symptoms (RRS) was obtained in 6/6 patients. 1 p. presented heparin induced thrombocytopenia and ATC was stopped and 1p presented retroperitoneal haematoma post thrombolysis. All patients received heparin, 5 received coumarins and one of these is on low molecular weight heparin (LMWH) (p6). 4 patients died during follow-up: 3 tumor related, (p2, 3 and 5), 1 sepsis (p4), with a mean survival of 6 months without recurrences, and 2 p are still alive: p1: 80 month survival(ms) under coumarin treatment (she developed second tumor), p6: 16 ms with several in situ recurrences, treated with multiple ANG and currently with LMWH. **Conclusions:** 1. ANG is effective and safe in

RRS. 2. Survival is illness related. 3. ATC is necessary to avoid recurrence and recurrence might be conditioned by prothrombotic state.4. - Is long-term ATC necessary in survivors?

PO060

Chemotherapy-induced activation of haemostasis: the role of D-dimer

Siragusa S (1), Arcara C (2), Malato A (1), Anastasio R (1), Fulfaro F (2), Lucio LC (1), Dolce A (1), Gebbia N (2), Mariani G (1)*

(1) Thrombosis and Haemostasis Unit, Division of Hematology, University of Palermo, Italy
(2) Chair of Oncology, University of Palermo, Italy

Evidence of haemostatic activation has been demonstrated in cancer patients. The role of chemiotherapy as a risk factor for venous thromobosis has been reported during therapy for breast cancer (tamoxifen) and for Multiple Mieloma (thalidomide). Among the markers of thrombin activation, D-dimer test has been found increased after chemotherapy for breast and lung cancer (Weitz et al, Thromb Haemost 2002;88:213-20). However, the type of cancer and the regimen of chemotherapy give a different risk of thrombosis. Therefore, no definitive conclusions are present on the role of markers of thrombin activation for identifying patients, on chemotherapy, at high risk of thrombosis. In ongoing clinical trials, we assessed D-dimer levels in patients on chemotherapy for cancer of the colon. **Materials and methods**. Consecutive patients receiving adjunctive chemotherapy for colon neoplasm were considered eligible. D-dimer test was tested at the beginning and at the end of any cycle of chemotherapy. Standard chemotherapy consists in Campto (CPT11) 180 mg/mq, and Fluororacile (400 and 600 mg/mq) for 2 days. D-dimer was furnished by Dade Behring (D-dimer PLUS, turbidimetric methods, normal value < 192 µL). D-dimer variation before and after chemotherapy was assessed by Wilcoxon test. Objective test for deep vein thrombosis (DVT) and/or pulmonary embolism (PE) were performed in symptomatic patients during the follow-up. **Results**. At the interim analysis, 29 patients were evaluated; D-dimer levels did not vary between the beginning and the end of chemotherapy (1st cycle p= 0.8, 2nd cycle p=0.9, 3rd cycle 0.67, 4th cycle 0.79). None of the patients developed symptomatic DVT and/or PE. **Conclusion**. At the present, our study does not confirm a significant increase of D-dimer levels in patients on chemotherapy for cancer of the colon.

PO061

Coagulation derangements in oral and maxillofacial surgery in patients with a documented cancer: a follow-up study after surgery

De Lucia D, Napolitano M, Misso M, Sessa M, Tagliaferri A, De Francesco F, Borriello C, Colella G*

Faculty of Medicine

Introduction ypercoagulability is normally due to derangements in the blood coagulation cascade, both genetic and acquired, which may predispose to abnormal clotting activation or deficiency in natural inhibitors' control. Thrombophilia is usually caused by aberrant coagulation and by cell activation, but it is also related to such specific factors as oral contraceptives, pregnancy, puerperium, trauma, prolonged immobilization, cancer, and surgery. **Aims** The aim of our study was to determine the mechanism by which cancer could cause or favour the development of a thrombo-embolic state in patients who had undergone surgery. **Materials and methods** Fifteen patients with a documented diagnosis of cancer and 30 healthy subjects, blood donors at our University matched for sex, age, body mass index, height, and social background were enrolled. The protocol was approved by an Institutional Review Board, and patients gave informed consent. Plasma samples for determination of PT, APTT, Fibrinogen (Fg), coagulation factors (II, VII, VIII, IX, X, XI, XII), coagulation inhibitors (ATIII, PC, PS, and APC resistance), fibrinolysis (PLG, t-PA, PAI-1), antiphospholipid antibodies (ACA beta 2GPI IgG and IgM, Lupus Anticoagulant), and activation peptides (D-Dimers and F1+2) were executed immediately after entry and then daily one day before and two days after surgery. All parameters were carried out according to International Laboratory Techniques. Normal plasma levels for PT, APTT, natural clotting inhibitors, and coagulation factors were documented in all patients. During the observational surgery period, no changes in all of these parameters were observed. High basal values of Fg, PAI-1, F VIII, F1+2, and D-Dimers were found in all patients compared with healthy subjects. The plasma levels rapidly increased before surgery reaching the highest values after surgery. Moderate titles of IgG anticardiolipin antibodies b2-glycoprotein type I were found in eight of 15 patients. **Results** Analysis of our data suggests a state of hypercoagulability in cancer disease associated with maxillofacial surgery. The significant increase of plasma fibrinogen levels and the activation peptides show a hypercoagulability state in this setting associated with endothelial cell activation and dysfunction, with thrombin formation and fibrin deposition. **Conclusions** Analysis of our data demonstrates a hypercoagulable state during the follow-up period of maxillofacial surgery associated with cancer disease. Our report gave considerable information on the clinical situation when surgeons cause patients to become thrombophilic by removing their cancer. The mechanism that causes these coagulation derangements is still unknown.

PO062

Budd Chiari syndrome in patients with myeloproliferative disorders (MPD) and high platelet count: evidence for an endothelial pathology

*Randi ML (1), Luzzatto G (1), Cella G (2), Tezza F (1), Fabris F (1)**

(1) Internal Medicine, Dept of Medical and Surgical Sciences, University of Padua Medical School
(2) Chair of Hematology, Dept of Medical and Surgical Sciences, University of Padua Medical School

Introduction: Budd-Chiari syndrome (BC) is a rare but dramatic complication in patients with high platelet count. BC more commonly occurs in females younger than 50 years, usually complicating MPD with just a mild increase in platelet count. **Aims**: to evaluate the possible association of MPD with prothrombotic conditions other than high platelet count and/or with endothelial disfunction that may contribute to thrombotic complications. **Material and methods**: We studied 7 patients (5 females, 2 males, mean age 35±3.2 years) with MPD and BC. We evaluated PT, PTT, AT III, protein C (activity and antigen), protein S (activity, antigen and free), protein-C-resistance, plasminogen, PAI-1 (activity and antigen), antiphospholipid autoantibodies, homocystein, vWF (factor VIII activity FvW antigen, vWF binding to collagen and vWF:FVIIIBA) serum P, E and L selectin, NO_2/NO_3, tissue factor pathway inhibitor (TFPI), thrombomodulin (TM), PECAM-1 and ICAM-1. **Results:** TM (98,36 ± 59,80 ng/ml) and ICAM-1 (1228,78 ± 237,32 ng/ml) were markedly elevated in our MPD patients. 1/7 patient (14%) had an identifiable prothrombotic factor (homozygous Factor V Leiden). No other alteration was observed in any of the other investigated factors. **Conclusions**: The high levels of soluble adhesion molecules in these patients may be an expression of endothelial alteration, possibly related to inflammation. However, TM is known to be higher in young ET patients like ours are. ICAM-1 has been reported to be elevated in clonal MPD. More study are needed to elucidate the endothelial function in MPD patients with hepatic veins thrombosis.

PO063

Endothelial damage/dysfunction and thrombogenesis in diabetes: positive effects of multi-factorial intervention

Lim S, Blann AD, Lip G*

Haemostasis, Thrombosis and Vacsular Biology Unit, City Hospital, Dudley Road, Birmingham, UK

Background: Endothelial abnormalities and a hypercoagulable state may contribute to increased cardiovascular risk in diabetes mellitus, particularly in patients with overt cardiovascular disease (CVD). We sought to determine if a 'package of care' of intensified multi-factorial cardiovascular risk intervention could improve parameters of endothelial abnormality and hypercoagulability in diabetes, and if diabetic patients with overt CVD would derive similar benefit as compared to those without. **Patients and Methods**: We measured plasma von Willebrand factor (vWf, an index of endothelial damage/dysfunction), soluble E-selectin (sE-sel, marking endothelial activation) and tissue factor (TF, an initiator of coagulation) by ELISA in 94 patients with diabetes mellitus (38 with CVD and 56 without overt CVD and 38 comparable controls. Of these, 33 patients with CVD and 31 without overt CVD then participated in multi-factorial cardiovascular risk intervention over one year. **Results** *[Data as mean (SD)]*: As expected, plasma levels of vWf, sE-sel and TF were significantly higher in patients compared to controls, with TF highest in patients with overt CVD ($p<0.001$). Intensive multi-factorial intervention resulted in significant reductions in total cholesterol (from 5.2 (1.2) to 4.1 (0.5) mmol/l) and HbA1c (from 7.7 (1.2) to 6.9 (0.9) %) (both $p<0.001$) and this was associated with significant reductions in vWf (by 27% and 46%) in patients with and without overt CVD (both $p<0.01$). TF was reduced (by 45%) only in patients without overt CVD (p=0.03). There was no significant change in sE-sel levels in either group. **Conclusion**: Patients with diabetes demonstrate endothelial perturbation and a hypercoagulable state, which can only be partially improved by a 'package of care' of intensified multi-factorial cardiovascular risk intervention. Earlier intervention prior to the development of clinically overt CVD may confer additional benefit in these patients.

PO064

Inhibitory mechanisms of YC-1 and PMC in the induction of iNOS expression by lipoteichoic acid in RAW 264.7 macrophages

Hsiao G, Huang H, Sheu J*

Graduate Institute of Pharmacology, Taipei Medical University, Taipei, Taiwan

Introduction. PMC is the most potent derivative of α-tocopherols in antioxidation and inhibits the activation of NF-κB. On the other hand, YC-1 has been described as an NO-independent activator of sGC. **Aims**. In the present study, the signal pathways involved in NO formation and iNOS expression in RAW264.7 macrophages stimulated by LTA were investigated. **Matreials and methods**. We compared the relative inhibitory activities and mechanisms of PMC, a novel potent antioxidant of α -tocopherol derivatives, with those of YC-1, an sGC activator, on the induction of iNOS expression by LTA in cultured macrophages *in vitro* and LTA-induced hypotension *in vivo*. **Results and conclusions**. LTA induced concentration (0.1-50 µg/mL)- and time (4-24 h)-dependent increases in nitrite (an indicator of NO biosynthesis) in macrophages. Both PMC (50 µM) and YC-1 (10 µM) inhibited NO production, iNOS protein, mRNA expression, and IκBα degradation upon stimulation by LTA (20 µg/mL) in macrophages. On the other hand, PMC (50 µM) almost completely suppressed JNK/SAPK activation, whereas YC-1 (10 µM) only partially inhibited its activation in LTA-stimulated macrophages. Moreover, PMC (10 mg/kg, *i.v.*) and YC-1 (5 mg/kg, *i.v.*) significantly inhibited the fall in MAP stimulated by LTA (10 mg/kg, *i.v.*) in rats. In conclusion, we demonstrate that YC-1 shows more-potent activity than PMC at abrogating the expression of iNOS in macrophages *in vitro* and reversing delayed hypotension in rats with endotoxic shock stimulated by LTA. The inhibitory mechanisms of PMC may be due to its antioxidative properties, with a resulting influence on JNK/SAPK and NF-□B activations. YC-1 may be mediated by increasing cyclic GMP, followed by, at least partly, inhibition of JNK/SAPK and NF-□B activations, thereby leading to inhibition of iNOS expression.

PO065

An improved assay for the enumeration of circulating endothelial cells

Woywodt A, Goldberg C, Scheer J, Regelsberger H, Haller H, Haubitz M*

Division of Nephrology, Hannover Medical School

Introduction: Circulating endothelial cells have been established as markers of vascular disease, such as small-vessel vasculitis, acute vascular rejection in renal transplant recipients and cyclosporine-induced endothelial damage. Enumeration of these cells by immunomagnetic isolation and acridine staining remains the gold standard but necessitates considerable experience and expenditure. A simpler test would therefore be of great utility. **Aim**: to develop an improved simple assay to enumerate endothelial cells in peripheral blood. **Materials and Methods**: We studied the use of immunomagnetic isolation and a variety of subsequent stains, such as CD 31 and von Willebrand factor (vWF) immunocytochemistry and lectin stains using Ulex Europaeus lectin 1 (UEA-1). **Results and conclusions**: We devised a simple protocol for immunomagnetic isolation with subsequent UEA-1 lectin stain. We evaluated the use of this protocol in parallel to immunomagnetic isolation and acridine counting alone in 92 renal transplant recipients who underwent renal biopsy. Recovery of various concentrations of human umbilical vein endothelial cells from blood was also studied. Immunomagnetic isolation and subsequent UEA-1 staining permits reliable enumeration of circulating endothelial cells in peripheral blood. The assay is simple and easy to use, thus allowing for a more widespread use of circulating endothelial cells as a marker of vascular damage.

PO066

Circulating endothelial cells as a marker of endothelial damage in allogeneic hematopoietic stem-cell transplantation

Woywodt A (1), Scheer J (1,2), Hambach L (2), Buchholz S (2), Ganser A (2), Haller H (1), Hertenstein B (2), Haubitz M (1)*

(1) Division of Nephrology, Hannover Medical School
(2) Division of Haematology/Haemostaseology/Oncology, Hannover Medical School

Introduction: Damage to endothelial cells is the common feature of vascular disorders associated with hematopoietic stem-cell transplantation (HSCT). Elevated numbers of circulating endothelial cells reflect the extent of endothelial damage in a variety of disorders **Aim**: To investigate the role of circulating endothelial cells in HSCT **Materials and Methods**: We studied 39 patients undergoing allogeneic HSCT with different conditioning regimens and 22 healthy controls. Circulating endothelial cells were enumerated with immunomagnetic isolation during the course of HSCT. **Results and conclusions**: After conditioning, cell numbers were significantly elevated (median 44 cells/ml) compared to baseline (median 16 cells/ml) and controls (median 8 cells/ml). Patients who received radiation had an earlier peak when compared to patients with chemotherapy. Patients with reduced intensity conditioning had significantly lower cell numbers (median 24 cells/ml) than those who received standard conditioning. These observations provide a novel marker to investigate microvascular endothelial damage and the effects of different conditioning regimens in patients undergoing HSCT.

PO067

Assessment of endothelial damage in atherosclerotic vascular disease by quatification of circulating endothelial cells

Blann AD, Makin A, Chung N, Silverman S, Lip G*

Dept of Medicine, City Hospital, Birmingham, UK

Background *In*creased numbers of CD146-defined circulating endothelial cells (CECs), as are present in the peripheral blood of patients suffering acute coronary syndromes, imply injury to the endothelium. Endothelial damage can also be assessed by the measurement of plasma levels of von Willebrand factor (vWf). Increased levels of procoagulant plasma Tissue Factor (TF), arising from monocytes/macrophages and endothelial cells, is present in atherosclerosis. We hypothesised increased CECs in patients with ischaemic rest pain (IRP) of the lower limb due to peripheral atherosclerosis and comparable to that seen in patients with acute myocardial infarction (AMI), when compared to patients with intermittent claudication (IC) or healthy controls that would correlate with vWf and TF. **Patients and Methods** We recruited 20 patients in each of four groups: (i) IRP of the lower limb; (ii) AMI; (iii) 'stable' IC; and (iv) healthy controls. CD146-expressing CECs were measured by immumomagnetic separation and counting under a fluorescence microscope; plasma vWf and TF by ELISA. **Results** In IRP, median (IQR) CEC levels were 3.5 (2.0-5.8) cells/ml, in IC were 1.1 (0.6-2.9) cells/ml, and in healthy controls were 1.0 (0.5-1.7) cells/ml ($p<0.001$). The levels of vWf ($p=0.034$) and TF ($p=0.007$) were also significantly different between the groups, with the highest levels in patients with IRP. Levels of CECs correlated with vWf ($r_s=0.4$, $p=0.002$) and TF ($r_s=0.296$, $p=0.021$). In AMI, CEC levels were higher than those in IRP at 4.9 (3.6-8.4) cells/ml ($p=0.0385$). **Conclusion** This study demonstrates evidence of direct endothelial cell injury (i.e. raised CECs) in patients with IRP that correlated with vWf and TF, but that this is less severe than in AMI.

PO068

Hemorheology, hemostasis and antiaggregate activity of endothelium in patients with borderline hypertension

Maximova M (1), Ionova V (1), Suslina Z (1), Tanashian M (1), Lutova L (2), Karabasova M (2)*

(1) Institute of Neurology of Russian Academy of Medical Sciences; Moscow, Russia
(2) Moscow State University; Moscow, Russia

It is likely that factors other than increased blood pressure contribute to the residual risk of cerebrovascular complications in essential hypertension. **The aim** of our study was to evaluate the hemorheological and hemostasis alterations and functional activity of endothelium in patients with borderline hypertension (AH). **Materials and methods**: We studied 37 patients with BH (age, 28 to 45 years). The hypertensive group had SBP 140-160 mm Hg and/or DBP 85 to 95 mm Hg. In all patients were performed MRI and DS extra- and intracranial arteries. We evaluated the following parameters of blood: total blood viscosity (BV), red blood cell agregability (RBCA), red blood cell deformability (RBCD), platelet aggregation (PA) and prostanoids (TxA_2, PGI_2 by detecting stable analogues of this substances – 6-keto$PGF_{1\alpha}$ and TxB_2), hematocrit (Ht), fibrinogen (FG), ATIII, PrC, PrS, tissue-type plasminogen activator (t-PA) antigen and plasminogen activator inhibitor (PAI-1) antigen, fibrinolytic activity and time of lysis euglobulin fraction (FAEF and TLEF), D-dimer (D-d), resoluble complex fibrin monomer (RCFM). Antiaaggregative reserve of the vascular wall was assessed with the help of «cuff»-test. **Results**: In the patients with BH there were increased following parameters: BV (10 c^{-1}), RBCA, TxA_2, PGI_2, t-PA and there were decreased RBCD, ratio of PGI_2/TxA_2. There were no significant differences in PA, Ht, FG, ATIII, PrC, PrS, FAEF, TLEF, RCFM, D-d and PAI-1 antigen. The functional «cuff»-test demonstrated insufficiency of antiaggregative potential of the vascular wall in patients with BH, since PA, PGI_2, ratio of PGI_2/TxA_2 after was unchanged. Some patients had an inverted response, characterized by elevation of aggregate activity of platelets. **Conclusion**: The obtained results are significant for a better understanding of hemorheological and hemostat mechanisms that disturb the microcirculation during development of the BH.

PO069

Gene expression profiling of endothelial cells from normal and systemic sclerosis patients

Giusti B (2), Fibbi G (1), Rossi L (2), D'Alessio S (1), Poggi F (2), Margheri F (1), Del Rosso A (1), Matucci-Cerinic M (1), Abbate R (2), Del Rosso M (1)*

(1) Department of Medical and Surgical Critical Area; Department of Experimental Pathology and Oncology;
(2) Department of Medical and Surgical Critical Area; Thrombosis Centre, University of Florence, Azienda

Systemic sclerosis (SSc) is a clinically heterogeneous, systemic disorder which affects the connective tissue of the skin, internal organs and the walls of blood vessels. Defective angiogenesis resulting in tissue ischemia is prominent in the diffuse form of SSc, but its pathogenetic basis is unknown. **Aims**: We isolated microvascular endothelial cells (MVEC) from the dermis of healthy individuals (N-MVEC) and patients with diffuse SSc (SSc-MVEC) in order to identify differences in the gene expression profiling. For this purpose we used a 14,000 gene oligonucleotide array (70-mers oligonucleotide, Operon technologies). Total RNA was isolated from cultured MVEC by RNeasy Kit (QIAGEN). Pooling of MVEC total RNA from patients and controls was performed. One hundred and ninety nine genes showed altered expression levels between SSc-MVEC and N-MVEC: 153 were up regulated and 46 were down regulated. More than 25 of the genes (e.g. MIF, LAMR1, IL-8, CTGF, CFL1, PEA15, PGAR, KLKs, PLAT, PLAU, etc), which were differentially expressed in SSc-MVEC are directly or indirectly involved with angiogenesis. Interestingly, in contrast with the clinical data indicating a vascular desert-like pattern, many proangiogenetic genes were found to be over-expressed in SSc. These results suggest that an epigenetic event, which occurs in SSc, may be able to vanish the angiogenic attitude of MVEC. Preliminary data indicate that the truncation of the urokinase-plasminogen activator receptor (uPAR) in SSc-MVEC may account, at least in part, for defective angiogenesis.

PO070

Comparison of platelets' and endothelium function between diabetics and normal subjects

Makris P (1), Koukourikou M (3), Girtovitis F (1), Boutou A (1), Giannoulis E (2), Pithara E (1), Spartali A (1), Karamitsos D (3)*

(1) Haemostasis and Thrombosis Unit, A' Propedeutic Clinic, AHEPA, Aristotle University of Thessaloniki,
(2) Department of Diabetology, A' Pathologic Clinic, AHEPA, Aristotle University of Thessaloniki, Greece
(3) Department of Diabetology, B' Propedeutic Clinic, Ippokrateio Hospital, Aristotle University o

Introduction: Type I diabetes is a life long metabolic disorder that initiates in young ages and can lead to serious complications, affecting the blood vessels of the whole body, where it induces atherosclerosis. **Aim:** The aim of this study is to investigate into a) the function of platelets and b) the functional state of blood vessels' endothelium in diabetic patients. **Material-Methods:** We studied 58 patients with type I diabetes (D), 30 normal subjects (control group1-CG1) in order to compare the function of their platelets with the one of the diabetics and 20 normal subjects (control group 2-CG2) in order to compare their plasma levels of thrombomodoulin (TM) and Willebrand factor (vWFAg) with the ones of the diabetics. We evaluated the aggregation of platelets with 4 stimulators: Ristosetine (RISTO), ADP, Collagen (COLLA) and Adrenaline (ADR), using the PICA® aggregometer of Chronolog co, and following directly the instructions for use given by its manufacturer. TM and vWFAg were determined using an immunoenzymatic method (ELISA). **Results:** The results are recorded in Table I

Table I: Mean Values (MV) and Standard Deviations (SD) all of the determined haemostatic parameters both in patients and in control groups.

	RISTO	ADP	COLLA	ADR	vWFAg	TM
	%	%	%	%	%	Mg/ml
D: MV	71.04	65.2	63.7	45.5	106.2	5.2
SD	13.3	19.4	27.6	29.7	25.2	5.7
CG1,2: MV	89.7[1]	78.8[1]	83.3[1]	79.8[1]	119.6[2]	3.7[2]
SD	11.8[1]	6.01[1]	9.6[1]	6.4[1]	20.3[2]	0.9[2]

Conclusions: 1) The comparison of MV between normal subjects and diabetics did not reveal any statistical significant difference. 2) However, in 8 out of 58 diabetics there were extremely high levels of TM; this fact together with the clinical manifestation of complications (diabetic nephropathy, neuropathy or retinopathy) in those patients implies a modification of the function of their endothelium.

PO071

The evaluation of disfunction of endothelium in patients with hypertensive small deep infarcts

Maximova M, Suslina Z, Ionova V, Tanashian M*

Institute of Neurology of Russian Academy of Medical Sciences, Moscow, Russia

Of late, the role of disfunction of endothelium in the pathogenesis of the cerebrovascular diseases has been widely discussed. The aim of the study was the assessment of the antiagregation potential of the vascular wall in patients with hypertensive small deep infarcts (SDI). **Materials and methods**: 80 patients with SDI in the carotid system due to hypertension were under study, mean age 60.9 ± 8.9 years. MRI verified the diagnosis. Laboratory investigations were made on the 1st day of the lacunar stroke. All data were compared with those of 20 healthy persons. Platelet aggregation (PA) was assessed by method suggested by Born. ADP was used as the indicator of PA in concentration 1.2 mkM. The evaluation of PGI_2 and TxA_2 concentrations was carried out with the use of radioimmune analysis by detecting stable analogues of this substances – 6-keto PGF_{1a} and TxB_2. Antiaaggregative reserve of the vascular wall was assessed with the help of «cuff»-test. **Results**: In the patients with hypertensive SDI ADP induced PA slightly increased in comparison the healthy subjects. The level of prostaglandins was different due to decrease of PGI_2 ($p<0.01$). The ratio of PGI_2/TxA_2 was reduced ($p<0.01$) that is the predominant of proaggregant components of prostanoid system took place. The functional test showed lack of reaction of the vascular wall since PA, PGI_2 and ratio of PGI_2/TxA_2 after «cuff»-test was unchanged. Some patients had an inverted response, characterized by elevation of aggregate activity of platelets. Thus, we conclude that our study has demonstrated insufficiency of antiaggregative potential of the vascular wall in patients with hypertensive SDI.

PO072

The influence of melagatran on thrombin generation, comparison with other anticoagulant drugs

Al Dieri R, Hemker H, Béguin S*

Synapse BV, Cardiovascular Research Institute (CARIM), Maastricht University, Maastricht, Netherland

Introduction All antithrombotics influence thrombin-generation, anticoagulants in both PPP and PRP, antiplatelet agents in PRP only. The influence on area under the curve (ETP), peak height and lag-phase is not identical for different drugs. Direct thrombin inhibitors significantly prolong the lag time because they inhibit the feedback activation by thrombin. **Aim** We wanted to compare the effect on thrombin generation of reversible (melagatran) and an irreversible (hirudin) thrombin inhibition and compare it to that of other anticoagulant drugs, both as to its effect on thrombin generation in PPP and PRP as to the interindividual variation. **Material and methods** In vitro addition of anticoagulant drugs melagatran, hirudin, different heparin(-likes) to pooled and individual plasmas and measuring calibrated automated thrombin generation as described in Pathophysiology of Haemostasis and Thrombosis Vol: 33 (2003) pp 4-15. **Results and conclusions** Because of its immediate irreversible binding hirudin does not significantly affect the ETP unless at doses equivalent to the concentration of prothrombin in plasma, whereas the reversible inhibitor melagatran simultaneously inhibits the ETP and prolongs the lag-time. In this respect it resembles the effect of oral anticoagulation. In PRP, melagatran also inhibits thrombin mediated feedback activation of platelets. Platelets release PF4, which does not affect melagatran action but strongly dampens the effect of unfractionated heparin and also attenuates that of low molecular weight heparins. The interindividual variation of the uninhibited ETP (CV= 15-19%) is high as compared to the intra-individual variation (CV= 4.5-7.5%) and the experimental error (CV<3%). This strongly suggests that standard dosage of any anticoagulant will not result in a standard effect. This conclusion is reinforced by the observation that the interindividual variation in the anticoagulant response to heparins is high as well. It can be expected that drugs that influence thrombin itself- and not the physiological mechanisms that make thrombin appear and disappear will show less interindividual variation.

PO073

Melagatran is efficiently eliminated by hemodialysis in uremic patients

Eriksson UG (1), Samuelsson O (2), Attman PO (2), Lepkowska M (1), Ohlsson L (1), Carlsson S (1), Fager G (1)

(1) AstraZeneca R&D Mölndal, Mölndal, Sweden
(2) Sahlgrenska University Hospital, Göteborg, Sweden

Introduction: Melagatran is the active form of the oral direct thrombin inhibitor ximelagatran, developed for the prevention and treatment of thromboembolic disorders. Renal excretion is the major route of elimination for systemic melagatran. **Aim**: The efficiency of melagatran elimination via hemodialysis in uremic patients was investigated. **Methods**: Uremic patients (glomerular filtration rate <8 ml/min; n=10) on chronic hemodialysis received melagatran 1 mg as an intravenous bolus during a dialysis session and also while not undergoing dialysis. To assess the elimination of melagatran via hemodialysis, pharmacokinetic parameters of melagatran during dialysis were compared with those between dialysis sessions. **Results**: Between dialysis sessions, mean±SD melagatran area under the concentration-time curve (AUC) and maximum plasma concentration were 2.79±0.91 μmol·h/l and 0.49±0.28 μmol/l, respectively. The corresponding values for melagatran administered during the dialysis session were 0.33±0.04 μmol·h/l and 0.17±0.04 μmol/l, respectively. Melagatran was rapidly excreted during hemodialysis with a 7-fold higher clearance than that observed between dialysis sessions. Mean±SD clearance of melagatran between dialysis sessions was 0.93±0.36 l/h compared with 7.20±0.76 l/h during the dialysis session. Mean±SD half-life was 14.1±3.7 h between dialysis sessions compared with 2.0±0.3 h during the dialysis session. The mean dialysis clearance for the 8 patients having data both between dialysis sessions and during the dialysis session was 104±10 ml/min. Melagatran was well tolerated, with no adverse events that were suspected to be causally related to the study drug. **Conclusion**: The elimination of melagatran is accelerated by hemodialysis in uremic patients.

PO074

No influence of food on the pharmacokinetics, pharmacodynamics, or tolerability of the 36mg oral tablet formulation of ximelagatran

Ersdal E, Schutzer K, Eriksson UG, Lönnerstedt C, Ohlsson L, Wall U*

AstraZeneca R&D Mölndal, Mölndal, Sweden

Introduction: Ximelagatran—an oral direct thrombin inhibitor that is rapidly converted to its active form, melagatran—is being developed for the prevention and treatment of thromboembolic disease. It is anticipated that a 36mg bid dose will be introduced for clinical use; therefore, a 36mg tablet of commercial composition was tested in this food interaction study. **Aim**: The potential effects of food on the pharmacokinetics, pharmacodynamics, and tolerability/safety of ximelagatran given as a single 36mg oral tablet were assessed in an open, randomised, 3-way crossover study. **Methods**: Healthy volunteers (n=50; mean age 27 years, male/female ratio 27/23, mean weight 70 kg) received 3 treatments separated by 2- to 14-day washout periods. The 3 treatments were a single 36mg ximelagatran oral tablet under fasting conditions, a single 36mg ximelagatran oral tablet after a high-fat and high-calorie breakfast, and a single oral dose of ximelagatran 36 mg solution under fasting conditions. **Results**: The 90% confidence intervals (CIs) and least squares mean estimates for the ratio of ximelagatran oral tablet given with food to ximelagatran oral tablet given under fasting conditions fell within the predefined bounds demonstrating no interaction for area under the melagatran concentration-time curve (AUC; 1.07 [90% CI, 1.03–1.11]) and maximum plasma concentration (C_{max}; 1.05 [90% CI, 0.98–1.12]). In addition, food did not alter the melagatran-induced prolongation of the activated partial thromboplastin time of ximelagatran. The relative bioavailability of melagatran for the tablet formulation versus oral solution given under fasting conditions demonstrated equivalent bioavailability (AUC 0.98 [90% CI, 0.94–1.01]) and maximum plasma concentration (0.97 [90% CI, 0.91–1.04]). Ximelagatran 36mg was well tolerated regardless of whether it was taken with food or under fasting conditions. No serious adverse events or adverse events judged to be caused by study medication were reported. No clinically significant laboratory abnormalities or changes in vital signs were observed. **Conclusion**: The pharmacokinetics, pharmacodynamics, and tolerability/safety of the oral 36mg ximelagatran tablet are not affected by food.

PO075

Efficacy and safety of postoperative ximelagatran for prevention of thromboembolism across different orthopaedic surgery patient groups

Dahl OE (1), Eriksson BI (2), Agnelli G (3), Cohen AT (4), Mouret P (5), Rosencher N (6), Panfilov S (7), Andersson M (7)*

(1) Department of Orthopaedics, Section for Joint Implants and Medical Science, Buskerud Central Hospita
(2) Sahlgrenska University Hospital/Östra, Göteborg, Sweden
(3) University of Perugia, Perugia, Italy
(4) Guy's, King's and St Thomas' School of Medicine and Dentistry, London, UK
(5) Frankfurt-Höchst Clinic, Frankfurt, Germany
(6) Cochin University Hospital, Paris, France
(7) AstraZeneca R&D Mölndal, Mölndal, Sweden

Introduction: Ximelagatran (Exanta™, AstraZeneca) is an oral direct thrombin inhibitor for the prevention and treatment of venous thromboembolic events (VTE). In the METHRO III study, postoperative subcutaneous (sc) melagatran 3 mg (active form of ximelagatran), followed by oral ximelagatran (24 mg bid), showed comparable efficacy to sc enoxaparin (40 mg od) in reducing total VTE, proximal deep vein thrombosis (DVT) and/or pulmonary embolism (PE) in patients undergoing total hip (THR) or knee replacement (TKR) surgery (1). Proximal DVT is of high clinical significance because of its potential to cause subsequent PE. It is recommended that proximal DVT be a primary endpoint in non-inferiority studies comparing anticoagulant agents for the prevention of VTE (2). **Aims**: A subgroup analysis was conducted on the intention-to-treat population to examine the efficacy and safety of the drug regimen in patients with different risks of either VTE or bleeding complications (gender, age > 65 years, obesity, reduced creatinine clearance, general anaesthesia, or type of surgery). **Methods**: The incidence of each binary outcome variable (proximal DVT/PE, severe bleeding, blood transfusion) was assessed by the above factors of potential prognostic significance in a logistic regression model, controlling for treatment, factor, and interaction between these. **Results**: No statistically significant interactions were found between treatment and potential prognostic factors for any of the efficacy variables (including the risk of proximal

DVT/PE), or for the risk of severe bleeding. The risk of blood transfusion was lower with ximelagatran than with enoxaparin (61.8% vs 66.2%, respectively; P = 0.016). **Conclusions**: The efficacy and safety of postoperatively initiated prophylactic treatment with sc melagatran followed by oral ximelagatran was consistent across different subgroups of orthopaedic surgery patients, suggesting that ximelagatran may be a useful alternative to the standard European regimen of enoxaparin in a wide range of patients. 1. Eriksson BI, Agnelli G, Cohen AT, Dahl OE, et al. Thromb Haemost. 2003;89:288-96. 2. Committee for Proprietary Medicinal Products, European Agency for the Evaluation of Medicinal Products. http://www.emea.eu.int/pdfs/human/ewp/070798en.pdf.

PO076

Effect of the oral, direct Factor Xa inhibitor, BAY 59-7939, on thrombin generation after tissue factor pathway activation

Gerotziafas G (1,2), Depasse F (2), Chakroun T (1), Elalamy I (1), Samama M (1,2)*

(1) Service d'Hématologie Biologique, Hôpital Hôtel-Dieu de Paris, France
(2) LCL Laboratory, Ivry sur Seine, France

Introduction: Factor Xa (FXa) is central to the blood coagulation process. Free FXa is thought to be responsible for generation of the first trace amounts of thrombin. FXa bound to prothrombinase induces the propagation phase of thrombin generation. Inhibition of FXa is an emerging strategy for the development of new antithrombotics, and new specific antithrombin-dependent and direct FXa inhibitors are being developed. **Aim:** To investigate the effect of BAY 59-7939 – an oral, direct Factor Xa inhibitor – on the inhibition of thrombin generation (TG) after triggering the tissue factor (TF) pathway in platelet-poor plasma (PPP) and platelet-rich plasma (PRP) of healthy human volunteers. **Methods:** The following parameters were studied: lag time (LT) of TG onset (min), time to peak (T_{max}; min), thrombin peak (C_{max}; nM) and endogenous thrombin potential (ETP; nM·min). TG was stimulated in the presence of a low concentration of TF that may have physiological relevance (1/1000 final dilution; Hemoliance® Recombiplastin, Instrumentation Laboratory, Italy) in both PRP and PPP. Plasma was spiked with BAY 59-7939 (Bayer HealthCare AG, Germany) at concentrations ranging from 0.0025 to 1 µM. TG was measured by the cleavage of a fluorogenic substrate (Z-Gly-Gly-Arg-AMC) using a Fluorimeter (Ascent, Thermolabsystem) and the Thrombinoscope™ software (Synapse, Maastricht). PPP and PRP were obtained from seven healthy volunteers. PRP platelet count was adjusted to 300 000/µl using homologous PPP. **Results:** In both PRP and PPP, BAY 59-7939 significantly inhibited TG. BAY 59-7939 prolonged LT and T_{max}, and reduced C_{max} and ETP in a concentration-dependent manner. All parameters were similarly affected in PRP and PPP. In the presence of 25 nM BAY 59-7939, LT and T_{max} were doubled, compared with the control. C_{max} was reduced with an IC_{50} value of 25 nM. Nearly complete reduction (90%) was achieved at 50 nM BAY 59-7939. The ETP was similarly inhibited with an IC_{50} value of 25 nM. The maximum decrease of the ETP obtained was 90% in the presence of 80 nM BAY 59-7939. **Conclusions:** This study clearly demonstrates that the direct FXa inhibitor BAY 59-7939 prolonged the initiation phase of TG and potently reduced TG occurring via the TF pathway in human PPP or PRP plasma. The results indicate that BAY 59-7939 is a promising antithrombotic drug that merits further investigation.

PO077

Studies on the mechanism of action of BAY 59-7939 – an oral, direct Factor Xa inhibitor

Fareed J (1), Hoppensteadt D (1), Maddenini J (1), Schultz C (1), Nevelle B (1), Iqbal O (1), Perzborn E (2), Misselwitz F (3)*

(1) Department of Pathology, Loyola University Medical Center, Maywood, Illinois, USA
(2) Cardiovascular Research, Bayer HealthCare AG, Wuppertal, Germany
(3) Global Medical Development, Bayer HealthCare AG, Wuppertal, Germany

Introduction: Currently, several Factor Xa inhibitors are in development. Despite comparable inhibitory actions on Factor Xa, these agents exhibit distinct effects on global clotting, antiprotease, and protease-generation assays. BAY 59-7939 is an oral, direct Factor Xa inhibitor in clinical development for the prevention and treatment of thromboembolic disorders. **Aim:** To study the mechanism of action of BAY 59-7939 in the inhibition of Factor Xa and thrombin generation (TG). **Methods:** The effects of BAY 59-7939 were assessed using plasma-based tests (PT, aPTT, HepTest, thrombin time and Russell's viper venom time). To investigate the relative effects of this agent on the generation of Factor Xa and thrombin in plasma-based systems, a modified method utilizing diluted fibrinogen-deficient plasma with thromboplastin (extrinsic) and ellagic acid (intrinsic) was used. Activation processes were measured kinetically, employing substrates specific for Factor Xa and thrombin. **Results:** BAY 59-7939 produced a concentration-dependent anticoagulant effect in all tests except the thrombin time, suggesting that, via inhibition of Factor Xa, BAY 59-7939 interacts with multiple sites in the coagulation cascade. In the extrinsic pathway, BAY 59-7939 strongly inhibited Factor Xa generation, with an IC_{50} of 0.14 µM, and an IC_{50} for TG of 0.28 µM. In the intrinsic system, BAY 59-7939 inhibited Factor Xa with an IC_{50} of 0.44 µM, and an IC_{50} of 0.32 µM for TG. These observations clearly indicate that BAY 59-7939 inhibited not only formed Factor Xa, but also its generation. These effects of BAY 59-7939 were independent of antithrombin III and heparin cofactor II. BAY 59-7939 also had anticoagulant effects on native normal human blood, as measured by activated clotting time and thromboelastographic methods. At concentrations up to 23 µM, BAY 59-7939 did not have any effect on agonist-induced aggregation (epinephrine, ADP, collagen, and arachidonic acid); however, it blunted the tissue factor-mediated activation of platelets in whole blood, as shown by flow cytometry. In the same system, BAY 59-7939 also inhibited the generation of prothrombin fragment $F_{1.2}$ (IC_{50} = 16.3 µM) and FPA (IC_{50} = 11.7 µM). **Conclusion:** These studies suggest that BAY 59-7939 modulates protease generation and the amplification processes in the control of thrombogenesis by mechanisms that are distinct from those described for other Factor Xa inhibitors.

PO078

Effects of BAY 59-7939, an innovative, oral, direct factor Xa inhibitor, on thrombin generation in healthy volunteers

Harder S (1), Graff J (1), v. Hentig N (1), Misselwitz F (2), Kubitza D (3), Zuehlsdorf M (3), Wensing G (3), Mueck W (3), Becka M (4), Breddin HK (5)*

(1) Institute of Clinical Pharmacology, University Hospital, Frankfurt am Main, Germany
(2) Global Medical Development, Bayer HealthCare AG, Wuppertal, Germany
(3) Institute of Clinical Pharmacology, Bayer HealthCare AG, Wuppertal, Germany
(4) Department of Biometry, Pharmacometry, Bayer HealthCare AG, Wuppertal, Germany
(5) International Institute of Thrombosis and Vascular Diseases, Frankfurt am Main, Germany

Introduction: BAY 59-7939 is an oral, direct Factor Xa inhibitor in development for the prevention and treatment of thromboembolic diseases. Factor Xa inhibitors exert their antithrombotic effects through inhibition of thrombin generation (TG). **Aim**: To evaluate the effect of BAY 59-7939 on TG in healthy subjects. **Method**: In this placebo-controlled, randomized, crossover study, 12 healthy volunteers received a single 5 mg or 30 mg dose of BAY 59-7939. Several assays were used to measure TG, including endogenous thrombin potential (ETP), platelet-induced thrombin-generation time (PITT) and platelet-induced clotting time (PICT). ETP is based on the cleavage of a chromogenic substrate by thrombin after ex vivo stimulation of platelet-rich plasma (PRP) by tissue factor (TF) (1.4 nM) or collagen (5 µg/mL). In contrast to ETP, no activator is used in the PITT assay, in which aggregation and coagulation of PRP are photometrically recorded in a rotating plastic cuvette in the presence of low concentrations (0.1 µg/mL) of hirudin. The PICT assay in platelet-poor plasma uses Russell's viper venom to activate TG via the Factor Xa pathway. **Results**: BAY 59-7939 exhibited dose-dependent inhibition of TG both in platelets and plasma, using either extrinsic (TF) or intrinsic (collagen) stimuli for platelet activation. A single 30 mg dose exerted a sustained effect on TG for up to 24 hours. Factor Xa was inhibited dose dependently after administration of BAY 59-7939. Maximum inhibition, observed 2 hours after drug administration, was 28% and 56% for the 5 mg and 30 mg doses, respectively. ETP was reduced significantly from baseline by 5 mg and 30 mg BAY 59-7939; the maximal effect was achieved at 2–4 hours. Significant prolongation of PITT was produced by the 30 mg dose and was sustained over 12 hours; maximal prolongation of 4-fold from baseline was observed 2–4 hours after administration. PICT was prolonged significantly by 5 mg and 30 mg BAY 59-7939, with maximal effect observed 2 hours after administration. PICT was prolonged over 12 hours with both doses. There was close correlation between BAY 59-7939 plasma concentrations and inhibition of Factor Xa activity, as well as with decreases in ETP; the correlation was modest with PITT. BAY 59-7939 had no effect on the actual thrombin content of the plasma. **Conclusion**: These data suggest that BAY 59-7939 effectively inhibits TG via both intrinsic and extrinsic pathways.

PO079

Biochemical and pharmacologic properties of BAY 59-7939, an oral, direct factor Xa inhibitor

Perzborn E (1), Strassburger J (1), Wilmen A (1), Lampe T (2), Pernerstorfer J (2), Pohlmann J (2), Roehrig S (2), Schlemmer K (3), Straub A (2)*

(1) Cardiovascular Research, Bayer HealthCare AG, Wuppertal, Germany
(2) Chemical Research, Bayer HealthCare AG, Wuppertal, Germany
(3) Preclinical Pharmacokinetics, Bayer HealthCare AG, Wuppertal, Germany

Introduction: BAY 59-7939 is an oral, direct Factor Xa (FXa) inhibitor in development for the prevention and treatment of thromboembolic diseases. **Aims:** To evaluate the biochemical properties of BAY 59-7939 in purified systems and plasma, and its effects on coagulation assays and platelet aggregation *in vitro*. **Results:** BAY 59-7939 inhibited human FXa with a K_i of 0.4±0.02 nM, and showed selectivity of more than 10 000-fold over thrombin, Factor VII, Factor IX, Factor XI, plasmin, urokinase, activated protein C, and trypsin. Kinetic studies demonstrated that BAY 59-7939 is a competitive inhibitor of human FXa. In a coupled enzyme assay measuring conversion of prothrombin to thrombin, using platelets as the phospholipid source, BAY 59-7939 blocked thrombin generation with an IC_{50} of 2.1±0.4 nM. In human plasma, FXa activated by Russell's viper venom, was inhibited with an IC_{50} of 21±1 nM. In rabbit plasma, the IC_{50} value of 21±2 nM was similar to that in human plasma, but 10-fold higher concentrations were needed in rat plasma (IC_{50} = 290±18 nM). The anticoagulant effect was compared in human, rabbit and rat plasma. BAY 59-7939 prolonged both prothrombin time (PT) and activated partial thromboplastin time (aPTT) in a concentration-dependant manner; its effect on PT was more pronounced than on aPTT. The concentrations required for doubling PT were 0.23±0.02 μM (human), 0.12±0.01μM (rabbit) and 0.3±0.02 μM (rat). The concentrations required for doubling aPTT were 0.69±0.09 μM (human), 1.97±0.49 μM (rabbit), and 2.09±0.19 μM (rat). Doubling of thrombin time (TT) was observed only at 26±1 μM in human plasma, indicating that BAY 59-7939 is highly selective against thrombin. BAY 59-7939 did not impair platelet function in platelet-rich plasma. Neither γ-thrombin-, collagen-, U46619-, ADP-, nor TRAP-6 (thrombin receptor activated peptide)-induced platelet aggregation were affected. **Conclusions:** These data show that BAY 59-7939 is a highly selective and potent FXa inhibitor, and has potential for the prevention and treatment of thromboembolic diseases.

PO080

Multiple dose escalation study investigating BAY 59-7939 – an oral, direct factor Xa inhibitor – in healthy male subjects

Kubitza D (1), Becka M (2), Wensing G (1), Voith B (1), Zuehlsdorf M (1)*

(1) Institute of Clinical Pharmacology, Bayer HealthCare AG, Wuppertal, Germany
(2) Department of Biometry, Pharmacometry, Bayer HealthCare AG, Wuppertal, Germany

Introduction: BAY 59-7939 is an innovative, oral, direct Factor Xa inhibitor in development for the prevention and treatment of thromboembolic diseases. **Aim:** To evaluate the pharmacodynamics, safety, and pharmacokinetics of multiple doses of BAY 59-7939 in healthy male subjects. **Methods:** In this parallel-group, randomized, single-blind, placebo-controlled trial, 64 subjects received multiple oral doses of BAY 59-7939: 5 mg once daily, twice daily, or three-times daily, or 10 mg, 20 mg, or 30 mg twice daily for 5 days with food. Full profiles of all pharmacodynamic (PD) parameters (Factor Xa inhibition, PT, aPTT, HepTest) were performed on days 1 and 7. In addition to standard safety assessments, bleeding time was also measured. Pharmacokinetics were assessed using standard parameters. **Results:** At steady state of the highest dose, maximum Factor Xa inhibition was 70%, with maximal changes of PT up to 2.6 times the individual baseline value. Similarly, maximal changes from baseline peaked at 2.7 for HepTest and 1.7 for aPTT. There were no differences between the PD effects on day 1 versus day 7 at any dose step. Comparable profiles were observed for all PD parameters. Relevant changes in the PD parameters were still present after 12 hours. BAY 59-7939 inhibited Factor Xa activity in a dose-dependent manner, with maximum effects 2–3 hours after administration. Effects were maintained for 8–12 hours at the 5 mg dose, and ~12 hours at the 10, 20, and 30 mg doses. Standard safety parameters were unaffected and no signs or symptoms of bleeding were observed across the dose range. In addition, BAY 59-7939 did not affect bleeding time at any dose. A dose-proportional increase in AUC was seen after the first dose and at steady state. C_{max} was reached after 2.5–4 hours; the terminal half-life was 4–6 hours. No severe drug-related adverse effects were reported, and all other adverse events resolved by the end of treatment. There was no indication of undue accumulation of drug beyond steady state for all six-dose regimens. **Conclusions:** This study demonstrated that BAY 59-7939 has predictable dose-dependent pharmacodynamics and pharmacokinetics without signs or symptoms of bleeding. Oral administration of BAY 59-7939 was safe and well tolerated in doses up to 30 mg bid.

PO081

Single dose escalation study of BAY 59-7939 – an oral, direct factor Xa inhibitor – in healthy male subjects

Kubitza D (1), Becka M (2), Wensing G (1), Voith B (1), Zuehlsdorf M (1)*

(1) Institute of Clinical Pharmacology, Bayer HealthCare AG, Wuppertal, Germany
(2) Department of Biometry, Pharmacometry, Bayer HealthCare AG, Wuppertal, Germany

Introduction: BAY 59-7939 is an oral, direct Factor Xa inhibitor in development for the prevention and treatment of thromboembolic diseases. **Aim:** To evaluate the pharmacodynamics (PD), pharmacokinetics (PK), and safety of a single dose of BAY 59-7939 in healthy male subjects. **Methods:** In this single-blind, placebo-controlled, dose-escalation trial, 103 healthy men received 1.25–80.0 mg of BAY 59-7939 under fasting conditions as a tablet, or a 5 or 10 mg dose as an oral solution. Full PD profiles (Factor Xa inhibition, PT, aPTT, HepTest) were determined for 24 hours after drug administration. Bleeding-time evaluation and Rumpel–Leede test were also performed. PK were assessed using standard parameters. **Results:** All PD profiles were dose dependent; BAY 59-7939 showed a rapid onset of action, with maximal inhibitory effects observed after 45 minutes with the solution and after 1–2 hours with the tablet. At the highest dose (80 mg), maximum Factor Xa inhibition was 60%, and maximal changes of PT were up to double the individual baseline values. Individual maximal changes from baseline in HepTest peaked at 2.3, and 1.5 for aPTT. Factor IIA and ATIII were not affected by BAY 59-7939. The inhibitory effect of BAY 59-7939 was almost completely reversed after 24 hours, and Factor Xa activity returned to within the normal range (0.7–1.2 U/mL) for doses up to 40 mg. PT prolongations also reverted to baseline after 24 hours. Standard safety parameters were unaffected, with no signs or symptoms of bleeding. Bleeding time was not prolonged at any dose. After administration of the oral solution, maximal plasma levels were observed after about 30 minutes, followed by a fairly rapid decline; the terminal half-life was 3–4 hours. Lower peak concentrations of approximately 50% were observed 2 hours after administration of the tablet, compared with the solution. However, the two formulations were comparable in terms of AUC. Increases in AUC and C_{max} were less than dose proportionate at higher tablet doses, likely due to incomplete absorption as a consequence of low solubility of the drug. PD and PK time profiles showed a close relationship, with a correlation coefficient between 0.6 and 0.9 depending on the parameters used. **Conclusions:** In this study, BAY 59-7939 was safe and well tolerated across a wide range of oral doses, with predictable dose-dependent PD and PK. These data suggest that BAY 59-7939 offers predictable anticoagulation with an excellent safety profile.

PO082

The oral direct thrombin inhibitor ximelagatran shows bioequivalence when administered as whole or crushed tablets or in solution via nasogastric tube

Schützer K (1), Lönnerstedt C (1), Wall U (1), Ohlsson L (1), Sarich T (2), Teng R (2), Eriksson UG (1)*

(1) AstraZeneca R&D Mölndal, Mölndal, Sweden
(2) AstraZeneca LP, Wilmington, DE, USA

Introduction: The oral direct thrombin inhibitor (oral DTI) ximelagatran (Exanta™, AstraZeneca) is currently under development for the prevention and treatment of thromboembolic disorders. Following oral administration, ximelagatran is rapidly absorbed and bioconverted to its active form, melagatran. In some patients, for instance those who are unable to swallow a tablet or swallow anything at all, it may be necessary to dose ximelagatran by a different method. **Aim**: To investigate if the pharmacokinetic profile of ximelagatran is affected by the alternative administrations of crushed or dissolved tablets compared to whole tablet. **Methods**: In an open, randomized, 3-period, 3-treatment, crossover study, healthy volunteers (n = 40; aged 20-50 years) received a single 36 mg, immediate-release ximelagatran tablet on 3 study days, separated by washout periods of 2 to 14 days. Tablets were: (I) swallowed whole, (II) crushed, mixed with apple sauce, and ingested, and (III) dissolved in water and administered via nasogastric tube. Plasma concentrations of melagatran were measured for determination of the area under the plasma concentration vs time curve (AUC) and maximum plasma concentration (Cmax) values. **Results**: Thirty-nine volunteers completed the study (n = 38 for treatment III). For melagatran the least-squares estimates (with 94% confidence interval [CI]) of the between-treatment ratios (crushed tablet: whole tablet and dissolved tablet: whole tablet) for AUC were 1.01 (0.965-1.06) and 0.970 (0.924-1.02), respectively; and for Cmax were 1.04 (0.972-1.11) and 1.02 (0.955-1.10), respectively. These ratios and their CIs were within the 94% CI predefined to demonstrate no pharmacokinetic interaction (0.80-1.25). The time to Cmax (tmax) of melagatran (~ 2 h) did not vary significantly with administration route. Ximelagatran was well tolerated, and tolerability was unaffected by administration route. **Conclusion**: The pharmacokinetics of the oral DTI ximelagatran as an immediate-release tablet were not significantly altered whether crushed and mixed with applesauce and given orally, or dissolved in water and given via nasosgastric tube.

PO083

The pharmacokinetics and pharmacodynamics of the oral direct thrombin inhibitor ximelagatran when administered with erythromycin

Dorani H (1), Schützer K (1), Sarich T (2), Wall U (1), Ohlsson L (1), Eriksson UG (1)*

(1) AstraZeneca R&D Mölndal, Mölndal, Sweden
(2) AstraZeneca LP, Wilmington, DE, USA

Introduction: Ximelagatran (Exanta™, AstraZeneca), an oral direct thrombin inhibitor for the prevention and treatment of thromboembolic disorders, is rapidly absorbed and bioconverted to its active form melagatran. The metabolism of ximelagatran is independent of CYP450 enzymes and hence it has a low potential for drug interactions. **Aim**: This study evaluated the effect of erythromycin on the pharmacokinetics (PK) and pharmacodynamics (PD) of melagatran. **Methods**: An open, sequential, single-centre study in healthy volunteers (n = 16; mean age 24 years, range 20-32 years) with ximelagatran 36 mg on Day 1, then erythromycin 500 mg tid on Days 2-5 followed by ximelagatran 36 mg plus erythromycin on the morning of Day 6 and a dose of erythromycin in the evening. Plasma concentrations of melagatran were measured for determination of the mean area under the plasma concentration vs time curve (AUC) and the maximum plasma concentration (Cmax) values. Time to Cmax (tmax) and terminal elimination half-life (t½) of melagatran were also determined. Activated partial thromboplastin time (aPTT) was also measured. **Results**: For melagatran, AUC and Cmax geometric mean ratios for combined therapy (Day 6) relative to monotherapy (Day 1) were 1.82 (90% confidence interval [CI], 1.64-2.01) and 1.74 (90% CI, 1.52-2.00), respectively, (n = 15), falling outside of the predefined bounds for no interaction (0.8-1.25 for AUC and 0.7-1.43 for Cmax). Geometric mean ratios for tmax and t½ of melagatran were 1.14 and 0.93, respectively. The erythromycin-associated elevation in plasma melagatran concentrations increased the peak aPTT prolongation from 41s to 44s (mean values). Ximelagatran was well tolerated alone, and in combination with erythromycin. **Conclusions**: This study showed evidence of a pharmacokinetic interaction between ximelagatran and erythromycin with respect to melagatran PK, which is being investigated, but only a small effect on aPTT.

PO084

Effect of malondialdehyde modified low density lipoproteins on platelet adhesion

Suttnar J, Otahalova E, Dyr JE, Cermak J*

Institute of Hematology and Blood Transfusion, Prague, Czech Republik

Low-density lipoproteins (LDL) affect the functions of blood cells and this plays an important role in atherosclerosis and its complications. Mounting evidence has shown that oxidized LDL (oxLDL) are involved in the early development of atherosclerosis through recruitment of monocyte-macrophages in vessel walls and accumulation of esterified cholesterol in the cells with the formation of foam cells. Lipoproteins are oxidatively modified by hydroxyl radicals produced by various systems (e.g. in the presence of transition metals) or modified by reactive aldehydes formed from oxidized lipids and lipoproteins. Since platelets also play a role in advanced atherosclerotis of blood vessels modified lipoproteins were tested on their ability to influence platelet functions. In the current study we have ivestigated the influence of native LDL, malondialdehyde (MDA) modified LDL, and LDL obtained from sera of patients overloaded with iron on platelet adhesion. LDL were isolated from human sera using a hydroxyapatite column (1). The purity of preparations was assessed by both agarose gel electrophoresis and SDS PAGE. MDA used for modification of LDL was obtained by acidic hydrolysis of tetraethoxypropane. MDA modification of LDL was measured by high-performance liquid chromatography method. Washed platelets in Tyrode's buffer were used for static adhesion studies performed according to the modified method of Bellavite (2). Agarose electrophoresis characterization of both LDL obtained from sera of iron overloaded patients and from MDA modified LDL's revealed that an increasing MDA content in lipoprotein led to increased relative electrophoretic mobility as compared with native LDL. It was probably due to blocking of free amino groups in lipoprotein species. The amount of adhered platelets on MDA modified LDL was enhanced and was dependent on a degree of MDA content via S-shaped saturation curve. These LDL's contained lower amounts of both witamin E and A as compared with normal LDL. The adhesion of platelets to LDL isolated from sera of patients overloaded with iron was also significantly enhanced as compared with native LDL. In this report we could demonstrate that both MDA modified LDL and LDL of iron overloaded patients enhanced platelet adhesion and thus exhibit proatherogenic potential with respect to platelet interaction. This work was supported by grants GACR 303/03/0249, IGA NA/7616-3, and VZ UHKT 237360001. References 1. Shibusazawa Y.: J. Chromatogr. 1997; 699: 419-37. 2. Bellavite P., Andrioli G., Guzzo P., Arigliano P., Chirumbolo S., Manzato F., Santonastaso S.: Anal. Biochem. 1994; 216: 444–50.

PO085

Lipoprotein (a) as a marker of diffuse coronary artery disease in young survivors of myocardial infarction

*Zorio E (1), Falcó C (2), Palencia M (1), Arnau MA (1), España F (2), Ramón L (2), España F (2), Castelló R (2), Almenar L (1), Estellés A (2)**

(1) Cardiology Department, Hospital Universitario La Fe, Valencia, Spain.
(2) Research Center, Hospital Universitario La Fe, Valencia. Spain.

Introduction: The establishment of biochemical markers of diffuse coronary lesions may improve the non-invasive risk stratification. High levels of lipoprotein(a) [Lp(a)] and small apolipoprotein(a) [apo(a)] isoforms have been found in patients with myocardial infarction (MI) and other locations of atherothrombosis but its association with diffuse coronary lesions remains controversial. **Aims:** The objective of the present study was to assess the usefulness of Lp(a) levels and apo(a) isoforms as markers of diffuse coronary disease and early MI. **Material and methods:** Lp(a) levels and apo(a) isoforms were determined in 119 (89% men) young MI survivors (under 51 years) and 135 matched healthy controls. The distributions of both parameters were analysed according to the number of coronary vessels diseased in the subgroup of patients without clinical atherosclerotic involvement of other arterial territories who underwent coronary angiography (79 patients). **Result:** Lp(a) levels and percentage of subjects with small apo(a) isoforms were higher in patients than in controls (median and range 11.0, 0.1-58.0 mg/dL versus 5.5, 0-35.0 mg/dL, $p<0.01$, respectively; percentage with small apo(a) isoform 30% versus 15%, $p<0.05$). Lp(a) levels>30mg/dL were more frequent among patients with 3-vessel disease than with 1- or 2-vessel disease (OR 4.3, $p<0.05$), normal or non-significant coronary lesions (OR 15.4, $p<0.05$) and controls (OR 31.4, $p<0.05$). No correlation was found between small apo(a) isoforms and the extension of coronary lesions. **Conclusions:** In young MI patients as the only expression of arterial disease, high levels of Lp(a) (specially>30mg/dL) may be a marker of diffuse coronary lesions. Our results suggest that high Lp(a) levels and the presence of small apo(a) isoforms may be useful markers of premature MI. (FIS PI020136 and PI020125 and Agencia Valenciana de Ciencia y Tecnología-Generalitat Valenciana Grupos03/010).

PO086

The effect of the new Russian food supplement "Eiferol" on the hemostasis and lipid metabolism in patients with disease of the liver

Vjacheslav I (1), Valentina P (2), Galina A (2), Margarita K (2), ludmila L (2)*

(1) Institute high-active substanses, Moscow, Russia
(2) Moscow State University, Moscow, Russia

Introduction. It is well known that the arising of the liver diseases may be depended on alcoholic and diabetic pathology. The search of the hepatoprotectors is very actual problem. **Aims**.The effect of the new Russian food supplement Eiferol on the functional state of the liver, lipid metabolism, hemocoagulation and fibrinolysis in patients suffering from alcoholism /AL/ and in patients with diabetes mellitus 2 type /DM 2/ was studied. **Materials and methods**. All patients had liver diseases /hepatitis, hepatosis or early stages cirrosis/ and the disfunction of the hemostasis-fibrinolysis system. Blood examples were investigated before and two month after of using Eiferol at 6 g daily. Eiferol is the complex of polyunsaturated fatty acids (eicosapentaenoic and docosahexaenoic acids) and such antioxidants as A, D, E vitamins. **Result**.Patients with AL had various disorders of the liver: alanin and asparagin transferases and γ-glutamintranspeptidase was significant higher that normal data. The lipid metabolism was insignificant changed. Patients with DM 2 had disturbances of lipid metabolism and small changes of the liver function. In both groups, hemocoagulation and fibrinolysis alterations were observed but patients with DM 2 had more deep fibrinolysis depression. The using of the Eiferol leaded to the positive changes of the liver functional data in patients with AL and to improvement of lipid metabolism data in DM 2 patients. Hemostasis and fibrinolysis indicates had the tendency to normalization more cleared in patients with DM 2. **Conclusion**. Thus the using of the new Russian food supplement Eiferol had more effective positive action on such physiological functions, which had more important pathological changes from its basal level.

PO087

Atorvastatin affects thrombosis/fibrinolysis system during the acute phace of unstable angina

Kotsopoulou M (1), Bosinakou E (1), Tousoulis D (2), Antoniades C (2), Fostira E (1), Pitsavos C (2), Stefanadis C (2)*

(1) Hematology Department, Hippokration Hospital
(2) Athens University Medical School, Athens

Background: Evidence suggest that lipid-lowering treatment with statins reduces mortality and morbitity in patients with coronary artery disease. The effects of lipid-lowering treatment during the early phase of the acute coronary syndromes are unknown. **Aims.** In this study we investigated the effect of atorvastatin treatment on plasma levels of tissue plasminogen activator (tPA), von Willebrand factor (vWF) and factors V (fV) and VII (fVII), in patients with unstable angina. **Methods**: Forty-six patients (34 males 12 females, aged 64+/-8 years old) with unstable ungina, were randomly divided into 2 groups and received atorvastatin 10 mg/day (n=23, ATR group) or no statin treatment (n=23, ATR group) for 6 weeks during and after admission. Plasma levels of tPA, vWF, fV and fVII were measured at baseline, at 1 week and at 6 weeks after the admission. Levels of the above thrombotic markers were determined by ELISA. All values are expressed as means+/-SEM. **Results:** At baseline, levels of tPA, vWF, fV and fVII were not significantly different between ATR (10.03±0.78 ng/ml, 107±6.5%, 125±7.8% and 92±4.4%) and the control group (10.8±1.0 ng/ml, 109.3±9.2%, 126±8.1% and 90.7±6.7%, p=NS for all). After 1 week, serum levels of tPA, vWF, fV and fVII were significantly increased in control group (13.3±1.3 ng/ml p<0.01, 127±8.5% p<0.05, 152±7.4% p<0.001 and 104±8.6% p<0.05 respectively, compared to baseline). This increase was prevented in ATR group (12.7±1.8ng/ml, 125±9.7%, 134±5.8% and 109±7.7% respectively, p=NS compared to baseline). However, at 6 weeks, plasma levels of tPA, vWF, fV and fVII returned to their baseline values in both ATR group (11.2±0.9ng/ml, 91.6±8.9%, 125.3±7.8% and 94.8±6.7% respectively, p=NS for all compared to baseline) and control group (11.4±0.95ng/ml, 98.8±10.6%, 118±6.9% and 114±31%, p=NS for all compared to baseline). **Conclusions:** During the first week of treatment, atorvastatin decreases the levels of factors V, VII, von Willebrand factor and tissue plasminogen activator in patients with unstable angina. These findings suggest that early administration of atorvastatin in patients with unstable ungina may be beneficial by affecting the thrombotic/fibrinolytic process.

PO088

Effects of atorvastatin on thrombosis/fibrinolysis system and endothelial function, in patients with heart failure

Kotsopoulou M (1), Antoniades C (2), Tousoulis D (2), Bosinakou E (1), Cheimona A (1), Pitsavos C (2), Stefanadis C (2)*

(1) Hematology Department, Hippokration Hospital, Athens
(2) Cardiology Department, Athens University Medical School

Introduction. Congestive heart failure (CHF) is characterised by endothelial dysfunction and increased thrombogenecity. **Aims.** We investigated the effect of atorvastatin on endothelial function and on plasma levels of antithrombin III (ATIII), proteins C and S, factors V and VII, von Willebrand factor (vWF), tissue plasminogen activator (tPA) and plasminogen activator inhibitor 1 (PAI-1) in patients with CHF. **Methods.** Thirty-five patients with CHF (NYHA II-IV) were randomized to receive atorvastatin 10mg/day (n=17) or no statin (n=18) for 4 weeks. Forearm blood flow was measured by venous occlusion strain-gauge plethysmography. Endothelium dependent dilation (EDD) and endothelium independent dilation (EID) were expressed as the % change of flow from baseline to the maximum flow during reactive hyperemia or after sublingual nitroglycerin administration respectively. Plasma levels of thrombosis/fibrinolysis components were determined with ELISA. **Results.** Atorvastatin improved EDD (42.44±4.5 to 83.7±8.5%, p<0.01), decreased plasma levels of tPA (15.5±2.2 to 12.3±1.6 ng/ml p<0.05), ATIII (82±3 to 74±4%, p<0.05), prtC (88±6 to 64±6%, p<0.01), fV (126±8 to 95±7%, p<0.01) and PAI-1 (3.02±0.39 to 1.96±0.34 IU/L, p<0.05), while it did not affect EID (65±8 to 53±6% p=ns) and levels of fVII (81±8 to 66±7% p=ns), vWF (135±13 to 123±19% p=ns) and prtS (93±5 to 95±8% p=ns). EDD and EID remained unchanged in controls (from 48±5 and 67±8 to 45±5% and 61±7% respectively p=ns for both). In control group, no significant change was observed in levels of ATIII (85±4 to 88±3%,p=ns), prtC(84±6 to 84±5%,p=ns), fV(131±10 to 122±9%,p=ns), fVII(78±12 to 69±9%,p=ns), vWF (151±19 to 135±38%, p=ns), prtS (100±8 to 96±6%, p=ns), tPA(13.2±1.5 to 11±2 ng/ml, p=ns) and PAI-1(2.64±0.38 to 3.25±0.34, p=ns). **Conclusions.** Short-term treatment with atorvastatin improves endothelial function and reduces plasma levels of tPA, PAI-1, antithrombin III, protein C and factor V, in patients with CHF, suggesting that atorvastatin may affect the expression of both endothelium- and liver-derived components of thrombosis fibrinolysis system, beyond its effect on vascular endothelium in these patients.

PO089

The t-PA and PAI-1 activities under treatment by thrombolytic and anticoagulant medicaments in patients with acute myocardial infarction

Krasnobryzha I (1), Savchuk O (2)*

(1) Taras Shevchenko Kiev National University, Kiev, Ukraine
(2) Palladin Institute of biochemistry NAS of Ukraine, Kiev, Ukraine

Introduction. Much attention is paid to plasminogen activators and their inhibitors because of their important role in fibrinolysis in a wide variety of biological function including tissue remodelling, cell migration, carcinogenesis and neoplasia. Fibrinolysis, which keeps the vascular compartment patent, is regulated by the activities of both tissue type plasminogen activator (t-PA) and its inhibitor (PAI-1). **Aims.** The aim of our study is to determine the plasma levels of t-PA and its inhibitor activity in patients with acute myocardial infarction (AMI) under treatment by thrombolytic and anticoagulant medicaments. **Materials and methods.** We studied fibrinolytic system in 58 patients with acute myocardial infarction treated by streptokinase (Sk) and heparin or fraksiparin. The parameters of fibrinolytic system were studied before thrombolytic therapy (TLT) and on several stages of treatment (in 2 hour after treatment by Sk, on 3, 7 and 30 days). Particularly we were interested in study of the main fibrinolytic system parameters such as t-PA, PAI-1, plasminogen, α_2-antiplasmin activities. We studied the activities of these parameters with used of chromogenic substrate S_{2251} and enzymeforesees the level of t-PA was also determined by ELISA. **Results.** Before treatment the mean activity of t-PA in a patient group with AMI was 0,87 ± 0,09 IU/ml compared to normal 2,05 ± 0,06 IU/ml. The influence of treatment by Sk on activity of t-PA has been found. In 2 hours after treatment by Sk activity of t-PA was significantly increased in a group of patients with AMI 7,89 ± 3,5IU/ml. The data achieved in a patient group with AMI without TLT revealed low activity of t-PA 0,5 ± 0,07 IU/ml. On following stages experimental data obtained from a patient group with AMI treated by heparin displayed the significant increase of t-PA activity on 24% and

184% (3 and 7 days of treatment) comparative to the t-PA activity before treatment. The data achieved in the second group of patient with AMI treated by fraksiparin revealed lower increasing of t-PA activity on 38% and 53% (comparative to the same parameter on the 3, 7 days) than in the group treatment by heparin. We found greatly elevated level of PAI-1 activity in a group of patients with AMI before treatment 63 ± 4,4 IU/ml. After treatment by Sk PAI-1 activity in blood plasma fell almost back to its original activity 37 ± 5,3 IU/ml average normal activity 0,5 - 40 IU/ml. In addition, it has been determined an increased consumption of plasminogen and α_2-antiplasmin. **Conclusion.** Thus, one of the reasons of AMI is dysfunction of fibrinolytic system cause by low activity of t-PA and high activity of PAI-1. The injection of Sk caused the significant increase of t-PA activity possibly due to the direct or/and indirect effects on endothelial cells. The heparin cause gradual and strong increase of t-PA activity and consequently fibrinolytic activity in contrast from fraksiparin may due to physiological effect of heparin such as synthesis and/or secretion of t-PA by endothelial cells.

PO090

Relationship between global fibrinolytic capacity and cardiovascular risk factors in obese patients

Turgut B (1), Guldiken S (2), Demir M (1), Ugur-Altun B (2), Gerenli M (3), Vuralo O (1), Tugrul A (2)*

(1) Trakya University Medical School, Department of Medicine, Division of Hematology, Edirne-Turkey
(2) Trakya University Medical School, Department of Medicine, Division of Endocrinology, Edirne-Turkey
(3) Trakya University Medical School, Department of Medicine, Edirne-Turkey

Aims: Obese patients are at particularly risk of cardiovascular complications, possibly related to haemostatic and fibrinolytic system. The aim of this study was to determine the effects of obesity on global fibrinolytic capacity (GFC, Diagnostica Stago, France), which is a new test used to assess fibrinolytic activity. We evaluate the relationship between GFC and cardiovascular risk factors in obese patients. **Materials and methods:** The study population consisted of 50 obese patients (36 women, 14 men, mean age; 30±7 years, mean BMI 34±3 kg/m^2) and 30 non-obese healthy subjects (19 women, 11 men, mean age, 30±6 years, mean BMI 22±2 kg/m^2). Anthropometric measurements (weight, height, hip and waist circumferences) of all participants were recorded. Plasma fasting glucose, insulin, lipid profiles, fibrinogen levels, D-dimer and GFC were measured. Insulin resistance was calculated by homeostasis model assessment (HOMA-R). **Results:** There were no significant differences between obese and non-obese groups regarding gender and age. Mean plasma levels of fasting glucose (p< 0.05), insulin (p< 0.001), HOMA-R (p< 0.001), fibrinogen (p< 0.001) in obese group were higher than control group. There was no significant difference between mean D-dimer levels of the two groups. Mean GFC was significantly lower in obese patients than controls (7.6± 7.5 μg/mL, 16.3±11.9 μG/mL, p< 0.001). GFC showed inverse correlation with mean levels of insulin (r= -0.2, p< 0.05), triglyceride (r= -0.3, p< 0.05) in obese patients. **Conclusions:** These data suggest that the GFC assay may be used to measure the fibrinolytic system in obese patients. We conclude that the increased cardiovascular risk observed in obese patients could in part be explained by the diminished fibrinolytic capacity in hyperinsulinemia and dyslipidemia.

PO091

Tissue plasminogen activator plasma levels is an independent predictor of in-hospital major events in patients with unstable angina

Gougopoulou D (1), Theodoridis T (1), El Ali M (1), Koulouris S (2), Karabinos I (2), Gianoulis T (2), Exadaktylos N (2), Christopoulou-Cokkin V (1)*

(1) Haematology Lab. Evangelismos Hosp. Athens, Greece
(2) 1st Cardiology Dept. Evangelismos Hosp. Athens, Greece

Purpose: Activation of various coagulation mechanisms contributing to thrombus formation following atherosclerotic plaque rupture represents a crucial step in the pathogenesis of unstable angina (UA) The aim of our study was to investigate the value of different coagulation markers [von Willebrand Factor (vWF), Factor VII (FVII), Thrombomoduline (TM) and Factor VIII (FVIII)] and markers of fibrinolysis [tissue plasminogen activator (t-PA) and plasminogen activator inhibitor -1 (PAI-1)] to predict in-hospital major events in patients (pts) with UA. **Methods**: We studied 119 pts with UA, aged 61±7 years. All pts had blood sampling on their admission, before the administration of any medication. We assessed plasma levels of t-PA (normal range=1-12ng/ml), PAI-1 (normal range<10U/ml), and TM (normal range= 30-55ng/ml), with ELISA and we measured % plasma activity of vWF (Ristocetin co- factor activity, normal range=50-140%), FVII (normal range=50-130%) and FVIII (normal range=60-150%). The presence of coronary artery disease risk factors, diabetes mellitus, hypercholesterolaemia, hypertension, smoking, and severe obesity (body mass index>30 kgr/m2) was recorded in all pts. A major in-hospital event was considered the development of one of the following: myocardial infarction, heart failure, major arrhythmias, conduction disturbances, mechanical complications, refractory angina or death. **Results**: 21 out of 119 pts experienced an in-hospital major event (3 deaths), during their 62 days hospitalization. Only plasma levels of t-PA were found statistically significantly higher in pts who developed a major in- hospital event (18,06 – 20,09) compared to the rest (6,27 - 10,8) (t-test: t=3,17, p=0,002). However, stepwise multivariate logistic regression analysis revealed that admission t-PA plasma levels is the only marker that can predict in-hospital major events (exp (b)=1,25, CI=1,02-1,53, p=0,02) in pts with UA, independently from age (p=0,2), sex (p=0,46), TM (p=0,31), PAI-1 (p=0,67), FVII (p=0,69), FVIII (p=0,89), vWF (p=0,93), ejection fraction (p=0,58), and the presence of CVD risk factors (p=0,07-0,91). **Conclusions** Paradoxically increased admission plasma levels of t-PA in UA pts who develop an adverse in-hospital outcome may reflect an inappropriate endothelial activation, which further enhances thrombus formation and recurrence of myocardial ischemia. The admission t-PA plasma levels are an independent predictor for the development of major in-hospital events in pts with UA and could be used to identify the pts who are at greatest risk.

PO092

D-dimer promotes endothelial dysfunction in diabetes mellitus

Yevdokimova N, Lugovskij E, Komisarenko S*

Institute of Biochemistry, Kyiv, Ukraine

Introduction: Previously we have demonstrated that D-dimer (DD) decreased the accumulation of pericellular heparan sulphate (HS) in endothelial cells and reduced HS anticoagulant ability via the suppressing of endogenous NO. Simultaneously, DD up-regulated PAI-1secretion. Since, diabetes mellitus is accompanied by the increased DD level, we supposed that DD per se may affect endothelial function, and may be the additional factor to disorganize extracellular matrix (ECM). The interaction of DD with endothelial cells is realized through the binding of its gamma 117-133 fragment to ICAM-1. However, it remains unclear, whether DD affects the above-mentioned properties of endothelium through the binding of gamma 117-133 sequence to ICAM-1. **Aims**: Our aim was to determine the role of gamma 117-133 - ICAM-1 interaction in DD-induced deterioration of endothelial ECM. Materials and methods: ECV30 cells were incubated with DD, D-fragment (D), synthetic peptide gamma 117-133 (gamma 3) and scrambled peptide. Some cells were preincubated with antibody, which blocks ICAM-1. We measured NO production, 14-C-acetate incorporation into pericellular HS, HS binding to antithrombin (AT) and PAI-1 secretion. **Results**: DD, D, gamma 3 decreased NO production, HS accumulation and HS binding to AT, whereas scrambled peptide had no effect. The most effective was gamma 3 (~2-fold decrease). Unlike DD and D, 3 did not alter PAI-1 secretion. Preincubation with blocking antibody canceled the effect of DD, D and gamma 3 on NO production, HS accumulation and HS binding to AT, but was ineffective concerning DD stimulation of PAI-1. High glucose increased ICAM-1 expression, increased the sensitivity of ECV30 cells to DD in terms of HS accumulation, and the joint action of high glucose and DD intensified HS reduction. **Conclusions**: The interaction of ICAM-1 with gamma 117-133 fragment is responsible for the decreased content and impaired anticoagulant properties of HS, but does not mediate DD-induced PAI-1 stimulation. Thus, the increased concentration of DD in diabetes mellitus may promote endothelial dysfunction by means of two independent mechanisms: (a) impairment of anticoagulant properties and accumulation of pericellular HS against the background of NO shortage; (b) up-regulation of PAI-1 secretion.

PO093

Pretreatment PAI-1 levels and streptokinase thrombolysis in Iranian patients with acute MI in spite of negligible antistreptokinase antibodies

Shemirani H, Tajmirriahi, Rezaei A, Oresi A*

Background: The risk for unsuccessful reperfusion after streptokinase therapy may be caused by the antifibrinolytic effect of platelet-derived type 1 plasminogen activator inhibitor (PAL-1) and streptokinase antibodies. This study aims to show the relation of pretreatment PAI-1 levels of patients with reperfusion in acute myocardial infarction treated with streptokinase therapy with and without considering pretreatment antistreptokinase antibodies. **Methods**: Pretreatment PAI-1 and antistreptokinase antibodies levels of 61 patients with acute myocardial infarction, treated with streptokinase, were determined by enzyme- linked immunosorbent assay kit methods. Failure of thrombolysis with streptokinase was present when reperfusion was unsuccessful as assessed by noninvasive reperfusion criteria. **Results**: Mean pretreatment PAI-1 level of patients was 29.72 ± 4.74 ng/ml; span 17.20 ng/ml to 41.20 ng/ml l. Thrombolysis with streptokinase failed significantly with higher pretreatment PAI-1 levels ($p < 0.05$) in all patients and patients with negative pretreatment antistreptokinase antibodies. **Conclusion**: we showed that higher pretreatment PAI-1 levels were associated with significant failure of streptokinase therapy in patients with acute myocardial infarction, with and without considering pretreatment antistreptokinase antibodies (anti-SK) with the emphasis on reperfusion.

PO094

Elevated levels of methylglyoxal may contribute to the development of thrombotic complications in diabetes mellitus

Léránt I, Kolev K, Machovich R*

Department of Medical Biochemistry, Semmelweis University, Budapest, Hungary

Introdutcion: Nonenzymic modification of proteins by 2-oxoaldehyde methylglyoxal (MeG) may influence the coagulation and fibrinolytic reactions. Blood levels of MeG increase 5 fold in Diabetes Mellitus (DM). This reactive □-ketoaldehyde modifies cysteine, lysine and arginine side chain residues of various proteins in the circulation and in the hepatocytes. *In vitro* MeG modification of plasminogen results in decreased rate of plasminogen activation and lower fibrinolytic activity of plasmin formed. *In vivo* MeG may interact with several additional factors within the same compartment. In our present study we evaluated the consequences of *in vitro* MeG treatment of human plasma and isolated coagulation factors. Plasminogen and antithrombin were isolated from plasma of diabetic patients and their fibrinolysis and inhibitor activity were also tested. **Results and conclusions**: Short time - 3 hours – incubation of prothrombin with MeG at physiological concentrations did not affect the rate of the prothrombin – thrombin conversion, only MeG at high concentrations inhibited the prothrombin activation. *In vitro* MeG treatment of antithrombin decreased the rate of thrombin – antithrombin reaction by 10 – 30 %. *In vitro* MeG treatment of human plasma decreased its thrombin inhibiting potential. Antithrombin isolated from patients with DM was less effective in thrombin inactivation and showed the same inhibitor potential in the plasmin – antithrombin reaction as the antithrombin isolated from healthy patient of control subjects. Plasminogen prepared from patients with DM showed lower fibrinolytic potential, its activation rate by streptokinase is decreased the fibrinolytic activity of the plasmin formed is lower compared to the control plasmin(ogen). Our data suggest several proteins may be modified in DM and as a result their biological activity is altered. Inhibition of the fibrinolytic activity of plasmin, the decrease in in the rate of thrombin – antithrombin reaction may contribute to the elevated risk of thrombosis in DM.

PO095

Plasma flow velocity and fibrin specificity of thrombolytic agent promote thrombolysis of non-retracted and retracted whole blood clots

Tratar G (1), Blinc A (1), Štrukelj M (1), Mikac U (2), Serša I (2)*

(1) Dept. of Vascular Medicine, Ljubljana Medical Center, Slovenia
(2) J. Stefan Institute, University of Ljubljana, Slovenia

We studied *in vitro* how thrombolysis of non-occlusive blood clots depended on flow velocity of plasma containing thrombolytic agents–0.2 µg/ml rt-PA or 250 IU/ml streptokinase (SK)–and magnetic resonance contrast agent Gd-DTPA (at 1 mmol/L) through an artificial reperfusion channel. Non-retracted or retracted whole blood clots were pierced lengthways and connected to a perfusion system. The initial flow of plasma through the channel was either rapid and turbulent (426±13 cm/s, est. shear rate of 48700/s in non-retracted and 137±88 cm/s, est. shear rate of 9100/s in retracted clots), or slow and laminar (31±4 cm/s, est. shear rate of 3500/s in non-retracted and 8±2 cm/s, est. shear rate of 500/s in retracted clots). Serial spin-echo MRI was used for measuring penetration of plasma and the remaining clot size. Penetration of plasma into clots was faster with rapid than with slow flow: after 6–10 min of exposure to turbulent flow, Gd-DTPA-containing areas were found inside non-retracted clots at a distance of 2.11 (1.86-2.30) mm, but at only 0.39 (0.32-0.51) mm from the channel border in clots exposed to laminar flow ($p<0.001$). In retracted clots, the distances were 1.65 (1.05-3.60) mm with turbulent and 0.71 (0.30-1.35) mm with laminar flow ($p<0.05$). The remaining undissolved cross-sections of non-retracted clots treated with rt-PA after 40 min were 3 (2-8)% for turbulent and 84 (82-88)% for laminar flow ($p<0.05$). The corresponding values for SK were 33 (18-49)% for turbulent and 95 (94-96)% for laminar flow ($p<0.05$). In retracted blood clots treated with rt-PA the remaining cross-section after 40 min was 66 (30-72)% with turbulent vs. 95 (94-98)% with laminar flow ($p<0.01$). Virtually no lysis was achieved in retracted clots with SK after 40 minutes: 93 (91-99)% with turbulent flow vs. 99 (98-100)% with laminar flow (p=NS). Conclusion: rapid turbulent flow of plasma along non-occlusive clots causes rapid exchange of serum inside the clot with outer plasma by convection, which promotes blood clot lysis by fibrin-specific rt-PA. In retracted blood clots, no lysis can be achieved in 40 min with non-fibrin-specific SK regardless of flow velocity.

PO096

Coagulation/fibrinolysis system parameters are affected by smoking cessation

Hatzizacharias A, Makris T, Krespi P, Stavroulakis G, Paizis J, Tsoukala C, Mandalaki T, Votteas V*

LAIKO General Hospital, Athens, Greece

Introduction: Smoking is one of the primary modifiable risk factors for coronary artery disease and is estimated to be the cause of approximately 20% of all deaths of cardiovascular origin. Smoking cessation seems to have a favourable effect on cardiovascular morbidity and mortality. Aim of our study was to examine the smoking cessation effect on the coagulation/fibrinolysis system parameters, in healthy smokers. **Methods:** Thirty healthy, male smokers mean age (MA) 40±5 yrs., and BMI 23,7±1,2 Kg/m², without any other risk factor, were studied. Plasminogen activator inhibitor-1 antigen (PAI-1 Ag), tissue plasminogen activator antigen (tPA-Ag), thrombomodulin (TM), fibrinogen (F) and factor VII (FVII) fasting plasma levels were determined (ELISA method) in the whole population at six different periods day 1 (0), 1st, 2nd, 3rd, 4th and 5th yrs., after smoking cessation, respectively. It is to be noticed that there were no other predisposing to CADrisk factors, during the follow-up period (ie hypertension, diabetes or dyslipidemia). **Results:** The mean values of the hemostatic parameters and the differences between them are shown in the Table.

Time (yr)	PAI-1 Ag (ng/ml)	tPA-Ag (ng/ml)	TM (ng/ml)	F (mg/dl)	FVII (%)
0	10±3	3,6±1,3	40±15	350±40	145±33
1	9,8±2,6	3,7±1,5	38±14	348±38	143±30
2	9,5±2,7	4±1,7	37±14	345±36	142±32
3	9±2,6	4,1±1,7	35,6±12	340±37	140±27
4	7,6±3	4,5±1,5	30±13	330±28	128±28
5	6,8±2,3	4,7±1,4	25±9	315±30	120±26
	0-4 p<.01	0-4 p<.05	0-4 p<.01	0-4 p<.05	0-4 p<.01
	0-5 p<.001	0-5 p<.01	0-5 p<.001	0-5 p<.001	0-5 p<.001

Conclusion: The results of our study suggest that smoking cessation has a favourable effect on the hemostatic parameters, which starts 4 yrs., and it is stabilized 5 yrs., after cessation, in healthy smokers.

PO097

Plasminogen activator inhibitor (PAI) 4G/5G polymorphism in patients with coronary artery disease

Apergis G, Bellia M*, Bratsas A*, Pavlou E*, Brilli S*, Gagou A*, Georgopoulos J*, Andrioti E**

1st Transfusion and Hemophilia Center, University Unit of Cardiology*, Hippokrateion Hospital of Athens

Purpose. We studied the association of PAI-1 polymorphism with coronary artery disease and AMI in a prospective series of patients who underwent coronary angiography. **Material and methods**: We investigated 46 patients, 14 females and 32males (mean age: 67+/-9years old) with heart disease. By means of coronary angiography our patients were divided into subjects without any detectable coronary artery disease or with no vessel disease and patients with single, double or triple vessel disease and acute myocardial infarction (AMI). The PAI-1 4G/5G gene polymorphism was analysed in all patients by using PCR.We also measured PAI levels by using Chromogenics substrate. **Results**: Eight patients out of 46 had no vessel disease (17.4%), 15 suffered from three vessel disease (32.6%), 8 from two vessel disease (17.4%) and 15 from one vessel disease (32.6%). The PAI-1 4G allele was found in 34 patients. Nineteen patients out of 25 with AMI were carriers while 8 out of 21 with no AMI had this allele (p~0.01). Twenty-eight patients out of 38 (73.6%) with one or more vessel disease were carriers of 4G allele while 3 out of 8 with no vessel disease carried this allele but this difference was not statistically significant. PAI levels were higher among patients with acute myocardial infarction (mean13,5+/-5UI/ml with normal range<10UI/ml) than among patients without but with no statistical difference. Seventeen patients with additional presence of risk factors had also increased PAI levels 12.7+/-4UI/ml. **Conclusion:** The present study indicate that the 4G allele of PAI gene polymorphism is an additional risk factor for coronary artery disease and AMI. The presence of other major cardiovascular risk factors increases the risk for the above disease.

PO098

The relationship between Ins/Del (I/D) polymorphism in ACE gene with t-PA I/D and PAI-1 4G/5G polymorphisms in PE

Altinok B (1), Oner F (2), Numanoglu N (2), Oguzulgen K (3), Ekim N (3), Akar N (4)*

(1) Ankara University Biotechnology Institute, Ankara, Turkey
(2) Department of Pulmonary Diseases, School of Medicine, Ankara University, Ankara, Turkey
(3) Department of Pulmonary Diseases, School of Medicine, Gazi University, Ankara, Turkey
(4) Department of Pediatric Molecular Genetics, School of Medicine, Ankara University, Ankara, Turkey

Introduction: Renin angiotensin system (RAS) is associated with the regulation of blood pressure,blood volume and electrolyte balance as an endocrine system. Angiotensin converting enzyme (ACE), which plays an important role in the renin angiotensin system. Angiotensin I is converted into angiotensin II by ACE. This is the key reaction in the RAS pathway. Angiotensin II, which is a potent vasoconstrictor,stimulates aldosterone-vasopressin secretion and the retention of sodium,increases blood pressure. ACE inactivates the vasodilator peptide bradykinin which stimulates the production of tissue plasminogen activator (t-PA) and supports to the protective effects of ACE inhibitors. ACE contributes the fibrinolytic balance between t-PA and PAI-1(plasminogen activator inhibitor 1); Ang I is converted to ang II by ACE,the production of PAI-1 increases. The bradykinin degradation and ang II formation is blocked by ACE inhibitor,the production of t-PA increases. The higher levels of ACE in plasma is associated with DD genotype and the conversion of ang I to ang II by ACE is faster than II genotype. This study was performed to determine the relationship between ACE I/D polymorphism,t-PA I/D and PAI-1 4G/5G polymorphisms in pulmonary embolism patients. **Materials and Methods**: After the DNA extraction,I/D alleles of ACE gene; I/D alleles of t-PA gene and 4G/5G alleles of PAI-1 were amplified by PCR as previously described. **Results and Conclusion**: One hundred thirty five pulmonary embolism patients and seventy one individuals were taken as the control group.Ace,t-PA,PAI-1 polymorphisms have been analysed. The frequency of ACE (intron 16) 190 bp D(deletion)allele 64.08 and 61.1% in control and pulmonary embolism;t-PA(intron 8) 112 bp D allele 69.01 and 54.07% ;PAI-1(-675) 98 bp 4G allele 50 and 53.3% respectively. (This study is supported by Ankara Universite research Fund.)

PO099

PAI-1 levels, 4G/5G genotype and insulin resistance in severe and morbid obesity. Effect of weight loss and influence of 4G/5G genotype

*Solá E (1), Vayá A (2), Castelló R (2), España F (2), Hernández A (1), Aznar J (2), Estellés A (2)**

(1) Hospital Universitario Dr Peset, Valencia, Spain
(2) Hospital Universitario La Fe, Valencia. Spain

Introduction. An association between increased plasminogen activator inhibitor type 1 (PAI-1), insulin resistance syndrome (IRS) and obesity has been described in adults, which may contribute to increased risk of vascular disease. It has also been suggested that a decrease in adiposity has beneficial effects on fibrinolytic parameters. However, less information is available regarding morbid obesity and fibrinolysis. **Aims.** The aim of the present study is to evaluate the effect of weight loss and the influence of the PAI-1 promoter 4G/5G genotype on PAI-1 levels and metabolic parameters in severe and morbid obesity. **Material and methods.** 48 obese patients were studied, 14 with severe obesity (body mass index, BMI >35 and <40 kg/m^2) and 34 with morbid obesity (BMI ≥40 kg/m^2). Patients were studied before and three months after a weight reduction program, with hypocaloric diet. 53 controls (BMI >20 and < 30 kg/m^2) of similar age and sex distribution were studied as well, in the same moments that the obese patients. The controls did not undergo diet treatment. In both groups, we measured PAI-1 antigen and activity levels, PAI-1 4G/5G genotypes, glucose, insulin and lipidic profile. **Results.** A significant increase in PAI-1 antigen and activity levels was observed in the patient group in comparison with the control group (PAI-1ag: 44±23 *vs* 15±11 ng/ml; PAI-1act: 27±16 *vs* 8±8 U/ml). The highest PAI-1 levels were obtained in the morbid obesity group. No significant differences in PAI-1 levels between the PAI-1 4G/5G genotypes were obtained. After a three-month treatment period of diet, a significant decrease in PAI-1ag (p=0.03), PAI-1act levels (p=0.001), BMI (p<0.001) and glucose levels (p=0.014) were observed and no significant variations in the other metabolic parameters were obtained. A significant inverse correlation between previous PAI-1 levels and variation in PAI-1 levels was also observed. Therefore, the largest decrease in PAI-1 levels was observed in patients with the highest previous PAI-1 levels. In the control group, no variation in BMI and in the remaining parameters analysed was observed after a three-month period. **Conclusions**. A decrease in BMI in severe and morbid obesity shows a favourable effect on the fibrinolytic system due to a decrease in PAI-1 levels. However, no influence of 4G/5G genotype on PAI-1 levels has been observed. (FIS PI020136 and Agencia Valenciana de Ciencia y Tecnología-Generalitat Valenciana Grupos03/010).

PO100

Abstract withdrawn

PO101

Troponin concentration in NSTEMI patients depends on intensity of prothrombotic reactions

Wachnicka-Truty R, Korzeniowski A, Birkholz-Gołaszewska A, Kliz J, Flasiński J, Dmochowska-Wróblewsk W*

Clinic of Internal D

Aim of our study was to define if in NSTEMI patients the intensity of prothrombotic state (expressed as the degree of thrombin generation and platelet adhesion) influences profoundness of myocardial injury (measured by troponin level). Thrombin generation was determined by the concentrations of thrombin-antithrombin III complexes (TAT) and prothrombin fragment 1+2 (F1+2) with ELISA commercial kits, blood platelet adhesion-with Roshopf's method, troponin concentration (T) - with luminescentic method in two groups of NSTEMI patients:30-with T<0,2ng/ml and 32with T from 2,1 to 17,2 ng/ml (mean 6,0 +/- 2,7 ng/ml). **Results**:

T ng/ml	platelet adhesion %	TAT ng/ml	F1+2 umol/l
<0,2	3,3+/-0,9	5,4+/- 1,5	1,8+/-0,7
6,0+/-2,7	5,2+/-1,9*	8,3+/-1,9*	2,3+/-0,9

* $p<0{,}05$; positive correlations: platelet adhesion-T and TAT-T

Conclusion: NSTEMI patients with more evident signs of prothrombotic state have myocardium more profoundly injured than those with lower thrombin generation and less intensive platelet adhesion.

PO102

D-dimer and soluble fibrin at ischemic heart disease and acute impairment cerebral circulation

Lugovskoy E, Kolesnikova I, Gritsenko P, Lugovskaya N, Komisarenko S*

9 Leonyovicha Str., Palladin Institute of Biochemistry, 01601 Kyiv, Ukraine

Introduction. D-dimer is a product of cross-linked fibrin degradation by plasmin. D-dimer is a useful molecular marker of the activation of blood coagulation system, fibrin formation and fibrinolysis. D-dimer concentration in blood is increased greatly at various diseases, especially in DIC, deep vein thrombosis and pulmonary embolism. **Aims**. On the base of our monoclonal antibody (mAb) III-3b to D-dimer we planned to carry out the Sandwich-ELISA method for quantification of D-dimer in human blood plasma. This method was used for the determination of D-dimer level in ischemic heart disease (IHD) and acute impairment cerebral circulation (AICC). We planned also to quantify soluble fibrin in blood plasma in these pathologies and to determine the correlation between two molecular markers. We studied the molecular composition of soluble fibrin in these pathologies. **Materials and methods**. MAbs were obtained by usual hybridoma techniques. Quantification of soluble fibrin was performed by its precipitation with phosphate salts. Molecular composition of soluble fibrin was determined by SDS-electrophoresis. **Results and conclusions**. Our mAb III-3b has strong specificity to its antigen – human D-dimer (KD = 1,43x10-10 M) without cross-reaction with fibrinogen. This mAb proved to react also with bovine, rat and rabbit D-dimers without cross-reaction with appropriate fibrinogens. The mAb III-3b was used as a catch-mAb in Sandwich ELISA method for D-dimer quantification in human blood plasma. Another mAb to D-dimer (II-4d) was used as a tag-mAb. The developed method allows D-dimer quantification from 0.10 mkg/ml till 10 mkg/ml. We investigated the concentrations of D-dimer and soluble fibrin at IHD and AICC. It has been found that normal concentration of D-dimer (< 0.5 mkg/ml) was in 43% of 53 patients, the elevated concentrations (0.65 – 1.25 mkg/ml) in 42% and high level (2.00 – 4.50 mkg/ml) – in 13% at IHD. There was no normal level of D-dimer in 15 patients at AICC, but elevated concentrations (0.65 – 1.25 mkg/ml) in 51% patients and high concentrations (2.00 – 4.50 mkg/ml) – in 46% patients. The concentrations of soluble fibrin at IHD vary from 10 - 30 mkg/ml (27%), through 30 –35 mkg/ml (36%), 65 –75 mkg/ml (21%), 90 –100 mkg/ml (10%) till 120 – 150 mkg/ml (6%). There were no correlations between D-dimer concentrations in human blood plasma and the quantities of soluble fibrin at IHD (r = - 0,10459). The SDS-electrophoretic data showed that the soluble fibrin precipitations at IHD consisted mainly of fibrin non cross-linked by factor XIIIa, E1-fragment and D-fragment, when we took blood samples without adding Aprotinin and epsilon-aminocaproic acid. But with Aprotinin (20 u/ml) and epsilon-aminocaproic acid (0,002 M) the soluble fibrin precipitations consists practically only of fibrin non cross-linked by factor XIIIa and no E1-fragment and respectively – no D-fragment.

PO103

D-dimer levels in long term anticoagulated patients

Gafou A, Tsevrenis V, Nomikou E, Bellia M, Paulou E, Andrioti E*

1st Regional and Haemophilia Center, Hippokration Hospital, Athens, Greece

Introduction: Recent studies indicate that D-dimer assays may play a role in management strategies for the prevention of thrombosis recurrences. **Aim**: Validation of prevalence of patients with positive D-dimer results with 2 assays. **Methods**: 1. D-dimer plus (Dade Behring, BCT), 2. VIDAS D-dimers new (Biomerieux) The central 96% interval was established in 29 blood donors (median age 42,5 years, range 22-59) and the cut-off for the method 1 and 2 are 301 and 506ng/ml respectively. **Patients**: 42 patients, anticoagulated for >3 months, were studied (20 men/ 22 women, median 52 years, range 21-83). **Statistical analysis**: Mann-Whitney rank test, x2 ($p<0{,}05$), and kappa coefficient were used as needed. **Results**: 30 patients (70%) were anticoagulated for venous and 16 for arterial thrombosis. 92,5% of the patients had >50% of INR results in the last 3 months, in the therapeutic range. Distribution of results in patients and controls. The percentage of positive D-dimer results were 7.1% and 16.7% for method 1 and 2, respectively. The k-value for the agreement was 0,333. For the method 2., there was a significant difference in the D-Dimer value only in elderly (>60 years, $p=0{,}001$), and in women ($p=0{,}007$), but not in the percentage of INR measurements in therapeutic range ($p=0{,}563$). The k-values in 10 retested patients were 1 and 0,375 for the methods 1 and 2, respectively. **Conclusions**: The agreement of patients classification by each of the methods was defined as moderate. The k-value for the repeated D-Dimers values was quite different between the 2 methods. The natural history of positive value of D-Dimers assays must be validated in a larger study.

PO104

A normal Wells´s score and a normal D-dimer test safely exclude pulmonary embolism

Söderberg M (1), Brohult J (2)*

(1) Dept of Medicine, Division of Internal Medicine, Stockholm Söder Hospital, SE 118 83 STOCKHOLM, Sweden

(2) Dept of Medicine, Division of Internal Medicine, Stockholm Söder Hospital, SE 118 83 STOCKHOLM, Sweden

Introduction: The diagnosis of pulmonary embolism (PE) is difficult. You often get both false positive and false negative results in ordinary clinical work. Recently it has been showed that computed tomography of the pulmonary arteries (CTPA) safely diagnos PE with a sensitivity of 91% and a specificity of 96%. Still there is often a need for radiological investigations to exclude PE. Several studies have shown that a normal D-dimer has a high negative predictive value in the diagnosis of PE. **Aims**: To compare the accuracy of a pretest probablility score (Wells´s score) and a D-dimer test to safely exclude acute pulmonary embolism in order to decrease the need for radiological investigations. **Material and Methods**: 123 hemodynamically stable patients with suspected acute PE underwent clinical scoring according to Wells´s pretest probability score, a rapid latex agglutination D-dimer test and contrast medium enhanced spiral CTPA. The Wells´s pretest probability score for prediciting the risk of PE consist of: clincal signs of deep vein thrombosis (DVT): 3 p, an alternative diagnosis deemed less likely than PE: 3 p, heart rate >100 beats/min: 1.5 p, immobilisation or surgery in the previous 4 weeks: 1.5 p, previous DVT or PE: 1 p, hemoptysis: 1 p and malignancy: 1 p. Maximum points are thus 12.5 All investigation were made within 24 hours and the patients were between 18-79 years old. We used the cut-off levels of 0.5 mg/L in the D-dimer test and a result below 6 in the Wells´s scoring system. **Results**: 47/123 (38%) of the patients were diagnosed having PE with CTPA. 76/123 (62%) had a non-diagnostic CTPA. 52/123 (42%) had a non-diagnostic CTPA, a normal D-dimer and a Wells´s score <6. 24 patients diagnosed not having PE had a normal CTPA, a positive D-dimer (i.e. >0.5 mg/L) and/or a Wells´s score more than or equal to 6. Twenty-one of these 24 patients had a D-dimer >0.5 mg/L and three had a Wells´s score above 6. In a chi-square test patients with PE and non-PE were compared with the different results of the D-dimer test and Wells´score. The negative predictive value for the 52 patients with normal CTPA and D-dimer and a score below 6 was 93,4% ($p<0{,}001$). **Conclusions**: We conclude that in patients with a normal D-dimer and a Wells´score <6 you can exclude acute PE without further radiological investigations.

PO105

D- dimer in the diagnosis of pulmonary embolism

Škrgat-Kristan S, Meško Brguljan P*, Košnik M, Šorli J*

University Clinic of Respiratory and Allergic Diseases Golnik, 4204 Golnik, Slovenia

Introduction and aims: D-dimer concentration is increased in pulmonary embolism (PE), deep vein thrombosis (DVT) and in many other diseases. The usefulness of plasma D-dimer concentration was assessed in differential diagnosis in patients with dyspnoea and suspected pulmonary embolism. **Materials and methods**: In retrospective analysis 144 patients were included who had been examined due to dyspnoea. We measured plasma D-dimer with immunoturbidimetric test Turbiquant D-dimer (Behring Diagnostics GmbH). Values above 250 µg/L were considered increased. Forty-one patients had also their plasma D-dimer measured with SimpliRED D-dimer (AGEN Biomedical) test simultaneously. **Results**: Among 144 patients there were 38 (26.4 %) with D-dimer concentration of 250 mg/L or less. Two of them had pulmonary embolism. 106 (73.6 %) patients had D-dimer > 250 µg/L. There was no statistical difference in concentration of D-dimer between the PE group and other groups of patients (p > 0.05). In 19 patients with negative SimpliRED D-dimer but positive Turbiquant D-dimer test, concentration of D-dimer was between 253 and 2640 µg/L. **Conclusions**: D-dimer above the cutoff value is of no help in differential diagnosis in patients with dyspnoea and suspected pulmonary embolism. Values of D-dimer concentration below cutoff value exclude pulmonary embolism with 95% probability. Cutoff value of SimpliRED D-dimer test is probably higher than cutoff value of Turbiquant D-dimer test.

PO106

The usefulness of D-dimer in hospitalized patients with lung diseases

Fijalkowska A (1), Piwek A (1), Wiatr E (2), Kurzyna M (1), Kuca P (3), Burakowski J (1), Kober J (1), Szturmowicz M (1), Tomkowski W (3), Torbicki A (1)*

(1) National Research Institute of Tuberculosis and Lung Diseases, Dep. of Chest Medici, Warsaw, Poland
(2) National Research Institute of Tuberculosis and Lung Diseases, Pulmonary Dep., Warsaw, Poland
(3) National Research Institute of Tuberculosis and Lung Diseases, Intensive Care Unit, Warsaw, Poland

Recently, the use of D-dimer testing has simplified the diagnosis of suspected venous thromboembolism (VTE) in outpatients. However, in hospitalised patients many various conditions can elevate D-dimer level and it has been suggested that D-dimer could have lower utility in this population. We sought to determine the proportion of normal D-dimer level in patients with lung diseases hospitalised at the chest or pulmonary department. Differential diagnosis of pulmonary embolism (PE) in this group during hospital stay is very difficult and D-dimer use could be very helpful. **Material and methods**: In 619 consecutive patients mean aged 54,9 (±15,4) hospitalized at the chest or pulmonary department, with different lung diseases (lung cancer 172 (27%), acute venous thromboembolism (VTE) 96 (15%), VTE in the past 70 (11%), COPD 65 (10%), pneumonia 39 (6%), sarcoidosis or lung fibrosis 30 (5%), connective tissue disease 28 (4%) and other) plasma D-dimer concentration was measured with rapid ELISA assay (VIDAS D-dimer New, bioMerieux). The cutoff value according to the manufacturer was 500ng/ml. **Results**: Overall, mean value of D-dimer was 1859 ng/ml (±3659) with 226 (37%) normal results (<500ng/ml). The highest level of D-dimer was observed in acute VTE (mean 5151ng/ml ±5867). Mean values of D-dimer concentration in other groups were: in lung cancer 1785ng/ml ±1990, in COPD 527ng/ml ±575, in pneumonia 2214ng/ml ±2950 and in connective tissue diseases 1324ng/ml ±1689. **We conclude** that D-dimer measurement could be contributed to the PE diagnostic strategy in patient hospitalized at pulmonary or chest department because about 40% of them have normal initial D-dimer level. Such algorithm requires confirmation in clinical studies.

PO107

The characteristic of the soluble fibrin-monomer complexes fraction

Savchuk O (1), Volodymyr C (2), Tatyana P (3)*

(1) Palladin Institute of biochemistry NAS of Ukraine
(2) Taras Shevchenko Kiev National University
(3) Palladin Institute of biochemistry NAS of Ukraine

The DIC-syndrome development and coagulation system activation degree is determined by accumulation of the soluble fibrin-monomer complexes (SFMC), D-D fragments of fibrin, fibrinopeptide A, thrombin-antithrombin (TAT) complexes, protrombin fragment 1+2 (F1+2). SFMC accumulation indicates the activation of coagulation system and the disbalance between fibrinolytic and coagulation systems. The aim of our work was to characterize the blood plasma proteins composition included to the soluble fibrin-monomer complexes. The plasma level of fibrinogen (Fg), factor X, antithrombin III (AT III), protein C (PC), SFMC, APTT were measured in patients with acute myocardial infarction (n=32), severe burn (n=17), operation (Caesarian section) (n=45). The characteristic of the soluble fibrin-monomer complexes was made by disc-electrophoresis and western-blot methods. Analysis displayed the activation of the coagulation system: high level of soluble fibrin, decreased activity of physiological inhibitors – protein C and AT-III. Electrophoresis of SFMC fraction achieved the presence of bands corresponding to 400-200 kDa, 110-85 kDa, 70-50 kDa molecular weight. Western-blot with used of fibrin/fibrinogen antibody demonstrated presence in SFMC fraction of the DD-, D-, E- fragments. The investigation shown that the simultaneous determination of soluble fibrin with analysis of fibrin/fibrinogen degradation products allows to diagnose the hemostasis system disbalance degree in patients. Analysis of SFMC permits to determine possible non-physiological influence mechanisms of fibrin/fibrinogen fragments on hemostasis system and also on all organism in general.

PO108

Management of coagulopathy and associated severe bleeding in immediate post-partum period

Gonçalves L, Oliveira G, Pereira R, Cunha-Ribeiro L*

Center of Thrombosis, Haemostasis and Vascular Biology, Department of Transfusion Medicine and Blood

Introduction: Disseminated intravascular coagulopathy (DIC) is a disorder characterized by the system activation of coagulation, which can result in organ failure as a result of thrombosis in the small vessels. It can also produce severe bleeding by the depletion of coagulation factors. DIC is associated with many conditions including obstetric complications, such as pré-eclampsia, acute fatty liver of pregnancy, abruptio placentae or amniotic fluid embolism, due to release of thromboplastin intravascularly or endothelial damage. In most patients, the disease can be ameliorated easily in early stages. **Aims**: In this report we present fives cases of DIC in immediate post-partum period, which were successfully treated with a prompt administration of blood components and derivatives with correction of coagulopathy. **Patients and Methods**: We describe 5 cases of severe acute coagulopathy in immediate post-partum period. Patients presented severe uterine bleeding, hemodynamic unstability, low levels of haemoglobin and abnormal coagulation parameters (prolongation of activated thromboplastin time and prothrombin time, low levels of plasmatic fibrinogen and antithrombin and high levels of D-dimers). Together with other supportive measures, red blood cells (RBCs), fresh frozen plasma (FFP), platelets (PLTs), antithrombin concentrates (ATc) and fibrinogen concentrates (FGc) were administrated according to the laboratory results and clinical judgement. All patients had normal haematologic and coagulation laboratory parameters within normal ranges before delivery. **Results**: All patients were successfully treated with a prompt administration of blood components and derivatives with rapid correction of coagulopathy. **Conclusions**: In obstetric patients, if any suspicion of DIC arises from either clinical or laboratory findings, it is imperative to monitor the patient carefully with clinical and laboratory tools. When coagulopathy is present, it has to be corrected in early stages, together with other supportive measures, to prevent a catastrophic ending.

PO109

Increased thrombin-antithrombin III levels in preeclampsia and disseminated intravascular coagulation on two different ELISAs

Simpson D, Whittier A, Andrews J, Fink C, Lopez L

Corgenix, Inc.

Introduction: Elevated plasma levels of thrombin-antithrombin III (TAT) complex are associated with active thrombosis. **Aim:** To compare the Dade-Behring TAT ELISA, with incubations at 37°C in a water bath, and the Corgenix TAT ELISA, with ambient incubations, in healthy individuals (n=33), patients with at a history of least one thrombotic event (n=10), DIC (n=10) and preeclampsia patients (n=10). **Materials and_Methods**: The assays were performed according to manufacturer's instructions. The Dade-Behring ELISA total time was 1 hour with incubations in a 37°C water-bath while the Corgenix ELISA total time was 2 hours with all incubations at ambient temperature (18-26°C). Separate TAT standard curves were used for each assay and results were interpolated from a log-log graph with a 60 ng/ml assay limit for both methods. **Results:** The normal cut-offs of the assays were determined with data generated from the healthy blood donors. The cut-off (mean plus 3 standard deviations) was 15.5 ng/ml for the Dade Behring kit and 15.4 ng/ml for the Corgenix kit. Patient subgroup mean values for the Dade Behring kit were 12.0 for DIC patients, 5.0 for thrombotic patients and 286.9 ng/ml for preeclampsia patients. Patient subgroup mean values for the Corgenix kit were 14.2 for DIC patients, 5.3 for thrombotic patients and 66.1 ng/ml for preeclampsia patients. None of thrombotic patients tested above the normal cut-off on either kit, probably because these patients did not have active thrombosis. Of the DIC patients, 20% on the Dade Behring kit and 40% on the Corgenix kit tested above the normal cut-off. 40% of preeclampsia patients on both assays tested above the normal cut-off. The mean TAT values for all patient groups in both ELISA tests were elevated compared to the control group. However, only the preeclampsia (P=0.0001) and DIC (P=5.1 x 10^{-6}) groups were significantly different from the healthy controls in both assays. **Conclusions**: Elevated TAT levels in the preeclampsia and DIC patients suggest the presence of an active state of coagulation. The TAT complex may be useful as a diagnostic and/or monitoring tool in patients in an active state of thrombosis. Furthermore, the Corgenix ELISA correlates well with the Dade-Behring ELISA kit (r=0.96) while having a user-friendlier format wherein all incubations are at ambient temperature.

PO110

Effect of parnaparin, a low molecular weight heparin, on platelet-leukocyte interaction

Maugeri N, de Gaetano G, Donati MB, Cerletti C*

Research Laboratories. Center for High Technology Research and Education in Biomedical Sciences, Campobasso, Italy

Introduction Recent evidence suggests that the antithrombotic effect of heparin may be partly due to its anti-inflammatory properties, mediated by effects on adhesive proteins involved in leukocyte- platelet-endothelium interactions. **Aims** To test the effects of parnaparin (PNP, Alfa Wassermann, Bologna, Italy), a low-molecular weight heparin, on human platelet-leukocyte (PMN) adhesion and on leukocyte function. **Methods** Platelets and PMN were isolated from venous blood of healthy volunteers and washed by standard procedure. PMN were incubated with PNP (0.3-3 IUaXa/ml) or unfractionated heparin (UH, 0.3-3 IU/ml) as reference drug, for 5 min (time course 0-20 min) at 4°C before assay. As an index of PMN activation, the shedding of L-selectin (CD62L) following PMN treatment with purified P-selectin (5ug/mL, 5 min, 37 °C) was measured by flow-cytometry, using a PE-labelled MoAb against CD62L. Platelet-PMN mixed cell aggregates (MCA) were determined using thrombin-activated and fixed platelets, which fully express P-selectin on their surface. Thrombin-stimulated, fixed platelets were labelled with FITC anti-CD61 MoAb and co-incubated (platelet/PMN ratio of 20) with PMN labelled with PC5-anti CD45 for 5 min under constant stirring at 37°C. MCA was expressed as the percentage of PMN with double fluorescence: PC5 anti-CD45 and FITC anti-CD61. All reactions were stopped by addition of an equal volume of 2% paraformaldehyde. **Results** PMN activation was expressed as % of control (amount of CD62L expressed on PMN incubated for 5 min without stimulus in stirring conditions, corresponding to 28±12%, means ± SEM; n= 6). PNP (0.3-3 IUaXa/ml) completely prevented the shedding of CD62L induced by P-selectin, corresponding to about 60% of unstimulated PMN. This effect was independent of the incubation time (from 5 to 20 min). PNP also effectively prevented the shedding of CD62L occurring during PMN stirring in the absence of agonist. Similar effects were observed with UH. CD61 co-fluorescence in PMN cluster (% of MCA) was 54±13 percent of total PMN population. PNP reduced in a concentration-dependent way the formation of MCA up to 70% inhibition at 3 IUaXa/ml, an effect shared at lower degree (40% inhibition at 3 IUaXa/ml) by UH. **Conclusions** The process of fractionation to obtain low molecular weight PNP, while reducing the anti-coagulant profile of this drug, did not remove the anticoagulant-independent effects on leukocytes and platelet-leukocyte interaction, previously described for UH and other glycosamino-glycans. Thus, if the overall anti-thrombotic properties of heparin were partly due to a leukocyte-mediated anti-inflammatory effect, PNP would share a similar mechanism at comparable concentrations as UH.

PO111

Paradoxical action of the synthetic pentasaccharide (Arixtra®)

Makris P, Boutou A, Tsoukas D, Papmichos S, Sarridou D, Triantafyllou A, Psatha V, Chasilidis A, Anestakis D, Girtovitis F*

Heamostasis Unit, A' Medical Propedeutic Clinic AUTH, Greece

Introduction: Synthetic pentasaccharide (Arixtra) has a particular anti-Xa activity. It impels thrombin's generation by forming a complex with antithrombin, which neutralizes FXa. This is an expected result, for which the drug was initially combined. With these characteristics of Arixtra, a major antithrombotic and a partial anticoagulant result is achieved (without any hemorrhagic complications). It seems paradoxical Arixtra to influence the platelets' function. However, accidentally, during the laboratory investigation of some patients, we studied the aggregation in a patient who was treated with Arixtra, to find out that there was a relative reduction of platelets' activation with ADP and Ristosetin (Risto). **Aim:** To study this paradoxal activity of platelets after the appliance of the synthetic pentasaccharide in vivo and ex vivo. **Material-Methods:** The aggregation of platelets with ADP and Risto was studied in 4 patients and 2 normal subjects. In patients a dose of 5mg/10kgr B.W. Arixtra was applied subcutaneous and periumbilical. In normal subjects Arixtra was added in vitro in their platelet rich plasma (PRP), (300,000/μl). Mixture was then incubated for 10 min at 37°C. The final concentration of the synthetic pentasaccharite in the mixture was 1μgr/ml, which corresponds to in vivo appliance of 5mg. The platelets' function under the effect of Arixtra was studied for 2 min, using the aggregometer PICA of Chronolog co. **Results:** There is a about a 10-15% reduction of the platelets' aggregation in all of the 4 patients. These findings were confirmed with the ex vivo incubation of PRP of normal subjects with Arixtra. The ex vivo activity of Arixtra is presented in Diagram I. The effect of Arixtra on patients after an 8-day long treatment is shown in Diagram II. **Conclusion:** Theoretically, Arixtra's only action is the antithrombotic one. However, by blocking the generation of thrombin, it directly impels the activation of platelets, since thrombin is one of their major stimulators. It also inhibits the production of prothrombinase, by blocking factor's Va and factor's Xa ability to turn prothrombin into thrombin, bringing the same anticoagulant result. This is how Arixtra can lead to a lack of platelets' activation, but not to the reduction of their aggregation. Possibly, the synthetic pentasaccharide affects the membrane receptors, leading to a decline of their function.

PO112

Influence of the original low molecular weight heparin on the rabbits plasma anticoagulant activity

Drozd N, Bannicova G, Sukhanova P, Miphtakhova N, Makarov V, Varlamov V, Vikhoreva G*

Introduction: Low molecular weight heparin (LMWH) possesses anticoagulant activity. It was used for prevention and treatment of venous thromboembolism. Due to manufacturing differences, there are marked structural variations between LMWH that exhibit distinct pharmacological and biochemical profiles. The potency of the LMWH is not less than 70 IU of anti-factor Xa activity (aXa) per milligram; the ratio of anti-factor Xa activity to anti-factor IIa activity (aIIa) is not less then 1.5. **Aims**: We investigated rabbit plasma anticoagulant activity after low molecular weight heparin 4.7 kDa (LMWH-1) intravenous injection. LMWH-1 obtained with the enzyme hydrolysis help of the unfractionated heparin (UFH). For this purpose used chitinolytic complex from Streptomyces kurssanovii. **Materials and methods**: For determination of antithrombin specific activity of the heparins and plasma activity used a method based on thrombin abilities to split synthetic oligopeptide amidous substrates. As a standard we took 5-th International UFH standard. Heparin specific activity against factor Xa and plasma activity determined with the help of the 1-st International LMWH standard. **Results**: aIIa activity of the was obtained heparin has made 72±9 IU/mg. aXa activity has made 430±40 IU/mg. aXa/aIIa ratio has made 5.4. Mongrel rabbits of both sexes weighing 2.5 –3.5 kg fed on a standard diet were given a bolus injection of LMWH-1 in a marginal ear vein at doses varying from 333 to 800 IU/kg. It was marked doso-dependent aIIa modification from 0.30±0.05 UI/ml for want 333 □/kg to 0.80±0.15 IU/ml for want 800 □kg on 5-th minute after injection. It was marked doso-dependent aXa modification from 0.80±0.04 UI/ml for want 333 □/kg to 3.00±0.60 IU/ml for want 800 □kg on 5-th minute after injection. **Conclusion**: LMWH-1 was obtained with the ensyme hydrolisis (chitinolytic comlex from Streptomyces kurssanoviii) help has ratio aXa/aIIa necessary for antithrombotic preparations (5.4). For want of intravenous LMWH-1 injection the plasma requaired aXa/aIIa ratio is saved. So, for want of smaller of used dozes, it was 2.7, and for want of greater – 3.8. The work is maintained by RFIF grant № 02-04-49850.

PO113

Different response of bone turnover markers during venous thromboembolic prophylaxis with LMWH or oral anticoagulants

Wawrzyńska L (1), Przedlacki J (2), Hajduk B (1), Tomkowski W (3), Torbicki A (1)*

(1) Department of Chest Medicine, National TB and Lung Diseases Research Institute, Warsaw, Poland
(2) Department of Radiology, Medical University, Warsaw, Poland
(3) Intensive Care Unit, National TB and Lung Diseases Research Institute, Warsaw, Poland

Background Bone turnover markers during the treatment with low-molecular-weight heparins (LMWH) or with oral anticoagulants (OA) are poorly investigated. Data on osteoporosis associated with LMWH and Vit.K antagonists are contradictory. **Aim** To estimate of bone turnover markers during secondary prophylaxis of venous thromboembolism (VTE) with low-molecular-weight heparins or with oral anticoagulants **Materials and methods** 31 patients mean age 40.1 years (range: 20 - 72), 15 women and 16 men entered our study. In all cases VTE was confirmed by objective method (compression ultrasound and/ or helical CT). There were 10 cases with deep venous thrombosis (DVT), 6 cases with pulmonary embolism (PE) and 15 cases with DVT and PE. In all patients bone densitometry was performed on the beginning of the study and 6-12 month (mean: 9months) during prolonged secondary prophylaxis of VTE.

There were 15 cases treated with enoxaparin (1 mg/kg of body weight once time daily) and 16 patients treated with acenocoumarol, administered to keep INR between 2-3. The group of patients treated with LMWH consisted of patients with contra-indications to administration of OA. At the same day as performed densitometry serum total alkaline phosphatase activity, serum concentration of N Mid- Osteocalcin and bCrossLaps were assessed. **Results** Comparing beginning values of bone turnover markers with values assessed during prophylaxis we observed substantial differences. Bone mineral density (BMD) decreased in both groups. In patients treated with LMWH mean decrease of BMD during prophylaxis was 1.97% while in patients using OA was 1.42%. Serum activity of alkaline phosphatase decreased differently 18.8 IU/dl ($p<0.003$) and 10.1 IU/dl ($p<0.02$) respectively. Osteocalcin serum concentration decreased by 3.89 ng/ml ($p<0.009$) in LMWH group and 4.51 ng/ml ($p<0.005$) in OA group. Serum concentration of bCrossLaps increased substantially in both group of patients. **Conclusions** During the treatment with LMWH and OA substantial changes in bone density are observed. Values of bone turnover markers in LMWH and OA groups were different. Mechanism of observed changes in bone turnover markers is probably different in patients treated with LMWH and OA.

PO114

The aPTT paradox of the bridging process

Volteas S, Bossinakou I, parigoti A, Kalatzopoulos D, Mattheou S, Nikolakeas M, Sikiotis K*

Hippocration Hospital, Athens Greece

Introduction While conducting a pilot study of replacing acenocoumarol with the low molecular weight (LMWH) Tinzaparin sodium in unselected patients undergoing general surgery operations, we had a surprisingly prolonged aPTT in certain phases of the study. **Aim** The aim of the present communication was to present this paradox finding and discuss its aetiology and clinical significance. **Material and Methods** According to our bridging protocol, 4-6 days pre-operatively acenocoumarol administration is stopped and the LMWH Tinzaparin sodium (Innohep®, Leo Pharma) is given subcutaneously at an adjusted daily dose (175 anti-Xa IU/Kg body weight); 2-3 days later complete haemorrheology tests are performed. Acenocoumarol restarts 2-4 days post-operatively and is co-administered with Tinzaparin for 2 days or as long as needed to achieve therapeutic INR levels; complete haemorrheology tests are also performed during that phase. **Results** From a total of 30 bridging processes, in 6 (20%) prolonged aPTT (above 90 seconds) was seen. The same happened in 2 patients during the post-operative co-administration of acenocoumarol and Tinzaparin. When firstly identified, the operation was postponed; blood-clotting time however was found normal (as it was in all cases of prolonged aPTT) and all operations thereafter were performed as scheduled. No major bleeding complications during or after the operations occurred: in our study we had only two cases of relatively large post-operative haematomas, but these patients were not among those with prolonged aPTT. The reason for this paradox result remains unclear, although a technical error during laboratory specimen preparation cannot be excluded. **Conclusions** Although the reason for the prolonged aPTT seen during the co-administration phase of acenocoumarol and Tinzaparin remains unclear, this paradox is of no clinical significance. According to the results of our study, the bridging process using the LMWH Tinzaparin sodium is a safe and effective procedure in patients undergoing general surgery operations.

PO115

Pharmacoeconomic analysis of bemiparin vs. enoxaparin as prophylaxis for venous thromboembolism in total knee replacement surgery

Honorato J (1), Gómez-Outes A (2), Navarro-Quilis A (3), Martínez-González J (2)*, Rocha E (1), Planès A (4)*

(1) University Clinic of Navarra, Pamplona, Spain
(2) Laboratorios Farmacéuticos ROVI, S.A., Madrid, Spain
(3) Hospital Vall d'Ebrón, Barcelona, Spain
(4) Clinique Radio-Chirurgicale du Mail, La Rochelle, France

Introduction: Low-molecular-weight heparins are effective and safe as a first-line prophylaxis of venous thromboembolism (VTE) in total knee replacement (TKR) surgery. However, pharmacological inequivalence within the class could lead to differences in cost-effectiveness ratios. **Aims:** To quantify the potential economic impact of bemiparin 3,500 IU/d compared to enoxaparin 40 mg/d during the in- and out-hospital prophylaxis of VTE in patients undergoing TKR. **Material and methods:** We performed a cost-effectiveness analysis by using a decision modelling approach. We expressed our results in terms of costs and incremental cost-effectiveness in euros (€). We considered for this analysis the treatment costs and costs derived from complications: proximal deep vein thrombosis (DVT) and/or pulmonary embolism (PE), bleeding events, wound haematoma and thrombocytopenia. The study perspective was the Spanish National Health System. The time horizon chosen was 6 weeks. **Results:** Bemiparin provided cost-savings of €144 per patient compared to enoxaparin when considering costs derived from treatment and complications during the 6-week post-operative period (€4,677 vs. €4,821). Bemiparin pharmacy costs per patient were lower than enoxaparin during hospitalisation (€43 vs. €50) and out-hospital prophylaxis (€69 vs. €88). Bemiparin avoided 102 clinically important VTE events (44 PEs and 58 proximal DVTs) per 1,000 patients treated, whereas enoxaparin avoided only 66 clinical important VTE events (32 PEs and 34 proximal DVTs) per 1,000 patients treated. The expected cost of PEs avoided per 1,000 patients treated was €100,669 for bemiparin compared to €138,497 for enoxaparin; the expected cost of proximal DVTs avoided per 1,000 patients treated was €76,294 for bemiparin compared to €130,350 for enoxaparin. The sensitivity analysis confirmed the cost-effectiveness of bemiparin in all the ranges tested for complications and costs. **Conclusions:** Bemiparin 3,500 IU was more cost-effective than enoxaparin 40 mg in patients undergoing TKR surgery, providing cost savings of €144 per patient treated. Cost savings were mainly attributable to fewer clinically important VTE events and, to a lesser extent, to lower acquisition costs for bemiparin.

PO116

Comparative profile of tinazaparin and a sulfaminoheparosan of bacterial origin: a possible potential alternate for low molecular weight heparins

Maddineni J (1), Manoni M (2), Cornelli U (3), Hoppensteadt D (1), Fareed J (1)*

(1) Loyola University Chicago, Maywood, IL, USA, 60153
(2) R.S.M., Montale, Italy, 51037
(3) Corcon, Milano, Italy, 20129

Introduction: Heparin and low molecular weight heparin (LMWHs) are the conventional drugs used to treat thrombotic disorders. They are produced from the mammalian tissues such as porcine lung and bovine intestine. Because of the widespread usage of LMWHs these sources are nearly depleted, necessitating the development of alternate approaches to produce heparin like anticoagulants. A series of heparin analogues derived from capsular polysaccharide of *E.coli* have been developed and found to exhibit similar properties as heparins. These compounds are called sulfaminoheparosans (SAHs). SAHs can be produced by deacetylation followed by N-sulfation and controlled O-sulfation and epimerization of N-acetyl heparosan. The molecular profiling of a low molecular weight sulfaminoheparosan (LMW-SAH) revealed that it has a similar profile as a commercially available LMWH, tinzaparin of MW=6,000D. Both the agents were produced by the similar means of depolymerization (nitrous acid digestion) from the high molecular weight components and exhibited similar anticoagulant profiles. **Objective:** To compare the biologic and pharmacologic effects of a LMW-SAH (Q93C/239) with a commercially available LMWH, tinzaparin. **Materials and Methods:** The following assays were used: global clotbased, antiprotease, protease generation and platelet activation assays to compare these agents. **Results:** Both of the tinzaparin and LMW-SAH produce a concentration dependence effect in the global anticoagulant assays, such as the APTT, heptest and thrombin time comparable results were obtained. In the anti-Xa and anti-IIa assays, LMW-SAH was somewhat weaker than tinzaparin; however, in the protease generation inhibition assays (Xa and IIa) utilizing intrinsic and extrinsic activators, marked differences were noted between tinzaparin and LMW-SAH. In these assays, LMW-SAH was found to be 2 to 50 times more potent than tinzaparin. Protamine sulfate neutralization profile of both tinzaparin and LMW-SAH were similar in terms of a complete neutralization of anti-Xa and partial neutralization of anti-IIa actions. In the platelet activation assays both agents produced no effect. Tinzaparin produced a positive screening in HIT assay but LMW-SAH did not produce these effects. **Conclusions:** This data clearly suggest that LMW-SAH produces anticoagulant and antiprotease actions, which are similar to tinzaparin. Due to its relatively stronger actions on protease generation inhibition, this agent may be more effective than tinzaparin. Furthermore, the optimized forms of LMW-SAH may potentially substitute LMWHs in various hematologic indications.

PO117

Partial results of the incidence of heparin induced thrombocytopenia

Oliveira S, Rached R, Cavalheiro-Filho C, Chamone D*

InCor-S.P Brazil

Introduction: Heparin Induced Thrombocytopenia (HIT) type II is an important immune-mediated disorder that occurs between 2 and 5% of the patients exposed to unfractionated heparin (UFH). In our routine the number of patients that receive heparin is often, mainly cardiac patients, however the report of heparin-induced thrombocytopenia is rare. **Aim**: To know the real incidence of heparin induced thrombocytopenia in our institution. **Material and Methods**: At the moment, we have studied 74 patients treated with unfractionated heparin or low molecular weight heparin for 5 or more days. Known causes of thrombocytopenia were excluded. Platelet count was monitored pre and post heparin therapy, after inclusion in the protocol all patients were tested for detection of "anti – heparin/PF4 antibodies" by ID – Card "Heparin/PF4 antibody test" (DiaMed – ID PaGIA). **Results**: Amongst the studied patients, 28 (37,8 %) developed a reduction in the platelet count below 30%, regarding the platelet count pre heparin therapy, whereas, 46 (62,2 %) did not show significant reduction. Among the 28 thrombocytopenia patients, 4 were tested positive for anti – heparin/PF4 antibodies. Among the 46 patients without thrombocytopenia, 2 were tested positive for anti – heparin/PF4 antibodies. **Conclusion**: The partial data suggests that 6 (8 %) patients developed anti – heparin/PF4 antibodies, from this 4 (5.4 %) patients developed thrombocytopenia with presence of anti – heparin/PF4 antibodies.

PO118

Confirmation of the pathogenic role of Ig M and Ig A anti-heparin-PF4 antibodies in patients with heparin-induced thrombocytopenia

Tardy-Poncet B (1), Tardy B (2), Piot M (1), Reynaud J (1), Campos L (1), Decousus H (2)*

(1) Laboratoire d'Hématologie, CHU St Etienne, Franc
(2) Groupe de recherche sur la thrombose, CHU St Etienne, Franc

Antibodies to heparin-platelet factor 4 (PF4) complexes are generally observed in patients with heparin-induced thrombocytopenia (HIT) syndrome. These antibodies may be of various isotypes, which differ with respect to their ability to activate platelets. We explored the pathogenic role of Ig M and Ig A anti heparin-PF4 antibodies in patients with HIT. Over a 7 years period (from 1996 to 2002), we determined 127 isotypes of antiheparin-PF4 antibodies detected in patients who developed thrombocytopenia during heparin therapy. Out of these 127 plasmas, 36 contained only Ig M and /or Ig A. For 29 out of these 36 patients, clinical HIT diagnosis was defined as sure or probable using a clinical score. Among these 29 plasmas, a positive platelet aggregation test was observed for only 5 plasmas which contained either Ig M and Ig A (2 patients), or Ig M alone (2 patients), or Ig A alone (1 patient). In 4/5 cases, the specificity of the aggregation induced by anti H-PF4 antibodies was verified. Among these patients with clinical HIT and isolated IgM or Ig A antibodies, 15 presented a thrombotic complication either arterial (7) or venous (8). Our results indicate that type II HITT (HIT with thrombosis) may be induced by Ig A and/ or Ig M anti-H-PF4 antibodies even in the absence of Ig G isotypes. It means that Ig A and Ig M play a significant role in the pathophysiology of HIT syndrome. It is therefore of great importance to use ELISA technique able to detect all the anti H-PF4 antibodies whatever their isotypes are. The final diagnosis of HIT will take into account the results of functionnal and ELISA tests as well as the clinical context in which thrombocytopenia occured.

PO119

Plasma pro and anticoagulant factors in the early stages of Buerger's disease

Sokolowska B (1), Dmoszynska A (1), Walter-Croneck A (1), Nowaczynska A (1), Skwarzynski A (2), Chrapko M (1), Soroka-Wojtaszko M (1), Gernand W (3), Grzebisz A (1), Trzesniowska W (1)*

(1) Department of Haematooncology and BMT, Medical University in Lublin, Poland
(2) Department of Vascular Surgery, Country Hospital in Lublin, Poland
(3) Institute of Laboratory Diagnostics, Medical University in Lublin, Poland

Pathogenesis of Buerger's disease is not completely understood. However, development of thrombosis in the course of the disease is undisputed. It has been suggested in the recent years that increased activity of plasma coagulation factors, such as factor VII, VIII, XI, hyperhomocysteinemia and disturbances concerning natural anticoagulants, such as e.g. anexin V, may play an important part in pathogenesis of vascular diseases characterized by an increased tendency to thrombosis. The aim of the study was to assess the activity of plasma coagulation factors VII, VIII, XI and the concentration of anexin V, and to relate these values to recognized prognostic factors in Buerger's disease, and also to look for relationship between the activity of these factors and the concentration of different lipid fractions and homocysteine. The study comprised 37 patients with thrombangiitis. The study group consisted of 8 women (21.6%) and 29 men (78.4%) aged 20 – 50 years, mean age 39.5. The duration of the disease was 1 - 22 years, mean 5.5 years. The low degree of ischaemia as evaluated by Fontaine scale (I+II) was found in 34 patients, the high degree of ischaemia was observed in 3 patients (III+IV). The history of the disease revealed habitual smoking in 23 patients, 12 stopped smoking at the time of diagnosing the disease, and 2 did not smoke at all. Among biochemical parameters being assessed were: total concentrations of lipids, cholesterol, HDL and LDL fractions, apolipoprotein A and homocysteine. We evaluated the activity of plasma coagulation factors VII, VIII, XI and the concentration of anexin V - the protein which shows anticoagulant properties and additional anti-inflammatory action. In comparison with the control group, a statistically significant increase in the activity of factors VIII and XI and in the concentration of anexin V was found (factor VIII 119.85 vs 60.19%, factor XI 108.72 vs 78.54%, anexin V 8.27 vs 3.39 ng/ml) and a statistically significant increase in homocysteine concentration was noted (11.53 vs 9.86 μmol/l). The activity of factor VII was within the normal range. No positive correlation between the activity of factor VII and VIII, homocysteine and anexin V concentrations and tobacco smoking was found in the whole group of patients. A group with a particularly high activity of factor VIII, exceeding 150%, was isolated among the patients. In this group, a positive correlation between homocysteine concentration and drinking coffee was found. Our study showed that factors VIII, XI, anexin V and homocysteine may play a part in pathogenesis of Buerger's disease.

PO120

Oxidative stress, cardiovascular disease and CC-chemokine levels in haemodialyzed patients

Pawlak D (1), Pawlak K (2), Mysliwiec M (2)*

(1) Department of Pharmacodynamics, Medical University, Białystok, Poland
(2) Department of Nephrology and Transplantation, Medical University, Białystok, Poland

Introduction. Accelerated atherosclerosis plays an important role in the development of cardiovascular disease (CVD) in haemodialyzed (HD) patients and there is evidence of its link with oxidative stress (SOX). Chemotactic cytokines (CC-chemokines) involved in leukocyte trafficking and activation, and their role in atherosclerosis is well documented. **Aims**. We hypothesized that SOX may participate in pathogenesis of atherosclerosis in HD patients via production of CC-chemokines. **Materials and methods**. The levels of 3 distinct SOX markers: Cu/Zn superoxide dismutase (Cu/Zn SOD), total lipid peroxide and autoantibodies against oxidized LDL (OxLDL-Ab), as well as those of 4 CC-chemokines: monocyte chemoattractant protein-1 (MCP-1); macrophage inflammatory proteins (MIP-1α, MIP-1β); regulated upon activation, normal T cell expressed and secreted (RANTES); and tumor necrosis factor-α (TNF-α) were measured pre and post HD session in 15 HD patients with CVD, 12 HD patients without CVD and 17 controls. **Results**. Cu/Zn SOD levels were elevated in HD patients (both before and after HD) compared to controls ($p<0.001$). Total lipid peroxide levels were similar in the controls in pre-dialysis samples, but were increased after an HD session ($p<0.001$). Pre-dialysis OxLDL-Ab levels were increased only in the HD group with CVD compared to controls ($p<0.05$). The pre-dialysis plasma levels of TNF-α ($p<0.001$), MCP-1 (p<0.001) and MIP-1β (p<0.01) were increased both in all HD patients and subgroups with CVD when compared to the controls, and remained significantly elevated when measured after HD. Dialysis increased MCP-1 (p<0.05) and MIP-1β (p<0.001) levels as compared to the controls also in patients without CVD. Plasma RANTES was significantly lower before HD and after HD in all HD patients when compared to controls (all p<0.001). A positive relationship existed between plasma Cu/Zn SOD levels and those of MCP-1, MIP-1β and TNF-α (all p<0.001). RANTES levels negatively correlated with Cu/Zn SOD (p<0.0001). TNF-α positively correlated with MCP-1 (p<0.01), MIP-1β levels (p<0.01) and an identifiable association exists between MCP-1 and MIP-1β levels (p<0.01). **Conclusions**. Our data indicate for the first time a probable functional relationship between oxidative stress and CC-chemokine levels in hemodialyzed patients, particularly in those with CVD. This relationship may represent one of the mechanisms involved in the progression of atherosclerosis in these patients.

PO121

Possible vascular-bed-specific role of interleukin-6 in young women with a history of three different types of thrombosis

Salobir B, Šabovič M*

University Clinical Center, Department of vascular diseases, Zaloška 7, 1000 Ljubljana

Introduction and aim: There is growing evidence that interleukin-6 (IL-6), a cytokine with prothrombotic properties might represent a novel, non-classical risk factor in different atherothrombotic diseases, especially in patients who suffer thrombotic events in the absence of (pronounced) classical risk factors, as occurred in young adults, especially young women in whom it was not studied yet. Thus the aim of our study was to evaluate level of IL-6 and its interactions with metabolic, coagulation and fibrinolytic parameters in young women with three different types of thrombosis. **Methods and materials:** The level of interleukin-6 (IL-6), and associations of IL-6 to metabolic, coagulation and fibrinolytic parameters, was investigated in 68 young women (23 to 49, mean 40 years old) half to six years after myocardial infarction (MI, N=22), lacunar cerebral infarction (LACI, N=16) and deep vein thrombosis (VT, N=30); all women were in the reproductive periode, aged <45 years at the time of acute thrombotic event. Forty-seven age-matched women comprised a control group. **Results:** Basic and multivariate analysis disclosed different patterns of IL-6 increase in all three groups of patients. In the MI group IL-6 was significantly elevated independently of factors known to increase IL-6 levels, the increase was most pronounced in patients with high lipoprotein(a). This result suggests a pro-thrombotic association of lipoprotein(a) with IL-6. In the whole LACI group IL-6 was not significantly increased. However, patients with elevated levels of IL-6 had abdominal obesity and elevated fibrinogen, suggesting the possibility that this combination might represent a specific risk profile. In VT group elevated IL-6 level was found in the group of previous users of oral contraceptives (OC). This might be relevant, since it is known that OC could importantly increase (previously elevated) IL-6 level in selected woman. **Conclusions:** Our results suggest the hypothesis that the role of IL-6 might be vascular-bed-specific and further propose that increased IL-6 level might represent a novel, non-classical risk factor for development of MI, LACI and VT in specific subgroups of young women, what have to be clarify in further studies.

PO122

Haemostatic abnormalities and inflammatory cytokines in patients with chronic obstructive pulmonary disease

Ferroni P (1), Martini F (1), Guadagni F (2), Roselli M (3), Bertazzoni G (1), Basili S (4)*

(1) Dept. of Experimental Medicine & Pathology, La Sapienza University, Rome, Italy
(2) Laboratory of Clinical Pathology, Regina Elena Cancer Institute, Rome, Italy
(3) Dept. of Surgery, "Tor Vergata" University, Rome, Italy
(4) Dept. of Medical Therapy, La Sapienza University, Rome, Italy

Introduction Inflammatory cytokines are involved in activation of the haemostatic system. IL-6, for example, causes an increased sensitivity of platelets to thrombin activation and enhances tissue factor expression, while TNF-α is thought to play a direct role in the activation of fibrinolysis. Both cytokines are enhanced in chronic obstructive pulmonary disease (COPD), a clinical setting characterized by a prothrombotic state due to platelet activation and/or abnormalities in blood coagulation. **Aims** The present study was aimed at analyzing the possible association between inflammatory cytokines (TNF- α, IL-6) and platelet (sCD62P) or coagulation/ fibrinolysis (TATc/D-dimer) activation markers in patients with COPD to better characterize the link between inflammation and haemostatic abnormalities in this clinical setting. **Materials and methods** Sixty-five COPD patients (51 males 14 females, 67±9 years, 11 current and 33 ex-smokers) and 65 healthy controls (51 males 14 females, 61±14 years, 12 current and 25 ex-smokers) were evaluated. No subject was on anti-inflammatory, anticoagulant or antiplatelet drugs in the 2 weeks preceding the study. Informed consent was obtained from each subject. TNF- α, IL-6, sCD62P (R&D Systems), TATc (Dade-Behring) and D-dimer (Roche Diagnostics) levels were determined on citrated plasma samples. **Results** Median levels of all 5 variables were higher in COPD patients compared to controls (TNF- α: 4.0 vs. 0.4 pg/ml, p<0.0001; IL-6: 4.7 vs. 1.5 pg/ml, p<0.0001; sCD62P: 87 vs. 49 pg/ml, p<0.0001; TATc: 5.7 vs. 1.8 μg/L, p<0.0001; D-dimer 1.1 vs. 0.3 μg/ml, p<0.0001), but did not show any difference according to the smoking habit. Multiple regression analysis including age, sex, smoking status, inflammatory cytokines, blood gas levels and coagulation parameters showed that blood carbon dioxide tension (p<0.05), sCD62P (p<0.005) and IL-6 (p<0.02) were independently related to TATc levels, which, in turn, were predictive of sCD62P levels (p<0.002). TATc (p<0.03), but not TNF- α levels, were independently related to D-dimer. **Conclusions** The present study demonstrates that TNF- α is not responsible for a direct activation of fibrinolysis in COPD. Conversely, we may hypothesize that increased IL-6 levels might be responsible for increased thrombin generation leading to platelet activation and secondary fibrinolysis.

PO123

Inflammatory markers and C-IMT in patients with previous myocardial infarction. The atorvastatin effect. MIAMI Study

Cortellaro M, Tremoli E on behalf of of the MIAMI Study Group*

Milan University, Italy

Introduction Plasma levels of Hs-CRP may be useful to select subjects at high risk of cardiovascular events. This inflammatory marker also helps identify patients most likely to respond to statins. **Aim**: A prospective clinical study was designed to investigate: a) the regression of CRP levels and other soluble inflammatory markers; b) the correlations between levels of C-IMT and soluble markers at different times; c) the influence of Hs-CRP levels on C-IMT regression; d) the utility of Carotid Intima Media Thickness (C-IMT) as an additional marker to identify patients likely to respond to statins. **Materials and methods**: MIAMI is an open, multicenter, independent study. In 100 patients with previous MI (> two months), in stable clinical conditions, with normal cholesterol and blood glucose, receiving atorvastatin (20 mg/daily) for 0, 12, or 24 months, the following variables were measured: VCAM, ICAM, E-selectins, IL-6, -8, -10, -18, TNF-alpha, hs-CRP, MMP-9, TF, TFPI, Fg, TC, HDL, LDL, TG, urinary isoprostanes. C-IMT was measured blind by computerised determination of images recorded in three examinations. The study started in January 2003 and is scheduled to end in December 2005.

PO124

Haemodialysis patients have more prominent non-classical than classical cardiovascular risk factors

Vujkovac B (1), Lavre J (1), Šabovič M (2)*

(1) Dept. of Nephrology and Dialysis, General Hospital Slovenj Gradec, Slovenia
(2) University Medical Centre, Department for Vascular Diseases, Ljubljana, Slovenia

In haemodialysis (HD) patients cardiovascular morbidity is 10 to 20 times higher than in general population. There is growing evidence that beside classical risk factors (dyslipidemia, arterial hypertension, diabetes mellitus, smoking), the non-classical risk factors are responsible for facilitated atherosclerosis. Among different non-classical factors the systemic »low grade« inflammation state (microinflammation), homocystein and lipoprotein(a) (Lpa) might have substantial role. We investigated the presence of classical and non-classical (microinflammation, Lp(a), homocystein) risk factors in our cohort of chronic haemodialysis patients (N=22, age 62.8±12.8, average duration of treatment with HD: 5±3 y). All patients had appropriate nutritional status (BMI: 26.32±4.34 kg/m2) and no signs of acute illness. The values of serum lipids were within normal range (no patient used lipid-lowering drug): total cholesterol (4.31±0.88 mmol/L), LDL cholesterol (2.43±0.53mmol/L), triglycerides (1.77±1.1 mmol/L), and HDL cholesterol (1.09±0.35 mmol/L). Twenty patients had arterial hypertension, and were all adequately treated (arterial pressure≤140/90 mmHg). Two patients had non insulin dependent diabetes mellitus (treated only with diet), one patient was smoker. Accordingly, all patients had low risk for cardiovascular events. In the contrast to classical risk factors, the patients had significantly (p<0.01) elevated values of serum markers of microinflammation: CRP (10.6±12.6 mg/L; normal values: <3 mg/L), IL-6 (1.49±1.66 pg/ml; normal values: <0.4 pg/ml), and TNFα (7.26±5.52 pg/ml; normal values: <10 pg/ml). Similarly, the levels of Lpa (0.17±0.15 g/l; normal values: <0.3 g/L) and homocystein (37.6 umol/L; normal values: 5.0-15,0) were also significantly (p<0.01) elevated. **In conclusion**, our results suggest that in optimally treated HD patients non-classical risk factors are more pronounced (and possibly more important) than classical risk factors. It seems likely that control and treatment of non-classical risk factors might be beneficial for slowing atherosclerosis in HD patients.

PO125

The most important factor for cardiovascular morbidity in hemodialysis patients is microinflammation

Lavre J (1), Vujkovac B (1), Šabovič M (2)*

(1) Dept. of Nephrology and Dialysis, General Hospital Slovenj Gradec, Slovenia
(2) University Medical Centre, Department for Vascular Diseases, Ljubljana, Slovenia

In hemodialysis patients cardiovascular (CV) morbidity is 10 to 20 times higher than in general population. Dyslipidemia, malnutrition and non-traditional CV risk factors are well known important determinants in the increased CV morbidity. So we measured levels of serum high-sensitivity C-reactive protein (CRP), interleukin 6 (IL-6), tumor necrosis factor–α (TNF- α), albumin, ferritin, cholesterol (CHOL), triglyceride (TG), HDL, LDL, lipoprotein(a) (Lpa) and body mass index (BMI) in 22 HD patients (age 62.8±12.8) on maintenance HD for 65.16±33 months. All patients received standard dietary guidance with an average protein intake of 1.2 g/kg/day, 35 kcal/kg, phosphate and potassium restriction. 20 of 22 patients had well treadted high blood pressure. Two patients had non insulin dependent diabetes mellitus treated only with diet. The patients were not treated with lipid lowering drugs, and ony one patient was smoker. The mean values of serum CHOL (4.31±0.88 mmol/L), TG (1.77±1.1 mmol/L), HDL (1.09±0.35 mmol/L) and LDL (2.43±0.53mmol/L) wer normal. The patients had elevated values of serum CRP (10.63±12.56 mg/L), IL-6 (1.49±1.66 pg/ml), TNF-α (7.26±5.52 pg/ml) and Lpa (0.17±0.15 ug/dl). The mean value of serum albumin (41.03±2.38 g/L)was also normal, the mean value of BMI (26.32±4.34 kg/m2) was mild elevated. The patients had elevated serum ferritin (518±342 mmol/L), but in expeted range. The mean value of Kt/V (1.86±0.23) was hig normal. Our patients have elevated CRP, IL-6 and TNF-α. On contrary with other studies our patients had normal lipid status and also normal nutritional status. No significant relationships were found between CRP, IL-6, TNF-α or ferritin and age, history of dialysis, albumin and BMI. There was only significant correlation between months on dialysis and HDL (r= -0.46, p=0.048), but no significant correlations between months on dialysis and albumin, BMI, CHOL, TG, LDL and Lp(a). We concluded that in our HD patients the most important factor for high CV morbidity was microinflamation. Dyslipidemia and malnutrition are well controlled in optimally treated HD patients and seems to be only a minor factor for CV morbidity.

PO126

Circulating plasma levels of annexin V in venous thromboembolism (VTE)

González-Ordóñ A (1), Macías D (2), Arias A (1), Ramas C (2), del Blanco JM (2), Morán M (2)*

(1) Department of Hematology. Hospital S. Agustín. Avilés, Spain
(2) Department of Internal Medicine. Hospital S. Agustín. Avilés, Spain

The annexin A5 (annexin V, ANV) is the most relevant member of the annexins, a group of highly homologous proteins that associate with anionic phospholipids in the presence of Ca^{++} developing functions of placental and vascular anticoagulant. ANV binds to membrane phospholipids when they become exposed during the cellular activation process (e.g. in platelets or erythrocytes) precluding the organization of prothrombinase and tenase complexes and producing a strong antithrombotic effect on cellular surfaces. By contrary, the circulating free ANV represents the short interval between the release and binding from blood and vascular cells. Recently, a functional C>T genetic variation in the Kozak sequence of the ANV gene was described so the -1C/T genotype increases translation efficiency (and their plasma levels) protecting younger patients from myocardial infarction *(Blood 2002; 100: 2081-6)*. Although the plasma concentrations of ANV could be independent of this polymorphism *(Blood 2003; 101: 4223-4)* the eventual protective role of a raised circulating ANV seems exciting. **Population and Methods.** We measured the free circulating ANV concentrations in citrated plasma from 244 subjects: 122 consecutive patients objectively diagnosed of venous thromboembolism (VTE) and 122 age and gender-matched controls [62.1(12.3) years, 49.2% males] by ELISA. **Results.** In the overall series ANV levels were age-related (r= 0.13, p<0.05) and independent of gender (NS p). Among the patients ANV was similar [1.96(1.55) ng/ml] to the controls [1.69(1.20) ng/ml](p=0.2). However, a trend to higher ANV values appears among female patients [2.15(1.84) vs. 1.55(1.02) ng/ml](p=0.06, Mann Whitney test). Even in women, the 90th percentile (3.1 ng/ml) was not significantly associated with the VTE [OR: 1.8 (95%CI 0.6-5.1)](p=0.3). The circulating ANV was similar in recurrent (n=32) and non-recurrent cases [2.52(2.29) vs. 1.76(1.14) ng/ml](p=0.19). The ANV values were also similar in deep vein thrombosis (DVT) and pulmonary embolism (PE) and independent of the existence of antiphospholipid antibodies (anticardiolipin or lupus anticoagulant). **Conclusion.** The free circulating ANV levels observed in citrated plasma are similar between VTE patients and controls. This preliminary report seems inconsistent with an obvious protective role attributable to the nonbound fraction of this anticoagulant protein. *This work was supported by the grant FIS # 031553.*

PO127

Lupus ratio (LR) and correction ratio (CR) applying to dRVVT results

Gennari L, Blanco A, Grosso S, Dominguez M, Lazzari M*

Haemostasis Division, National Academy of Medicine, Buenos Aires, Argentina

Intoduction: The laboratory detection of lupus anticoagulant (LA) is sometimes troublesome not only due to the heterogeneity of the antibodies but also because of the phospholipid (PL)-reagent employed and the way the results are expressed. The APTT-based Lupus Ratio (LR), on 1:1 mixture of patient (P) plasma and normal (N) pool, has been described as a single test that includes screening, mixing and confirmatory procedures. This integrated test appeared to be not only less time consuming, but also increases the specificity (SP=100%) and the sensitivity (S=95%) in comparison with the use of separate screening and confirmatory assays. Aim and objective: We wondered if the dRVVT results expressed as LR (dRVVT-LR=[(PN DilutePL/PN HighPL)/(N DilutePL/N HighPL)] improves the SP and S for the LA detection in comparison with the results expressed as prolonged screening test (P/N>1,12), not corrected by normal plasma and neutralized by PL (Delta dRVVT=[(P/N)DilutePL-(P/N)HighPL] ≥ 0,10). Moreover, we also expressed confirmatory results as a ratio (dRVVT-Ratio (R)=[(P DilutePL/P HighPL)/(N DilutePL/N HighPL)] or dRVVT-CR=[(P DilutePL/N DilutePL)-(P HighPL/N HighPL)]/(P DilutePL/N DilutePL) x100. **Materials and methods**: 160 controls were analized in order to define cut-off values for each expression, in addition to 54 LA+ samples, applying a home made dRVVT (Sigma). **Results**: Similar S and SP results were obtained with any of the employed expressions: LR (76%/84%); R (81%/85%) and CR (89%/79%); giving an overall accuracy of 82%, 84% and 81% respectively. **Conclusions**: This results shows that LR is as good as other expressions of the results that considered the SSC-ISTH criteria and suggests that detection of LA is perhaps more dependent of the (PL)-reagent employed than the mode of expression.

PO128

Antiphospholipid antibodies in young women without autoimmune diseases and suffering from arterial or venous thromboses

Salobir B (1), Šabovič M (1), Hojnik M (2), Čučnik S (2), Kveder T (2)*

(1) Department of vascular diseases, University Medical Centre, Ljubljana, Slovenia
(2) Department of rheumatology, University Medical Centre, Ljubljana, Slovenia

Background: The exact prevalence and role of antiphospholipid antibodies (aPL) in patients with thrombosis in the absence of autoimmune diseases remains incompletely understood. They might be important in groups of patients with otherwise a low risk according to their classical risk profile such as young women are. **Methods**: We investigated the aPL (anti-β2-GPI IgM, IgG and IgA; aCL IgM and IgG; aPS IgM and IgG) in 68 young women (aged<45 years at onset of the event, without autoimmune diseases and with otherwise a low risk of thrombosis) in the stable periode following myocardial infarction (MI), lacunar cerebral infarction (LACI) or deep vein thrombosis (DVT) and in 37 healthy age-matched controls. **Results**: Patients had significantly increased anti-β2-GPI IgM and aCL IgG compared to controls (36.0, 11.5 - 49.5 vs. 17.50, 3.50 - 30.0 arbitrary units (AU), $p<0.001$ and 0.17, 0.13 - 0.21 vs. 0.14, 0.09 - 0-17 optical density units 405nm, $p<0.005$). Subgroup analysis revealed increased levels of anti-β2-GPI IgM and aCL IgG in DVT and LACI, but not in MI. Further, anti-β2-GPI IgM was higher in lean (BMI<25 kg/m^2, N= 26) compared to overweight (BMI>25 kg/m^2, N=42) patients (45.5, 30-61 vs. 30, 11.0-39.9 AU, $p<0.005$). In patients anti-β2-GPI IgM significantly negatively correlated with BMI (r=-039, $p<0.005$) and other parameters of polymetabolic syndrome. **Conclusions**: In young women with thrombosis in the absence of autoimmune diseases , predominantly anti-β2-GPI IgM are increased in stable phase after the acute event, especially post LACI and DVT. Negative correlations between anti-β2-GPI IgM, and the parameters of polymetabolic syndrome suggest the existence of two distinct risk profiles of thrombosis in young women: aPL and polymetabolic syndrome.

PO129

Autoantibodies to B2GPI/OxLDL complexes: a novel risk factor for thromboembolic disease in Systemic Lupus Erythematosus?

Lopez L (1), Garcia De La Torre I (2), Matsuura E (3)*

(1) Corgenix, Inc. Westminster, Colorado 80234, USA
(2) Hospital General de Occidente, Univ. of Guadalajara, Jalisco 45170, Mexico
(3) Okayama University Graduate School of Medicine and Dentistry. Okayama 700-8558, Japan

Introduction: We have demonstrated that β2-glycoprotein I (β2GPI) binds *in vitro* to oxidized low-density lipoprotein (oxLDL) via oxLDL-derived ligands (oxLig-1) forming complexes, and shown that circulating β2GPI/oxLDL complexes were present in systemic lupus erythematosus (SLE) patients with and without antiphospholipid syndrome (APS). Autoantibodies to these complexes were reported mostly in SLE patients with APS, and shown to have a stronger association with arterial than venous thrombosis and pregnancy morbidity, implicating oxLDL/β2GPI complexes as thrombogenic and possibly as atherogenic autoantigens. **Aims:** To evaluate the association of circulating β2GPI/oxLDL complexes and antibodies to β2GPI/oxLig-1 complexes with various clinical and serologic measures of disease activity in a group of SLE patients followed for a period of 12 months. **Material and Methods:** Serum samples were obtained at various time intervals from 6 SLE patients, 4 with active and 2 with inactive disease. Clinical (SLE-DAI) and serologic (anti-DNA, C3, C4, ESR) disease activity measures were recorded for each patient. Antiphospholipid antibodies, anticardiolipin (aCL) and anti-β2GPI, as well as β2GPI/oxLDL complexes and anti-β2GPI/oxLig-1 antibodies were measured by ELISA. **Results:** Circulating β2GPI/oxLDL complexes were found in all 6 SLE patients and their levels fluctuated widely with time regardless the disease activity status. Two patients with inactive disease (SLE-DAI scores 0-3, normal serologic measures) did not have anti-β2GPI/oxLig-1 antibodies at any time. Three of the four patients with active disease (SLE-DAI scores >5, abnormal serologic measures) had elevated levels of anti-β2GPI/oxLig-1 antibodies. IgG aCL and anti-β2GPI antibodies remained within normal levels in both active and inactive patients throughout the study. **Conclusions:** Serum levels of β2GPI/oxLDL complexes fluctuated widely in SLE patients with both active and inactive disease. In contrast, autoantibodies to β2GPI/oxLig-1 complexes were present only in SLE patients with active disease. The coexistence and the pattern observed between complexes and antibodies in SLE patients with active disease suggest a causal relationship i.e. β2GPI/oxLDL complexes may serve as autoantigens triggering autoantibody production, possibly representing a risk factor for thromboembolic disease and APS.

PO130

Protein C inhibitor, isolated together with β2-glycoprotein I (β2GPI). A possible player in anti-β2GPI antibody mediated thrombosis?

Čučnik S, Rozman B, Kveder T, Božič B*

Department of rheumatology, University Medical Centre, Ljubljana, Slovenia

Introduction: The pathogenic autoantibodies in the antiphospholipid syndrome were identified as anticardiolipin antibodies (aCL). In 1990 it was demonstrated that pathogenic aCL were in fact anti-β_2GPI antibodies. Isolation of pure, intact β2GPI is believed to be of crucial importance for subsequent detection of anti-β_2GPI. The physiological importance of β_2GPI as a regulator of coagulation is disputable and the mechanism of thrombosis in patients with anti-β_2GPI is still unclear. The exact mechanism by which pathogenic antiphospholipid antibodies induce thrombosis in vivo is not fully understood. **Aim:** To evaluate the isolation procedure of β_2GPI with special emphasis on the composition and antigenic properties of different fractions, and possible presence of other plasma proteins in complexes with β_2GPI. **Methods:** Isolation from pooled plasma apparently healthy blood donors was initiated by perchloric acid precipitation for either 3, 18 or 50 minutes, followed by heparin affinity and cationic exchange chromatography. The properties of isolated proteins were tested by rocket electrophoresis, ELISA, reducing and non-reducing poly-acryl amide gel electrophoresis, immunoblotting and N-terminal sequencing. To isolate anti-β_2GPI by affinity chromatography, purified β_2GPI was bound to CNBr activated agarose. **Results:** The isolation procedure yielded 3 distinct protein peaks containing β_2GPI, regardless of the duration of perchloric acid precipitation. Immune complexes with β_2GPI were found in the fractions of the first peak in all three cases. The second peak following 18-minute precipitation gave the best yield of unnicked β_2GPI. In the fractions of the third peak, protein C inhibitor (PCI) was identified next to β_2GPI under all 3 time conditions of precipitation. The antigenic properties of β_2GPI from the second peak were retained after coupling to agarose activated with CNBr. The bound anti-β_2GPI from patients' sera of low as well as of high affinity were identified by specific elution conditions and by ELISA using different buffers/solutions. **Conclusions:** The described isolation procedure proved to yield pure nondegraded β_2GPI under controlled conditions. Co-isolation of PCI with β_2GPI suggested a novel link of anti-β_2GPI with the coagulation cascade and thrombosis: high affinity anti-β_2GPI could bind to the β_2GPI/PCI complex, resulting in dissociation of PCI from the complex. Free PCI would then inhibit APC, thereby increasing coagulation tendency.

PO131

Thrombosis risk in systemic lupus erythematosus

Sallai K, Nagy E, Gergely P, Bodó I*

Central Laboratory of Immunology, Semmelweis Medical University, Budapest, Hungary

Introduction: The diagnosis of Systemic Lupus Erythematosus (SLE) carries an increased risk of venous and arterial thrombosis. The main predictor of a thrombo-embolic event in SLE is the presence of antiphospholipid antibodies as detected by an immunoassay (aPL), and/or by coagulation testing (lupus anticoagulant, LA). The relative contribution to the thrombosis risk of other factors known to be associated with thrombo-embolism is, however, unknown. **Aim**: of our study was to determine the contribution to thrombosis risk in SLE of the following factors: aPL (ELISA for: anticardiolipin IgG and IgM, anti-β_2-Glicoprotein-I, and anti-Phosphatidyl-Serine; complex coagulation studies to detect the lupus anticoagulant), factor V Leiden, prothrombin G20210A, protein C, protein S, antithrombin, plasma homocystein, factor VIII and von Willebrand factor (vWF) levels. **Methods**: We analyzed data from 110 patients with SLE followed by the Division of Immunology at Semmelweis University. **Results**: Patients were devided into two groups: those positive (n = 49) and negative for aPL. Within each group, two subgroups were defined: patients with and without a history of either arterial or venous thrombosis, or recurrent fetal loss (considered a pregnancy-specific thrombotic event). 20 patients from the aPL, and 1 patient from the non-aPL group had a thrombotic event. **Conclusion**: a detailed thrombophilia workup is helpful in determining thrombosis risk in SLE patients.

PO132

Management of pregnancy in patients with autoimmune diseases and antiphospholipid syndrome

Makatsaria A, Muravieva I, Kusainova V*

Chart of Obstetrics and Gynecology of Moscow Medical Academy

We observed 92 patients, aged 19-38 years, with different autoimmune diseases. 28 women suffered from rheumatoid arthritis (RA), 30 - from systemic lupus erythematosus (SLE), 18 - from autoimmune thrombocytopenic purpura (ATP), 16 - from autoimmune thyroiditis (AT). Based on our data, the frequency of pregnancy and labor complications in women with RA composed: fetal loss syndrome - in 10,7%, gestosis - in 32,1%, preeclampsia - in 3,6%, early postpartum bleeding - in 7,1% of patients. The obstetric complications of SLE were habitual abortion in 26,6%, gestosis - in 53,3%, premature labor - in 33,3%, weakness of pains - in 16,6%, fetal growth retardation - in 56,6%, antenatal death - in 6,7% of patients. Women with AT had fetal loss syndrome in 56,3%, infertility - in 31,25% in anamnesis. Intrauterine fetal hypoxia was observed in 43,7%, threatening abortion - in 56,25%, gestosis - in 50%, premature birth - in 12,5% and weakness of pains - in 18,75% of patients. In patients with ATP fetal loss syndrome was observed in 5,6%, menorrhagia - in 16,6% of cases. Pregnancy was complicated by gestosis in 22,2% of women. Fetal growth retardation was diagnosed in 22,2% and threatening abortion - in 11,1% of patients. In 11,9% of women antiphospholipid antibodies (APA) were revealed, in 19,6% of women secondary antiphospholipid syndrome (APS) was diagnosed. In 58,6% of women treatment with low molecular weight heparin (LMWH) Fraxiparin was prescribed: in the dose of 0,3 ml per day 10 injections for the course in APA circulation and in the dose of 0,3-0,6 ml per day during the total pregnancy from it's early terms in APS development. The frequency of pregnancy and labor complications in this group of women was the same as in women with autoimmune diseases without APA. There were no thrombotic or hemorrhagic complications. 41,4% of women didn't receive anticoagulant therapy due to late income. And they had severe obstetric and perinatal complications - gestoses, preeclampsia, placental insufficiency, placentae abrupcio, antenatal death, postpartum hemorrhages. Presence of APA in women with autoimmune diseases is the risk factor for obstetric and perinatal complications. Anticoagulant therapy with Fraxiparin from early terms of gestation can help to prevent severe pregnancy complications.

PO133

Prediction value of several functional examinations for the identification of antiphospholipid-antibody syndrome

Pecka M, Maly J, Slezakova E, Dulicek P*

Charles University, Second Department of Medicine, Department of Clinical Haematology, Hradec Kralove, Czech Republic

Antiphospholipid antibodies (APA) represent a heterogenous group of antibodies (immunoglobulins – mostly IgG and IgM), which form complex compounds either with negatively charged phospholipids (cardiolipin, phophatodylserin, phosphatidylethanolamin) or their complexes with macromolecular substance – cofactor mostly of protein nature. They are often called antiphosphoprotein antibodies. These are mainly antiphospholipid antibodies of Lupus Anticoagulans type (LA). In LA a group of immunoglobulins is taken into account which interfere with one or more coagulantive tests dependent on phospholipids. These are autoantibodies directed against phospholipid components of a coagulative cascade protrombine complex. These autoantibodies enter the coagulation at different levels of the coagulative process. They react with procoagulative phospholipids and cause abnormal findings in blood coagulative tests, especially in the Activated partial thromboplastin test – APTT. The result is not only the interference with endothelial activation of protein C system but also the interferences at the level of primary haemostasis, or at other sites where active phospholipid surfaces are applied in coagulation. The functional tests were used for the laboratory identification of APA, because of their ability to affect coagulative tests dependent on phospholipids. If the tests are abnormal, a dilution study is carried out (patients´ plasma and standard plasma mixture). We used the following functional tests: the Thromboplastin test (Prothrombine time – PT), APTT, APTT – LA sensitive to LA type antibodies and the dilution test with use of Russel´s viper poison (Russel Viper Venom time – RVVT). For identification, commercially available diagnostic tests were used (in PT: Grifols, Spain, in APTT, APTT-LA and d RVVT: Stago, France) All coagulative studies were carried out on the apparatus Compact, STAGO, France, which operates on the magnetic principle of moving marble and thusidentifies the end of coagulative process. In this study, we observed mentioned above functional tests with the test, which directly determines the hexagonale phospholipids levels in plasma (STACLOT LA, STAGO, France). We made an effort to find out a prediction value for the presence of LA type antibodies for both individual functional tests and for some of their mutual ratios. In the course of hexagonal phospholipids identification, the two groups were made with positive (25 respondents) and negative results (173 respondents). These two groups were compared with each other. The correlation relationships dependences between STACLOT LA and individual tests were not confirmed. A statistically significant increase ($p<0,01$) was proved in all functional tests. An interesting result was observed in comparing a ratio APTT-LA/APTT (r) for identification of hexagonal phospholipids – STACLOT LA (positive test: $r = 1,39 \pm 0,29$, negative test: $r = 1,02 \pm 0,12$, $p<0,01$. This finding shows that the ratio r could be a certain predictive factor in selection of tests used for the examination of antibodies against lupus anticoagulans.

PO134

Antiphospholipid antibodies enclosed to diagnosis of venous thrombosis

Kostovska S (1), Neceva V (1), Pockova L (2), Pejceva J (1), Dejanova V (1)*

(1) Institute of Blood Transfusion, Skopje, Republic of Macedonia
(2) Medical Center, Veles, Republic of Macedonia

Specificity of antiphospholipid antibodies (APA) is to plasma proteins (beta2 glycoprotein I, B2GPI), which bind to phospholipids of cell plasma membranes and play the important role in the regulation of mechanism of haemostasis. Recent evidence suggests one potential pathophisiologic mechanism for thrombosis involving the ability of APA to inhibit the anticoagulant effect of B2GPI and to activate the process of haemostasis or thrombosis. The major problems in the fields of APA have been the laboratory identification of these antibodies. **Aim** To determinate of concentration of three classes of APA (IgG, IgA and IgM) in patient with deep venous thrombosis (DVT) and their correlation with current state. **Material and methods**: 70 patients with DVT were examinee for the concentration of three classes of APA with micro – ELISA test kits, prepared and standardised in laboratory for thrombosis and haemostasis, Institute of Blood transfusion, Skopje. **Results**. Concentration of APA was expressed in standard units (SU). From 70 patients with DVT, at 13 patients (18 %), the concentration of IgG APA was the elevated (28.46 $\pm$2.34 SE v.s. 8.64 $\pm$11.29 SE, $p < 0.01$), at 27 patients (38 %) the concentration of IgA APA was the elevated (71.96 $\pm$84.45 SE v.s. 32 $\pm$61 SE, $p < 0.01$) and the concentration of IgM APA was the elevated at 19 patients (27 %) (38 $\pm$16.14 SE v.s. 13.98 $\pm$17.53 SE). **Conclusion**. Obtain Results stated the hypothesis that elevated level of APA are cause for development of thrombothic episodes. A proper protocol and algorithm for treatment and therapy (heparin, aspirin alone or together) of antiphospholipid syndrome was introduced.

PO135

Thrombin concentration and clotting time

Savushkin A V

Chita State Medical Academy, Chita, Russia

Blood coagulation is an unique ferment reaction cascade which results in the change of the aggregate state of blood. Fibrin formed in it is the only component possessing non-liquid quality of clot and thrombin is the main ferment of this conversion. It is surprising that in spite of so long investigation of blood coagulation it is impossible today to calculate or forecast thrombin concentration for real blood sample. It is due to the complexity of this process, the number of components and feed-backs. Statistical methods are useful in such situation. It is possible to find dependence between start conditions and final results without features. Dependence between thrombin concentration and clotting time was the aim of our study. Experiments were carried out with artificial model clots formed with bovine preparations. Clots were formed after mixing of equal volumes of thrombin and fibrinogen solutions. The final fibrin concentration was approximately physiological one (186 g/l). The final concentrations of thrombin were used: 0.15, 0.3, 1.5, 3 and 15 (thrombin IU/ mg fibrinogen). These concentrations corresponded to the next relation of thrombin molecules to fibrinogen molecules: 13/100; 26/100; 130/100; 260/100 and 1300/100. 18-25 samples were tested in group with every thrombin concentration. Clotting time was registered with Burger`s method. It reflects the lose of its liquid property by solutions. The regression equation was calculated on the base of 106 experiments. $T = 31.9 / C + 3.8$; T – coagulation (fibrin formation) time (sec), C – relationship between thrombin and fibrinogen concentrations (thrombin IU/mg fibrinogen). We suppose that substrate (fibrinogen) dominants in zone of lesser thrombin concentrations (0.15 and 0.3). Therefore there is no significant effect of thrombin concentration on clotting time. The ferment is prevailing and its influence is sizable in zone of high thrombin content. Moreover, as fibrin is antithrombin 1 so it adsorbs the ferment on forming surface and inactivates it. This effect mostly manifests itself in small thrombin concentrations. These experiments show that there is hyperbolic regression function between thrombin concentration and clotting time.

PO136

The comparison of clotting and colorimetric assay of quantitative measurment of the functional protein C level

Slezakova E, Pecka M, Maly J*

Department of Haematology, Teaching Hospital Hradec Kralove, Czech Republic

Protein C belongs to the group of vitamin K – dependent proteins. It is synthesized mostly in the liver. In the activated state protein C regulates the coagulation process by neutralizing the procoagulant activities of the factors Va and VIIIa in the presence of protein S (cofactor of activated protein C and also a vitamin K – dependent protein). In inhibiting the factors Va and VIIIa protein C helps to limit thrombus extension, and thus acts a major regulator of the coagulation process. In our study, we measured the function of protein C level quantitatively by clotting assay and by colorimetric assay. Test principle: 1. Colorimetric assay: The specific activator based on the venom from Agkistrodon c. contortrix activates protein C. The quantity of enzyme thus formed is measured by its amidasic activity on the synthetic chromogenic substrate (paranitroanilin release at 405 nm). The intensity of the colour produced is directly proportional to the level of protein C initially present in the test plasma. 2. Clotting assay: The presence of specific activator extracted from Agkistrodon c. contortrix venom activates protein C. The resulting activated protein C inhibits the factors Va and VIIIa, and thus prolongs the APTT of a system in which all the factors are present, constant and in excess, except the protein C, which is derived from the sample being tested. In the first part of our study, we tested 50 samples of plasma. The range of functional protein C level was from low (27 %) to normal values (130 %). We did not detect any significant diversions between comparisons methods. There was relatively close dependence between colorimetric and clotting assay (coefficient of correlation = 0,95; slope = 0,8; intercept = ?6,85). Generally, we found very small differences in the area of low levels, but in the area of normal levels, we measured a little bit higher values by clotting assay than colorimetric assay. Occasionally we obtained significantly higher values by colorimetric assay. The reason is probably that some of the PIVKA – protein C that is present in the plasma of patients receiving oral anticoagulant therapy is measured by the colorimetric assay. We verified this hypothesis in the second part of our study, when we tested 20 samples of plasma of patients receiving oral anticoagulant therapy (Warfarin). The results declared, that the colorimetric assay is sensitive to the presence of some PIVKA protein C. The both methods are insensitive to heparin up to 1 IU/ml. It has been reported that very elevated levels of factor VIII (greater than 250 %) may lead to an over-estimation of the protein C level measured by clotting assay. There is also LA/and or APA interference of clotting assay. Colorimetric assay is insensitive to the principal coagulation factors (i.e., XII, XI, IX, VIII, X, V...) and to protein S. In conclusion, the results determined by the clotting and colorimetric assay are comparable, but only in plasmas of the patients without oral anticoagulant therapy.

PO137

Effect of platelet factor 4 on laboratory tests of the protein C system

Van Dreden P, Rousseau A, Woodhams B*

Serbio SAS (Diagnostica Stago), Gennevilliers, France.

Introduction: Recently Slungaard et al (Blood: (2003):102:146-151) described a new in vivo function for PF4 - binding to protein C and modifying the activity of the protein C pathway. This raises the question on whether PF4 in plasma could have an ex vivo effect on diagnostic assay that are used to investigate or include components of the protein C pathway. All plasma samples preparations (a platelet poor plasma should contain $<10x10^6$ platelets/ml) will contain some platelets and thus PF4. If it is poorly prepared much higher levels are possible. A series of experiments were performed to assess the level of PF4 interference in diagnostic assays for the protein C pathway. **Methods:** Two plasma pools were prepared spiked with different levels of a recombinant PF4 that retains full function. One pool was prepared with concentrations of PF4 that could be expected in normal plasma (0 to 0.01µg/ml PF4) and the other with levels up to 6µg/ml PF4. We studied the influence of this added PF4 on the clotting time on the STA Staclot PS, STA Staclot PC, STA Staclot APC-R and in the Stachrom PC (all assays from Diagnostica Stago, Asnieres, France). All assays were performed according to the manufacturer procedures. **Results:** The results obtained show no significant interference in these assays with concentration of PF4 up to 0.5µg/ml. With higher concentrations the clotting times are increased significantly with differences at 2 and 6µg/ml of 13.5 and 29.7, 3.2 and 9.9 and 11.9 and 24.0 seconds respectively for Staclot PS, Staclot PC and Staclot APC-R assays. The Stachrom PC assay does not show any interference even with these very high concentrations in PF4. **Conclusion:** Based on these data PF4 does not affect functional PC, PS, and APC-R assays at level that could be expected in a properly prepared plasma sample. However with higher doses of PF4 we can observe an effect that could, according to assay type, lead to either spuriously low or high assay results. We can conclude that the functional assays for PC, PS, APC-R we tested in this study are insensitive to PF4 in platelet poor plasma. Interference will only be seen at PF4 concentrations >0.5µg/ml that would be found in plasma samples heavily contaminated with platelets or if assays were performed on platelet rich plasma or whole blood.

PO138

Influence of fibrin polymerization on citrated whole blood thromboelastography profile

*Chakroun T, Gerotziafas, Samama M, Elalamy I**

Service d'Hématologie Biologique Hôtel-Dieu Hospital Paris France

Introduction: The recent introduction of the computerized Thromboelastography (TEG), at a time when the understanding of the mechanism of blood coagulation *in vivo* has made substantial progress, lead us to reconsider the significance of TEG parameters and specially those related to the maximal amplitude and the velocity of clot formation. **Aims:** In this *in vitro* study we have assessed the effect of fibrin polymerization (FP) on whole blood tissue factor-triggered TEG profile. **Materials and methods:** Whole blood TEG profile employing minimal tissue factor pathway activation was performed as previously described (1). Samples were supplemented with buffer (control), or a FP inhibitor (Pefabloc® FG, Pentapharm) (1; 2 and 5 mg/ml; final concentrations). Five parameters were analyzed, *r* (min; clotting time), *k* (min; achievement of certain clot firmness), α *angle* (degree; kinetics of clot development), *ma* (mm; maximal amplitude) and *G* (dyn/cm^2; shear elastic modulus strength). **Results:** Pefabloc® at 1 mg/ml had significantly prolonged the *r* and *k* times (1.5 fold) and decreased the α *angle* (26%) but *ma* and *G* values were not affected. At 2 mg/ml concentration, a 60% reduction of α *angle* and 3 to 5 fold prolongation of *r* and *k* times was observed, whereas *ma* and *G* values were only decreased by 20 and 34%, respectively, as compared to control values. Clot formation was completely abolished at 5 mg/ml of Pefabloc®. Interestingly, a linear decrease of α *angle* was observed (R^2 = 0.996). These results demonstrate that FP clearly influences *k* and *α angle* values which are related to the rate of clot strength increase once clotting starts. In contrast, FP involvement seems less important regarding *ma* and *G* values which measure the maximum clot strength. **Conclusion:** Our original findings determine the more reliable TEG parameters to explore quantitative and/or qualitative fibrinogen deficiencies and FP process. 1. T. Chakroun, G. T. Gerotziafas, I. Elalamy & M. M. Samama. Effect of Fondaparinux on clot formation after tissue factor pathway activation. A thromboelastography study. *(Abstract P0716: Supplement to the Journal of Thrombosis and Haemostasis), ISTH Birmingham* July 2003.

PO139

Is the Light Cycler - real time PCR as reliable as the conventional PCR? Our experience

Saour T (1), Sheereen A (1), Saour B (1), Saour J (2), Mammo L (1)

(1) King Faisal Specialist Hospital & Research Center , Biological and Medical Research
(2) King Faisal Specialist Hospital & Research Center , Department of Medicine

Introduction: The distribution of Factor V Leiden (FVL) among healthy population is reported to be 3-7% whereas that for prothrombin G20210A is 2-3%. These two factors are gaining momentum among clinicians caring for patient with thrombotic problems. Speed and reliability in delivering results both clinically and economically is very important. A minimum of three days is needed to obtain results using the conventional polymerase chain reaction (PCR), whereas results can be obtained in 30 minutes when the Light Cycler

(Roche) real time PCR (LC) is used. **Objective**: In this work the same samples are tested for FVL and for the prothrombin G20210A mutation using PCR and the LC. The results are comparedfor conformity. **Method**: DNA extracted from 860 subjects was tested for FVL and for the prothrombin G20210A mutations using PCR and the LC. **Results**: We performed 8600 tests to detect the presence of FVL and prothrombin G20210A mutation using the conventional PCR and the real time PCR using Light Cycler (Roche). Results obtained for FVL using the conventional PCR method showed that 821 tests carried the wild type variant, 26 were heterozygous and 12 were homozygous. Results for the prothrombin G 20210A mutation showed that 848 tests carried the normal allele, 14 were heterozygous and none were homozygous. Results obtained from analyzing the melting curves produced by the LC showed that 821 tests carried the wild type variant for FVL, 26 were heterozygous and 12 were homozygous for the mutations. Results for the prothrombin G20210A mutation showed that 848 tests carried the normal allele, 14 were heterozygous and none were homozygous. Discussion : The setup of the polymerase chain reaction (PCR) typically requires thawing of the various reagents, setting up a master mix, and then distributing the mix to the individual reaction tubes. The various handling steps can cause pipetting mistakes, experimental error(s), bear the risk of contaminating the amplification reaction and is time consuming. Whereas these factors are eliminated when the LC is used. Each DNA sample was tested three times by the conventional PCR and twice using the LC to confirm initial results. Samples that tested positive for the mutation on the conventional PCR showed exactly the same mutation on the light Cycler. Hence, our results show 100% correlation. **Conclusion**: Based on our results, we hereby conclude that the LC ® provide fast and reliable results.

PO140

Evaluation of the Dialab APC sensitivity assay

Coen D, Milos M, Zadro R*

Clinical Institute of Laboratory Diagnosis, Zagreb Clinical Hospital Centre, University School of Medicine

Introduction: Activated protein C resistance (APCR) has become a well-established part of the thrombophilia screening profile in most laboratories due to a high frequency of Factor V Leiden (FVL) mutation. As several commercial assays of modified APCR (with predilution in FV deficient plasma) are now available, the goal of every coagulation laboratory is to find a sensitive and specific assay that will be suitable for routine work. **Aim**: The aim of our study was to evaluate the Dialab APC Sensitivity Assay for the laboratory determination of APCR in comparison with DNA analysis. **Materials and methods**: Plasma samples were obtained from 24 carriers of FVL (19 heterozygotes and 5 homozygotes) and 62 non-carriers, as identified by DNA analysis. Among tested patients 3 heterozygotes and 12 non-carriers were receiving OAT (INR range: 1.61-3.59). APCR was performed on BCT (Dade Behring) coagulation analyzer and the results were expressed as APC ratios. **Results**: By using a cut-off value of 2.1 we were able to identify all carriers of FVL. No difference in APC ratios was observed between non-carriers receiving OAT or not (p=0.71). There was no overlap of APC ratios between heterozygotes (mean: 1.80, range: 1.62-1.99) and normal controls (mean: 2.85, range: 2.18-3.37) even with elevated F VIII:C levels (181-452 %). There was a clear discrimination between heterozygotes and homozygotes (mean APC ratio: 1.39, range: 1.30-1.48) when a cut-off value of 1.5 was used. **Conclusions**: Based on our results this test appears to be highly sensitive and specific for the diagnosis of APCR associated with FVL. Furthermore, the test is easy to perform and fulfills the criteria for a screening assay.

PO141

A practical von Willebrand disease screening method using ELISAs

Whittier A, Andrews J, Fink C, Lopez L*

Corgenix, Inc., USA

Introduction: Von Willebrand Disease (vWD) is the most common inherited bleeding disorder with an estimated prevalence of 1%. Von Willebrand Disease subtypes may be qualitative or quantitative. Therefore, in order to correctly distinguish subtypes, activity as well as antigenic tests are necessary. The ristocetin cofactor assay is normally used as the initial test for von Willebrand Factor (vWF) activity. However, this assay is technically limited. Aim: The aim of the study was to determine if the three ELISA assays, could be used to screen vWD samples and discriminate type 1 from type 2. **Materials and methods:** A vWF antigen ELISA, a collagen binding ELISA and a vWF activity ELISA were used. The vWF activity ELISA uses a purified monoclonal which recognizes the portion of vWF that binds platelet glycoprotein Ib. Fourteen type 2 (subtype 2A, 2B and 2M) and seventeen type 1 vWD samples were evaluated on all three ELISAs. **Results**: Using the activity ELISA, thirteen of fourteen type 2 samples tested below the 50% cutoff, one sample tested near the cutoff (59.8%), with a mean result of 21%. Fourteen of seventeen type 1 samples tested below the 50% activity ELISA cutoff, three samples tested near the cutoff (71.9, 65.7 and 52.8%), with a mean result of 36.4%. Using the antigen ELISA, twelve of fourteen type 2 samples tested below the 50% cutoff, two samples tested near the cutoff (56 and 76.9%), with a mean result of 32.1%. Sixteen of seventeen type 1 samples tested below the 50% antigen cutoff and one sample tested near the cutoff (51%), with a mean result of 34.7%. Using the CBA ELISA, fourteen of fourteen samples tested below the 50% cutoff, with a mean result of 11.1%. Thirteen of seventeen type 1 samples tested below the 50% cutoff, with a mean result of 40.9%.. Using the CBA/antigen ratio to further evaluate the samples, the mean ratio for the type 2 vWD samples was 0.29 compared to the mean ratio for the type 1 samples of 1.20 (P<0.001). In all cases, where the sample tested as borderline or above the deficient cutoff on any of the assays, the CBA/antigen ratio supported the previous vWD classification of the sample. **Conclusions**: The vWF activity, collagen binding and the vWF antigen ELISAs individually detect deficient samples in the majority of vWD patient samples. The CBA/antigen ratio provides the best discrimination of type 1 and type 2 vWD samples.

PO142

Iliofemoral deep vein thrombosis in childhood; developing a management protocol

Brightwell R, Osman I*

Objective: Iliofemoral deep vein thrombosis (IDVT) in childhood is rare. Having recently treated a seven-year-old child with this problem we set out to develop an evidence-based protocol for the management of this condition. **Methodology**: An electronic search of the literature was undertaken. All publications pertaining to IDVT in childhood were analysed and then categorised according to their level of evidence. Recommendations were then made on the basis of this. **Results**: 52 papers were identified in the literature. The commonest presenting symptoms were pain and swelling in the affected limb (evidence level 2). Predisposing risk factors of special significance in children included the recent use of venous access device, malignancy, prothrombotic disorders, infection, surgery and congenital venous anomalies (evidence level 2). The most frequently described imaging modalities were compression B-mode ultrasonography, Duplex ultrasonography, venography, and helical CT (evidence level 3). The mainstay of treatment is anticoagulation with LMWH alone or followed by warfarin (evidence level 1). Early clot removal through catheter-directed thrombolysis or surgical thrombectomy has been shown to be beneficial (evidence level 2/3). There is little evidence for the benefit of early mobilisation and compression therapy in childhood. **Conclusion**: Level-1 evidence relating to IDVT in childhood is sparse. The possibility of IDVT should be considered when examining a child with a swollen and painful limb. Imaging should be with Duplex ultrasound, followed by spiral CT to include assessment of the IVC. A thrombophilia screen should be taken prior to anticoagulation with LMWH (and warfarin). Thrombolysis should be considered in cases of extensive IDVT.

PO143

Prothrombin gene 20210 G→A heterozygote mutation in a patient with multiple thrombosis - a case report

Ileri T (1), Uysal Z (1), Azik F (1), Ertem M (1), Akar N (2), Kologlu M (3), Dindar H (3), Gozdasoglu S (1)*

(1) Department of Pediatric Hematology, School of Medicine, Ankara University, Ankara, Turkey
(2) Department of Pediatric Molecular Genetics, School of Medicine, Ankara University, Ankara, Turkey
(3) Department of Pediatric Surgery, School of Medicine, Ankara University, Ankara, Turkey

Introduction: Although thrombosis is relatively rare in children, reports of young children with thrombosis are becoming more frequent with time. Genetic and acquired multifactorial disorders are associated with an increased risk of thrombophilia. A decrease in the natural anticoagulants (protein C, protein S and antithrombin III), factor VIII elevation or mutations of the factor V Leiden and prothrombin 20210 G-A are known as predisposing factors for thrombophilia.

Screening these disorders may be useful for prophylactic treatment. This article highlights a case of a child with severe hepatic vein and recurrent right atrial thrombosis. Seven months old girl patient was admitted to our hospital with abdominal distention which was followed by diarrhea and dehydration. Findings on examination were growth failure, abdominal distention, hepatosplenomegaly and severe ascites. Venous Doppler USG demonstrated thrombosis in hepatic vein and vena cava inferior. Thrombophilic analysis confirmed that the patient was carrier of the heterozygotic 20210G/A variant of the prothrombin gene. To control severe ascites, peritonovenous shunt was placed. After placing, right atrial thrombosis was detected by echocardiography at the end of the catheter. Fibrinolytic and anticoagulant treatment lead to thrombolysis, but thrombosis recurrent due to catheter. Response to recurrent thrombolytic treatment was insufficient. The patient is sill clinically stable with oral anticoagulant therapy. **Conclusion**: The data obtained from this patient suggest that the synergy of inherited factors and transient risk conditions could play a key role in the occurrence of thrombotic accidents.

PO144

Study of haemostasis in neonates with intrauterine growth retardation (IUGR)

Makris P (1), Eydoridou I (2), Mitsiakos G (2), Girtovitis F (1), Stathopoulou T (2), Boutou A (1), Kremenopoulos G (2)*

(1) Haemostasis Unit of A΄ Prop. Pathological Clinic
(2) Neonatal Clinical AUTH.

Introduction: It is known that pregnant women with thrombophilic predisposition often display complications of gestation such as hypertension and proeclampsia, which result to their foetuses disturbance of body weight gain. **Aim:** We tried to appreciate the presence or not of disorders of haemostasis in IUGR neonates. **Material and Methods:** We studied 34 neonates with Birth Weight=2276,8±771,3gr and Gestation on Age (GA)=37,5±3,29 weeks (19 males with GA=35,97±3,37 weeks and 15 females with corresponding GA=37,87±3,53 weeks). Among these neonates, 29 presented IUGR and the 5 rest had normal growth. We determined 1) the plasma levels of factors II, V, VII, VIII, IX, XII and Willebrand, of protein C, plasminogen, antithrombin and a2-antiplasmin using a synthetic chromogenic-substrate method and 2) the presence or not of APCr using a modified method. **Results:** The Mean Values (MV) and Standard Deviations (SD) of the haemostatic parameters which were determined in the normal neonates are referred in table 1, while in table 2 there are the corresponding MV and SD among the IUGR neonates. The comparison of mean values between the two groups did not reveal any statistically significant difference.

Table 1. MVs and SD of haemostatic parameters of the normal neonates.

(%)	FII	FV	FVII	FVIII	FIX	PrC	AT	PLG	A_2PL	FXII	VWF	APCr*
MV	43,2	61	44,8	73,4	39,6	20	40	42	62	165,1	45	132
SD	8,42	24	13,1	25,2	8,19	8,6	12	6,2	8,4	17,05	13,2	10,8

Table 2. Mean values and standard deviations of the IUGR group .

	FII	FV	FVII	FVIII	FIX	PrC	AT	PLG	A2PL	FXII	VWF	APCr*
MV	49,4	67	63	64,6	39,5	25	46	44	68	178,4	43	136
SD	10,6	24	17,9	16	10,2	7,9	11	7,3	12	34,01	9,19	9

In one IUGR neonate which presented ischemic stroke there is an obvious decline in the levels of coagulation inhibitors:

Table 3 .Levels(%) of haemostatic parameters in one neonate with ischemic stroke.

FII	FV	FVII	FVIII	FIX	PrC	AT	PLG	A2PL	FXII	VWF	APCr*
38	21	68	81	46	20	28	28	56	250	37	141

(APCr*: fixed as pathologic when <120)

Conclusions: 1) There is no data in the literature and conclusions are difficult to be reached. All neonates have lower levels of several factors of haemostasis, due to their immaturity. In what extent these levels of haemostatic factors are further affected by the disturbance of body weight gain, it is not known. 2) The established presence of ischemic stroke in one neonate allows us to investigate which factors are related with the thrombotic episodes in these neonates and in what levels.

PO145

Is long term prophylaxıs in pediatric stroke necessary?

*Unal O, Uysal Z, Ocal G, Akar N, Deda G**

Ankara University Faculty of Medicine, Pediatric Neurology, Hematology, Endocrinology and Molecular

Introduction: We evaluated 29 pediatric patients (mean age 10,11± 0,70), with arteriel ischemic stroke between 1993 - 2003. **Materials and methods**: The diagnosis was confirmed with cranial imaging and magnetic resonance angiography. Patients aged 1 to 23 years; 19 were males (%67). Mean symptom age was 3,71±0,49. **Results**: Hemiparesis was the most common symptom (N:20) following cranial nerve involvement in 7 and seizures in 11. There were several acquired risk factors among patients (encephalitis(7), prematurity (1), non Hodgkin's lymphoma (1), pylosytic astrocytoma (1), VSD operation (1) congenital adrenal hyperplasia (1) and isolated glucocorticoid deficiency (1), antiphospholipid antibody syndrome (1) and Moyamoya syndrome (1). Thrombophilic factors were as follows: PT 20210A in (3), FV 1691A in (8), PC deficiency in 2 , PS deficiency in 3 , elevated FVIII levels in 15, elevated lipoprotein(a) levels in 6, elevated homocysteine level in 1 patient. We found 1 genetic risk factor in 5 patients, 2 genetic risk factors in 11 patients, 3 and more genetic risk factors in 6 patients. Two of our patients died of antiphospholipid antibody syndrome at fourth ischemic stroke attack under anticoagulant therapy and other of lymphoma. In mean 6,48 ± 0,35 years of follow up period (1–17 years) recurrence was not seen in 27 patients. Time interval between the first attack and admission to our department was over three months for the rest. Because of this reason, we didn't give prophylaxis to 26 patients. We had given prophylaxis to a 16-year-old patient who was being followed up for seven years with congenital adrenal hyperplasia-and stroke. When we determined 6 heritable risk factors (FV 1691A, MTHFR 677 TT, elevated FVIII, FIX, homocystein and lipoprotein (a) levels), we started her 100 mg/day aspirin, but 2 months later she referred with headache; cranial MRI was consistent with intracranial microbleeding. Aspirin prophylaxis was interrupted and bleeding disappeared. **Conclusions**: Patients with hereditary or acquired prothrombotic states should receive prophylactic anticoagulation therapy during high-risk situations. However our data brings out the question whether long-term prophylactic treatment has efficacy in pediatric stroke. (This study is supported by Ankara University Research Fund).

PO146

Cervical artery dissection: long term outcome after anticoagulant therapy

Quintavalla R, Paganelli E, Pattacini C, Rossetti A*

Azienda Ospedaliera, Thromboembolic Unit Medical Department 3, Italy

Dissection of the internal carotid and vertebral arteries in the neck accounts for about a fifth of strokes in the young (second cause of stroke in patients younger than 45 years), compared with about 2.5% in older patients. The main mechanism of stroke is the arterioarterial embolism, whereas hemodynamic mechanisms play a minor role. Early anticoagulation may improve the outcome, although no randomized trials comparing anticoagulants (usually unfractionated heparin-UFH plus vitamin K antagonists-VKA) with antiplatelet drugs and both with controls have been performed. Nonrandomized studies didn't show any difference between the two treatments. Some authors recommend carotid angioplasty followed by stent implantation but the rationale is lacking. Since 2000 we routinely treat patients affected by extracranial cervical artery dissection with low molecular weight heparin-LMWH 100 UI/kg b.i.d. for a week, followed by VKA.After three months a magnetic resonance angiography is performed: if the recanalization is near complete the therapy is stopped, if not the VKA continues for three other months. Neurological follow up is based to Barthel Index-BI and Modified Rankin Scale-MRS. From March 2000 to December 2003 we have treated 7 patients (3 women, 4 men; mean age 43 y., range 30-53) affected by artery dissection (3 vertebral, 4 internal carotid, initial MRS ranging from 3 to 5). The mean follow up was 30 months (range 4-45). No adverse events related to therapy or recurrence of dissection was observed during follow up. Neurological recovery was complete in 5 patients (MRS 0), uncomplete in 2 patients (MRS 2). The grade of improvement seems to be age-related. In our opinion anticoagulation with LMWH followed by VKA is an effective and safe therapy in the cervical artery dissection, however which is the best treatment (antiplatelet drugs, anticoagulation, catheter-based revascularisation) is still debated, and large randomized trials are needed.

PO147

Homocysteine in pediatric patients with migraine

Katsadze Y, Tadtaeva Z, Shmeleva V*

Hyperhomocysteinemia (HHcy) is known to be associated with cerebral disorders, including stroke. C677T polymorphism in the 5,10-methylene-tetrahydrofolate reductase (MTHFR) gene is well known genetic factor predisposing to mild and moderate hyperhomocysteinemia. Literature dates about homocysteine (Hcy) levels in migraine are rare and controversial, particularly in pediatric patients. The aim of our study was to determine Hcy levels in pediatric patients with migraine. **Materials and methods**: Genotyping was performed by PCR and restriction digest. Fasting plasma Hcy levels were determined by HPLC with HHcy defined as > 10 μmol/l. The diagnosis of migraine in these patients was established according to the International Headache Society Classification of Headache (1988). **Results**: Our study involved patients with migraine. Among studied patients (age range 9-16 years) 15 cases with MTHFR C677T substitution was selected for Hcy detection: (11 patients with migraine aura (MA) and 4 patients with tension-type headache (TH). HHcy was detected in 45% (5/11) cases with MA. They had Hcy levels from 10.3 to14.75 μmol/l. Patients with TH had Hcy levels < 10 μmol/l. **Conclusion**: Our results suggest that hyperhomocysteinemia could contribute to pathogenesis of migraine.

PO148

Frequency and association between polimorphism MTHFR gene, folic acid, vitamin B12 and mild hyperhomocysteinemia in pediatric stroke

Lenicek Krleza J (1), Bronic A (2), Ferencak G (3), Kusec V (3), Duranovic V (4), Zizic V (1), Nakic M (1), Mejaski Bosnjak V (4)*

(1) Dep.for Laboratory Diagnostics, Children's Hospital Zagreb, Croatia
(2) Dep.for Laboratory Diagnostics, Trauma Clinic Zagreb, Croatia
(3) University School of Medicine, Clinical Institte of Laboratory Diagnosis Zagreb
(4) Dep. of Neuropediatric, Children's Hospital Zagreb, Croatia

Introduction: In pediatric stroke, the cause of brain infarction remains unexplaines in 20–40%. Hypercoagulability may account for a significant proportion of unexplained strokes. Homocystein (Hcy) and him many-sided effect on hypercoagulability are good established in adults and children with different illness. For beginning mild hyperhomocysteinemia mostly responsible are inadequate taken with low folic acid and vitamin B_{12}. Mutation for methylenetetrahydrofolate reductase (MTHFR) gene, too. **Aim**: Establish frequency of decrease values for folic acid and vitamin B_{12}, increase values for Hcy and incidence mutation for MTHFR gene. Answer to which degree disorder folic acid pathway have effect on remetilation Hcy and beginning mild hyperhomocysteinemia in children with ischemic stroke. **Materials and methods**: Frothy-five children (0-18 years) with ischemic stroke studied. Diagnosis of stroke was established after evidence of cerebral infarction on brain with computed tomography scan. Hcy was determined on Abbott IMx analyzer with FPIA method. Folic acid and vitamin B_{12} were determined with competitive LIA method on Vitros analyzer. DNA was prepared from peripheral blood leukocytes using a method described by Miller SA, et al. Point mutation MTHFR was determined with polymerase chain reaction (PCR-RFLP) method described by Frosst P, et al. **Results**: Increase concentration Hcy was present in 15,6%, decrease concentration folic acid was present in 31,1%, normal concentration vitamin B_{12} was present in all children (N=46). C677T polymorphism of MTHFR gene was present like genotype T/C in 26,7% and genotype T/T in 8,9%. High Hcy, low folic acid and present T/C or T/T genotyp for MTHFR in same time not found. In five cases we found low folic acid and MTHFR polymorphism in same time (11,1%). **Conclusion**: No association was observed between folic acid pathway and mild hyperhomocysteinemia in our group of children with ischemic stroke. Polymorphism C677T MTHFR only in 11,1% cases can be cause of decrease folic acid but not increase of Hcy.

PO149

The role of cathepsin G (N125S) and TNF-α (-308G/A) polymorphisms in the Turkish pediatric cerebrovascular attack (CVA) patients

Hasipek M (1), Karahan Z (2), Deda G (3), Akar E (2), Akar N (2)*

(1) Biotechnology Institute, Ankara University, Ankara, Turkey.
(2) Department of Pediatric Molecular Genetics, School of Medicine, Ankara University, Ankara, Turkey.
(3) Department of Neurology, School of Medicine, Ankara University, Ankara, Turkey.

Introduction: Cathepsin G (CTSG) is a 26 kDa serin protease expressed in the promyelocyte stage of polymorphonuclear leukocytes. The 2,7 kb CTSG gene has been localized to chromosome 14q11.2 and consists of 5 exons and 4 introns. CTSG has been shown to induce thrombosis by inducing the release and surface expression of fibrinogen and release of plasminogen activator inhibitor-1, suppressing prostacylin production, and cleaving the glycoprotein (Gp) Ibα subunit of the GP Ib/IX receptor complex. Tumour necrosis factor alpha (TNF-α) plays an important role in the clot formation by activating platelets, monocytes and endothelial cells and inducing procoagulant substances such as negatively charged phospholipids or tissue factor. There is a genetically controlled inter-individual variation of TNF-α production, and patients carrying the TNF2 allele have shown to have higher levels of TNF-α. **Aims**: In this study, we aimed to evaluate the role of CTSG N125S and TNF-α 308 G/A polymorphisms in the Turkish pediatric cerebrovascular attack (CVA) patients. **Materials and methods**: Eighty-six CVA patients and 53 healthy age and sex matched controls were included in the study. DNA was extracted by conventional methods. CTSG N125S and TNF-α 308 G/A genotypings were performed by Sdu I and BspHI digestion following PCR as previously described. **Results**: In the patient and control groups, CTSG N125S (G) frequencies were 0.03 and 0.04 (p=0.98) and TNF-α 308 A frequencies were 0.18 and 0.10 (p=0.95) respectively. In TNF-α 308 G/A carriers, CTSG N125S G frequency was found 0.16 in the patient group, and 0.125 in the control group (p=0.72). **Conclusions**: These results show that, CTSG N125S and TNF-α 308 G/A polymorphisms are not associated with CVA in pediatric patients. (This study is supported by Ankara University Biotechnology Institute).

PO150

Homozygous factor V G1691A mutation in Turkish children with thrombosis

Ulu A, Yildiz Z, Akar E, Akar N*

Department of Pediatric Molecular Genetics, School of Medicine, Ankara University, Ankara, Turkey

Introduction: Factor V (FV) G1691A mutation is one of the most common inherited risk factor for the occurrence of thrombosis. Homozygous for FV G1691A mutation in children is rarely reported. **Aim**: The aim of this study was to evaluate the clinical manifestations of children with thrombosis who were homozygous for this mutation. **Materials and methods**: Previously reported molecular techniques and Light Cycler (Roche Diagnostics, Germany) were used. **Results**: Six patients (3 male/3 female; mean age 10.7 years; age range 2-15 years) with FV 1691AA mutation among 297 consecutive children with thrombosis (2.02%) were reported. Three of the 6 patients had CVA with arterial origin. Of these, one girl had systemic lupus erythematosus at the same time. One had portal vein thrombosis; one patient had beta thalassemia major and postsplenectomy thrombosis. One had hemaphagocytic syndrome lost with a sudden death. None of the patients had familial history of thrombosis. Further, we screened 368 normal healthy individuals and only one of them had homozygous FV 1691A. Of the 368, 32 (8.7%) were heterozygous for Factor V G1691A. None of these patients had prothrombin G20210A mutation or homozygous MTHFR C677T polymorphism. **Conclusion**: Our data indicate that homozygous Factor V G1691A mutation is also an important risk factor with a risk of 7.43 fold, may lead to thrombotic event during childhood. (This study is supported by Ankara University Research Fund).

PO151

Prothrombin G20210A and A19911G in Turkish pediatric stroke patients

Yildiz Z, Akar N, Deda G*

Department of Pediatric Molecular Genetics, School of Medicine, University of Ankara, Ankara, Turkey

Introduction: The incidence of cerebral infarction in children has been reported to be 1.2 cases per 100.000 children per year. Although several causes or potential risk factors exist for the occurrence of stroke in children, in about one third of these patients, no obvious cause or underlying disorder can be diagnosed. Inherited gene defects related to the coagulation system were reported as risk factors for stroke. Genetic and/or environmental factors could influence the prothrombotic role of hereditary mutations. Recently, another polymorphism located in the PT gene at 19911 A-G associated with slightly increased plasma prothrombin levels. We aimed to study the effect of PT19911 A-G site in children with the diagnosis of pediatric stroke. **Materials and methods**: The case-control study included 107 patients with stroke. Eighty three healthy unrelated individuals from the same geographical area without any familial history of thrombosis, and stroke were selected as a control group. DNA was extracted by conventional methods and polymerase chain reaction (PCR) of the 20210 A allele in the prothrombin gene was performed according to previously described PCR method using the primers 5' TCTAGAAACAGTTGCCTGGC 3' and a mutagenic primer 5'

ATAGCACTGGGAGCATTGAAGC 3'. Hind III was used to determine the mutation. FV1691 G-A mutation was analysed according to previously described technique. PT19911 A-G polymorphism was analysed according to previously described PCR method using the primers 5' AGGTAAGCTTCTCTAAAGCCCAGG 3' and 5'. **Results**:When we searched the combined effect of PT20210A carriers and PT19911 A-G alleles, our data revealed no significant difference between the groups (p: 0.69). Twenty four (22.4%) of the pediatric stroke group carried FV1691A allele which was found to be a significant risk factor (OR:4.5 CI 95% 1.63-12.40) (p:0.01). When we excluded FV1691A and/or PT20210A patients from the main group; PT19911G allele also does not reveal a significance (p:0.23). (This study supported by Ankara University Research Fund.)

PO152

Successful immune tolerance therapy with vWF/FVIII concentrate in a hemophilic child with inhibitor

Unuvar A, Saribeyoglu E, Anak S, Devecioglu O*

Istanbul University, Istanbul School of Medicine, Division of Pediatric Hematology-Oncology, Istanbu

The development of inhibitors is one of the most serious complications of hemophilia, and the rate of inhibitor development is high in severely affected hemophilia A patients, and immune tolerance therapy (ITT) is the treatment of choice. However, the success of this therapy is limited (63-87%). Recently, Kreuz et al. gained successful results using vWF containing FVIII concentrates in high doses. On the contrary, we present severe hemophilic child with inhibitor who immune tolerance was achieved with vWF/FVIII concentrate with a lower dose. FVIII inhibitor was detected when he was 13 months old (1.5 B.U.), and he was using high purity plasma-derived FVIII concentrate assuming this as transient inhibitor. However, one month later, inhibitor level increased to 7.5 B.U together with his bleeding symptoms. Fifteen days later, inhibitor level was 7.5 B.U. , again, and ITT was initiated with the same FVIII concentrate in a dose of 50 U/kg, three times in a week. However, inhibitor level continued increasing to 16 B.U. in a 8-month period, and the factor concentrate was changed to vWF/FVIII concentrate in the same dose and schedule. One month later, inhibitor level was 3.5 B.U. only, and five months later his inhibitor was negative, and then FVIII recovery was normal. In **Conclusion**, vWF/FVIII concentrate may play an important role in the immune tolerance therapy even in low doses.

PO153

Alterations of coagulation pathway parameters in children with sickle cell disease (SCD)

Hatzipantelis E (1), Athanassiou-Metaxa M (1), Taparkou A (2), Kleta D (3), Gerotziafa S (3), Gombakis N (2), Tsatra I (1), Koussi A (1), Garipidou V (3)*

(1) Thalassemia Unit
(2) 1st Paediatric Department
(3) General Haematologic
(4) 2nd Internal Medicine

Introduction: Endothelial inflammation together with destruction of cellular membranes may activate several coagulation factors, which also bring a local coagulation phenomenon into play. Several studies have shown that in children with SCD there is a decrease of the levels of coagulation inhibitors and increased endogenous thrombin generation. **Aim**: Based on that knowledge, the aim of this study was to determine the levels of coagulation pathway parameters in children and adolescents with SCD during steady state and thrombotic crisis, targeting in their possible prognostic value and therapeutic intervention. **Materials and methods**: Forty-one patients with SCD were studied (38 S/β-thalassemia and 3 S/S), aged 2-22 years old (mean age: 14,3 years), 22 girls and 19 boys. In 38 patients during steady state and in 16 during thrombotic crisis, as well as, in 28 healthy individuals the levels of laboratory parameters of coagulation pathway (Platelets, PT, APTT, TT, Fibrinogen, D-dimers, ATIII, PC, PS, FVLeiden-APCR, LA, tPA, PAI-1, VWF, Plasminogen, A2-antiplasmin, A2-macroglobulin, thrombomodulin) were determined. **Results**: From all parameters determined abnormal findings were as follows: a) in patients during steady state we found significantly increased levels of D-dimers (432,1μg/lt, $p<0,001$), and decreased levels of A2-antiplasmin (67,78%, $p<0,05$), compared with healthy controls and b) in patients during thrombotic crisis we found significantly increased levels of D-dimers (825, 24 μg/lt, $p<0,001$), increased levels of VWF (186,97%, $p<0,001$), and decreased levels of TT (14,86 sec, $p<0,05$) compared with healthy controls and patients in steady state. **Conclusion**: Abnormal values of some parameters determined confirms the serious dysfunction of coagulation pathway during thrombotic crisis, while pathologic values in some of them during steady state shows the presence of chronic inflammation of vascular endothelium and activation of coagulation in SCD patients.

PO154

The role of inherited hypercoagulable abnormalities in pediatric hematopoietic stem cell transplantation

Ertem M, Azık F, Ileri T, Akar E, Ulu A, Akar N*

Ankara University Pediatric BMT Unit, Ankara, TURKEY

Introduction: Recent reports from different groups pointed predisposing factors in the development of thrombotic processes after hematopoietic stem cell transplantation (HSCT) in adults. **Aim**: In this prospective study, we aimed to investigate the effect of inherited hypercoagulable abnormalities on HSCT outcome in children. **Materials and methods**: The laboratory evaluation included functional anticoagulant assays for protein C, protein S, antithrombin III (AT III), factor VIII and factor V Leiden and prothrombin 20210 G-A were performed before conditioning therapy. Patient characteristics, thrombotic processes(catheter related thrombosis, pulmonary embolism, deep venous thrombosis) and veno-occlusive disease (VOD) were evaluated. In this ongoing study, 33 children (median age:10 years, range:1,1-17 years) who underwent HSCT for leukemia (n:13), hemoglobinopat (n:11), aplastic anemia (n:3), MDS (n:2), JCMML (n:2), CML (n:1) and FHLH (n:1) were included. **Results**: Laboratory evaluation of inherited hypercoagulable abnormalities indicated a patient had heterozygote protein C deficiency. Protein S and AT III levels were normal in all of the patients. Factor VIII levels were elevated in five (%15.1) patients. Factor V Leiden heterozygosity was seen in 7 (%21.2) patients, but none of the patients had prothrombin gene 20210 G-A mutation. Thrombotic complications were diagnosed in 8 (%24.2) patients. There were 6 (%18.1) cases of VOD and 2 (%6) cases developed catheter related thrombosis. VOD was diagnosed on the basis of clinical criteria as previously described by Seattle. 2 patients had severe and 4 patients had moderate VOD. 3 of the 6 VOD had factor V Leiden heterozygosity. Catheter related thrombosis was not associated with inherited hypercoagulable abnormalities in our 2 cases. **Conclusions**: Hereditary thrombophilia did not increase the risk of thrombosis in pediatric HSCT patients except VOD. We recognise that the number of patients in this study is small to draw a conclusion. However, we believe that factor V leiden mutation may increase the risk of VOD in HSCT patients and early intervention for VOD should be considered for patients with this mutation.

PO155

Importance of HDL-Cholesterol determination for the diagnosis of hypercholesterolemia during childhood

Lafita M (1), Yolanda S (1), Narvaez I (1), Vacas M (1), Saez de Lafuente J (2), Sagastagoitia J (3), Santos M (1), Molinero E (3), Sabino E (2), Iriarte J (1)*

(1) FIDEC, Bilbao, Spain
(2) UPV/EHU, Bilbao, Spain
(3) Hospital de Basurto, Bilbao, Spain

Introduction: High blood cholesterol in childhood associated with early development of atherosclerotic plaques has been well stablished, but the strategy to be used to detect hypercholesterolemia during childhood remains controversial. **Objectives**: The purpose of this study was to determine the prevalence of hypercholesterolemia and evaluate HDL-c values and their relation to high total cholesterol values during childhood. **Patients and Methods**: We studied 984 children of both sexes (513 boys and 471 girls) aged between 6-7 years representative of that aged school population in our province. Total cholesterol (TC) and HDLcolesterol (HDLc) values were obtained by capillary puncture using Cholestech LDX (Menarini SA) to calculate the atherogenic index TC/HDLc. For sample descriptions we have used mean values (X) with standard deviation (sd) and frequencies distribution. Our data were processed using the SPSS/V10.1 statistical package **Results**: The following mean values ± standard deviation were obtained: for TC 164.22±34.64 mg/dl (CI 95%: 162.26÷166.18), HDLc 62.31±14.7 mg/dl (CI 95%: 61.37÷63,.25) and TC/HDLc ratio 2.75±0.76 mg/dl (CI 95 %: 2.70÷2.80). Only 2.1% of the sample had HDLc values below 35 mg/dl, 68.2% had HDLc values over 50 mg/dl and of those, 86.1% had HDLc values over 60 mg/dl. A total of 118 (12%) children were hypercholesterolemic according to criteria described in the literature, where hypercholesterolemia is considered as TC values ³ 200 mg/dl. When evaluating HDLc we found that 96 (81.6%) had HDLc values over 60 mg/dl and only 39 (23.8%) had a TC/HDLc index >3.5 (proposed value to evaluate cardiovascular risk). **Conclusion**: HDLc values constitute an important part of TC in children, for that reason, high TC values must be evaluated carefully, as this elevation is most often due to an increase in HDLc concentrations.

PO156

Thrombogenic parameters in hypercholesterolemic children

Saez Y (1), Lafita M (1), Narváez I (1), Vacas M (1), Saez de Lafuente J (2), Sagastagoitia J (3), Magro A (2), Caso R (1), Gandarias JM (1), Iriarte J (1)*

(1) FIDEC, Bilbao, Spain
(2) UPV/EHU, Bilbao, Spain
(3) Hospital de Basurto, Bilbao, Spain

Introduction: Atherosclerosis is a process that is initiated in the earlier stages of life. Thromboenic risk factors in hypercholesterolemics play an important role in atherosclerosis genesis. The **aim** of our study was to determined D-Dimer, Fibrinogen, PAI 1 and Lp(a) concentrations in hypercholesterolemic children. **Material and Method**: We studied 115 children, 51 girls and 64 boys (40% with TC ³ 200 mg/dl) aged between 6-7 years. Peripheral blood extraction after fasting has been carried out to each of the attendants to determine Total Cholesterol (TC), PAI 1, D-Dimer, Fibrinogen and Lp(a). We divided the sample in two groups according to the TC level (below or over/equal to 200 mg/dl) to evaluate the influence of high TC levels in thrombogenic factors. **Results**: Children with Total Cholesterol ³ 200 mg/dl presented the following mean values of thrombogenic risk factors: Lp (a) 14.79±19.19 mg/dl, PAI 1 4.42±6.53 AU/ml, D-Dimer 313.5±204.04 ng/dl and for Fibrinogen 275.47±53.53 mg/dl. When Total cholesterol values were < 200 mg/dl, mean values were respectively 11.28±13.82 mg/dl, 3.92±4.13 AU/ml, 274.77±167.87 ng/dl and 246.46±42.35 mg/dl. Hypercholesterolemic children presented higher concetrations of all the thrombogenic risk factors studied, in the case of fibrinogen the difference was statistically significant. **Conclusion**: If we consider that is not infrequent to find hypercholesterolemia during childhood, and that there is an additional burden if there are thrombogenic risk factors associated that can negatively influence in the future development of the atherosclerotic plaque, we think that is important the early detection in order to adopt rapid and efficacy preventive measures.

PO157

TFPI –33T→C polymorphism in Turkish children with crebral infarct

Donmez BN (1), Deda G (2), Sipahi T (3), Çaksen H (4), Cin Ş (5), Akar N (6)*

(1) Biotechnology Institute, Ankara University, Turkey
(2) Department of Pediatric Neurology, Ankara University, Ankara, Turkey
(3) Sami Ulus Children's Hospital, Ankara, Turkey
(4) Van Yüzyıl University, Turkey
(5) Department of Pediatric Diseases, Ankara University, Turkey
(6) Department of Pediatric Molecular Genetics, Ankara University, Ankara, Turkey

Introduction: Tissue Factor Pathway Inhibitor, a Kunitz-type serine protease inhibitor, is the main inhibitor of the factor VIIa-tissue factor pathway of blood coagulation. In intron 7 of the TFPI gene a T to C single-base polymorphism (-33T→C), which is strongly associated with total circulating TFPI antigen levels, was identified. CC genotype was associated with significantly higher total TFPI levels than the TT genotype. CC genotype of the TFPI intron 7 polymorphism is an independent protective factor for venous thromboembolism, an effect probably mediated by increased TFPI levels. **Aim**: The aim of this study was to search for an association between the –33T→C polymorphism of intron 7 and pediatric stroke. **Materials and methods**: The case-control study included 118 patients with cerebral infarct who were below the age of 18 years. All were clinically diagnosed and the infarction verified with cranial imaging of the brain. Patients with venous thrombosis are excluded. 100 healty unrelated age and sex matched individuals from the same geographical area without any familial history of thrombosis and stroke were selected as a control group. DNA was extracted by classic fenol-chloroform method and 86 bp region intron 7 of TFPI gene was amplified by PCR. To determine the mutation PCR products were digested by Nde1 restriction endonuclease enzyme as previously reported. **Results and Conclusion**: We found T and C allele frequencies as 48,5%-51,5% in control group and 49,6%-50,4% in patient group respectively. Our data revealed that, when C allele is combined with FV1691A, the risk of thrombosis decreases but TFPI gene –33T→C polymorphism doesn't have any effect in PT20210A carriers. (This study is supported by Ankara University Biotechnology Institute.)

PO158

Body mass index and atherothrombotic risk factors during childhood

Saez Y (1), Lafita M (1), Vacas M (1), Narváez I (1), Sagastagoitia J (2), Saez de Lafuente J (3), Magro A (3), Molinero E (2), Martinez B (1), Iriarte J (1)*

(1) FIDEC, Bilbao, Spain
(2) Hospital de Basurto, Bilbao, Spain
(3) UPV/EHU, Bilbao, Spain

Introduction: It is reported that obesity is associated with the development of cardiovascular disease (CVD). Factors that predispose individuals to CVD are thought to develop during childhood. **Objective**: To determine if there is any relationship between Body Mass Index (BMI) and fibrinogen, D-Dimer, PAI-1 and Lp(a). **Material and Methods**: We studied 110 children of both sexes aged between 6-7 years. These children came from an epidemiological study on the prevalence of hypercholesterolemia in children in the province of Biscay. To each child the following parameters were carried out: Weight and height to obtain BMI, and peripheral blood extraction after 12 hours' fasting to analyse fibrinogen (von Clauss), D-Dimer (enzymo-inmune sandwich method) PAI 1 (inmunoactive method) and Lp(a) (enzymo-inmune test). For the sample descriptions we have used mean values (X) with standard deviation and to measure the linear relationship between two variables we used Pearson correlation. Our data wee processed using the SPSS statistical package. **Results**: We found the following mean values for atherothrombotic risk factors: BMI Kg/m2 17.4±2.49 (lowest value 12.84 and highest value 26.51), Lp(a) mg/dl 12.07±15.35 (lowest value 0.170 and highest value 66), PAI 1 AU/ml 3.77±3.93 (lowest value 0.11 and highest value19.3), D-Dimer ng/ml 288±182.41(lowest value 94 and highest value 1095) and Fibrinogen mg/dl 268±48.59 (lowest value 170 and highest value 395). We have found a postive correlation coefficient statistically significant ($p<0.01$) between fibrinogen concentrations and BMI. This association is maintained if we correlate overweight-obesity degree with fibrinogen ($p<0.05$). We didn't found any correlation with the rest of the parameters studied and BMI. **Conclusion**: Our data suggest, that elevated BMI is associated with elevated fibrinogen levels. This means that they have a higher risk of atherosclerotic disease.

PO159

FXIII Val34Leu Gene Polymorphism in Turkish Children with Cerebral Infarct

Donmez BN (1), Deda G (2), Akar N (3)*

(1) Biotechnology Institute, Ankara University, Turkey
(2) Department of Pediatric Neurology, Ankara University, Turkey
(3) Department of Pediatric Molecular Genetics, Ankara University, Turkey

Introduction: FXIII catalyses the formation of covalent bounds between fibrin monomers, thus stabilizing the fibrin clot and increasing its resistance to fibrinolysis. A common G→T polymorphism in exon 2 of the FXIIIA gene which is characterized by a Val→Leu exchange at amino acid position 34, three amino acids from the thrombin activation side, has been identified. An increased FXIII activity has been reported in carriers of the Leu allele, with Leu homozygotes having the higher activities compared with Val homozygotes. In addition, the prevalence of the Leu encoding allele was found lower in adult patients with cerebral infarction.The **aim** of this case-control study was to determine whether there exist an association between FXIII Val34Leu polymorphism and pediatric stroke. **Materials and methods**: This study included 116 pediatric patients with cerebral infarct who were below the age of 18 years. All were clinically diagnosed and the infarction verified with cranial imaging of the brain. 100 healty unrelated age and sex matched individuals from the same geographical area without any familial history of thrombosis and stroke were selected as a control group. DNA was extracted by classic fenol-chloroform method and amplification of 192 bp region was performed by PCR. To determine the mutation PCR products were digested by Dde1 enzyme as previously reported. **Results and Conclusion**: We found G and T allele frequencies as 86,5%-13,5% in control group and 89,2%-10,8% in patient group respectively. Our data revealed that, FXIII gene Val34Leu polymorphism was not associated independently with pediatric stroke in our population and doesn't have any effect in PT20210 carriers. The risk of thrombosis decreases from 2 fold to protective side (OR 0,9)in patients carrying FV1691A. This may be an important clue and needs further study in FV1691A carriers with and without thrombosis. (This study is supported by Ankara University Biotechnology Institute.)

PO160

Deficiency of coagulation inhibitors in children with ischemic stroke and transient ischemic attack (TIA)

Lenicek Krleza J (1), Coen D (2), Zadro R (2), Stavljenic-Rukavina A (2)*

(1) Dep. for Laboratory Diagnostics, Children's Hospital Zagreb, Croatia
(2) Zagreb University School of Medicine, Clinical Institute of Laboratory Diagnosis Zagreb Cli

Introduction: Coagulation inhibitors antithrombin (AT), protein C (PC), and protein S (PS) represent an important barrier to thrombosis. These factors inhibit mechanisms that counteract hemostasis contributing to an increased state of hypercoaguability and thereby can play an etiological role in stroke. **Aim**: The aim of the study was to investigate the frequency of decreased AT, PC and PS activities in children with ischemic stroke and TIA and try to find out at which degree deficiencies of coagulation inhibitors participate in the etiology of pediatric ischemic cerebrovascular events. **Materials and methods**: Children less than 18 years age with radiological evidence of stroke (N=29) and TIA (N=45) were studied. Antithrombin and protein C activities were determined by using a chromogenic method (Berichrom AT (A) and Protein C, Dade Behring) on Sysmex CA–500 analyzer. Free protein S was determined with ELISA (Asserachrom Free Protein S, Stago Diagnostics). **Results**: In 38 of 74 investigated patients (51.4%), decreased activities of one coagulation inhibitor was present, decreased PC activity was present in 13.5%, free PS in 35.1% and AT in 2.7%. In children with ischemic stroke we found decreased PC activity in 10.3%, free PS in 31.0% and AT in 3.4% of patients, whilst the frequency of decreased activities in children with TIA was 13.3% for PC, 37.8% for free PS and 2.2% for AT. Combined PC and PS decreased activities were found in five patients (4 with TIA, and 1 with stroke). One child (2 years old with stroke) had combined PC and AT decreased activities. **Conclusion**: Half of our investigated group had at least one coagulation inhibitor deficiency being PS deficiency the most frequent. No significant difference of the frequencies of coagulation inhibitor deficiencies was found between children with stroke and TIA. Deficiency of coagulation inhibitors, especially PS, can participate in the etiology of pediatric ischemic cerebrovascular events, but it is very important to differentiate between congenital and acquired PC, PS and AT deficiencies.

PO161

Thromboembolic complication in children with oncologic disease - review of two cases

Vukelic-Damijani N (1), Smokvina M (2), Caser L (1), Vujaklija-Stipanović K (1)*

(1) Institute of Transfusion Medicine, Clinical Hospital Center, Rijeka, Croatia
(2) Division of Hematology/Oncology, Department of Pediatrics, Clinical Hospital Center, Rijeka, Croatia

Case 1: 10-year old boy with diagnosis non Hodgkin lymphoma of mediastinum gr. III MR. He has got Broviac catheter implanted at the right side and he was treated according to the protocol NHL-BFM 95. In the second week of hospitalization he was getting rightside bronchopneumonia, which was treated with antibiotics. In the fifth week of hospital's stay, after 6 dosis of L-asparaginase, has been developed symptoms of thrombosis of right brachial artery what was confirmed by color doppler ultrasonography. In the coagulogram result we found: APTT 135s, PT 77%, TT 55s, fibrinogen 0.58g/l, AT III 55%, D-dimers 22μg/l, platelet count 230×10^9/l. Along with therapy with fresh frozen plasma and supstitution with AT III concentrate we started anticoagulant therapy with low-molecular-weight heparin (LMWH) - nadroparin 2×0.3 ml sc for four days and then next ten days with nadroparin 0,3 ml once a day. After anticoagulant therapy symptoms of thrombotic process disappear and citostatic therapy was continued. The result of coagulogram three weeks after thrombotic episode was normal. **Case 2**: 9-year old girl hospitalized because of III hematologic recidive of acute lymphoblastic leucosis, resistant disease also after bone marrow transplantation. She is going to treatment for resistant leukemia. In the third week of treatment she have got respiratory symptomatology and by CT was proved pulmonary embolism. The results of coagulogram were: APTT 34s, PT 100%, TT 14s, fibrinogen 11,34 g/l, AT III 92 %, D-dimers 212 μg/l, platelet count 31×10^9/l. In the therapy was introduced LMWH (nadroparin 2×0,3 ml sc). Because of thrombocytopenia, which persist, anticoagulant therapy was temporarilly interrupted. Due to progression of basic disease, ten days later she died. **Conclusion**: thromboembolic disease in the children is rare and mostly is consequence of other disease or therapeutic procedure, which is tipically for these two cases too.

PO162

Normal ranges with PFA-100 (Dade-Behring) in healthy subjects

Vacas M (1), Narvaez I (1), Lafita M (1), Saez Y (1), Santos M (2), Longa M (2), Saez de Lafuente J (3), Magro A (3), Iriarte J (1), Gandarias JM (1)*

(1) FIDEC, Bilbao, Spain
(2) MEDIKOSTA, Bilbao, Spain
(3) UPV/EHU, Bilbao, Spain

Background: We can see in the literature that there are interlaboratory variations among normal ranges measured with PFA-100 (Dade-Behring) in healthy subjects. In the majority of the published data, these normal ranges are made in 10 healthy subjects, except one that has been made in 90 subjects. **Aim**: To determine normal ranges in the platelet function analizer PFA-100. **Material and Methods**: 30 healthy subjects (17 males and 13 females) with a mean age of 28.77±9.18 years has been studied. Nonfasting blood samples were all obtained between 9 and 12 a. m. They were withdrawn by antecubital venipuncture and the initial first milliliters of blood were discarded to avoid spontaneous platelet activation. Nine millilters of blood were collected in 0.129 M buffered sodium citrate tube (Vacutainer) for analysis by PFA-100 with col/epi cartridges (lot 569563) and 4.5 ml EDTA tube (vacutainer) for platelet and red blood cells count, hemoglobin and hematocrit. Duplicate measurements were performed to determine closure time. For sample descriptions we have used mean values with standard deviation, 95 % confidence interval and coefficient of variation for duplicates. Our data were processed using the SPSS/V10 statistical package. **Results**: Mean value for closure time was 124.78±24.08 seconds (lower value 86 and higher value 178). Coefficient of variation for duplicates was 1.92 %. For normal ranges, mean value ± 2 standard deviations was established and the interval obtained was 77-173 seconds. Platelet and red blood cells count, hemoglobin and hematocrit were all between normal ranges. **Conclusions**: Due to the different normal ranges that have been published, we consider that it is necessary that each laboratory should establish its own reference ranges.

PO163

Function of platelets: comparison of findings between the PFA-100 and the aggregometer in normal subjects

Makris P, Boutou A, Sarridou D, Papamichos S, Tsoukas D, Bougiouklis D, Zarmakoupis A, Papageorgiou I, Anestakis D, Girtovitis F*

Haemostasis –Thrombosis Unit, A' Medical Propedeutic Clinic Aristotle University of The

Introduction: PFA-100 is a relatively new platelets' function testing-device, which has not yet been fully evaluated for its accuracy. **Aim:** This study aims to control platelets' function in normal subjects by using both PFA-100 and aggregometer and to compare their findings to each other. **Material:** 21 normal subjects (9 women and 12 men) with a mean age of 39±13 years were studied. They had not taken any medication that affects platelets function for the previous ten days, they did not have any diagnosed pathologic condition or illness and they all had normal haematocrit and platelets count. Blood sample was taken by free flux, with butterfly 19G, in the morning after a whole-night fasting. Stimulating the platelets with ristosetin confirmed the lack of any platelet dysfunction of the subjects. **Methods:** 1) We calculated the bleeding time in vitro with PFA-100, using filters which were covered by collagen and ADP (ADP) or by collagen and epinephrine (EPI). 2) We studied the aggregation of platelets with the aggregometer PICA of Chronolog co, using as stimulators ADP or adrenaline (ADR). Applying the methods in the same sample for twenty times checked their repeatability. **Statistical analysis:** We calculated the Mean Value (MV) and the Standard Deviation (SD) of the above-mentioned parameters and then we accepted as normal range of platelets' function the limits of MV±3SD. Coefficient of Variation (CV) was determined to check the repeatability of the methods. **Results:** Table I: MV, SD and

MV±3SD of bleeding time and platelets' aggregation and CV of the two methods used to estimate these parameters.

	PFA (ADP) closure time (sec)	Aggregometer (ADP) (%)	PFA (EPI) closure time (sec)	Aggregometer (ADR) (%)
MV	84.30	69.3	105.06	78
SD	9.97	13.2	11.40	2
MV±3SD	54.4-114.2	29.7-108.9	34.2-139.06	72-84
CV	4.2%	1.3%	8.6%	3.7%

Conclusions: 1) The repeatability control of platelets' aggregation in aggregometer with ADP and ADR gave us a corresponding CV of 1.3% and 3.7%, which is statistically acceptable, since it is lower than the statistical limit of 5%. On the contrary, PFA-100 has an acceptable CV of 4.2% with ADP but a non-acceptable one (8.6%) with EPI. 2) Based on the strict limits, within which we have determined the normal range, none of the studied subjects had pathologic platelets' function.

PO164

PADA – Fast and quantitative monitoring of blood platelet adhesiveness

Nowak G (1), Bucha E (2), Wiesenburg A (1), Schumann A (2)*

(1) Friedrich Schiller University, Medical Faculty, Research Group "Pharmacological Haemostaseology", Jena
(2) HaemoSys Ltd., Jena, Germany

Background: Haemostatic balance in the circulation is mainly determined by activity state of blood platelets. By now, acquired platelet derived diseases (thrombocytopathies) can not be detected nor quantified as real time whole blood methods are still missing. Platelet aggregometry and similar methods can measure only the second, final step of platelet reactivity. However, first step of platelet activation, the platelet adhesion, is of more importance. A historical method, the platelet spreading test, can provide only qualitative results, but is not quantifiable. **Methods/Results**: We developed a new test named PADA (**p**latelet **ad**hesion **a**ssay) to quantify current platelet adhesiveness. PADA requires besides an automated cell counter only a low-cost minishaker and a maximum of 1 mL anticoagulated whole blood. Transit time between blood withdrawal and measurement of adhesion index (AI) should not exceed 1 h. To 200 µL anticoagulated blood a defined amount of specific surface-structured polymer particles is added. Following exactly 5 min of mechanical alteration by shaking the sample, adhesive platelets will adhere to the polymer surface. As control, to another blood sample saline is added instead of polymer particles and the sample is treated in the same manner. Thereafter, the number of platelets in both samples is determined and from these the adhesion index can easily be calculated. In healthy volunteers, a mean AI of 52± 10 is reached. In evaluation of this test with POCT-quality, no age-dependency could be proved. Variation of platelet count between 100 and 300 Gpt/ml does not affect measuring results. Furthermore, the method is insensitive to variation of fibrinogen level and other coagulation variables. **Summary:** PADA is the first POCT-capable quantitative test for monitoring of current platelet adhesiveness. It is suited for diagnostics of pathologically increased adhesion of platelets in patients (AI > 62) and can also be used as monitoring method of GPIIb/IIIa receptor antagonist or thienopyridine therapy.

PO165

Poly-APS induced thrombocyte aggregation is partly blocked by the combination of acetylsalicylic acid, clopidogrel and abciximab

*Šuput D, Bunc M**

University of Ljubljana, Medical faculty, Institute for pathophysiology, Ljubljana, Slovenia

Introduction In search for biologically active substances water-soluble polymeric 3-alkylpyridinium salts (poly-APS; MW 18900 and 5520 Da) were isolated from the marine sponge Reniera sarai. Poly-APS inhibited acetylcholinesterase (AChE), but this effect was not sufficient to explain the lethality of the substance. Intravascular plug formation was a typical finding on autopsy indicating that poly-APS either activated the coagulation pathway, induced platelet aggregation, or interfered with the endothelial function. **Aims** The aim of the study was to study the mechanism of action of poly-APS, and to evaluate possible therapeutic effects of antithrombotic drugs. **Materials and methods** Poly-APS was isolated as described previously. Spectrophotometric measurements showed that the speed and intensity of platelets aggregation was dose dependent. Data obtained on blood samples from animals treated with poly-APS also revealed numerous platelet aggregates. A quantitative assessment of the effects of poly-APS on platelets was performed by use of optical aggregometry. Washed platelets were incubated with the following final concentrations of poly-APS (mg/ml): 1.08, 0.1, 0.01, 0.001, 0.0001 and measured by means of optical aggregometry. Platelet aggregation due to different concentrations of poly-APS was modulated by addition of either acetylsalicylic acid (Aspegic), clopidogrel (Plavix) and abciximab (Reo-Pro) in 0.5 mg/ml, 0.5 mg/ml and 0.06 mg/ml concentrations, respectively or in combination of all the agents in the previously mentioned concentrations. At the highest concentration of poly-APS, Aspirin lowered the aggregation for 40 %, Plavix for 10% and ReoPro for 8%, and the combination of all three for 50%. The speed of aggregation is much slower when Aspirin is added than in case of Plavix or ReoPro. Tests of coagulation revealed that the toxin had no direct effects on coagulation rate. **Conclusion** Our data suggest that activation of cyclooxygenase pathway is substantially important in Poly-APS induced platelet aggregation. The data allow the conclusion that ADP-receptor activation and GP IIa/IIIb are important in the late phase of the Poly-APS induced platelet aggregation.

PO166

Influence of platelet activation agonists on lymphocyte-platelet adhesion

Solpov A, Vitkovsky Y, Kuznik B*

Chita Medical Academy, Chita, Russia

Our previous in vitro study showed that cytokine IL 1beta, IL 2 increased 2,5 fold number of lymphocyte-platelet co-aggregates. Contra-inflammatory cytokines IL 4 and IL 10 possessed inhibitory activity on lymphocyte-platelet adhesion. Similar effect was observed for IF gamma. These suggest important role of cytokines for regulation of lymphocyte functional activity to form co-aggregates with platelets. However importance of platelet activation in lymphocyte adhesion is unknown. Our aim was to study the influence of different platelet aggregation agonists on lymphocyte-platelet adhesion. Investigation was performed on healthy donors' blood. To preserve platelet aggregation the tirofiban in final dose 20 mg/ml into experimental samples and sodium chloride isotonic solution into control samples was added previously. Samples were incubated in 37°C during 10 minutes and different platelet aggregation agonists (ADP, collagen, platelet activating factor (PAF), adrenaline and arachidonic acid) were added. Lymphocytes pool was extracted from activated whole blood. It was established that control samples contented 13% lymphocyte-platelet aggregates (LPA). Presence of tirofiban increased the number of LPA up to 16% in experimental samples. If ADP, collagen, adrenaline, arachidonic acid, PAF were added the number of LPA increased up to 25-35 %. We observed that control lymphocytes adhered 4 ± 1 platelets on their surfaces. Tirofiban decreased number of trombocytes on lymphocytes 2 fold. Collagen activated platelets possessed increase ability to adhere of lymphocytes up to 7,1. Others agonists increased did not change count of platelets on cells. Thus, these results suggest that platelet functional activity influences on lymphocyte–platelet interaction.

PO167

Influence of recombinant interleukin 2 on platelet aggregation and lymphocyte-platelet adhesion

Vitkovsky Y, Solpov A, Kuznik B*

Chita Medical Academy, Chita, Russia

Earlier we have demonstrated the ability of lymphocytes carrying CD3+ and CD4+ markers to form co-aggregates with platelet spontaneously. Our findings showed that in vitro culturing of lymphocytes during four hours with interleukin (IL) 2 increased 4-fold the of rosette-forming cells in total lymphocyte pool. Stimulation of lymphocytes by IL 2 enhanced adhesive activity of CD4+ cells and induced ability of CD16+ lymphocyte to form co-aggregates with platelets. It was observed that ICAM molecules are ligand of cell-platelet adhesion. Our aim was to study the influence of recombinant IL 2 on platelet aggregation and ability of lymphocytes to adhere platelets in vivo. 12 patients who administered of recombinant IL 2 in dose 500000 U daily intravenously were investigated. Lymphocyte-platelet adhesion and ADP induced thrombocyte aggregation were tested three times: before and after administration of medicine and after 24 hours. It was established that lymphocyte-platelet adhesion enhanced up to 4-5% after administration of IL 2 and on 14-15% after 24 hours in comparison with before injection. In repeated administration of a medicine the parameter of lymphocyte-platelet adhesion was kept on a high level. But after first injection all patients had decreased platelet aggregation. However the next day before repeated injection of recombinant IL 2 the essential increase of parameters of aggregatogram was observed. The additional administration of IL 2 was accompanied by inhibition of platelet aggregation. We consider that IL 2 renders influence on platelets by means of activated lymphocytes.

PO168

The severity of peripheral arterial disease can influence plasma platelet microparticle levels

Tan K (1), Tayebjee M (1), Blann AD (1), Lynd C (2), Lip G (1)**

(1) HTVBU, University Department of Medicine, City Hospital, Birmingham B18 7QH, UK
(2) Department of Vascular Surgery, City Hospital , Birmingham B18 7QH, UK

Introduction Platelet microparticles (PMPs) are formed by microvesiculation from activated platelets. They are believed to play an important role in promoting thrombosis in various disease states, including hypertension, acute coronary syndromes and post-coronary angioplasty. **Aims** We hypothesize that the level of PMPs in the blood can be directly related to the clinical severity of atherosclerotic disease. **Materials and methods** We recruited patients with critical limb ischaemia (CLI), intermittent claudication (IC), and healthy controls. PMPs were detected in platelet poor plasma by flow cytometry after staining with anti-CD61-PerCP and anti-CD42-FITC monoclonal antibodies. 23 patients with CLI, 36 patients with IC, and 34 age and sex matched controls were recruited. The mean age for CLI, IC, and control groups were 66.5 (SD=11.2), 65.3 (SD=9.2), and 66.7 (SD=13.9) respectively (P=0.623). Mean systolic blood pressure (SD in brackets) for the CLI, IC, and control groups were 135 (28), 145 (18), and 130 (12) respectively (P=0.007). HDL (IQR in brackets) was 1.2(1.2-1.4), 1.4(1.2-1.7), and 1.5(1.3-1.7) among the three groups (P=0.001). 70% of CLI, 56% of IC, and none of the controls were on long-term aspirin therapy. **Results and Conclusion** The CLI, IC, and control groups (IQR in brackets) had significantly different PMP levels of 98650 (25720-192630)/ml, 39080 (20840-67460)/ml, and 17459 (9329-40885)/ml (P=0.02, Tukey's posthoc analysis). The presence of various risk factors in patients with atherosclerosis may lead to inappropriate platelet activation, resulting in high PMP levels that have a graded relationship to the severity of disease. Elevated PMP levels in atherosclerosis may be clinically important as they can further promote thrombosis, resulting in the acute presentation of atherosclerotic disease.

PO169

Patients with stable ischaemic heart disease have increased levels of platelet microparticles

Tan K, Tayebjee M, Blann AD, Lip G**

HTVBU, University Dept of Medicine, City Hospital, Birmingham B18 7QH, UK

Introduction Membrane vesicles derived from activated platelets, platelet microparticles (PMPs), may have important effects in promoting thrombosis, angiogenesis, and inflammation. It is likely that PMPs are elevated in stable coronary heart disease (CHD) as previous studies have shown that there is increased platelet activation, as measured by platelet surface P-selectin positivity, in atherosclerosis. **Aims** To support the hypothesis that there is increased PMPs in stable CHD. **Methods** We recruited 52 patients with stable CHD, as characterised by the presence of clinical symptoms and abnormal coronary angiography, as well as 34 age & sex matched healthy volunteers. The mean age of the CHD patients was 62.5(SD=8.0), whilst that of the controls was 65.5 (SD=14.5). HDL was 1.3 (IQR=1.1-1.4) in the CHD group and 1.5 (1.3-1.9) in the control group (P=0.0004). Systolic blood pressure was 138 (IQR=120-153) in the CHD group and 130 (120-140) in the healthy volunteers (P=0.11). Three indices of platelet activation, the percentage positivity of platelet surface P-selectin and CD63, as well as the number of platelet microparticles per cubic milimetre of plasma were established by flow cytometry (FACScan, BDBiosciences). **Results and Conclusions** There is increased platelet activation in the patients with CHD, as determined by percentage surface P-selectin positivity (7.3 (IQR=2.0-14.0) vs 2.7 (1.7-5.5), p=0.007), and CD63 positivity (12.2 (SD=8.7) vs 8.2(SD=5.1)). Patients with CHD also have increased levels of PMP/ml plasma (39700 (IQR=19000-91300) when compared to healthy controls (19400 (IQR=10900-40900) (P=0.0016). It is possible that PMPs may play a role in the pathophysiology of stable CHD. Further studies are needed to investigate the prognostic implication of elevated PMP levels.

PO170

Prevalence of aspirin resistance in cardiovascular patients using the PFA-100 diagnostic system

Narvaez I (1), Vacas M (1), Saez Y (1), Caso R (1), Martinez B (1), Sagastagoitia J (2), Molinero E (2), Santos M (1), Saez de Lafuente J (3), Iriarte J (1)*

(1) FIDEC, Bilbao, Spain
(2) Hospital de Basurto, Bilbao, Spain
(3) UPV/EHU, Bilbao, Spain

Introduction: Standard of care for the treatment of patients with coronary arterial disease (CAD) includes antiplatelet therapy with aspirin (ASA). However, the antiplatelet effect of ASA varies across the broad distribution of CAD patients. A new laboratory method to control this effect is the PFA-100 (Dade) an instrument and test cartridge system in which the process of platelet adhesion and aggregation is simulated in vitro. **Aim:** To evaluate the prevalence of aspirin resistance (AR) in CAD patients using the PFA-100 analyzer. **Patients and Methods**: 158 patients (116 men and 42 women) with an age range between 64.60±11.83 years underwent cardiac catheterism for coronary disease suspicion. All of them were treated with aspirin (100-300 mg.) Blood was drawn into Vacutainer tubes containing 3,8% (0,129M) buffered sodium citrate. Colagen/epinephrine test cartridges (Lot nº 569563) were used on the PFA-100. Following our range of normality, three groups were stablished: AR (Group A) with a range closure time of 77-173 sec, Moderate AR (Group B) with values between 174-300 sec, Non AR with values >300 sec. **Results**: A total of 102 patients (64.55%) were enrolled in Group C, 21 patients (13.29%) in Group B and 35 patients (22.15%) in Group A. **Conclusions**: The prevalence of aspirin resistance found is similar to the ones reported in other studies. Nevertheless considerable differences exist (11-50%) depending on the normality ranges used, indicating the need for standardization of the test to be able to carry out rigorous clinical studies, as already has been implemented in other coagulations tests like Prothrombin Time.

PO171

Clinical effects of combined tirofiban with LMWH in patients with acute coronary syndrome

Kim J, Jeong M, Kim W, Ahn YK, Cho JG, Park J, Kang J*

Chonnam National University Hospital, Gwangju, Korea

Background and Objectives: Platelet activation and aggregation with resultant arterial thrombus formation play pivotal role in the pathophysiology of acute coronary syndrome (ACS). We evaluated the efficacy of tirofiban, a specific inhibitor of the platelet glycoprotein IIb/IIIa receptor, combined with heparin or low molecular heparin (LMWH) in the management of ACS prospectively. **Subjects and Methods**: We divided 160 patients (60.9±11.1 years, 104 male) with unstable angina or non-ST elevation myocardial infarction, who had ST-T changes and elevated troponin, into 4 groups: Group I (n=40: heparin alone), Group II (n=40: LMWH, dalteparin alone), Group III (n=40: tirofiban combined with heparin) and Group IV (n=40: tirofiban with LMWH), and compared major adverse cardiac events (MACE) among 4 groups during 6-month clinical follow-up prospectively. **Results**: Percutaneous coronary intervention (PCI) or coronary artery bypass graft (CABG) was performed 32 in Group I, 29 in Group II, 28 in Group III and 31 patients in Group IV (p=0.72). Minor bleeding complication was developed 2 (5.0%) in Group I, 2 (5.0%) in Group II, 4 (10.0%) in Group III and 3 patients (7.5%) in Group IV (p=0.78). During six-month follow-up MACE after PCI or CABG occurred 10 (31.3%) in Group I, 9 (31.0%) in Group II, 4 (14.3%) in Group III and 4 patients (12.9%) in Group IV (p=0.02: Group I and II vs. Group III and IV). **Conclusion**: Tirofiban combined with LMWH is safe and may improve long-term prognosis in patients with ACS.

PO172

Thrombocytopenia in the intensive care unit. Case series

Duarte P, Grand B, Egozcue J, Fernandez J, Cacchione R, Riveros D*

Department of Internal Medicine, Hematology Section, CEMIC University Hospital, Buenos Aires, Argentina.

Objective: To determine the prevalence and outcome of specific causes of thrombocytopenia in medical intensive care patients. **Design**: A review of the medical records of patients admitted during a period of 4 years. **Setting**: The 11-bed medical intensive care unit of a university hospital. **Patients**: All consecutively admitted patients with normal platelet count at admission during a

4-year period (n: 3102). **Main outcome measures**: Prevalence of thrombocytopenia (defined by a platelet count < 100.000/mm^3), specific causes of thrombocytopenia (defined by those causes that would have only one mechanism involved) and death in thrombocytopenic patients with specific causes of thrombocytopenia. **Results**: Thrombocytopenia occurred in 293 patients (9,4%). Thrombocytopenia was multifarious in 272 patients (93%) and specific causes were identified with 21 patients (7%). The specific causes of thrombocytopenia were: thrombotic microangiopathy in 10 patients, hemophagocytic histiocytosis in 6 patients (confirmed with bone marrow aspirates) and heparin induced thrombocytopenia in 5 patients (confirmed with functional assays). The number of death in patients with thrombotic microangiopathy was 3, in patients with hemopahgocytic histiocytosis was 4 and no death occurred in patients with heparin induced thrombocytopenia. **Conclusion**: Thrombocytopenia in the intensive care unit is generally multifarious. Hemophagocytic Histiocytosis is associated with very high mortality despite any therapeutic measure. It is needed in our country, more accessible diagnostic assays for heparin induced thrombocytopenia.

PO173

Salvage plasmapheresis in case of pulmonary embolism caused by heparin-induced thrombocytopenia type II resistant to danaparoid sodium and lepirudin

Antonijevic N (1), Savic N (1), Perunicic J (1), Mikovic D (2), Kovac M (2), Stanojevic M (1), Calija B (1), Obradovic S (3), Milosevic R (4), Vasiljevic Z (1)*

(1) Institute of Cardiovascular Diseases, Clinical Centre of Serbia, Belgrade, Serbia and Montenegro
(2) Blood Transfusion Institute of Serbia, Belgrade, Serbia and Montenegro
(3) Military Medicine Academy, Belgrade, Serbia and Montenegro
(4) Institute of Haematology, Clinical Centre of Serbia, Belgrade, Serbia and Montenegro

The standard therapeutic regimen of heparin-induced thrombocytopenia (HIT) type II complicated by thrombosis, besides the discontinuation of further heparin administration, implies the use of danaparoid sodium, lepirudin or other alternative antithrombin drugs. An early plasmapheresis administration is an acknowledged adjunct therapeutic method for the aforementioned HIT type II. We report the case of 64-year-old female patient who, upon receiving low-dose unfractionated heparin throughout the period of 13 days, as a venous thromboembolism prophylaxis due to the right femur neck fracture, developed thrombocytopenia of 66x109/l, pulmonary embolism and bilateral femoropopliteal deep vein thrombosis,. HIT type II was diagnosed based on the positive high specificity heparin aggregation test and fast particle gel ID-HPF4 immuno-assay. The initially administered subcutaneous danaparoid sodium and full-dose intravenous lepirudin resulted in further aggravation of thrombocytopenia. The commencement of platelet count recovery was observed as late as after the one-off plasmapheresis administration. Intravenous lepirudin infusion was continued up to the platelet count normalisation and patient's significant clinical improvement, upon which an oral anticoagulant therapy was introduced. We place emphasis on the fact that danaparoid sodium was not selected for further administration, although the in vitro danaparoid sodium aggregation test was negative.

PO174

Prospective study of coagulability in pregnancy – a new approach to the early detection of preeclampsia and cardiovascular complications

Sylvest Andersen A (1), Berthelsen JG (2), Breindahl M (3), Fareed J (4), Rud Lassen M (1)*

(1) Clinical Trial Unit
(2) Gynecological-obstet
(3) Pediatric Department
(4) Loyola University Me

Introduction: At present, screening of preeclampsia and cardiovascular complications in pregnancy is based on clinical symptoms presenting late in pregnancy, such as proteinuria combined with hypertension and oedema. However, the development of preeclampsia starts between the 8th and18th week of gestation. Studies have suggested that hypercoagulapathy may be the underlying mechanism, leading to fibrin depositions in the vascular bed of different organ systems, such as the kidneys and the maternal part of the foeto-placental circulation. **Aims**: The aim of the study is: - to establish predictors for preeclampsia and cardiovascular complications in pregnancy before clinical symptoms develops in order to start treatment with anticoagulant drugs. **Material**: 600 pregnant women will be included consecutively and followed prospectively in a standardized manner until one month postnatal. Inclusion starts in January 2004, and the inclusion period is estimated to last 12 months. **Methods**: Each woman will be included during their first visit to the Midwife clinic (about the 16th week of gestation), and thereafter seen on a routine basis. Every 2 weeks 10 ml urine sampling will be mailed to the hospital for analysis of several coagulations factors, including Prothrombin Fragment 1+2. Blood samples will be drawn at each routine antenatal visit, approximately 7-8 times throughout the pregnancy. All known coagulation and fibrinolysis markers will be analysed. At delivery a blood sample from the umbilical cord will be taken and the pH and HCO^3 determined, and the placenta sent for histological and immuno-histochemical examination. For those developing obstetrical complications gene-typing coding for thrombophilia will be determined. As controls a random number of women without cardiovascular complications will be analysed. **Results** and **Conclusion**: The first preliminary results are expected 2005. Measuring Prothrombin fragment 1+2 in urine may be a promising new approach to the early detection of preeclampsia, eclampsia, HELLP (haemolysis, elevated liver enzymes and low platelets) and cardiovascular events in pregnancy as well as providing new opportunities for prophylactic treatment to patients at risk before the damage by fibrin depositions becomes symptomatic. One method of modulating a hypercoagulapathy could be administration of a low-molecular-weight heparin, which has already been proven not to cross the placental barrier due to the highly negatively charged molecule.

PO175

No need for laboratory monitoring during low dose LMMH thromboprophylaxis during pregnancy

van Rooijen M, Nord E, Lampén Mondzo K, Bremme K*

Dept of Womans Health, Karolinska Hosptial, Stockholm, Sweden

Introduction: The purpose of this study was to investigate how to monitor thromboprophylactic treatment with low molecular mass heparin (LMMH) during pregnancy in women with low risk for thrombotic events. Hitherto, thromboprophylactic treatment in these women has been monitored throughout pregnancy by measurement of anti factor Xa activity, antithrombin and aPTT together with platelet count. **Method:** Pregnant women (n=150) with one previous venous thrombosis were included in the study. Thromboprophylaxis started in early pregnancy, i.e. before 17th gestational week, with Dalteparin (Fragmin®) 5000 IU, once daily. The Fragmin® therapy was monitored by measurements of anti factor Xa activity. Antithrombin, aPTT, and platelet count were also regularly analyzed. Blood samples were drawn at several times during pregnancies. The aim of the treatment was to reach an anti factor Xa activity in plasma above 0.2 IU/L three hours after injection. At time of delivery, the dosage was changed to 2500 IU twice daily. Post partum the treatment continued with 5000 IU daily in a single dose for six weeks. **Results:** The plasma levels of antithrombin and aPTT together with platelet counts remained normal throughout pregnancy. Thus, these markers did not influence the thromboprophylactic regime. In only a few women the Fragmin® dosage was increased, due to too low anti factor Xa activity (below 0.2 IU/L). All of them were overweight at start of pregnancy. **Conclusion:** Assessment of anti factor Xa activity, antithrombin, aPTT, and platelet counts during LMMH thromboprophylactic treatment in low risk pregnancies is not necessary in normal weight women.

PO176

Factor VIII levels in the early postpartum period

Procházka M (1), Slavík L (2), Procházková J (2), Hrachovec P (1), Krčová V (2), Zielina P (1)*

(1) Dept. of Obstetrics and Gynaecology, Medical Faculty, Palacký University, Czech republic
(2) Dpt. of Hematooncology, Medical Faculty, Palacký University, Czech republic

Objective: Pregnancy is accompanied by changes in the coagulation and fibrinolytic systems. There is a marked increase in some of the coagulation factors, particularly fibrinogen and factor VIII. A high plasma level of coagulation factor VIII is an important risk factor for thrombotic complications during pregnancy and puerperium. The aim of the study was to determine changes of the VIII:C in the early postpartum period. **Design:** A longitudinal prospective study of 189 healthy women. Primi or multigravidas whose previous pregnancies had been uncomplicated, aged 18 – 41 years. All of the deliveries were spontaneous and vaginal. First samples were taken between 24 –72 hours postpartum. Women whose factor VIII plasma levels were higher than 160 (percentage of standard) were tested again after 6 weeks. Factor VIII:C was investigated by the one-step coagulation method. **Results:** Pregnancy is associated with increased levels of VIII:C. Mean 197,5 percentage of standards, (95% ranges 72 – 389). 119 (63%) of the tested women had VIII:C higher than 160%. The post-puerperal test showed similar values to those from formerly published data in age-matched non-pregnant group. Mean 70% (95% range 70 – 218). **Conclusion:** Normal pregnancy is connected with increased levels of factor VIII. However elevated plasma levels of VIII:C is not associated with poor pregnancy outcome. Supported by the grant from the Ministry of Health of the Czech Republic IGA NH/6986 – 3, 2002

PO177

Polymorphism of gene PAI-1 4G/4G and preembrionic losses

Bitsadze VO, Baimuradova SM, Makatsaria A*

Chart of Obstetrics and Gynecology of Moscow Medical Academy, Moscow, Russia

Early preembrionic losses are usually connected with defects of ovum implantation. Fibrinolysis plays an important role in this process. Desynchronization of fibrinolysis and fibrin formation due to thrombophylia can be the cause of preembrionic losses, IVF failure and thromboses during hormone therapy. We observed 38 patients, aged 30-41 years, with preembrionic losses, which were thought to be infertility of unknown genesis. 25 women had IVF failure in anamnesis. Thrombophilia was found in 27 patients (70%). Gene PAI-1 4G/4G polymorphism was revealed in 23 patients (59%), among them 12% had homozygous form 4G/4G, 8 patients (21%) had antiphospholipid syndrome (APS). Multigenous forms of thrombophilia (combination of gene PAI-1 4G/4G polymorphism with MTHFR C677T mutation, factor V/Leiden mutation or platelet glycoproteins polymorphism) were observed in 15 patients (39%). Antithrombotic prophylaxis from the fertile cycle helped to achieve pregnancy in 16 women (48%) and save it due to continuous Fraxiparine use during the whole pregnancy in the dose of 2850-5700 IU depending on thrombophilia severity (TAT, D-dimer). 12 from 16 women were delivered with cesarean section. Antithrombotic prophylaxis was continued in postoperation period during 2 months. There is a high persent of gene PAI-1 4G/4G polymorphism in early preembrionic losses.

PO178

Acute vascular violations in pregnant women with thrombophilias

Bitsadze VO, Baimuradova SM, Stuleva N, Makatsaria A*

Chart of Obstetrics and Gynecology of Moscow Medical Academy, Moscow, Russia

We observed 25 pregnant women, aged 20-35 years, with acute vascular violations in anamnesis (thromboses, thromboembolias, insults, abruptio placentae). The factors of genetic and acquired thrombophilias were evaluated. Thrombophilias were revealed in 100% of patients: 1 (4%) - AT III deficiency, 11 (44%) - APS, 2 (8%) - homozygous form of factor V/Leiden mutation, 3 (12%) - heterozygous form of FV/Leiden mutation, 1 (4%) prothrombin G20210A mutation, 6 (2,4%) homozygous form of MTHFR C677T mutation, 14 (56%) heterozygous form of MTHFR C677T mutation, 8 (32%) gene PAI-1 4G/4G polymorphism, 4 (16%) gene PAI-1 4G/5G polymorphism, 5 (20%) homozygous form of fibrinogene gene 455G/A polymorphism, 9 (36%) heterozygous form of fibrinogen gene 455G/A polymorphism, 3 (12%) homozygous form of polymorphism of platelet receptor GPIIIa 1565 T/C, 4 (16%) heterozygous form of polymorphism of platelet receptor GPIIIa 1565 T/C, 2 (8%) homozygous ACF I/D gene polymorphism, 4 (6%) heterozygous ACF I/D gene polymorphism, 3 (12%) homozygous polymorphism of angiotensine II I type 1166 A/C receptor, 5 (20%) heterozygous polymorphism of angiotensine II I type 1166 A/C receptor, 7 (28%) APS combined with genetic forms of thrombophilia, 22 (88%) - multigenic thrombophilias. From 25 women we observed 15 during the pregnancy. Antithrombotic prophylaxis was prescribed from the fertile cycle during the whole pregnancy and in postpartum period with LMWH Fraxiparin, Aspirin, Omega-3, Folic acid, vitamins of B-group. In all cases the pregnancy was successfully termed without any perinatal losses or recurrences of acute vascular violations. In postpartum period Fraxiparine was used during 2 months with further change to Warfarine for 6 months.

PO179

The effects of oral hormone replacement therapy on C-reactive protein and other inflammatory markers in women with previous venous thromboembolism

Eilertsen A (1), Høibraaten E (1), Sandvik L (2), Opstad Andersen T (1), Mowinckel M (1), Sandset P (1)*

(1) Department of Hematology, Hematological Research Laboratory, Ullevål University Hospital, Oslo, Norway
(2) Research Forum, Ullevål University Hospital, Oslo, Norway

Introduction: In a recent randomized, double-blind, placebo-controlled trial of postmenopausal women with a history of venous thromboembolism (VTE), we found that oral HRT containing estradiol was associated with strong activation of coagulation markers and increased risk of recurrent thrombosis (Høibraaten et al: Thromb Haemost 2000; 84: 961-7). ***Aims***: The aim of the present study was to evaluate whether this increased risk can be attributed to changes in levels of high sensitive CRP (hs-CRP) and other inflammatory markers. ***Materials and methods:*** 140 women with a history of at least one VTE were randomly assigned to receive continuous treatment for 24 months with once daily HRT tablets (n=71) containing 2 mg 17 β-estradiol and 1 mg norethisterone acetate or placebo (n=69). All assays were performed by using commersial kits from R&D Systems (IL-6, TNF-α, TGF-β, ICAM-1, P-selectin) and Kordia (hs-CRP). ***Results:*** HRT was associated with a significant increase in hs-CRP after 3 months as compared with placebo (median 79% [95% CI 36-119%] versus –4% [–13-10%], p=0.001). These changes sustained after 12 months. Among those allocated HRT the increase in CRP was non-significantly higher in women who subsequently developed recurrent thrombosis (median 328%, n=5, versus 54% n=60 in those who did not develop recurrence). TNF-α levels decreased significantly by mean –10% versus 3% (p=0.004), whereas IL-6 levels increased by median 16% versus –9% (p=0.04). Soluble VCAM-1 decreased in the HRT group compared to the placebo group (mean –13% versus 1%, p<0.001). There were no significant changes in levels of TGF-β and P-selectin. ***Conclusions:*** Our findings substantiate that oral HRT containing estradiol is associated with a marked and rapid increase in CRP. However, this increase is probably not mediated by increases in IL-6 or TNF-α. Since oral HRT was associated with no changes or even reductions of other inflammatory markers, the increase in CRP is of questionable physiological relevance. In another study we have recently found that transdermal HRT given to postmenopausal women with coronary artery disease is not associated with a change in CRP levels (unpublished). Therefore, the increase in CRP on oral HRT may be due to a "first pass" effect by which estrogen induce increased hepatic synthesis of several proteins.

PO180

Estrogen receptors and venous thrombosis

*Aléssio AM (1), Höehr N (1), Nogueira C (2), Mansur A (2), Ozello M (1), Siqueira L (1), Annichino-Bizzacchi JM (1)**

(1) Unicamp, State University of Campinas, Sao Paulo, Brazil
(2) Usp, University of São Paulo, Sao Paulo, Brazil

Common variants in estrogen receptor-alpha (ER-alpha) and receptor-beta (ER-beta) can alter clinical response to estrogen, with impact in the risk of venous thrombosis (VT). Estrogen and progestin medications can increase the level of procoagulant proteins (fibrinogen, VIII, II and VII), decrease anticoagulant proteins (protein S and antithrombin) and cause acquired protein C resistance. In this study the prevalence of three polymorphisms in ER (one in the ER-alpha identified by enzyme PvuII with alleles P/p, and two in ER-beta identified by enzymes RsaI and AluI, with alleles R/r and A/a, respectively) was investigated in 143 women with VT associated to acquired risk factors: oral contraceptive (OC) - 61, pregnancy - 36, puerperium - 20, hormonal replacement - 14, association of these risk factors - 12. The control group comprised 113 healthy subjects, 41 male and 72 female. The prevalence of homozygous for PvuII polymorphism was significantly higher in pacients (34,7%) than controls (22%) (P=0,01), and also in patients with OC risk (39%) than in controls (22%) (P=0,007). When patients (34,7%) were compared only to female controls (21%) the prevalence was significantly higher in the first group (P=0,01). Genotype distributions and allele frequencies of AluI polymorphism were not significantly different between patients and controls. The prevalence of heterozygous for RsaI polymorphism was significantly higher in patients with puerperium risk (15%) than those with pregnancy risk (0%), (P=0,04). Genotype distribution of RsaI polymorphism did not differ between patients and controls. These results suggested that women homozygous for PvuII polymorphism could have an increased risk of thrombosis, more pronounced in those under OC. Since hepatic expression of the genes for several coagulation and fibrinolytic proteins is regulated by estrogen through estrogen receptors, this polymorphism could interfere with this response.

PO181

The effect of norethisterone acetate on inflammatory markers in postmenopausal women receiving estradiol

Žegura B (1), Gužič-Salobir B (2), Šebeštjen M (2), Keber I (2), Koenig W (3)*

(1) Maribor Teaching Hospital, Clinical Department of Gynecology and Obstetrics, Maribor, Slovenia
(2) University Clinical Centre, Hospital of Internal Medicine, Department of Angiology, Ljubljana, Sl
(3) University of Ulm Medical Center, Department of Internal Medicine II-Cardiology, Ulm, Germany

The increase of C-reactive protein (CRP), an independent predictor of coronary events in apparently healthy women, after oral estrogen replacement therapy, could be one possible mechanism for the increased cardiovascular risk in the first year of hormonal replacement therapy. Androgenic progestins such as norethisterone acetate (NETA) may inhibit proinflammatory effects of estrogen. We compared the effects of oral estradiol and estradiol combined with NETA on markers of inflammation in a randomised double-blind study. **Methods**: Fifty one healthy women were randomised to receive 28 weeks of oral treatment, either with estradiol (2 mg E2) or estradiol combined with NETA (2 mg E2 plus 1 mg NETA). At baseline and after 28 weeks of hormonal replacement therapy, levels of CRP, serum amyloide A (SAA), fibrinogen and cytokines interleukin-6 (IL-6) and tumor necrosis factor alpha (TNF-α) were determined. **Results**: E2 significantly increased CRP from 2.15 (0.71-4.05) to 3.41 (1.12-5.92) mg/l (p=0.04) and from 1.12 (0.81-2.06) to 1.95 (1.34-3.38) mg/l (p<0.01) when E2 was combined with NETA. The addition of NETA influenced the change in CRP levels, as the increase in CRP was more significant after E2 without NETA (p=0.005). E2 significantly decreased fibrinogen levels: from 3.58 (2.81-3.77) to 2.58 (2.47-2.80) g/l (p= 0.002) while E2 combined with NETA showed no effect. The levels of SAA, Il-6 and TNF-α did not change significantly after both modes of hormonal replacement therapy. **Conclusion**: The addition of NETA to E2 decreased the proinflammatory effect of E2, but it also attenuated the favourable effect of E2 on fibrinogen, an independent predictor of cardiovascular disease.

PO182

The influence of hormone replacement therapy (HRT) on factor VIIa/antithrombin (FVIIa/AT) complex

Dahm A, Hoibraaten E, Morrissey J, Andersen T, Sandset P*

Introduction. In a recent randomised, double-blind, placebo-controlled trial on the effects of oral hormone replacement therapy (HRT)(Høibraaten et al, Thromb Haemost 2001; 85, 775-81), we found that combined 17-β- estradiol (2 mg) and norethisterone acetate (1 mg) induced a reduction in activated factor VIIa (FVIIa) by median 17-23%, but with no decrease in total FVII concentration. Free tissue factor pathway inhibitor (TFPI) decreased by 29-30%, whereas antithrombin (AT) decreased by 8-9%. Recently it has been shown that AT may inhibit FVIIa bound to tissue factor (TF), building a FVIIa/AT complex, which is then released from TF, and may potentially be a marker of TF activated coagulation. **Aims.** To investigate whether the reduction in FVIIa on HRT, but not in the total FVII concentration, can be explained by AT induced inactivation of FVIIa and the formation of FVIIa/AT complexes, and also to investigate whether FVIIa/AT covariates with markers of activated coagulation. **Materials and methods.** Patients were 140 post-menopausal women with a history of venous thrombosis who were randomized to receive HRT (n=71) or placebo (n=69). This study reports data at baseline and after 3 months. FVIIa/AT complexes were assayed with an ELISA developed by Dr. Jim Morrissey. **Results.** At baseline FVIIa/AT was median 160 pM (25th, 75th percentiles 102, 219) in placebo patients and 167 pM (103, 254) in the HRT group. Median relative changes from baseline to 3 months in placebo and HRT treated patients were: FVIIa/AT +5.1% and -8.9% (ns), respectively, FVII antigen +2.4% and -7.5% (ns), respectively, and FVIIa +7,9% and -14,9% (p<0.001). Simple linear regression within the HRT group with prothrombin fragments 1+2 (F_{1+2}) showed that an increase in the relative change in FVIIa/AT was weakly associated to the increase in F_{1+2} from baseline to 3 months. **Discussion.** The decrease in FVIIa on HRT cannot be explained by an increase in FVII/AT complexes, which suggest that the reduction in activated FVII is not mediated by AT. FVIIa/AT complexes were weakly associated with F_{1+2} suggesting that FVIIa/AT may be a potential marker of TF induced coagulation.

PO183

Thrombophilic mutations as inherited risk factors for myocardial infarction in postmenopausal women

Sirotkina O (1), Smirnova N (2), Rodygina T (1), Toperverg O (1), Churina S (2), Schwarzman A (1)*

(1) Petersburg Nuclear Physics Institute RAS, Russia
(2) Saint-Petersburg Hospital "Pokrovskaya", Russia

Introduction. Ischemic heart disease is the major causes of death and disability in industrial countries. It is known that individual variation or environmental factors, such as over-weight, diabetes mellitus, arterial hypertension, cigarette smoking and menopause in women are associated with a high risk for myocardial infarction (MI). In recent years, epidemiological studies have shown that abnormalities in some hemostatic parameters may help predict the risk for ischemic events and acute MI. **Aims.** The aim of our study was to determine the thrombophilic gene polymorphism associated with the increased risk for MI in postmenopausal women. **Materials and methods.** 128 females (mean age 59.6±0.8) with MI in postmenopausal period and 122 healthy control females before menopause (mean age 41.6±0.7) were taken into analysis. Factor V Leiden mutation, 20210GA polymorphism in the prothrombin gene, G-455A in the β-fibrinogene gene, the 4G/5G PAI-1, C677T in the MTHFR gene, PlA1A2 GP III polymorphism and A1/A2 insertion promoter polymorphism in the factor VII gene were analyzed by PCR and RFLP. **Results.** The tendency of the 5G5G PAI-1 genotype prevalence in patients with MI compared to controls was found. The frequencies of the 5G5G, 4G5G and 4G4G genotypes were 29.7%, 43.8% and 26.5% in MI group and 20.5%, 51.6% and 27.9% in controls, respectively (p=0.06). The risk of the development of MI in postmenopausal women was higher in carriers of 5G5G PAI-1 compared with 4G5G or 4G4G individuals (OR=1.64, CI 95% 1.0-2.69). No other differences between patients and controls were observed. **Conclusion.** The 5G5G genotype of the PAI-1 gene is associated with the development of MI in postmenopausal period in women and might be considered as inherited risk factors for the disease.

PO184

Heterozygous Factor V Leiden deficiency with venous thrombosis and pulmonary embolism in a woman with breast cancer

Kotsopoulou M, Apergis G, Bosinakou E, Sklabou S, Paylou E, Mantzourani A, Andrioti E*

Hematology Department, (2) 1st Regional Transfu, Greece

Factor V Leiden mutation is a well-established risk factor for venous thrombosis. We present here a 48 female, who had venous thrombosis of the right leg veins 10 years ago. She had a normal delivery at the age of 23. One year ago, she was diagnosed with breast cancer and underwent mastectomy. After the first round of chemotherapy, she suffered from pulmonary embolism. An extensive coagulation examination (including serum ATIII, PrC, FV, FVII, FVIII, FIX, FXI, FXII, PrS, –functional assays-, Plasminogen, Homocystein, APC-Resistance, platelet counts and Lupus anticoagulants) revealed only positive lupus anticoagulants with a normal APC-Resistance. The molecular analysis of FII 20210 G→A, FV Leiden mutations showed a heterozygosity for Factor V Leiden mutation. The same analysis has been performed to the daughter of the above subject (19 years old, free of any thrombotic episod). All the values were normal and the lupus anticoagulants were negative. The molecular analysis revealed a heterozygosity of Factor V Leiden mutation, inherited from her mother. The discrepancy between APC-R phenotype and genotype is subject to further studies, since this cases are rare and additional unknown genetic events may be present. A false normal APC-Resistance cannot be excluded, due to implications of her disease and treatment. Counseling regarding the risks of thrombosis is essential for the

PO185

Coagulation studies in patients with thrombosed prosthetic heart valves and intracardiac clots

Saour J (1), Saour T (2), Shereen A (2), Al Hamed M (3), Hawari S (2), Saour B (2), Shoukri M (4), Mamo L (2)*

(1) Department of Medicine, King Faisal Specialist Hospital and Research Center, Saudi Arabia
(2) Coagulation Unit, Biological and Medical Research, KFSHRC, Saudi Arabia
(3) Genetics, KFSHRC, Saudi Arabia
(4) Biostatistics, Epidemiology and Scientific Computing, KFSHRC, Saudi Arabia

Introduction: Valve thrombosis and systemic thromboembolism continue to be the most serious complication in patients with prosthetic heart valve on long-term anticoagulation therapy. While under treatment with oral anticoagulants is a recognized cause for these complication, other factors possibly play a role as not all patients under-treated develop a coagulation problem. Three genetic mutations recently described to be associated with thrombosis at the venous and possibly the arterial side. Factor V Leiden (FVL) prothrombin at position G20210A and the 5,10-methylenterahydrofolate-reductase C677T (MTHFR) mutation. No studies as to whether or not these factors are associated with valve thrombosis, intracardiac clots and systemic thromboembolism in patients with prosthetic heart valves are available to date. **Aims**: To study the association of FVL, FII and MTHFR mutation in patients with Thrombosed Prosthetic Heart Valves And Intracardiac Clots. **Material and Methods**: Blood from consenting healthy subjects, and patients with prosthetic heart valves, left ventricular clot and left Atrial clot was collected. The DNA was extracted and stored at –70°C until tested. **Results**: DNA from consenting healthy donors (400 males and 100 females) was tested for the for FVL, FII and MTHFR mutations. Seven subjects (1.4%) tested positive for FVL; two (0.4%)for F11; and 132 (26.4%) for MTHFR. Thirty-one patients were tested. Twenty-four with thrombosed prosthetic heart valves, five with left ventricular clot and two with left atrial clot. Two patients tested positive for FVL (6.4%), one for FII (3.2%) and twelve for MTHFR (38.7%). **Conclusion**: Our results suggest a possible association between FVL, FII and MTHFR and patients Thrombosed Prosthetic Heart Valves And Intracardiac Clots. More data is needed to confirm this observation.

PO186

Thrombosis and familial thrombophelia registry, preliminary report

Mammo L (1), Saour T (1), Hawari S (1), Sidiqui K (2), Shereen A (1), Saour B (1), Saour J (3)*

(1) Coagulation Unit, Biological and Medical Research, King Faisal Specialist Hospital and Research Cent
(2) Biostatistics, Epidemiology and Scientific Computing, KFSHRC, Saudi Arabia
(3) Department of Medicine, KFSHRC, Saudi Arabia

Introduction: Registries are potent tool in healthcare for workers and planners. They provide statistics, trends and data on which short and long term decisions can be made. Such statistics also help in assessing treatment outcomes for different diseases. The incidence and prevalence of venous thrombosis (VT) and venous thromboembolism (VTE) and their trends in Saudi Arabia is not known. However, there is a good reason to suspect that they will increase as the population ages; patients undergo and survive more major surgery and, survive chemotherapy, myocardial infarction and cerebro vascular accidents. The Venous Thrombosis and Familial Thrombophelia Registry (TAFT) was set up by the Coagulation Unit, Department of Biological and Medical Research in collaboration with Thromboembolic Diseases Service, Department of Medicine at King Faisal Specialist Hospital and Research Center, Riyadh in 1999. Currently it is a hospital-based registry for Saudi national. Patient acceptance was an initial concern. **Aims**: The Registry will be a tool to collect data on incidence, prevalence, trends and outcomes of VT, to identify and council patients with familial thrombophelia and asymptomatic carriers; enhance national awareness & collect data to facilitate clinical and basic research. **Material and Methods**: A professional health educator and/or a physician interviewed and consented Subjects. Printed patient education material dealing with thrombosis was given. We are using Microsoft Access 2000(R) as a front-end to the registry database, which is being maintained in the MS SQL Server 2000. Access to the registry data is limited to the authorized individuals only and is through password authentication at two levels. Database is regularly updated and backed up and physical security of the database server is ensured. DNA extracted from whole blood collected from consenting subjects is stored at –70°C until tested for thrombophelia factors. **Results**: All subjects and family members studied approached consented willingly. There was no refusal and no requests for withdrawal. Blood from 400 healthy consenting Saudi and 290 patients with confirmed diagnosis of VT was tested. About 90 data item per subject has been collected. Confidentiality is ensured. **Conclusion**: We encountered no resistance from all subjects to consent for inclusion in the TAFT Registry. We thus plan to develop a National Registry, which will be the first in the Gulf and in the Middle East.

PO187

Frequency of hereditary thrombophilia in Egypt population

Ulu A (1), Elsayed S (2), Yildiz Z (1), Cin S (1), Elsobky E (2), Akar N (1)*

(1) Department of Pediatric Molecular Genetics, School of Science, Ankara University, Ankara, Turkey
(2) Pediatric Hospital, Ain Shams University, Khaira, Egypt

Introduction: This study was conducted in order to evaluate the incidence of FV1691A, FV4070G, PT20210A, EPCR 23 bp insertion and ACE 300 bp deletion among healthy Egyptians. Seventy three healthy Egyptians were included to the study. **Materials and methods**: Previously reported molecular techniques were used for the determination of mutations. **Results**: Ten individuals had FV1691A (13.6%) mutation with a frequency of 0.06. R2 and R3 haplotypes were found in 7 (9.5%) and 2 (2.7%) individuals respectively. Only one healthy individual had EPCR 23 bp insertion in heterozygous form (1.3%). None of the 73 individuals had PT 20210A mutation. The distribution of angiotensin converting enzyme -300 bp del in homozygous state was present in 40 (54.7%) individuals. The frequency was 0.7397. **Conclusion**: Our preliminary data revealed that FV1691A mutation is an important risk factor for thrombosis in Egyptians. (This study is supported by Ankara University Biotechnology Institute)

PO188

Prothrombin G20210A mutation in patients with cerebrovascular disease

Ulutin T (1), Altinisik J (1), Somay G (2), Buyru N (1)

(1) Cerrahpasa Medical Faculty, Department of Medical Biology, Istanbul University, Istanbul, Turkey
(2) Haydarpasa Numune Hospital, Neurology Clinic, Istanbul, Turkey

Introduction: The coagulation factor prothrombin (factor II) is the precursor of thrombin, which is an enzyme in the coagulation cascade. It has procoagulant, anticoagulant and antifibrinolytic properties. A variant form of the prothrombin gene has been characterized by a guanine to adenine at nucleotide 20210 in the 3'-untranslated region. Carriers of the prothrombin G20210A mutation have higher plasma levels of prothrombin and a several fold increased risk of thrombosis. Although venous thromboembolism seems to be a clinical manifestation in patients with prothrombin G20210A mutation, it is not clear whether this defect could be associated with arterial thrombosis. The role of this mutation for arterial vascular events, in particular cerebrovascular disease is still under discussion. **Aim:** We conducted a study in patients presenting ischemic stroke and intracerebral hemorrhage to assess whether prothrombin G20210A mutation increases the risk of arterial thrombosis. **Materials and methods:** The study was performed on 49 patients, 29 of these patients have ischemic stroke, 20 have intracerebral hemorrhage. 20 healthy individuals were also enrolled in the study as a control group. **Results and Conclusion:** No mutation was detected in patients whereas 2 of 20 healthy subjects were having this mutation in heterozygote form. The prevalence of prothrombin G20210A mutation among control subjects in our study was 10%, a rate higher than that reported in several prior studies and our data shows no evidence between the prothrombin mutation and risks of ischemic stroke and intracerebral hemorrhage.

PO189

Prothrombin G20210 mutation and association with severe life threatening thrombosis among thrombophilic patients

Bellia M, Sklavou S, Theodosiadis G, Gafou A, Georgopoulos J, Andrioti E*

1st Regional Transfusion and Hemophilia Center, Hippokrateion Hospital of Athens, Greece

Purpose: Prothrombin mutation is a hereditary cause of venous and less commonly arterial thrombosis. We performed this study in order to investigate the association of this mutation with life threatening severe thrombosis among patients suffering from thromboembolism. **Material and methods**: We performed 750 tests in patients with history of thromboembolism 440 males and 310 females with mean age 45+/-5years old. They were all tested for PT, APTT, Fibrinogen, FS, ProtC, S, ATIII, Llasminogen, FXII, FVLeiden, APC-Resistance, LLA, ACA, and FII20210 PROTHROMBIN mutation by .DNA isolation PCR and allele specific hybridization. **Results**: Fifty-eight out of 750 patients were found carriers (heterozygotes) of prothrombin mutation FII20210. Forty-two out of 58 patients, heterozygotes for FII20210 were analyzed. Nineteen patients carriers of the mutation (45.2%) with mean age 39.2 years old, suffered from deep vein thromboses and pulmonary embolism while 12 patients (63.1%) had severe life threatening thrombosis. Six patients carriers, females with mean age 30 years old, had recurrent spontaneous abortions and fetal growth retardation. Fifteen patients, carriers, 8 females and 7 males, with mean age 41 years old, suffered from stroke .One patient carrier, 50 years old, had acute myocardial infarction and another one patient carrier, 30 years old, had severe pulmonary hypertension. Although the number of patients studied for the FII20210 allele is small, the appearance of multiple and life threatening episodes in the majority (69%) of the carriers of FII20210 who additionally are young patients show that this mutation increases the risk of life threatening thrombosis and death. **Conclusion**: All patients, especially the young individuals, with severe, unexplained and life threatening thromboembolic events must be investigated for FII20210 allele mutation.

PO190

Thrombosis associated with multiple hereditary prothrombotic risk factors and sepsis

Gozdasoglu S (1), Akar N (2), Sen Z (3), Ozakpinar R (3), Argun M (1), Emiroglu M (3)*

(1) Ankara University, Department of Pediatric Hematology, Ankara, Turkey
(2) Ankara University, Department of Pediatric Molecular Genetics, Ankara, Turkey
(3) Ankara University, Department of Plastic and Reconstructive Surgery, Ankara, Turkey

Introduction: Acquired and inherited prothrombotic risk factors increase the risk of thrombosis in neonates, infants and children as in adults. Nonhereditary risk factors such as infections, malignancy, congenital heart disease, Behcet disease, homocystinuria, thalassemia major, kidney diseases, polycytemia, travma, surgery, SLE, autoimmune disorders, liver and bone marrow transplantations, dehydration, hyperalimentation, the use of central lines contribute to the development of thrombosis. In this report, we present thrombosis associated with multiple hereditary risk factors in the child with septicaemia. **Case Report**: A 14 years old boy was referred to the Department of Plastic and Reconstructive Surgery with grade III decubital ulcers at his back, sacral region and heels. It was learned that the patient had been admitted to the local hospital with weakness, high fever and confusion two months ago and that he had been diagnosised of sepsis and disseminated intravascular coagulation (DIC). He had received medical therapy for the sepsis and DIC. Necrosis had been developed and necrosed toes had been surgically amputated. When he was referred to the Hematology Department, he was pale and weak. A complete blood count revealed hemoglobin 9,2 g/dl, leukocyte count $10.5x10^9$/L, platelet count: 796x 10^9/L. Coagulation tests were PT: 12,7 sec, aPTT:30 sec, INR.:1,16, fibrinogen:592 mg/dL, D-dimer: 1,6 µg/ml., F VIII: 225,2 %U/dl, F IX: 201,5 % U/dl and protein C: 75,4 %U/dl, factor V Leiden (+/-) and prothrombin 20210 A(-/-) were found. The sacral and heel ulcers were recovered without any surgical treatment. The cubital ulcers at the back were repaired surgically with Tensor Fascia Latal Hatchett Flaps. **Conclusion**: Congenital risk factors such as factor V Leiden and prothrombin 20210 A mutations, F VIII, FIX levels should be screened in the patients with sepsis associated with thrombosis. If the patient has these risk factors, the other members of the familly have to be screened and they should be warned about his hereditary risk factors.

PO191

Thrombophilia markers in venous thrombotic events

Canak V, Povazan L, Mitic G, Gnip S, Latinovic O

Clinical Center of Novi Sad, Institute for Laboratory Medicine, Novi Sad, Serbia and Montenegro

Introduction: Department for The Prevention of Thrombosis uses oral anticoagulative therapy and works on integrative principle of clinical and laboratory patient follow-up, realized by the teams of specialists. **The Aim**: Project is set to test the thrombophilia markers of patients with venous and arterious and venous thrombosis, who experienced their first thrombosis at age not exceeding 50. **Materials and methods**: The sample composed of 100 patients, during 2002 and 2003; 43% male and 57% female, average age 32. Venous thrombosis was present in 94%, arterious and venous thrombosis in 6%, and recidivist in 38% of the sample. The diagnosis of thrombosis were confirmed by clinical and laboratory examination in 31%, by Duplex scan in 48%, lung scintigraphy in 16%, MR 4% and CT in 1% of the patients. Family anamnesis was positive in 48% of the patients. Thrombosis followed traumas in 13%, surgery in 8% and physical activities in 1% of the patients. In the female part of the sample: oral contraception in 1.7%, surgery during pregnancy in 1.7%, pregnancy in 21%, childbirth in 15.7% and Sectio Cesaea in 12.2% of the patients. Blood samples were taken for thrombophilia marker test at most three months before the diagnostic of the thrombosis. In the time of the testing, 39% of the patients were taking no therapy, 15% were treated by antithrombocite therapy, 13% by LMW Heparin, and 33% of the patients by oral anticoagulative therapy. The following thrombophilia markers were tested: APC-R resistance, Antithrombin (AT), Protein C, Protein S (PS), Lupus anticoagulants (LA), Factor VIII (FVIII). All were done using IL reagents, on a coagulationmeter ACL-200. **Results and Conclusions**: APC-R was done on 96 patients, and 26% are resistant, that is they are F V Leiden carriers; AT on 92 patients where 7,6% are deficient; PC on 60 patients, 3.3% are deficient; PS on 56 patients, 10.7% are deficient; F VIII on 22 patients, 27.3% has a value above the upper limit; LA on 74 patients. Slightly positive was present in 8.1%, positive in 6.7%; APC-R and PS deficiency was found in 2% of the sample; APC-R and LA in 4%; AT and LA slightly positive in 2%; AT and PS deficiency in 1% and both PC and PS deficiency in 1% of the sample. Determination of thrombophilia markers in time is crucial in patients under 50 years of age, due to importance of adequate antithrombosis therapy, length of recovery, ongoing clinical disorders. All should be approached on individual basis. Testing of the family members for the purpose of prevention in special events such as surgery, trauma, pregnancy, childbirth and oral contraception are crucial.

PO192

Case report of a family with inherited combinant deficiency of protein C and antithrombin III

Trajkov A (1), Kostovska S (2), Neceva V (2)*, Pejceva J (2), Dimovska N (2)*

(1) Medical Centre, Kavadarci, R. of Macedonia
(2) Institute of Blood Transfusion-Skopje, R. of Macedonia

The inherited deficiency of natural inhibitors of coagulation: antithrombin III (ATIII), protein C (PC), protein S (PS) is potential risk factor for development of thrombosis. **Aim** To represent a characteristic family with combine deficiency of PC and ATIII. **Matherial and methods**: Two brothers-twins (I.M. and L.M.), borne from one mother and one daughter and two brothers (R.M.; N.M. and S.M.) borne from another mother. They all have same father. Twin's mother died during delivery. The twin's brothers have deep venous thrombosis and they are on oral anticoagulant therapy. One brother (S.M.) from another mother died, two years ago and he had recidivist's thrombosis. The other brother (N.M.) and daughter (R.M) are health. Different methods were used for determination of concentration of: 1. PC and PS (micro-ELISA method) 2. ATIII (immunochemical and biological activity) and 3. APCr-Quick test, Russell Viper Venom based screening test for the f.V Leiden defect and resistance of activated PC. **Results**: The concentration of PC was low at I.M. (6 %) and L.M. (7 %) and it increased to 16 % and 22 % at same patients after oral anticoagulant therapy; decreased at S.M. (42%) and normal at R.M. (104 /98 %). The level of PS was normal at all patients: I.M. (100/63/51 %); L.M. (60/61 %); R.M. (47/113%) and S.M. (114 %). Concentration of ATIII was decreased at all : I.M. (0.08 gr/L); L.M. (0.12 gr/L); R.M. (0.08 /0.11/gr/L); N.M. (0.11 gr/L) and S.M. (0.17 gr/L).After receiving proper therapy, concentration of AT III raised to 0.17 gr/L(I.M.) and 0.23 gr/L at L.M. The biological activity of AT III was normal at: I.M. (102 %), L.M. (84 %) and decreased at S.M. (53 %).L.M. and I.M. showed Leiden variant of f.V with ratio 0.98 and 1.26 (generally, rations less than or equal to 1.5). **Conclusion**: Low levels of PC and resistance of activated PC suggest to inherited heterozygous defects of PC or Leiden variant of f.V (absence of inhibition of activated f.V by PC). These patients should be investigated further with specific assays for PC and DNA tests to see from where coming genetic defects.

PO193

Combined congenital thrombophilia and essential thrombocythemia in patients with recidivous pulmonary embolisms and myocardial infarction

Antonijevic N (1), Stanojevic M (1), Vukcevic V (1), Kovac M (2), Mikovic D (2), Novakovic I (3), Milosevic R (4), Savic N (1), Jaukovic M (1), Vasiljevic Z (1)*

(1) Institute of Cardiovascular Diseases, Clinical Centre of Serbia, Belgrade, Serbia and Montenegro
(2) Blood Transfusion Institute of Serbia, Belgrade, Serbia and Montenegro
(3) Institute of Biology, School of Medicine, Belgrade, Serbia and Montenegro
(4) Institute of Haematology, Clinical Centre of Serbia, Belgrade, Serbia and Montenegro

The identification of acquired and congenital etiopathogenetic factors for venous thromboembolism (VTE) contributes to an effective risk stratification for the occurrence of VTE recurrent episodes, and, therefore, to the determination of an optimal therapeutic and prophylactic regimen. Even up to 24%-37% of patients with venous thromboembolism have some of the congenital risk factors, the most frequent finding among them being gene mutation for factor V Leiden, MTHFR, and F II 20210A. The combination of FV Leiden mutation and homocysteine gene mutation have an impact on a seven-fold increased relative risk of thromboembolic episodes occurrence compared with abnormalities found in respective mutations. It is well known that patients, especially those over 60 years of age, previously having thromboembolic events, with essential thrombocythemia themselves are at increased thromboembolic risk even in a preclinical phase. We present the case of a 63 year-old female patient, with a clearly positive family history, multiple VTE episodes and myocardial infarction. Due to the first episode of massive pulmonary thromboembolism in the fifth month of pregnancy at the age of 32 she underwent urgent embolectomy. This was followed by subtotal hysterectomy and left adnexatomy in the eighth month of pregnancy by reason of left ovarian venous plexus thrombosis. The second episode of submassive pulmonary embolism and left leg deep vein thrombosis occurred at the age of 51, upon the plaster cask immobilisation due to a bimaleolar fracture of the left cruris. At the age of 63, myocardial infarction of diaphragmal wall complicated by a new episode of left leg deep vein thrombosis was diagnosed. Coronarography findings showed a right coronary artery subocclusive stenosis. Thrombophilia examinations found resistance to the activated protein C. Genetic examinations detected heterozygous mutations for factor V Leiden and MTHFR 677 genes. Thrombocythemia occurred at her age of 60 (the platelet count 530-670x109/l). Bone marrow haematological analysis supported by stem cell culture positive findings diagnosed a chronic myeloproliferative disease of essential thrombocythemia type. Due to an increase in the platelet count to 924x109/l, the hydroxyurea therapy was employed, accompanied by an earlier oral anticoagulant and antiaggregation therapy.

PO194

The role of PT 20210 G-A, FVL 1691 G-A and FV 4070 A-G as thrombotic risk factors in the development of idiopatic sudden hearing loss

Yildiz Z (1), Incesulu A (2), Ozkaptan Y (3), Akar N (1), Tekin M (1)*

(1) Department of Pediatric Molecular Genetics, School of Medicine, Ankara University, Ankara, Turkey
(2) Department of ENT, Social Security Hospital of Ankara, Turkey
(3) Department of ENT, Military Medical School, Ankara, Turkey

Introduction: Idiopathic Sudden Sensorineural Hearing Loss (ISSHL) is a frequent disease in otolaryn-gology with an incidence of approximately 1-2/10.000 per year. Nevertheless, the etiology of suddden hearing loss is still unknown. Despite the most common mechanism of sudden hearing loss appearing to be impaired cochlear blood circulation, the scientific basis of this assumption has not yet been proven. In recent years, several inherited prothrombotic risk factors have been found. The three most common, FV 1691 G-A, PT 20210 G-A, FV 4070 A-G mutations are studied in Turkish population. If thromboembolic events play a role in SSHL, these inherited risk factors might also be found more frequently in patients with SSHL. **Materials and methods**:Genomic DNA was extracted from periferal blood by conventional phenol-chloroform method. A 345 bp fragment of the 3'untranslated region of the prothrombin gene and 241bp fragment of exon 10 of the Factor V gene were amplified as descreibed previosly. PCR products were digested with Hind III restriction endonuclease. Amplification of exon 13 of the factor V gene was performed and PCR products were restricted with RsaI. **Results**: Fifty patients (28 male, 22 female) with confirmed sudden sensorineural hearing loss and fiftythree (19 male, 34 female) individuals were taken as the control group, have been analysed. The frequency of FVL mutation in ISSHL was found to be 6 and 2% in control and ISSHL patient group; of Prothrombin 20210 G-A mutation 1,9 and 2%; FV 4070 A-G 6 and 12% respectively. **Conclusion**: Our study has shown that neither of the mutations are not significant risk factors for sudden hearing loss. These risk factors must be studied in large series of patient groups. (This study is supported by Ankara University Research Fund.)

PO195

Factor V Leiden mutation and blood coagulation at the site of microvascular injury in healthy and anticoagulated subjects

Undas A, Brzezińska-Kolarz B, Iwaniec T, Brożek J, Musiał J*

Department of Medicine, Jagiellonian University School of Medicine, Cracow, Poland

Introduction: Little is known regarding the in vivo course of coagulation reactions in subjects with factor (F)V Leiden (G1691A). **Aims**: Therefore, the study was designed to evaluate the effect of FV Leiden on blood coagulation at the site of microvascular injury. **Materials and methods**: By quantitative immunoblotting and enzyme linked immunosorbent assays, we studied 16 apparently healthy subjects and 16 patients on long-term anticoagulation with acenocoumarol (mean INR, 2.4), with 8 carriers of FV Leiden in each group. Thrombin formation, measured by levels of thrombin-antithrombin complexes (TAT) and thrombin B-chain proceeded at the similar rate in carriers and non-carriers of FV Leiden. **Results**: As expected, anticoagulation was associated with a significant impairment of thrombin formation (maximum TAT levels, 12.2±1.6 vs 25.7±3.0 nM, p=0.01, and maximum rate of increase, 0.06±0.01 vs 0.15±0.02 nM/s, p=0.002). FV Leiden did not affect FV activation, while inactivation of FVa by activated protein C (APC), evidenced by the detection of the 30 kD fragment of the FVa heavy chain (residues 307 to 506), was significantly delayed by 60 seconds and its rate was depressed by 49.4% in carriers of FV Leiden, compared with the data obtained in non-carriers. These differences were observed both in healthy and anticoagulated individuals. In contrast to healthy subjects, patients receiving coumadins showed a 26% decrease in the FVa heavy chain levels at the last minute of bleeding (p=0.04). Moreover, the 97 kD fragment of the FVa heavy chain (probably residues 1 to 643) was detected in all subjects, with a 60-second delay in the time of its appearance and relatively higher concentrations than those of the heavy chain in patients treated with coumadins. **Conclusions**: our results indicate that when blood clotting is triggered by vascular injury, FV Leiden has no effect on thrombin generation, but inactivation of FVa by APC is significantly attenuated. The degree of this effect is much less pronounced comparing with the data from purified systems.

PO196

Effects of enoxaparine for prevention of thrombosis and thromboembolias in patients with chronic heart failure

Olbinskaya L, Kochkareva J, Kolossova K

Introduction: Venosus thromboses and thromboembolias are common in patients with chronic heart failure (CHF). Studying prevention of venosus thmboses in patients witn CHF is an urgent and important task of current medicine. Analysis of a number of clinical studies has shown that enoxparine is an efficient and safe drug for prevention of venosus thromboses in medical patients. Aims: Evaluate effects of enoxaparine on hemostasis system in patients with CHF III-IV FC (NYHA) and optimize prevention of venosus thromboses and thromboembolias in this group of patients. **Mateial and methods**: 18 patients with CHF III-IV FC (NYHA) and with mean left ventricular ejection fraction 39% were included in the study. Enoxaparine was injected ubcutaneously at a dose 40mg, once daily, for two weeks. Dynamic of hemostatic system (fibrinogen, thrombin time, activated partitial thromboplastin time, prothrombin index, solube fibrin-monomer complexes and index of thrombodynamic potential) was compared at baseline and at two weeks. **Results**: No clinical symptoms of venosus thromboses and thromboembolias were found during 6 months of observation. After 14 days of enoxaparine therapy levels of solube fibrin-monomer complexes, fibrinogen and index of thrombodynamic potential were decreased. **Conclusions**: Enoxaparine diminished intravascular bloud coagulation. Therefore it may be useful in patients with CHF for prevention of venosus thrombosis and thromboembolias.

PO197

Multicentric, observational, cross-sectional study to evaluate the VTE risk factors and venous thromboprophylaxis use: a pilot study

Martins M (1), Caramelli B (1)*, Deheinzelin D (2)*, D'Amico E (1)*, Braga AL (1), Schettino G (3), Hernandes A (1), Yoshida W (4), Machado F (5), Birolini D (1)*

(1) Hospital das Clínicas da Faculdade de Medicina da Universidade de São Paulo, Brazil
(2) Hospital do Câncer ACCamargo, São Paulo, Brazil
(3) Hospital Sirio Libanês, São Paulo, Brazil
(4) Hospital das Clínicas da Faculdade de Medicina de Botucatu; São Paulo, Brazil
(5) Hospital Albert Einstein, São Paulo, Brazil

Introduction: Although effective and safe strategies of preventing venous thromboembolism (VTE) are now available, a significant proportion of patients still develop VTE because appropriate thromboprophylaxis is not correctly prescribed. **Aims:** This is a pilot study designed to estimate the risk profile for VTE and the use of adequate thromboprophylaxis procedures in patients admitted to hospitals in the State of São Paulo, Brazil. **Material and methods:** Five hospitals were included in this study. Data on risk factors for VTE and use of pharmacological and non-pharmacological thromboprophylaxis were collected on two consecutive days, Data were obtained from 324 randomly chosen patients' medical records and/or from nurses of the same units using a questionnaire. Three risk assessment models were used: ACCP guidelines, Samama and Caprini. The first two scores classify the patients according to five risk categories: no risk, low, moderate, high and highest. Caprini score assumes values from low to highest. Descriptive analyses of the variables by hospital and different medical specialties were done. Contingency tables were built presenting the joined distribution of the risk score and the use of thromboprophylaxis (yes or no), stratified by hospital and medical specialties. **Results:** According to the Caprini score 242 (77%) of the 315 patients were under the highest risk for VTE. From these, 82 (34%) did not receive any thromboprophylaxis. Considering ACCP guidelines and Samama scores, 48 and 34% of the patients under some risk did not receive thromboprophylaxis, respectively. The use of thromboprophylaxis was influenced by specialty of the physician. In contrast, patients that had no or low risk of VTE (depending on the risk stratification score used) were receiving thromboprophylaxis with either unfractionated or low-molecular-weight heparins. **Conclusion:** Despite the existence of several guidelines, adequate thromboprophylaxis is not correctly prescribed: high-risk patients were shown to be undertreated and sometimes low-risk were shown to be overtreated. This situation determines a need to ensure that guidelines are created in order to guarantee that patients receive the care they need. Supported by AstraZeneca, Brazil.

PO198

Thrombotic complications of peripherally inserted central catheters: a one year retrospective study

Perron S, Miron M*

Notre-Dame Hospital, Montreal, Quebec, Canada

Introduction Recent years have been marked by a considerable increase in ambulatory care and many patients now receive chemotherapy, IV antibiotics or other IV treatments without being hospitalised. Safe long-term venous access such as peripherally inserted central catheter (PICC) was developed and is now widely used. The rate of associated central venous catheter (CVC) deep vein thrombosis (DVT) ranges from 3.2 to 32% depending on the population studied and the diagnostic method. The PICC are believed to induce less DVT (1%-4%) but only a few studies were done. **The aim** of our study was to retrospectively determine the rate of PICC related DVT, the associated risk factors and the prophylaxis prescribed by physicians. A chart review of all patients in whom a PICC was installed during year 2002 was done. All catheters were installed at the radiology department of Notre-Dame Hospital, a University teaching tertiary care facility. No prospective follow up was done during the study. **Results**: Preliminary results on 442 patients are reported. Patient population is as follows: mean age 56 (18-92), men 48.6%, active cancer 173 (39%). PICCs were used for total parenteral nutrition (TPN), chemotherapy and antibiotic administration in 10%, 28% and 58.6% of cases respectively. The mean duration of PICC use was 36.5 days (1-278). Patients were already fully anticoagulated for other reason than PICC installation in 10.2% of cases or received prophylactic anticoagulation in 44.3% of cases (19.4% s/c heparin or LMWH, 24.9% warfarin 1 mg/d). All patients having chemotherapy by PICC (124 patients, 28%) had a DVT prophylaxis. Complications occurred in 24% of patients: superficial venous thrombosis 2.3%, DVT 3.4% (all symptomatic and proven with venous ultrasound), intra-catheter thrombosis 4.8%, technical problems (mostly broken catheter) 3.8% and catheter related infections 9.7%. Seventy two percent (124/173) of patients with cancer received chemotherapy through a PICC and 8% had a thrombotic complication, half of them being DVT. Only 57% patients with cancer had prophylactic treatment when PICC was used for other reasons than chemotherapy. In those without prophylaxis, 14.3% (3/21) had a DVT. Two patients out of 45 that received TPN had a DVT. Despite the fact that only 38% of patient had a DVT prophylaxis associated with the PICC insertion for antibiotic administration purpose, only 2.7% DVT occurred. **Conclusion**. The PICC are widely used and technically safer than other central venous catheters. DVT occurred mainly in cancer patients, in those receiving chemotherapy or TPN. Few thrombotic events were associated with PICC when these risk factors were absent. PICC related DVT in cancer patient receiving chemotherapy seems comparable to what is seen in the literature for other CVC when a prophylactic therapy is used.

PO199

True incidence of arterial and venous thromboembolic events in the THA patient?

Ryge C (1), Rud Lassen M (1), Solgaard S (2), Sonne Holm S (3), Borris L (4)*

(1) Clinical trial unit, Denmark
(2) Hillerød Univ, Denmark
(3) Hvidovre Univ. Hospital, Denmark
(4) Århus Univ. Co, Denmark

Background: Today's data on the incidence of all thromboembolic events (acute myocardial infarction, new angina, stroke, trancitoric cerebral ischemia, pulmonary embolism, deep venous thrombosis) in patients undergoing Total Hip Arthroplasty (THA) opration is derived from register studies, clinical trials on pharmacological products or extrapolated from other populations. During Major joint replacement a state of hypercoagulopathy is present resultion in increased formation of fibrin, which can result in clot formation. These clots may result in occlution in vessels both on the arterial and venous site of the vascular bed. Some clots might dislodge andembolise to other parts of the vascular system with potentially severe consequences. The aim of the ESMOS study is to predict the "true" incidence of all cardiovascular complications after THA operation in an observational setting. **Method**: A prospective, consecutive cohort study including 500 patients from 3 general hospitals in Denmark. All THA patients are asked to participate in the datacollection the day before the operation. They will have an objective examination and a formalised interview about their living and health. Their GP will be asked to give information about medication and known previous diseases. Information about the operation and changes in patient health will be registered in a database. Quality of life (QOL) will be measured with SF36 before and after 1 year after the operation. All patients will receive appropriate thromboprophylaxis according to the in-house protocols. Early mobilisation and physiotherapy according to the protocols of the participating centers. The patients will be followed for 1 year after operation. Before and after surgery all patients will have meassurement of thrombin formation by measuring thrombin Fragment 1 + 2 in urine (ActiWatch, BESST-TEST, Copenhagen, Denmark). **Main hypothesis**: 10% of the patients will have complications related to coagulopathy resulting in AMI, new angina, stroke, TCI, PE and DVT within the first postoperative year. The primary THA patient and the revision THA patient will have an equal number of cardiovascular events. Prediction of cardiovascular events will be related to the severness of the coagulopathy initiated by the surgical procedure and the patients' comorbidity. The design and hypothesis will be discussed at the congress.

PO200

Epidemiology of post-operative venous thromboembolism in Asian countries: preliminary results of the SMART venography study

Leizorovicz A, Study Group t*

Faculté R.T.H. Laennec, Lyon, France

Introduction: In Asia, the prevalence of postoperative venous thromboembolism (VTE) is traditionally thought to be lower than in Western countries. In the SMART study, a multicenter (11 Asian countries), observational study on a cohort of 2432 consecutive Asian patients undergoing major orthopaedic surgery and not receiving any pharmacological thromboprophylaxis, the rate of adjudicated symptomatic VTE at discharge was 1.2%. However, the rate of post-operative asymptomatic DVT remains uncertain in this patients' population. **Aims**: The main objective of the SMART Venography study was to estimate in patients undergoing hip or knee replacement surgery the incidence of objectively verified asymptomatic deep-vein thrombosis (DVT). **Materials and methods**: In 8 centers (4 from Korea, 3 from Taiwan and 1 from Bangladesh), 400 consecutive patients, aged ≥40 years were to be enrolled. The primary endpoint was the incidence of DVT detected by systematic bilateral venography performed between days 7-14 after surgery. All venograms were adjudicated by a central reading committee. Symptomatic events and mortality at 1-month follow-up were also evaluated. **Results**: Interim data from 246 patients were available at the time of submission of the abstract. Their mean±SD age was 62.4±10.9 yrs and their mean body-mass index (BMI) 27.02±19.7 kg/m^2, 66.7% of the patients being female. The percentage of patients with classical risk factors for VTE at entry was low: previous or active cancer: 4.1%; varicose veins: 1.6%; chronic heart failure: 3.7%; BMI ≥30 kg/m^2: 13.8%, and no patient had a personal or family history of VTE or known thrombophilia. The following median durations were observed: 12.1 days for hospital stay, 5.4 days for immobilization, and 138.2 min for surgery. Regional anesthesia was used in 30.3% of patients. From surgery to discharge, 43.9% of patients received graduated compression stockings and 72.4% received non-steroidal anti-inflammatory drugs. Overall, 88.6% of patients were followed up for a median of 36 days. At the time of interim analysis, venography was available and evaluable in 184 patients. DVT was detected in 62 (33.7%) patients, 19 proximal, 41 distal only, one vena caval and one not specified. Overall, 4 symptomatic events, all DVT, were reported at one month, 3 during hospital stay and 1 during follow-up. By 1 month, one patient had died from bleeding. Complete results will be available for presentation in June 2004. **Conclusions**: These preliminary results show that the rate of asymptomatic and symptomatic DVT in our Asian study population undergoing orthopedic surgery is not negligible, taking into account the initial low-risk profile of the included patients, and confirm the results of our systematic review of all published data from Asian surgical patients.[2] (1. Leizorovicz et al. J Thromb Haemost 2003; Suppl: P 1440.; 2. Leizorovicz et al. Intern J Angiology 2004, in press.)

PO201

Thrombolytic therapy in patients with phlegmasia cerulea dolens

Tardy B (1), Moulin N (2), Mismetti P (2), Decousus H (2), Laporte S (2)*

(1) Intensive Care Unit, Thrombosis Research Group, University Hospital of Saint-Etienne, France
(2) Clinical Pharmacology Dept., Thrombosis Research Group, University Hospital of Saint-Etienne, France

Introduction: *Phlegmasia cerulea dolens* is an uncommon, severe form of lower extremity deep-vein thrombosis (DVT) characterised by extremity swelling, pain and cyanosis (hence the other name, blue phlebitis). It can compromise the whole circulation of the limb, affecting both the veins and the arteries. Progression of such DVT may result in gangrene, amputation and death. The effect of thrombolysis in the treatment of this disease remains uncertain. **Aim:** A prospective cohort of patients with *phlegmasia cerulea dolens* who received a thrombolytic was followed in order to determine the effects of such treatment in this indication. **Materials and methods:** Since August 1994, 9 patients (5 females and 4 males) with *phlegmasia cerulea dolens* have been admitted with an indication for thrombolysis. Straightaway after venography, patients received streptokinase (bolus of at least 250,000 units followed by 100,000 units/h for 48-72 h) or alteplase (25 to 45 mg for 4 h). All were also treated with extremity elevation, fluid resuscitation and elastic stockings. In addition, curative regimens of heparin followed by vitamin K antagonists were administered for at least one year (six months in one patient). The effect of thrombolysis was blindly assessed by the change in the Marder score between the initial venography and the venography performed at the end of thrombolysis. **Results:** Predisposing risk factors of *phlegmasia cerulea dolens* included malignancy (2 patients), hormonal therapy (4 patients), hypercoagulable state (4 patients), personal or familial history of DVT (7 patients), ulcerative colitis (1 patient), and recent surgery (1 patient) (some patients had more than one condition). All the patients had an iliac DVT, 6 also had concomitant pulmonary embolism (PE). The average level of fibrinogen before treatment was 4.3 ± 1.3 g/L; this decreased to 1.0 ± 0.6 g/L after thrombolysis. Venography performed at the end of thrombolytic therapy showed no improvement in six patients, a partial repermeabilisation in two patients and an extension in one patient; no improvement in the lung scan was shown for patients with a PE. No complication directly due to *phlegmasia cerulea dolens* was observed. Finally, two patients died during the follow-up: one at one month and one at three years, both due to their malignancy. **Conclusions:** From a venographic viewpoint, no improvement was observed in terms of venous obstruction. However, thrombolytic therapy could be considered to be beneficial in these patients given the absence of gangrene or amputation.

PO202

Management of thrombophlebitis with two-layer short-stretch bandages

Planinšek Ručigaj T (1), Košiček M (2)*

(1) Department of Dermatology, University Clinical Centre, Ljubljana, Slovenia
(2) Ambulance of Dermatology, General Health Centre Kranj, Slovenia

Introduction: Thrombophlebitis is an aseptic inflammation of the superficial vein with formation of the adherent thrombus in the vein's lumen. The affected vein is painful, hard and the skin over the vein is red and worm. The most important treatment is compression. **Aim**: The aim of the study was to evaluate clinical effectiveness of two-layer system of short – stretch bandages comparing to "resting" therapy in management of thrombophlebitis. The "resting" therapy is frequently prescribed by general practitioners. **Materials and methods**: One patient with thrombophlebitis of upper limb and 119 patients with thrombophlebitis of lower limbs (24 male and 96 female) were included in the study between January 2000 and December 2003. Patients were selected according to their medical history, clinical tests and diagnostic procedures (Doppler, Duplex scan). Patients were allocated to one of the three groups retrospectively. In the group 1 short – stretch bandages (Varicex Fâ with zinc, Porealstâ, Panelastâ Lohmann&Rauscher GmbH) were reapplied weekly. In the group 2 patients where treated with "resting" therapy first and after that with short – stretch bandages. In the group 3 "resting" therapy was prescribed. "Resting" therapy (rest, antibiotics, cold compress, local heparin ointment) was done daily. Patients were observed until good clinical improvement (no pain, no redness, no hard vein). **Results**: Group 1: 70 patients were included (15 male, 55 female), mean age 56,1 years The mean duration of the treatment with short – stretch bandages was 12,7 days. Group 2: 31 patients were included (6 male, 25 female), mean age 59,7 years. Patients were treated with "resting" therapy first in mean duration of 45,7 days with no clinical improvement. After that, they were treated with short - stretch bandages 12,6 days. In this group patients were treated in average 58,3 days totally. Group 3: 19 patients (3 male, 16 female) with mean age 62,6 years were treated with "resting" therapy 55.4 days. **Conclusions**: The correct treatment of thrombophlebitis with short – stretch bandages is clinically more effective comparing to "resting" therapy. Bandages were well tolerated by patients in all three groups.

PO203

Haemorheological and haemostatic alterations in patients with Idiopathic Sudden Sensorineural Hearing Loss

Mannini L, Paniccia R, Cecchi E, Alessandrello Liotta A, Lari B, Bandinelli B, Betti I, Abbate R, Gensini GF, Prisco D*

Department of Medical and Surgical Critical Care, Thrombosis Centre, University of Florence, Aziend, Italy

Sudden Sensorineural Hearing Loss is a frequent disease in otolaryngology characterized by abrupt onset of deafness. Its incidence is approximately 20/100,000 persons per year, and young and otherwise healthy people are often affected. The aetiology of sudden hearing loss is still unknown in as much as 80% of patients. Some studies have suggested that both haemorheological changes and haemostatic alterations may be associated with Idiopathic Sudden Sensorineural Hearing Loss (ISSHL). Aim of this study was to evaluate if haemorheological changes and some parameters which are indexes of hypercoagulability and endothelial damage are associated with ISSHL. We studied 63 patients [30 M, 33 F; median age 54 yrs (19-78)] who referred to Florence Thrombosis Center with diagnosis of ISSHL and 67 healthy control subjects [27 M, 40 F; median age 50 yrs (25-78)], matched for age, sex and traditional cardiovascular risk factors. Haemorheological studies were performed by assessing whole blood viscosity (WBV) at 0.512 and 94.5 s^{-1}, plasma viscosity (PLV) at 94.5 s^{-1} and erythrocytes filtration test (EFT). WBV and PLV were studied with rotational viscosimeter Contraves LS 30 and EFT was assayed on washed red blood cells with erythrocyte filtrometer Myrenne MF4. A global investigation to assess whole blood coagulation and platelet function was performed by Sonoclot analysis. Sonoclot variables studied were Sonoclot activated clotting time (SonACT), Clot Rate (CR) and time to peak (TP). Fibrinogen was assayed according to Clauss method; ELISA test was used to determine PAI-1 antigen (ag) plasma levels; factor VIII was measured by a clotting method. WBV at both shear rates, PLV, SonACT, CR, PAI-1ag, factor VIII:C were significantly altered in patients in comparison with controls ($p<0.05$). At a multivariate analysis, adjusted for traditional cardiovascular risk factors, hematocrit and fibrinogen, WBV at 94.5 s^{-1}, EFT, Son ACT, CR, PAI-1ag plasma levels and factor VIII:C activity resulted significantly altered in ISSHL patients ($p<0.05$). Mild but significant correlations were found between both PAI-1ag and factor VIII:C plasma levels with both WBV 94.5 s^{-1} and CR. Our data show that ISSHL is independently associated with an increase of WBV at 94.5 s^{-1}, PAI-1ag and factor VIII:C plasma levels and with alterations in EFT, SonACT and CR values. High PAI-1ag and factor VIII:C plasma levels, may be an expression of both clotting activation and endothelial damage, probably due to an altered erythrocyte deformability. In conclusion, the alterations in blood viscosity and haemostasis may have a role in the pathogenesis of sudden deafness and its complications and may be a target of therapeutic approaches in these patients.

PO204

Thrombotic complication treated with defibrotide followed by central nervous system failure in a child after bone marrow transplantation

Dobaczewski G, Latos-Grazynska E, Wrobel G, Szmyd K, Chybicka A, Toporski J*

Department of Pediatric Oncology/Heamatology, Medical University, Wroclaw, Poland

Introduction: Defibrotide is a polydeoxyribonucleotide possessing antithrobotic and thrombolytic properties. The drug is considered to be an agent of high clinical benefit in the treatment of thrombotic complication after bone marrow transplantation (BMT). **Aim**: To evaluate the clinical course of the patient with vono-occlusive disease (VOD) treated with antithrombotic agents, complicated by various central nervous system (CNS) failure. **Case report**: The 14-year-old boy with nueroblastoma in stage IV, previously treated with conventional chemotherapy and abdominal tumour radiotherapy after autologous BMT, developed VOD about 4 weeks after transplantation with busulfan/melphalan pretransplant regimen. Ascites, rapidly increasing bilirubin concentration, hepatomegaly developed in a week. No other symptoms of organ failure were observed, and due to Baltimore criteria moderate VOD was diagnosed. Other initial symptoms of VOD developed: refractoriness to platelet transfusions, weight-gain, thickness of gall bladder wall (ultrasound) and marked jaundice. Initial treatment with low molecular heparin (Clexane®) was of no benefit. Bilirubin concentration rose up to 28 mg/dl; marked D-Dimers elevation and antithrombin activity fall was also observed. Defibrotide (Noravid-Aventis®) was administered with initial dose of 20 mg/kg bw/day subsequently increased to 40 mg/kg bw/day with rapid improvement- fall of hepatic failure parameters. Magnetic resonance imaging (MRI) revealed no obstruction in a bile flow. Doppler ultrasound of portal venous flow was in normal range. After discontinuation of defibrotide treatment (2 weeks) the patient's consciousness worsened, metabolic and endocrinological changes appeared. Laboratory examination revealed pituitary gland malfunction. No subsequent diagnostic evaluation explained its origin. Repeated MRI and cerebro-spinal fluid examination were also normal or slightly changed. Simultaneously, the patient developed severe neurologic changes from local muscle rigidity to profound coma. **Conclusion**: Thrombotic complication of BMT diagnosed as hepatic VOD may be effectively treated with defibrotide. The case described other distant organ failure of thrombotic or non-thrombotic origin, which might be potentially connected with administered medication.

PO205

Residual venous obstruction in patients wih a single episode of deep vein thrombosis (DVT) and in patients with recurrent DVT

Dentali F, Ageno W, Galli M, Mera V, Manfredi E, Steidl L, Venco A*

Internal Medicine, University of Insubria, Varese, Italy

Introduction: The presence of residual venous obstruction (RVO) in patients with deep vein thrombosis (DVT) of the lower limbs was recently suggested as an independent risk factor for recurrent venous thromboembolism (VTE). RVO could be a marker of a persistent prothrombotic state. To further support this hypothesis, we have compared the rate of RVO between patients who had a single episode of objectively confirmed DVT and patients with recurrent episodes of DVT. **Methods**: All patients underwent compression ultrasonography (CUS) of the lower limbs after 1 year from index DVT. In patients with recurrent DVT, the index event was defined as the last documented DVT. RVO was arbitrarily defined as a thrombus occupying, at maximal compressibility, more than 20% of the vein area in the absence of compression. Information on age, gender, cause of DVT and duration of anticoagulant treatment was collected. **Results**: We have enrolled 38 consecutive patients with recurrent DVT and 50 age matched patients with a single episode of DVT. Mean age in the former group was 63.4 years, males were 68.4%. Mean age in the latter group was 64.6 years, males were 62%. In the group with recurrent DVT, the index event was idiopathic in 57.9%, and secondary to a known risk factor in 42.1%, 4 patients had cancer. Among patients with a single episode of DVT, in 54% the event was idiopathic and in 46% it was secondary to a known risk factor, 5 patients had cancer. All patients with recurrent DVT were receiving oral anticoagulant treatment (OAT) after 1 year, whereas in the control group of patients with a single DVT 72% had OAT stopped after 3 or 6 months and in 28% the treatment was still ongoing. In 70.6% of patients with recurrent DVT the index event occurred in the contralateral leg or in a different segment of the homolateral leg. RVO was detected in 50% of patients with a single episode of DVT and in 84.2% of patients with recurrent DVT ($p=0.0009$). **Discussion**: The prevalence of RVO after one year from the index event is significantly higher in patients with recurrent DVT than in patients with a single episode. Because patients with multiple episodes of DVT are known to be at very high risk of further recurrences, this finding supports the importance of RVO as a potential marker of a persistent prothrombotic state or at least of a persistently increased risk of recurrent DVT.

PO206

Hydrofibre dressing versus ointments in the treatment of venous leg ulcers

Košiček M (1), Planinšek Ručigaj T (2)*

(1) Ambulance of Dermatology, General Health Centre Kranj, Slovenia
(2) Department of Dermatology, University Clinical Centre, Ljubljana, Slovenia

Introduction: Venous leg ulcers can be one of the signs of postthrombotic syndrome. Different dressings and ointments are used for the treatment of venous leg ulcers. The AIM of the study was to compare hydrofibre dressing and ointments in terms of effectiveness of each therapy and changes of microbial colonisation of venous leg ulcers. **Methods:**This trial included 20 patients with 35 venous leg ulcers, some of them postthrombotic. Patients were selected based on their medical history, clinical tests and diagnostic procedures. Exclusion criteria were an ankle-brachial pressure index < 0.8, severe concurrent diseases and immobility of patients. Two groups of patients were formed. Nine patients in group 1 were treated with hydrofibre dressing (Aquacelâ, ConvaTec) and hydrocolloid secondary dressing. Eleven patients in group 2 were treated with antibiotic and necrectolytic ointments. Patients in both groups were treated with long – stretch bandages. Dressings and ointments were changed when clinically indicated. Ulcer areas were measured in square cm and swabs were taken from leg ulcers at the beginning of the study, after 3rd and after 7th week of treatment in both groups. The microbial identification of ulcers and sensitivity tests were done. **Results**: The mean ulcer area at the baseline in the group 1 was 9.6 square cm, in the group 2 was 16.4 square cm. The mean ulcer area after 7th week of treatment in the group 1 was 8.8 square cm and in the group 2 was 19.5 square cm. The most frequently isolated bacteria at the beginning of the treatment in group 1 were: Staphylococcus aureus in 66.7%, Pseudomonas aeruginosa in 44.4% of patients; in group 2 were: Staphylococcus aureus in 53.3% and Pseudomonas aeruginosa in 53.3% of patients. The most frequently isolated bacteria after 7th week of treatment in group 1 were: Staphyloccocus aureus in 60%, Pseudomonas aeruginosa in 20% of the patients; in group 2 were: Staphylococcus aureus in 50% and Pseudomonas aeruginosa in 60% of patients. **Conclusion:** The small trial shows the decrease of mean ulcer area and the decrease of Pseudomonas aeruginosa isolation after 7th week of the treatment with hydrofibre dressing. The above findings suggest that the hydrofibre dressing has promising clinical benefits in ulcer care.

PO207

The floating thrombus: a fictitious actor on thromboembolic set (considerations about a clinical case)

*Lo Pinto G**

Thrombosis Center - Galliera Hospital, Genoa, Italy

Introduction: a floating thrombus is very often depicted as a high risk clinical situation concerning pulmonary embolism, but it is well known that about two thirds of proximal deep venous thrombosis of lower limbs occur at the same time as the asymptomatic pulmonary embolism. This clinical condition does not change the treatment. Instead the extensive use of cava filters may cause further clinical problems. The floating status is, actually, a physiological phase in the life of each thrombus as you can see in the clinical case described below. **Clinical case**: a woman aged 63 was operated because of a right middle fossa meningioma, later she was re-operated because of the relapse of the cancer with involvement of the cavernous sinus. Then she was treated with radiotherapy. In the following months she developed an hydrocephalus, therefore a ventriculoperitoneal shunt was placed. Because of the kinking of the catheter it was necessary a further operation with the replacement of the catheter. By consequence of the long staying in bed she developed a deep venous thrombosis involving the left poplitea, femoral, iliac and cava vein up to the right renal vein, with looking like a floating thrombus in cava when CT-scan with contrast medium was performed. We there decided to insert a caval filter, but due to technical difficulties we delayed the operation of three days. The cavography with contrast medium showed the thrombus sticked to the cava vein wall, therefore the filter was not installed. A perfusion lung scan with Tc-99m labelled macroaggregated serum albumin was normal, excluding pulmonary embolism. **Conclusions**: the use of the cava filters should be strictly limited when absolutely required: i.e. the life-threatening recurrent pulmonary embolism in spite of an optimal anticoagulant treatment, or absolute contra-indications to the above said treatment.

PO208

The influence of advanced age and immobility on physician practices for prescribing venous thromboembolism prophylaxis to medical patients

Decousus H (1), Tapson V (2), Chong B (3), Merli G (4), Kakkar A (5), FitzGerald G (6)*

(1) Centre Hospitalier Universitaire de Bellevue, Saint-Etienne, France
(2) Duke University Medical Center, Durham, USA
(3) St George Clinical School, Kogarah, Sydney, Australia
(4) Thomas Jefferson University Hospital, Philadelphia, USA
(5) Imperial College, London, UK
(6) Center for Outcomes Research, University of Massachusetts Medical School, Worcester, USA

Introduction: Advanced age and immobility are thought to contribute to the overall risk of venous thromboembolism (VTE) in medical patients. However, there is little published data on these risk factors and their influence on VTE prophylaxis (Px) practices. **Aims:** To examine the influence of age and immobility on VTE Px practices in IMPROVE, an international prospective cohort study of hospitalised acutely ill medical patients. **Materials and Methods:** Patients ≥18 years old and hospitalised for ≥3 days with an acute medical illness are enrolled consecutively. Exclusion criteria: therapeutic antithrombotic/thrombolytic agents at admission; major surgery or trauma during 3 months prior to admission; and VTE treatment within 24 hours of admission. Data are recorded at discharge and 3 months after discharge. A logistic regression model was used for multivariate analysis to calculate odds ratios (OR) and confidence intervals (CI). **Results:** Data from 1770 patients (from 25 hospitals in 10 countries) were analysed. 51% of patients were mobile, 12% were immobile prior to admission, and 37% were immobile only after admission. Only 37% of patients received Px. More patients ≥60 years old received Px than those <60 years old (42.9% vs 26.2%; OR 2.12; 95% CI 1.71–2.72). More patients immobile for ≥7 days received Px than those immobile for <7 days (61.4% vs 27.8%; OR 4.12; 95% CI 3.30–5.13). Patients immobile for <7 days were more likely to receive Px if they were ≥60 years than <60 years old (34% vs 19%; OR 2.17; 95% CI 1.67–2.83). However, the rate of Px use was equally high for patients immobile for ≥7 days and either <60 or ≥60 years old (62% vs 61%; OR 0.97; 95% CI 0.62-1.52). Adjusting for other known VTE risk factors in a multivariate analysis confirmed that age and immobility remain independent risk factors for physician Px patterns. **Conclusions:** Older patients were more likely to receive Px than younger patients, while patients immobile for ≥7 days were more likely to receive Px than those immobile for <7 days. Age did not influence the decision to give Px to patients immobile for ≥7 days. Only 61% of patients ≥60 years old and immobile for ≥7 days received Px. Further studies should aim to simplify the decision to give Px to medical patients based on only age, immobility and presence of clinical risk factors. Analysis of future data from IMPROVE may enable us to determine the influence of these risk factors on the development of VTE.

PO209

Prevention of venous thromboembolism: evaluation of the use of thromboprophylaxis guidelines in a teaching hospital

Grand B, Duarte P*, Orosco J, Gutierrez R, Oscar M, Riveros D**

Department of Internal Medicine and Hematology section. CEMIC University Hospital, Buenos Aires, Argentina.

Objective: To evaluate the results of the application of the use of thromboprofilaxis guidelines in a teaching hospital. Design: Prospective observational study. Setting: The 50-bed medical and surgical floors of a university hospital. **Patients**: All consecutively admitted patients during a 6-month period (n:567). **Methods**: The guide divided patients in risk groups. General surgical patients were divided in low,moderate, high and very high group according to age, number of risk factors and the duration of the surgery. Medical patients included for prophylaxis were those with myocardial infarction, congestive heart failure, pulmonary infection, stroke and acute spinal cord injury. Prophylaxis methods included: general measures, intermittent pneumatic compression, elastic graduated stockings, and either unfractionated heparin or low molecular weight heparin (enoxaparin). The type of prophylaxis suggested by the guide was defined according to international recommendations based on risk groups. Main outcome measurements: Adequacy of prophylaxis (correct application of the guide), sufficient prophylaxis (defined by an equal or superior prophylaxis than recommended) , continuity of adequacy of prophylaxis (comparison of adequacy of prophylaxis between the first and sixth month). **Results**: Adequacy of prophylaxis was noted in 306 patients (54%), sufficient prophylaxis in 334 patients (59%). The tromboprophylaxis guidelines were correctly applicated in 62% of the patients in the first month but only in 46% of the patients in the sixth month of the study **Conclusion**: The correct implementation of prophylaxis guidelines needs continuous medical education and institutional diffusion. This kind of guide and follow up allowed us to detect inadequacy of prophylaxis and take corrective measures.

PO210

Evaluation of the symptoms of acute venous thrombo-embolism

Rached R, De Piano L, Cavalheiro C, Chamone D*

Heart Institute - INCOR, School of Medicine, University of São Paulo, Brazil

Introduction: the diagnosis of deep venous thrombosis (DVT) and the pulmonary embolism (PE) has many difficult, mainly because less than 30% of the suspected subjects have the diagnostic confirmed. **Objective**: evaluation of the frequency of symptoms of acute venous thromboembolism. **Patients and Methods**: we studied 131 patients (age 13-95 years) that attended the emergency service with suggestive clinical picture of pulmonary emboli (PE) and/or deep venous thrombosis (DVT). Among the patients, 93 (71%) subjects didn't present acute venous thromboembolism, while, 38 (29%) presented. The symptoms were referred from the patients by specific questionnaire. **Results**: PE DVT PE + DVT thrombosis No yes no yes no yes N 45 18 35 14 13 6 mean age yo) 58ą17 40ą18 52ą19 55ą17 62ą17 64ą15 pain chest 69% 67% 54% 50% dispnea 67% 83% 77% 67% syncope 11% 6% 0% 0% cough 42% 50% 23% 17% hemoptysis 13% 28% 23% 0% leg pain 86% 93% 77% 67% leg swollen 86% 93% 85% 67% leg hyperemia 29% 14% 39% 17% The positive predictive value of clinical symptoms was 29%. **Conclusion**: the positive predictive value of the clinical symptoms is very low and the diagnosis confirmation of acute venous thromboembolism needs a complementary tests.

PO211

Progressive versus decreasing elastic stockings in patients presenting with mild venous insufficiency: a randomised clinical trial

*Couzan S (1, 3), Assante C (2, 3), Pouget J (1, 3), Prufer M (1, 3), Laporte S (2, 3), Mismetti P (2, 3)**

(1) BVSport, 16 cours d'Herbouville, Lyon, France
(2) Thrombosis Research Group, University Hospital of Saint-Etienne, France
(3) BOOSTER Study Group

Introduction: Prescription of conventional elastic stockings in venous insufficiency for the prevention of thrombosis in the post-operative period or after an episode of venous thrombosis is based on a decreasing compression concept, in which pressure is maximal at the ankles, and gradually decreases proximally. A new type of elastic stockings was developed using a novel elastic compression concept, with low pressure at the ankles and maximal pressure around the calf (where first symptoms of venous insufficiency occur). The efficacy of these progressive elastic stockings has already been assessed in athletes after physical efforts in terms of venous return [1]. They may improve compression efficacy, as well as the comfort, which would, in turn, improve compliance in venous insufficiency. **Aim:** To assess the efficacy and convenience of the new elastic stockings (BVSport® [2]) in comparison to conventional ones in patients presenting with mild venous insufficiency. **Materials and methods:** Patients presenting with mild insufficiency, i.e. class 1 in Porter's classification (corresponding to C0 or C1 in the CEAP or Hawaii classification), for which elastic compression by knee stockings was indicated were eligible for inclusion in a multicentre randomised double-blind clinical trial. They were assigned to receive either standard elastic stockings or BVSport® stockings. Patients with post-thrombotic syndrome, peripheral arterial disease, dermatological disease, renal or nephrotic or cardiac insufficiency were excluded. It was planned to enrol 120 patients in order to be able to demonstrate non-inferiority of the progressive compression concept in terms of efficacy (tiredness) and convenience (comfort) combined. Compliance was assessed as a secondary endpoint. The evaluation was carried out at 2 weeks. **Results:**To date, 83 patients have been enrolled by 15 French centres. Recruitment is scheduled to end in March 2004. The final results will be available and presented at the congress. **Conclusions:** To our knowledge, these are the first results from a randomised study evaluating a new compression concept in venous insufficiency. If the results are positive, this kind of elastic stockings could be considered in other indications (1. Couzan et al., Int Angiol 2000, 19 (suppl): 41; 2. http://www.bvsport.com/).

Author index